Prevention of
Coronary Heart Disease

Prevention of Coronary Heart Disease

Edited by

Ira S. Ockene, M.D.

Professor of Medicine, and Director
Preventive Cardiology Program
Associate Director, Division of Cardiovascular Medicine
Department of Medicine
University of Massachusetts Medical School
Worcester, Massachusetts

Judith K. Ockene, Ph.D.

Professor of Medicine, and Director
Division of Preventive and Behavioral Medicine
Department of Medicine
University of Massachusetts Medical School
Worcester, Massachusetts

Foreword by

Jeremiah Stamler, M.D.

Professor Emeritus
Department of Community Health and Preventive Medicine
Northwestern University Medical School
Chicago, Illinois

Rose Stamler, M.A.

Professor
Department of Community Health and Preventive Medicine
Northwestern University Medical School
Chicago, Illinois

Little, Brown and Company
Boston/Toronto/London

Library of Congress Cataloging-in-Publication Data

Prevention of coronary heart disease / edited by Ira S. Ockene, Judith K. Ockene; foreword by Jeremiah Stamler. — 1st ed.

     p. cm.

Includes bibliographical references and index.

ISBN 0-316-62214-1

1. Coronary heart disease — Prevention. 2. Coronary heart disease — Risk factors. I. Ockene, Ira S. II. Ockene, Judith K.

[DNLM: 1. Coronary Disease — prevention & control. 2. Risk Factors.]

RC685.C6P666 1992

WG 300 P9454 — dc20

DNLM/DLC

for Library of Congress   92-10336
                                       CIP

Second Printing

Printed in the United States of America

MV-NY

To our children, Lauren and Kim, who now teach us as much as we taught them; to our beloved parents; and to Frodo, Kelly, Odie, Mycroft, Kilroy, the Tooth Fairy, and all those other characters who make life interesting

Contents

Contributing Authors

Lynn Ahlquist, Ph.D.

Assistant Professor of Medicine, Division of Cardiovascular Medicine, Department of Medicine, University of Massachusetts Medical School, Worcester, Massachusetts

Richard C. Becker, M.D.

Assistant Professor of Medicine, Division of Cardiovascular Medicine, Department of Medicine, University of Massachusetts Medical School; Director, Thrombosis Research Center, University of Massachusetts Medical Center, Worcester, Massachusetts

Milo L. Brekke, Ph.D.

Clinical Assistant Professor, School of Public Health, University of Minnesota; President, Brekke Associates, Minneapolis, Minnesota

David R. Brown, Ph.D.

Assistant Professor of Medicine, Division of Cardiovascular Medicine, Department of Medicine, University of Massachusetts Medical School; Director, Exercise and Sport Psychology, Exercise Physiology and Nutrition Laboratory, University of Massachusetts Medical Center, Worcester, Massachusetts

Daniel Carlucci, M.D.

Fellow, Division of Cardiovascular Medicine, Department of Medicine, University of Massachusetts Medical School, Worcester, Massachusetts

David Chiriboga, M.D.

Fellow in Preventive Cardiology, Division of Cardiovascular Medicine, Department of Medicine, University of Massachusetts Medical School, Worcester, Massachusetts

Michael P. Eriksen, Sc.D.

Director, Office on Smoking and Health, National Center for Chronic Disease Prevention and Health Promotion, Centers for Disease Control, Atlanta, Georgia

Karen Glanz, Ph.D., M.P.H.

Professor, Department of Health Education, Temple University; Adjunct Professor, Department of Medicine, Temple University School of Medicine, Philadelphia, Pennsylvania

Robert J. Goldberg, Ph.D.

Professor of Medicine and Epidemiology, Division of Preventive and Behavioral Medicine, Department of Medicine, University of Massachusetts Medical School, Worcester, Massachusetts

James R. Hebert, Sc.D.

Associate Professor of Medicine and Epidemiology, Division of Preventive and Behavioral Medicine, Department of Medicine, University of Massachusetts Medical School, Worcester, Massachusetts

Jay Himmelstein, M.D., M.P.H.

Associate Professor of Family and Community Medicine, University of Massachusetts Medical School; Director, Occupational Health Program, University of Massachusetts Medical Center, Worcester, Massachusetts

Brian F. Johnson, M.B.

Professor of Medicine, University of Massachusetts Medical School; Director, Division of Clinical Pharmacology and Hypertension Clinic, University of Massachusetts Medical Center, Worcester, Massachusetts

Jon Kabat-Zinn, Ph.D.

Associate Professor of Medicine, Division of Preventive and Behavioral Medicine, Department of Medicine, University of Massachusetts Medical School; Director, Stress Reduction Clinic, University of Massachusetts Medical Center, Worcester, Massachusetts

Thomas Erling Kottke, M.D.

Associate Professor of Medicine, Department of Internal Medicine, Division of Cardiovascular Diseases and Internal Medicine, Mayo Medical School; Senior Associate Consultant, Mayo Clinic, Rochester, Minnesota

Robert J. Nicolosi, Ph.D.

Professor and Director of Cardiovascular Research, Department of Clinical Sciences, University of Massachusetts-Lowell, Lowell, Massachusetts

Ira S. Ockene, M.D.

Professor of Medicine, and Director, Preventive Cardiology Program; Associate Director, Division of Cardiovascular Medicine, Department of Medicine, University of Massachusetts Medical School, Worcester, Massachusetts

Judith K. Ockene, Ph.D.

Professor of Medicine, and Director, Division of Preventive and Behavioral Medicine, Department of Medicine, University of Massachusetts Medical School, Worcester, Massachusetts

Trevor J. Orchard, M.B.B.Ch.

Associate Professor of Epidemiology, and Medical Director, Nutrition Lipid Program, Graduate School of Public Health, University of Pittsburgh, Pittsburgh, Pennsylvania

Michael Pertschuk, J.D.

Co-Director, The Advocacy Institute, Washington, D.C.

James M. Rippe, M.D.

Associate Professor of Medicine, Division of Cardiovascular Medicine, Department of Medicine, University of Massachusetts Medical School; Director, Center for Clinical and Lifestyle Research, University of Massachusetts Medical Center, Worcester, Massachusetts

Ernst J. Schaefer, M.D.

Professor of Medicine, and Chief, Lipid Metabolism Laboratory, USDA Human Nutrition Research Center on Aging, Tufts University School of Medicine; Director, Lipid Clinic, New England Medical Center, Boston, Massachusetts

Leif I. Solberg, M.D.

Medical Director for Quality Improvement, Blue Cross, Blue Shield, and Blue Plus of Minnesota, St. Paul, Minnesota

Glorian Sorensen, Ph.D., M.P.H.

Associate Professor, Department of Health and Social Behavior, School of Public Health, Harvard University; Director, Community Based Programs, Division of Cancer Epidemiology and Control, Dana Farber Cancer Institute, Boston, Massachusetts

Pamela Ann Taylor, M.D.

Attending Cardiologist, Memorial Hospital and Penrose–St. Francis Hospitals, Colorado Springs, Colorado

Beti Thompson, Ph.D.

Assistant Professor, School of Public Health and Community Medicine, University of Washington; Assistant Member, Cancer Prevention Research Program, Fred Hutchinson Cancer Research Center, Seattle, Washington

Nicole Urban, Sc.D.

Assistant Professor of Health Services, School of Public Health and Community Medicine, University of Washington; Assistant Member, Cancer Prevention Research Program, Fred Hutchinson Cancer Research Center, Seattle, Washington

Ann Ward, Ph.D.

Associate Professor of Medicine, Division of Cardiovascular Medicine, Department of Medicine, University of Massachusetts Medical School, Worcester, Massachusetts

Bonnie H. Weiner, M.D.

Professor of Medicine, Division of Cardiovascular Medicine, Department of Medicine, University of Massachusetts Medical School; Director, Cardiac Catheterization Laboratories, University of Massachusetts Medical Center, Worcester, Massachusetts

Christine L. Williams, M.D., M.P.H.

Professor of Pediatrics, New York Medical College; Attending Pediatrician, Westchester County Medical Center, Valhalla, New York

Juan Carlos Zevallos, M.D.

Teaching Director, Central University — Quito; Attending Cardiologist, Centro Médico Quirurgico Pichincha, Quito, Ecuador

Foreword

Physicians' efforts to prevent coronary heart disease (CHD) have been in progress, with mounting intensity and scope, for more than a quarter of a century. As this book details, much has been accomplished; much more remains to be done. Mastery of this book's substance by M.D.s and their staffs — mastery especially of the in-depth "how to" chapters on clinical and public health intervention — will greatly enhance the capability and readiness of medical practitioners to respond successfully to the expanded challenges of the CHD preventive endeavor in the 1990s.

In the late 1950s and early 1960s, landmark statements — by cardiologists and cardiovascular researchers, and by the American Heart Association — spelled out the need for and possibility of CHD prevention. These were given wide currency. From the beginning the emphasis has been on the *epidemic impact* of CHD on the U.S. population, both for people in the prime of life and for older people. To curb this mass problem, treatment for those already ill, however necessary and useful, is not enough; it alone will not and cannot turn the tide, especially since more than 40 percent of first major coronary events are fatal, usually before medical care can be brought to bear. *Primary prevention,* the prevention of first episodes of CHD, is essential. And primary prevention requires breaking links in the chain of CHD causation, especially links early in the chain. That means dealing with the origins of the epidemic in twentieth-century lifestyles. Down this road lies the possibility of large-scale CHD prevention, both for the millions at higher risk and for the population overall.

From the start, the CHD preventive effort has had a solid scientific foundation. This has been continuously reinforced and enriched decade after decade by research findings from clinical-pathologic investigation, animal experimentation, and epidemiologic studies. The vast and coherent data base, reviewed at intervals, is comprehensively presented in this book.

The general theoretical framework of reference is the concept set down more than a century ago by Rudolph Virchow: epidemics occur as a result of "disturbances in human culture." The specific disturbances causing the CHD epidemic are well known to American physicians, other health professionals, policy makers, and the public. They are first and foremost the four major CHD risk factors: "rich" diet, diet-dependent elevated levels of serum cholesterol and blood pressure, and cigarette smoking. (These four major risk factors are aided and abetted by sedentary habits and adverse psychosocial factors.) The data are overwhelming in support of the conclusion that these four play a significant and decisive role in the causation of the CHD epidemic. They are appropriately designated *major* risk factors because of their established important etiologic role, because they are amenable to prevention and control, and because they are prevalent in the population. In fact, rich diet and diet-dependent elevations of serum cholesterol and blood pressure are manifest among the great majority of the population. And cigarette smoking continues to be an addiction involving a substantial minority of the population.

"Rich" diet is the pivotal mass exposure responsible for the coronary epidemic. Where rich diet does not prevail as a populationwide trait, there is no CHD epidemic. This is the case even when high blood pressure and cigarette smoking are prevalent (witness Japan). Physicians therefore need to understand thoroughly what a rich diet is, and what to do about it; this book serves them well in this regard.

A rich diet is an imbalanced diet excessive in cholesterol, saturated fats, and total fats; in calories for level of physical activity; in salt; in high-fat animal products; in visible fats; in other highly processed foods, including processed meats, dairy products, baked goods, "junk" foods, separated refined sugars. It is a diet of high caloric density — that is, a high ratio of calories to essential nutrients — and hence (along with sedentary lifestyle) it readily results in obesity while at the same time it is often relatively and even absolutely low in essential constituents (potassium, fiber, and antioxidant vitamins, for example). It is also too often a diet excessive in alcohol. It is a diet producing in the population a high mean level of serum cholesterol in youth, a steady substantial rise in that mean level from youth through young adulthood into middle age, high prevalence rates of dyslipidemia, and low prevalence of optimal low-normal lipidemia — effects induced largely by high intakes of cholesterol and saturated fats, calorie imbalance, and low fiber intake. It also produces in the population a high mean level of blood pressure in youth, a steady substantial rise in that mean level from youth through young adulthood into middle age, high prevalence rates of hypertension, and low prevalence of optimal low-normal blood pressure — effects induced significantly by excessive salt intake, a high ratio of dietary sodium to potassium, calorie imbalance, and excessive alcohol intake. It is a diet contributing to high prevalence rates of non-insulin-dependent diabetes mellitus among Americans age 55 and over. Because of its lipid composition, and especially its high cholesterol content, this diet adds independently to CHD risk over and above all of the foregoing adverse effects. It increases risk of both atherogenesis and thrombosis, as this book details.

Because of all these effects, "rich" diet is the *primary* and *essential* cause of epidemic CHD. Once this diet is operative over the long term, other mass exposures — first and foremost cigarette smoking — act as important secondary (adjuvant) causes.

The twentieth-century American diet is — like the twentieth-century mass use of cigarettes — a new and unprecedented exposure for the human species. It is radically different from previous eating patterns; there has been no basis in prior human experience for evolutionary adaptation to this exposure. Therefore the human genome does not include the biological resources to enable people to maintain optimal levels of such traits as serum lipids and blood pressure in the face of this dietary impact. Almost all of us are more or less at risk of its deleterious consequences, as is the case with such other unprecedented twentieth-century mass exposures as cigarette smoking and sedentary lifestyle.

It is this fact of the "nature-nurture" (heredity-environment) relationship that accounts for the populationwide impact of the coronary epidemic, and that determines the *fundamental thrust of strategy* for its control. As this book emphasizes, that strategic thrust — and physicians' efforts to implement it — is two-pronged: recommendations for improved lifestyles for the whole population from early childhood on, and special medical care efforts for individuals and families at particularly high risk. For such high-risk persons, physicians must emphasize the key role of improved lifestyles — better habits of eating, drinking, and exercise, and avoidance of tobacco. They need to make it clear to their patients repeatedly that drug treatment, prescribed when indicated for particular individuals, is adjuvant to lifestyle recommendations. Given the origins of the coronary epidemic in mass disturbances of human culture, it is clear that high-tech "magic bullets" are not and cannot be the solution, be they drugs, surgical procedures, gene splicing, or whatever. At most, such special approaches can contribute only if they are recognized — and utilized — as supplements to the main lifestyle efforts.

The two-pronged strategy, emphasizing improved lifestyles both for the whole population and for persons and families at higher risk, was originally set down in the pioneering initial statements of the American Heart Association in the early 1960s and the milestone reports of the Inter-Society Commission for Heart Disease Resources in the early 1970s. Over the years, a key prerequisite for a major disease prevention effort was achieved: this same two-pronged strategy for control of the CHD epidemic was progressively adopted as official national government policy. The policy began with the *Report to the Surgeon General on Smoking and Health* in 1964, and the recommendations of the White House Conference on Nutrition shortly thereafter. Its most current expressions are in reports of the National Cholesterol Education Program and National High Blood Pressure Education Program, and in *Healthy People 2000 — National Health Promotion and Disease Prevention Objectives,* from the Public Health Service. These recent reports serve as valuable supplementary reading for physicians who have mastered this book.

Despite all too limited resources for implementation and roadblocks from special commercial interests (the tobacco industry and sectors of the food industry), the message has gotten out, has been heard up and down the land, and has been acted on by tens of millions of American families, as this book documents. Critical mass has been achieved; the impact is registered in general national statistics reviewed in this book: per capita consumption of butter, total dairy fat, lard, high-fat beef and pork, and eggs are all down considerably, with consequent reductions in the population's mean intake of cholesterol and saturated fats, and in mean population serum cholesterol levels — all reflecting mass discovery of alternative, healthier paths to pleasurable eating, for example the Mediterranean and Far Eastern ways. Prevalence of cigarette smoking among men is down from about 55 percent three decades ago to less than 30 percent nowadays, and it's down, too, among women. And there has been mass adoption of leisure-time exercise as a health-maintenance, health-promotion, and pleasurable activity. As this book repeatedly documents, every survey probing reasons for these favorable trends comes up with a uniform answer: advice from physicians and other health professionals has been a key factor leading to improved lifestyles. Possibly we health professionals don't fully grasp our own powers of firm steady persuasion. This book is a big help in that regard.

Above all, there is the dramatic and exciting bottom line, set out in data also described in full detail here: CHD mortality is down more than 50 percent from its peak in the late 1960s; throughout the 1970s and 1980s, the United States set the pace for industrialized countries in declining CHD mortality rates; there have been absolute decreases in total numbers of CHD deaths despite increases in the size and median age of the population; evidence shows that the decline in CHD mortality reflects a fall in total incidence of "hard" major coronary events, nonfatal plus fatal; even steeper falls in stroke mortality rates have been seen, with substantial declines in death rates from all cardiovascular disease and from all causes, as well. Years have been added to life expectancy — not only for newborns, but also for adult Americans, a reversal of a previous unfavorable trend. Indeed it seems reasonable to infer that during these years of the unfolding coronary prevention effort, we physicians have apparently been engaged in "doing the right things"!

Awareness of these accomplishments needs to be tempered by sober understanding of the limitations in their extent, and therefore the scope of the challenges ahead. The flank of the CHD epidemic has been turned, but the epidemic still rages. CHD remains the most important producer of sickness, disability, and death among Americans, as this book amply documents. Internationally, U.S. death rates from CHD still rank in the top ten; that is, they are among the highest in the world. Largely as a consequence, life expectancy for both newborn and adult Americans still lags behind that of several countries — Costa Rica, Greece, and Japan, for example. In this regard, the chapter here giving the international perspective is both sobering and challenging for American physicians.

While progress has been made in improving lifestyles, stated national dietary goals have not been met, nor are we really close to their attainment: dietary cholesterol intake of less than 300 mg/day or less than 100 mg/1000 kcal; saturated fat intake less than 10 percent of kcal; and total fat intake less than 30 percent of kcal. Almost no progress has been made in controlling obesity among Americans; in fact, data from successive national health and nutrition surveys indicate that for most adult sex-race groups, body mass has on average increased. Given these trends, the pattern of population mean serum cholesterol change is an expected one: significant declines, modest in degree, falling well short of the 1990 health goal of an average adult level of less than 200 mg/dl. Similarly, given the lack of evidence for substantial declines in per capita consumption of salt, in body mass, or in percent of heavy drinkers in the population, trends of mean blood pressure and prevalence rates of hypertension are expected ones: little or no evidence of declines except among older Americans, these latter attributable almost certainly to the fact that a high proportion — possibly a majority — of Americans age 60 and over are taking antihypertensive drugs. Clearly the primary prevention of high blood pressure by safe nutritional-hygienic means is a challenge whose time has come. Further, as this book emphasizes, while the decline in prevalence of cigarette use is a substantial accomplishment, "hard core" problems confront us in this area with regard to very heavy smokers. And for many people who have taken up leisure-time exercise, involvement is sporadic and of a low order. All these experiences serve to drive home a key lesson for further sustained success of the CHD prevention effort: *we need to make primary prevention of the major risk factors a major priority*. This approach, emphasizing primary formation of favorable habits from early childhood on and not just changing habits later in life, is the way to the ultimate end of the epidemic.

All physicians, health professionals, and policy makers reading this book must also be seriously concerned that in regard to all aspects of lifestyle (eating, drinking, smoking, and exercise patterns), improvements have occurred at a much lower rate among the less educated and less affluent than among the more educated, more affluent. Correspondingly, and as predicted based on the concept that unfavorable lifestyles and lifestyle–related risk factors play a decisive role in causing the CHD epidemic, declines in CHD incidence and mortality have been significantly smaller among the less educated, less affluent strata of our population. It

is noteworthy that the decline in CHD mortality has been particularly steep among U.S. physicians. After all, don't doctors have the most ready access to knowledge about the major risk factors, and the most ready capability and motivation to act on this knowledge? In the light of such facts, the wealth of information for physicians in the Ockenes' book on the why and how-to of CHD prevention affords a splendid opportunity for all of us to do right by our patients and our community, with the fresh dedication and fervor essential for meeting current challenges.

How high, then, should we set our sights? How much more can we hope to accomplish? An illuminating guide for answering these questions is to be found in the unique data on 361,662 men aged 35 to 57 screened in 18 U.S. cities in the years 1973 to 1975 for the recruitment effort of the Multiple Risk Factor Intervention Trial (MRFIT). At present, 12-year follow-up data are available on the vital status of these men (24,013 are deceased). With these unprecedented large numbers, estimates of the impact of major risk factors can be made with great precision. With use of baseline findings, it is quickly apparent that men at very low risk are nonsmokers, free of a clinical history of diabetes and myocardial infarction, with serum cholesterol in the lowest quintile (20%) of the distribution of this major risk factor (less than 182 mg/dl), and with systolic and diastolic pressures under the medical profession's classical cut points of 120/80 mmHg. (No data on eating, drinking, or exercise habits were collected when these men were screened.) Use of these criteria identified 11,098 men at very low risk, only 3 percent of the total cohort. Given contemporary deleterious mass exposures, the very low risk American is a "rare bird"! The problem of risk factor levels being above optimal is indeed a populationwide problem and not "just" a problem for a minority at higher risk. The age-adjusted 12-year CHD death rate for these 11,098 men was only 10 percent of the rate for the rest of the cohort; that is, it was lower by 90 percent. All other death rates were also substantially lower, including those from stroke, cancers, and all causes. And these estimates must be underestimates of the potential for prevention, since they are based on only a one-time measurement of only three of the four major risk factors. Despite these limitations, the data demonstrate that the major risk factors are responsible for the vast majority of CHD deaths. They point the way to goals for the next stage of our coronary prevention effort.

Having contributed to the more than 50 percent fall in the CHD death rate already achieved, American physicians can proceed to intensify the decline, with the goal of its becoming 90 percent by the first decade of the twenty-first century. This they can do by enhancing the effectiveness of their preventive services for their patients and patients' families and for their communities, and — through their organizations — by ensuring at the national level the maintenance of a sound public policy and the allocation of necessary resources for its implementation. For this worthy purpose, the Ockenes' book is a valuable weapon indeed.

Jeremiah Stamler, M.D.
Rose Stamler, M.A.

Preface

Interest in the prevention of coronary heart disease has increased at a remarkable rate. It is unusual to pick up a copy of any popular weekly magazine or daily newspaper without finding at least one article dealing with this subject. The public is deeply concerned with cholesterol and dietary fat, overwhelmingly aware of the hazards of smoking, and very interested in information on such other coronary risk factors as stress and exercise. Book stores have devoted entire sections to these topics. Yet there are surprisingly few books on the prevention of coronary heart disease that are directed to the professional medical audience. In part this reflects a belief that physicians are interested only in treatment and care little about the prevention of disease. If this were ever true, it is no longer the case today. The majority of physicians and other health care workers now recognize the "why" of coronary heart disease prevention. What remains to be addressed are the feasibility of prevention and the "how to" in a busy clinical practice or in a community setting.

Prevention of Coronary Heart Disease brings together authors from clinical medicine and public health to address the how to of preventing coronary heart disease. We include considerable background information and scientific documentation to support a vigorous approach to prevention, and we focus on developing the individually oriented intervention skills that clinicians need to make a preventive approach work and to make it a standard of care. We also address the community setting in which the physician and health care provider work, to provide an understanding of how heart disease prevention extends beyond the clinical office practice.

Prevention of Coronary Heart Disease is written for general internists, family physicians, pediatricians, and gynecologists who have responsibility for the primary care of the patient, as well as for such subspecialists as cardiologists. Residents and medical students can also benefit from this book. In addition, the information and approaches provided can serve as a useful guide for the many other students, teachers, practitioners, and advocates interested in public health and the prevention of coronary disease: dietitians, psychologists, sociologists, and individuals in the media and politics. For the clinician, this book will be a tool for clinical prevention; for the researcher, it will provide data to support the preventive approach to medicine and to coronary heart disease in particular; and for the physician and the public health practitioner, it will provide a guide to prevention in the context of the community.

Prevention of Coronary Heart Disease addresses several correctable factors that have played an important role in keeping clinicians from practicing preventive cardiology. First and foremost, physicians and other health care practitioners often lack the skills they need to translate a desire to effect change into reality. Until recently, training in such areas as behavioral medicine, dietary modification, exercise prescription, and outpatient management of hyperlipidemia has not been part of either the medical school or the usual postgraduate curriculum. This book provides the information necessary to carry out the needed interventions. Second, physicians' days are filled with pressure, and they have few extra moments to spend in leisurely counseling. Therefore the methods presented in this book are efficient and require minimal time. In addition, techniques are included for organizing an office practice in a way that makes the practice of preventive cardiology flow smoothly and that efficiently integrates it into the everyday routine of patient care. Third and finally, information is provided to help the clinician develop a public health point of view that will allow him or her to think in terms of the health of society as a whole, as well as that of the individual patient.

Prevention of Coronary Heart Disease is divided into four sections:

I. **Introduction and Background**. We provide the necessary grounding in epidemiology, pathophysiology, and animal and human research to support our current philosophy of intervention. We also explore the international aspects of coronary heart disease.

II. **Clinical Intervention**. In the central section of this book, we summarize current thinking about counseling patients for risk-factor reduction, and then devote specific chapters to each of the major risk factors. In all of these chapters the emphasis is on giving the health care practitioner the tools needed to intervene effectively — including a chapter on organizing a prevention-oriented practice.

III. **Intervention: The Public Health Perspective**. For the clinician and for others, we broaden our focus to include areas outside the traditional medical practice — school, worksite, and community — where change must occur before we can truly affect the incidence of coronary heart disease. Many physicians do play a role in these areas, and we believe that others would also if provided with an appropriate base of information. In addition, we suggest methods by which the health care practitioner can work with the media and interact effectively with those in political life, so that he or she can be an effective advocate for the prevention of heart disease.

IV. **Other Issues Regarding the Prevention of Coronary Heart Disease**. In the last two chapters we deal with cost-effectiveness issues — a topic of great interest — and with methods that may be used effectively to incorporate prevention training in the training of medical students, residents, and fellows.

We owe much to our colleagues, family, friends and patients. They have taught us how to listen, how to teach, and how to learn. We are particularly indebted to three individuals who were role models to both of us and oriented our path toward the prevention of coronary heart disease. James E. Dalen, M.D., M.P.H., our mentor first at the Peter Bent Brigham Hospital and the Harvard School of Public Health and later as Chief of Medicine at the University of Massachusetts Medical School, and now Dean of the Medical School of the University of Arizona Health Sciences Center, had the vision to promote the concepts of preventive cardiology and behavioral medicine. In his own career he showed how well interests in clinical cardiology and cardiovascular epidemiology compliment each other. Jeremiah Stamler, M.D., Professor Emeritus, Department of Community Health and Preventive Medicine, Northwestern University, taught us the importance of believing strongly in a cause and dedicating oneself to that effort. Lewis Kuller, M.D., Dr.P.H., Professor and Chairperson, Department of Epidemiology, Graduate School of Public Health, University of Pittsburgh, was another wonderful role model who taught us the importance of continuing to question and explore. We are grateful to all of them.

This book is the result of the combined clinical, research, and teaching experience of many individuals. Our goal has been to introduce the clinician, researcher, public health practitioner, student, and teacher to the excitement and attainability of coronary heart disease prevention and to encourage greater efforts in this area, both for the public's health and for the personal rewards such efforts bring.

I.S.O.
J.K.O.

I

INTRODUCTION AND BACKGROUND

1

Coronary Heart Disease: Epidemiology and Risk Factors

ROBERT J. GOLDBERG

EDITORS' INTRODUCTION

To effectively develop methodologies for the prevention of coronary heart disease (CHD), it is necessary to understand the nature of the problem and the relationship of risk factors to the development of disease. This chapter reviews the epidemiology of CHD and provides the all-important groundwork for that which follows. Dr. Goldberg describes the magnitude of the problem and then introduces the large-scale epidemiologic studies, such as the Framingham Heart Study and the Seven Countries Study, that have provided much of the basis for our understanding of how population characteristics affect the incidence and course of the disease. The natural history of CHD is then described, and the manner in which risk factors may affect the pathophysiologic process is discussed. The remainder of the chapter introduces the known (and some of the speculated) CHD risk factors. The more important risk factors are individually addressed in subsequent chapters, but here the reader will find useful summaries of current knowledge.

Despite recent and encouraging declines in the mortality rates attributed to coronary heart disease, coronary atherosclerosis and its accompanying clinical manifestations remain the leading cause of death in the United States [1]. The consequences of this disease process exact an enormous economic toll and cause considerable personal suffering. Many of the adverse sequelae associated with coronary atherosclerosis could be prevented, or at least delayed, in those individuals at increased risk for coronary disease by careful and continued attention to the lifestyle and personal characteristics that may place them at high risk and that can be favorably altered through an increasing array of tailored intervention approaches.

A number of modifiable risk factors, as well as nonmodifiable risk markers, have been associated with the occurrence of coronary heart disease (CHD). Data collected from landmark prospective epidemiologic investigations and studies of migrant populations over the past several decades have established a clear relation between increased risk for the development of CHD and increasing levels of serum cholesterol, cigarette smoking, and blood pressure. These risk factors have been shown to be singly important and interactively multiplicative for CHD.

Given the extensive literature compiled on the risk factors for CHD [2,3,4], this chapter provides an introductory overview of the primary as well as secondary risk factors for CHD, with a particular focus on those factors that may be altered through lifestyle changes and/or pharmacologic interventions. Later chapters specific to individual risk factors provide information in greater depth, and the interested reader is also referred to the references cited. Given that the major risk factors for CHD are related to all the principal clinical manifestations of CHD, including angina pectoris, acute myocardial infarction (MI), and sudden cardiac death (although their predictive utility may vary according to the clinical condition examined as well as to age, sex, and other sociodemographic or comorbid factors), distinctions according to the specific clinical manifestations of CHD are made only in those instances where sufficient

data suggest an association of a presumed coronary risk factor to a specific manifestation of CHD.

The first section of this chapter reviews the magnitude of the problem of CHD in the United States and the landmark prospective, population-based studies that provided the initial insights into the concept of risk factors for CHD. Subsequent sections discuss the natural history and the descriptive epidemiology of CHD, ending with an overview of the epidemiology of the risk factors for CHD, including those for which the evidence is not yet well established. Temporal trends in these risk factors are specifically addressed in Chapter 2.

Magnitude of CHD in the United States

Since the early decades of the twentieth century, when the epidemic of coronary atherosclerosis first began to appear in the United States, cardiovascular disease has been the leading cause of death in this country, as well as contributing significantly to the disability of persons afflicted with its various clinical syndromes and accompanying symptomatology. As a group the cardiovascular diseases exact a considerable toll, as reflected by over 5.6 million hospitalizations for cardiovascular disease and approximately 975,000 deaths in 1987.

Of the various forms of cardiovascular disease, heart disease is the most prevalent, significantly affecting individual and community mortality rates and the use of health care resources. In 1987, over 3.7 million persons were hospitalized with a first-listed discharge diagnosis of heart disease. Over 760,000 persons died from heart disease that same year, leading to its unenviable position as the leading cause of death among all persons in the United States, causing approximately 36 percent of all deaths in 1987 [1]. Of the various manifestations of heart disease — rheumatic and hypertensive heart disease, diseases of the pulmonary circulation, heart failure, cardiomyopathies, and others — CHD, or atherosclerotic heart disease, is the principal disease entity discussed in this chapter. Indicative of the prevalence and seriousness of this condition in the United States is the fact that in 1987 approximately 2.2 million persons were hospitalized with a first-listed discharge diagnosis of CHD. These persons spent an average of 6.5 days in the hospital, and over 512,000 died as a result of CHD. In 1985 over 10 million visits were made to physicians' offices due to this disease [1]. Based on 1987 estimates, approximately 7 million persons, or 3 percent of the United States population, have atherosclerotic heart disease, and slightly over one-third of these persons are limited in their activities due to CHD. These data provide further reinforcement and rationale for research and clinical activities that are attempting to better understand the pathogenetic mechanisms involved in this disease process, to improve the efficacy and cost effectiveness of various prevention and treatment strategies, and to provide more effective delivery of acute care and rehabilitative services in order to limit the disability and improve the prognosis associated with CHD.

Landmark Studies of the Epidemiology of CHD

Beginning in the late 1940s with the establishment and screening of the first cohort of a general population sample of males and females in Framingham, Massachusetts [5, 6], a number of worksite and community-based studies investigating the determinants of cardiovascular disease were launched. These investigations included the Chicago Peoples Gas Company Study [7] and the Chicago Western Electric Company Study in Chicago, Illinois [8], the Tecumseh Health Study in Tecumseh, Michigan [9], the Albany Cardiovascular Health Center Study in Albany, New York [10], the Los Angeles Heart Study in Los Angeles, California [11], the Minnesota Business and Professional Men's Study in St. Paul and Minneapolis, Minnesota [12], and the Western Collaborative Group Study in the San Francisco-Oakland Bay area and Los Angeles, California [13]. The baseline demographic and descriptive characteristics of persons enrolled in these studies are shown in Table 1-1. These studies ranged from relatively small select samples of middle-aged men to more extensive community-based samples designed to provide a more representative appraisal of the risk factors for CHD and associated morbidity and mortality. This chapter examines one of these landmark studies, the Framingham Heart Study, in greater detail.

Since 1949 and continuing to the present, a general population sample of 5209 adult residents (2336 men and 2873 women) of Framingham, Massachusetts, between the ages of 30 and 62 years has received a routine, standardized examination for cardiovascular disease and for the risk factors for CHD on a biennial basis. The participants were selected from approximately 10,000 persons in this age range living in Framingham in 1949. The town of Framingham at the time of the initiation of the study was an industrial and trading center of approximately 28,000 persons slightly more than 20 miles west of Boston. The town was selected for a number of reasons: the first community study of tuberculosis was successfully undertaken there more than 30 years previously; the size of the town, which had a town-meeting form of government, would facilitate the ability to secure full cooperation and coverage for such a community-wide investigation; and the Massachusetts Department of Public Health and the Department of Preventive Medicine at Harvard Medical School were receptive to cooperating with the Heart Disease Demonstration Section of the United States Public Health Service in conducting such a study. Operationally an executive committee, which represented various community groups, and six subcommittees were established for this longitudinal study.

Prior to the formal acceptance of the Framingham Study by the National Heart Institute in 1949, a clinic was opened at the only hospital in Framingham, Framingham Union Hospital, for the express purpose of examining potential participants. By the time the study was transferred to the National Heart Institute, over 1500 volunteers had been examined for purposes of participating in the formal investigation. A sampling scheme was subsequently designed in

Table 1-1. Descriptive characteristics of landmark prospective epidemiologic investigations of coronary heart disease

Investigation	Geographic locale	Year of initiation	Sample size*	Sample characteristics	Age range, years
Framingham Study	Framingham, MA	1948	5127 men and women	Sample of town residents	30–62
Minnesota Business and Professional Men's Study	St. Paul and Minneapolis, MN	1948	281 men	Volunteers from local businesses	45–55
Los Angeles Heart Study	Los Angeles, CA	1950	1653 men 354 women	Stratified sample of local civil service employees	21+
Albany Cardiovascular Health Center Study	Albany, NY	1953	1843 men	Volunteer sample of civil service employees	<40–55+
Chicago Peoples Gas Company Study	Chicago, IL	1954	3203 men	Complete sample of employees of a large public utility company	25–59
Chicago Western Electric Company Study	Chicago, IL	1957	1989 men	Random sample of long-term employees of a large manufacturing corporation	40–55
Tecumseh Health Study	Tecumseh, MI	1959	2328 men 2592 women	Sample of town residents	16–70+
Western Collaborative Group Study	San Francisco Bay Area and Los Angeles, CA	1960	3154 men	Recruited from ten companies in California	39–59

*Participants were free from CHD where such information was available.

which two-thirds of the Framingham residents between 30 and 59 years of age would be selected for further study. The lower age limit was decided on because of the small number of CHD events expected in younger persons and because their mobility would make repeat examinations difficult; the upper age limit was selected because of the large expected prevalence of CHD in an older sample. Families were considered eligible and were recruited for this study. From the adult residents of the town, 6532 were originally sampled, and 4469 were examined and completed the initial screening assessment. Approximately 68 percent of those invited to participate did so. The baseline cohort was further supplemented by 740 volunteers, thereby making the original cohort sample size

of 5209 persons. Comprehensive cardiovascular and CHD risk-factor histories were taken from each participant; all also underwent a cardiovascular physical examination, multiple blood pressure measurements, and a variety of blood chemistry measurements, including cholesterol, lipoproteins, and blood sugar. Among the original sample, 5127 men and women were found to be free from cardiovascular disease at the time of study entry.

Follow-up of this cohort has been excellent: over 80 percent of the study subjects have undergone each biennial exam, and less than 5 percent had been lost to mortality follow-up at the time of the fourteenth biennial examination. Recent efforts to improve the long-term follow-up rates have reduced those lost to mortality follow-up to less than 1 percent of the original study sample. The most recent examination of this cohort was carried out in 1990, the twenty-first biennial examination. This cornerstone prospective epidemiologic study has identified a host of nonmodifiable risk factors (family history, male sex, advancing age) and modifiable risk factors (elevated total cholesterol, low levels of high-density lipoprotein cholesterol, cigarette smoking, elevated blood pressure, diabetes mellitus, physical inactivity, and obesity) associated with the development of cardiovascular disease and has also provided a systematic framework for the assessment of the magnitude of risk associated with these risk factors singly and in combination. Reflecting the successful achievements of this prospective study, the children of the original Framingham Study cohort have been administered a detailed clinical and noninvasive evaluation for CHD since 1972, forming the Framingham Offspring Study [14]. This cohort is reexamined every four years to determine changes in cardiovascular health status and in the predisposing risk factors for CHD. The two primary goals of this cohort study are to examine secular changes in the major CHD risk factors between the two generations of Framingham enrollees and to understand the role of familial factors in determining the levels of these risk factors.

The landmark prospective epidemiologic investigations of CHD in the United States were complemented by additional cohort studies in other parts of the world, including Great Britain [15], men of Japanese descent living in Hawaii [16], Israel [17], Japan [18], and Scandinavia [19]. These key investigations have been followed by numerous case-control and longitudinal investigations of CHD in these and additional countries. A particularly ambitious undertaking of the study of the determinants of CHD was the Seven Countries Study [20]. This multicohort study, initiated in the mid 1950s, examined the morbidity and mortality rates of CHD, as well as host and environmental factors associated with its occurrence, among over 12,000 middle-aged (40–59 years) men assembled from seven countries and differing in their cultural and lifestyle habits. The countries studied were Finland, Greece, Italy, Japan, the Netherlands, the United States, and Yugoslavia. As can be seen in Table 1-2, a diverse array of countries and population samples were selected to provide contrasts in lifestyle and dietary factors associated with the development of CHD. A careful personal, occupational, and medical history was taken from each of the participants in the Seven Countries Study, and all underwent a physical examination, as well as having a 12-lead electrocardiogram, respiratory function tests, height, weight, skinfold thickness, and blood pressure measurements, and a blood sample for hematocrit and cholesterol determinations. Dietary surveys of the cohorts were also carried out. The men were followed and reexamined after five years, and the period of follow-up was subsequently extended. Standardized criteria were utilized for the various endpoints assessed. As further seen in Table 1-2, among the 12,511 men judged to be free from CHD at the outset of the study, the annual incidence rates of CHD differed considerably among the various cohorts. The incidence rates of CHD were highest in Finland and the United States and lowest in Japan and Greece; differences were also observed both between and within the cohorts in terms of the risk factors for CHD, with the Japanese, in general, having lower prevalence rates for most of the examined principal risk factors with the exception of cigarette smoking.

These national and international prospective epidemiologic investigations established a framework for the study of cardiovascular disease and its natural history from a broad population-based perspective and furnished clues to those factors associated with its occurrence and ultimately its prevention. In addition they also firmly established the credibility and usefulness of the epidemiologic approach to the study of cardiovascular disease.

The findings from five of these studies — the Albany Cardiovascular Health Center Study, the Chicago Peoples Gas Company Study, the Chicago Western Electric Company Study, the Framingham Heart Study, and the Tecumseh Health Study — were considered sufficiently comparable to have their data collectively ana-

Table 1-2. Descriptive characteristics of population samples participating in the Seven Countries Study (n = 12,763)

Geographic cohort	Year of cohort initiation	Sample size at entry*	Study sample	Prevalence rates (%)					Age-adjusted average annual CHD incidence rates (per 10,000)
				Regular smokers of ≥10 cigarettes/day	Cholesterol >250 mg/dl	Systolic bp ≥160 mmHg	Relative weight >110%	Sedentary	
United States	1958–1960	2571	Employees of selected railroad companies	51	39	16	32	60	177
Yugoslavia	1958	1367	Residents of Dalmatia, on the coast, and Slavonia, on the plains						
	1962–1964	1565	Residents of Velika Krsna (a rural village) and Zrenjanin (a small agricultural market town) and faculty of the University of Belgrade	49	7	11	19	30	53
Finland	1959	1677	Residents of rural areas of east and west Finland	50	56	19	15	10	198
Italy	1960	1712	Residents of the rural agricultural villages of Crevalcore and Montegiorgio	43	13	18	22	14	100
	1962	768	Railroad men from Rome						
Netherlands	1960	878	Residents of the commercial town of Zutphen	44	32	21	13	24	139
Greece	1960, 1961	1215	Residents of the islands of Crete and Corfu	49	14	13	11	18	32
Japan	1958, 1960	1010	Residents of the rural agricultural village of Tanushimaru and the fishing village of Ushibuka	59	7	14	2	6	15–20

*Participants were free from CHD where such information was available.

lyzed and reported in the findings of the Pooling Project Research Group [21]. The essential findings of this seminal publication, based on information derived from white middle-aged men free from CHD at the time of their baseline screening examinations, were that increasing age and an array of potentially modifiable risk factors (e.g., cigarette smoking and elevated cholesterol and blood pressure levels) were associated with the subsequent development of CHD.

Further support for the role of environmental factors in the occurrence of CHD was provided by migrant studies carried out in Israel, New Zealand, and Japan [22, 23, 24]. Perhaps the most compelling of these studies was the Ni-Hon-San (from *Nippon*, *Honolulu*, and *San* Francisco) Study of middle-aged Japanese men who had migrated to Honolulu and to San Francisco. In comparison to those remaining in Japan, the CHD death rates of the migrants came to resemble those of their country of adoption [24] (Figure 1-1). As seen, the age-specific mortality rates from CHD were two to three times greater for Japanese migrating to a country with epidemic rates of CHD (the United States) compared to those persons remaining in Japan, whereas the mortality rates were in between for those Japanese men who had migrated to Hawaii. The differences in these death rates were attributed to likely changes in dietary habits and the adoption of adverse lifestyle factors associated with an increased risk for the development of and/or the risk of dying from CHD among those migrating to the United States compared to those Japanese remaining in their native country. In a further long-term (12-year) follow-up of the men of Japanese ancestry in Japan and Hawaii free from CHD at the time of their baseline examination, the mortality rate from CHD was found to be approximately 40 percent higher among Japanese men in Hawaii than in Japan [25].

Each of the factors described in subsequent

Figure 1-1.   Death rates from CHD in the Ni-Hon-San Study.

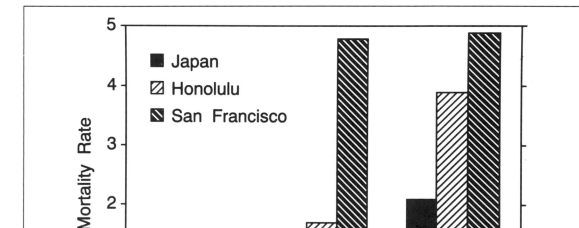

sections is associated with selected clinical manifestations of coronary atherosclerosis. However, these predisposing factors may or may not have a causal relationship to CHD, although their presence increases the likelihood that a person has or will develop CHD within a defined period of time. It may very well be that there is a single causal risk factor (perhaps a lipid abnormality, such as elevated low-density lipoprotein levels) and that all other known or suspected risk factors are accelerators, namely agents that cannot by themselves initiate the atherosclerotic process but that hasten its course once it is present. On the other hand, it should not be inferred that persons free of the coronary risk factors or risk markers identified to date are immune from the risk of developing CHD. In the United States many individuals have none of the currently identified and established risk factors for CHD, yet the incidence of CHD in groups of such individuals is much higher than that in similar groups in other parts of the world. Moreover, it is widely accepted and generally acknowledged that CHD is a multifactorial disease and that a multiplicity of interacting factors are involved in its development. It is also possible that risk-factor levels we consider normal, e.g., serum cholesterol levels of 180 to 200 mg/dl, are abnormal on a worldwide scale and in a range where CHD can develop. Chapter 4 examines this concept more fully.

The following section is an overview of the natural history of CHD. The section after that describes the epidemiology of CHD and examines the incidence and mortality rates of CHD according to the host characteristics of age, sex, and race. The chapter ends with a discussion of the classic primary and secondary risk factors associated with CHD.

Natural History of Atherosclerotic Heart Disease

CHD is the end result of underlying atherosclerosis. The disease process has a multiple-decade-long latent period, which starts in the relatively young and culminates in the onset of clinically detectable disease most typically in the

fifth through seventh decades of life. The etiologic factors involved in the development of coronary atherosclerosis include genetic and environmental factors as well as constitutional factors related to the circulation and the arterial wall.

The three focal lesions of coronary atherosclerosis, which primarily affect the intimal layer of normal arteries, are fatty streaks, fibrous plaques, and complicated lesions [26, 27]. The fibrous plaques and complicated lesions are collectively referred to as *raised lesions*. As the raised lesions increase in size, they may impede or cut off blood flow in affected coronary arteries and be responsible for the clinical signs and symptoms of CHD. In contrast, the fatty streak is not associated with significant obstruction of the coronary vessel and is therefore not associated with clinical disease. While some debate continues concerning the relation of the fatty streak to the more advanced lesions of coronary atherosclerosis, the fatty streak is, in general, considered to be the precursor lesion to the more clinically significant lesions. There is no definitive agreement concerning the precise progression of change from the earliest recognizable lesions of coronary atherosclerosis to the raised or calcified lesions and the eventual onset of clinically recognizable disease, but the *response to injury hypothesis*, originally formulated by Ross and colleagues [28] and subsequently modified and updated based on more recent findings [29], places the probable sequence of events in an understandable and working context (Figure 1-2). (Chapter 3 discusses the pathophysiology of atherosclerosis in detail.)

The primary significance of the atherosclerotic process in the coronary vessels is that the lesions of atherosclerosis, alone or in association with acute coronary occlusion, are the primary cause of myocardial ischemia. In turn, myocardial ischemia is responsible for the various clinical states that result from underlying coronary atherosclerosis. These clinical manifestations, including angina pectoris, myocardial infarction, and sudden cardiac death, were elegantly described by Herrick at the turn of the twentieth century:

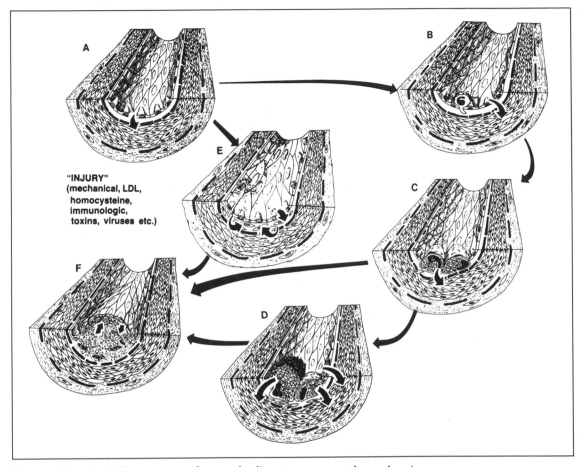

"INJURY"
(mechanical, LDL,
homocysteine,
immunologic,
toxins, viruses etc.)

Figure 1-2. Probable sequence of events leading to coronary atherosclerosis.

The clinical manifestations of coronary obstruction will evidently vary greatly, depending on the size, location and number of vessels occluded. The symptoms and end-results must also be influenced by blood-pressure, by the condition of the myocardium not immediately affected by the obstruction, and by the ability of the remaining vessels properly to carry on their work, as determined by their health or disease. No simple picture of the condition can, therefore, be drawn. All attempts at dividing these clinical manifestations into groups must be artificial and more or less imperfect. Yet such an attempt is not without value, as it enables one the better to understand the gravity of an obstructive accident, to differentiate it from other conditions presenting somewhat similar symptoms, and to employ a more rational therapy that may, to a slight extent at least, be more efficient [30].

The well-established risk factors for CHD may become involved in the pathway to atherosclerosis in a number of ways. They may be intimately involved in leading to the earliest lesions of coronary atherosclerosis (e.g., cholesterol); they may facilitate changes in the earliest lesions to the more complicated or raised lesions (e.g., cholesterol, blood pressure); and they may be involved in transforming the underlying subclinical state to that of overt, clinically detectable disease (e.g., cigarette smoking).

As a further means to conceptualize the interplay of risk factors and the onset of clinical events of CHD, a working theory recently has been proposed by which the activities of daily living, with a particular focus on the role of physical and mental stressors, may trigger coronary thrombosis in a susceptible host [31] (Figure 1-3). These investigators essentially propose that, in persons with underlying atherosclerosis

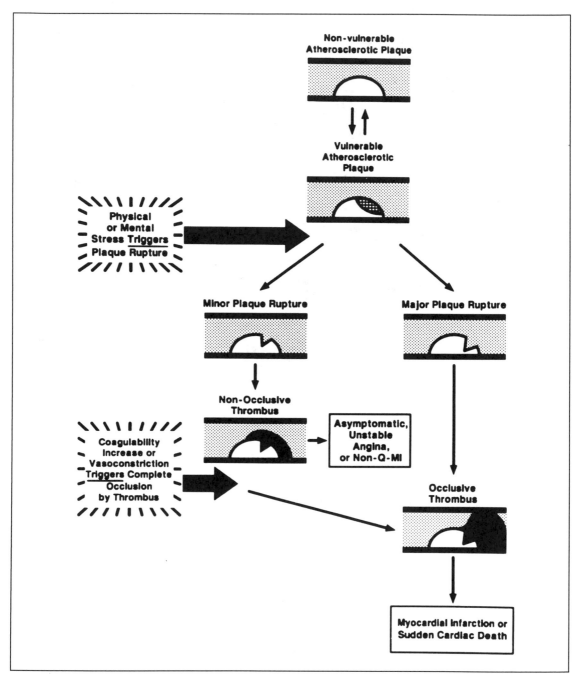

Figure 1-3.   Potential triggering of coronary thrombosis.

and vulnerable atherosclerotic lesions that may be susceptible to minor or major plaque rupture, atherosclerotic thrombosis and its disease sequelae may be set into motion through a complex and incompletely understood interaction of stressor agents and accompanying hemodynamic changes. While few data support or refute this interesting hypothesis, the theory places into further perspective the role of potential acute triggers in the development of myocardial necrosis and provides a fertile base from which further investigative and intervention activities might arise. Indeed, these and other investigators have fostered work in the identification of the possible short-term, transient risk factors that may trigger the onset of coronary disease. The existence of triggers for acute myocardial infarction is suggested by a prominent circadian rhythm, with an increased rate of onset of acute myocardial infarction in the morning hours [32, 33, 34, 35]. Additional evidence also suggests circadian variation in the onset of silent myocardial ischemia and sudden cardiac death [36, 37]. A recent report further extends these findings by observing a marked increase in the frequency of the symptoms of acute myocardial infarction within the first hour after awakening [38]; these observations can be viewed as a special case of the proposed mechanism for the triggering of the onset of acute myocardial infarction [31].

Epidemiology of CHD

This section is an overview of the descriptive epidemiology of CHD, with a primary focus on the relation of age, sex, and race to the attack and mortality rates of CHD.

Age

Every major prospective epidemiologic investigation carried out in the United States over the past several decades has shown a marked increase in the risk of CHD with increasing age. This finding should not be unexpected, given the well-known association of age with the development of the chronic diseases of major public health importance and the decades-long latency period for CHD. During the first 14 years of follow-up in the Framingham Study, among those found to be initially free from CHD every eighth man 40 to 44 years of age at the time of study entry had developed some form of coronary artery disease; the percentage of men developing CHD increased with age to approximately every sixth man aged 45 to 49 years at entry, every fifth man aged 50 to 54 years at entry, and every fourth man 55 years of age or older at entry [39]. Among women free from CHD at the time of their baseline examination, women under 50 years of age experienced about one-sixth the CHD incidence rate as that among men, with the incidence of CHD rising dramatically after the menopause. By 60 years of age, approximately every fifth man and every seventeenth woman in the Framingham Study had developed CHD during the first 14 years (Figure 1-4).

Death rates from CHD rise in an essentially linear fashion with increasing age, and heart disease is the leading cause of death among males by their fourth decade of life and among females by their sixth and seventh decades [1] (Figures 1-5 and 1-6). Increasing age has also been shown to be related to an unfavorable prognosis among those hospitalized with acute myocardial infarction during the acute hospital phase as well as among discharged hospital survivors [40, 41, 42]. In the population-based Worcester Heart Attack Study, the risks of dying during the acute hospital phase for those with an initial acute myocardial infarction, adjusted for a variety of demographic, clinical, and therapeutic factors of prognostic importance, were 1.1, 2.9, and 7.5 times greater for patients 55–64 years, 65–74 years, and 75 years and older, respectively, relative to the referent group of patients less than 55 years of age [42].

Sex

CHD is a major health concern for both men and women. In the United States males typically exhibit higher age-specific incidence rates of CHD than women throughout life, though the difference in attack rates of CHD tends to narrow after the menopause, with CHD be-

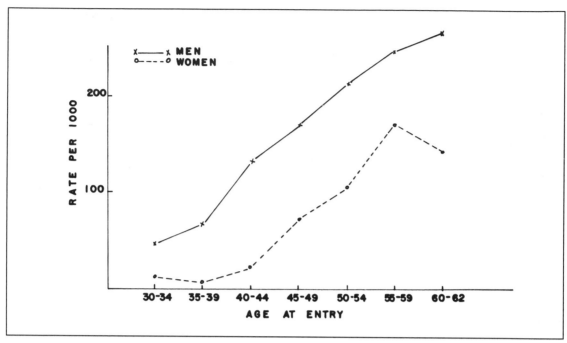

Figure 1-4.   Risk of coronary heart disease by age and sex (Framingham Heart Study).

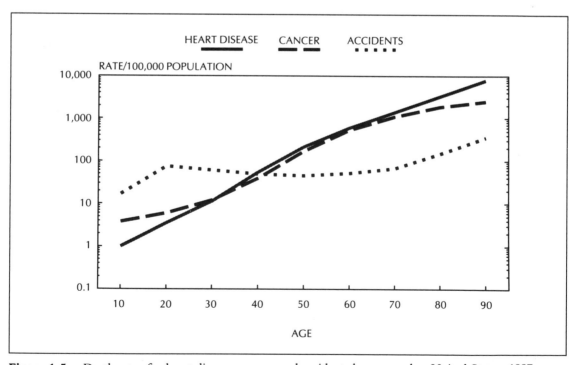

Figure 1-5.   Death rates for heart disease, cancer, and accidents by age: males, United States, 1987.

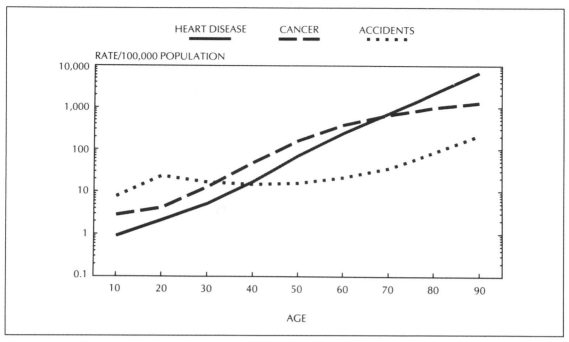

Figure 1-6. Death rates for heart disease, cancer, and accidents by age: females, United States, 1987.

coming a major cause of morbidity and mortality among women beyond their mid- to late 50s [43]. Whether the menopause in and of itself, however, is responsible for the increased attack rates of CHD in females remains controversial. As noted previously, in the Framingham Study the incidence rates of CHD increased in both sexes with advancing age, with the rates greater among men than women; these gender-related differences diminished, however, with incremental increases in age [44].

In general the recognized risk factors for CHD tend to be operative in both sexes, although obesity and diabetes mellitus appear to have a relatively greater effect in women. The presenting symptomatology of CHD in women is typically that of angina pectoris. Data from the Framingham Heart Study have shown that the proportion of unrecognized myocardial infarctions, among all myocardial infarctions occurring, is higher among women than among men [45]. Women suffering acute myocardial

infarction are older than men (on average eight to ten years older) and exhibit higher crude in-hospital case-fatality rates [46, 47, 48, 49, 50]. On the other hand, when age and other potentially confounding prognostic factors are controlled for, gender differences in short-term prognosis following acute myocardial infarction generally disappear [46, 47, 49]. Studies among discharged hospital survivors have shown conflicting results: some studies show women to have increased long-term mortality rates following acute myocardial infarction; in other studies women have higher long-term survival rates; and in still other studies no differences were observed between the sexes in long-term prognosis [46, 48, 49, 50, 51, 52].

Race

Limited data exist that examine differences in the predisposing risk factors for CHD as well as the incidence rates of and mortality from CHD in blacks compared to whites in the United States. In terms of mortality rates from

CHD, death rates from CHD were lower in black men than in white men in the United States in the 1940s but then increased rapidly until the late 1960s, after which time marked declines have been observed [53]. In 1987 the age-adjusted death rates from CHD were slightly higher in white males than black males and higher in black females than in white females [1]. The mortality rates from CHD were approximately twice as high in males as in females irrespective of race. With regard to the age-specific death rates from CHD, mortality tends to be slightly greater in black males than in white males until approximately 60 years of age, after which the death rates from CHD rise to a greater degree in whites than in blacks (Figure 1-7). The death rates from CHD tend to be consistently higher in black females than in white females from 35 to 64 years of age, after which the death rates tend to run an essentially parallel course.

Despite ongoing questions about the relevance of the usual risk factors for CHD in black populations, there is a dearth of investigative activity in this area. Black adults tend to have higher prevalence rates of elevated blood pressure and cigarette smoking, though the prevalence rates of heavy smoking are less among blacks than whites [54]. The incidence of hypercholesterolemia tends to be relatively similar between the races, whereas obesity is highly prevalent among black women. On the other hand, black males tend to have a more favorable lipoprotein profile than white males, as reflected by higher plasma levels of high-density lipoprotein cholesterol and lower levels of low-density lipoproteins; these differences are less striking among females. In an attempt to explain some of the paradoxical observations with regard to the distribution of risk factors in blacks and the occurrence rates of CHD, it has been suggested that blacks may have higher levels of those risk factors that protect against CHD, including higher work-related patterns of physical activity, lower triglyceride levels, higher alcohol intake, and possibly familial and other factors that may protect them from cor-

Figure 1-7.   Death rates for CHD by age, race, and sex: United States, 1987.

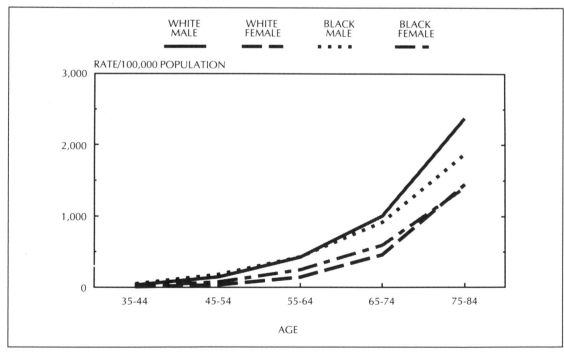

onary atherosclerosis [55]. Differences in hemostatic factors between blacks and whites have not been systematically examined. In the NHANES II Survey (1976 to 1980) 20 percent of black males and 15 percent of black females had at least two of the three primary risk factors for CHD, compared to 13 percent of white males and 10 percent of white females. However, black adults also showed substantial and encouraging decreases in the prevalence of elevated blood pressure and cigarette smoking between the initial NHANES Survey (1971 to 1974) and its successor survey [56].

Few incidence data exist that would allow a systematic determination of differences in the annual incidence or hospitalization rates for acute myocardial infarction in blacks compared to whites [53]. In general the incidence rates of acute myocardial infarction have tended to be lower in black males compared to white males, with inconsistent trends observed in black females relative to white females, in part explained by the small number of cases studied among women. Data from the National Hospital Discharge Survey show essentially identical hospital discharge rates for myocardial infarction among whites and nonwhites for the period 1973 to 1984 with no apparent differences in these rates between the sexes [57]. Blacks in the Coronary Artery Surgery Study were shown to have considerably less coronary artery disease than their white counterparts, including multivessel and left main coronary artery disease [58], despite having higher levels of modifiable risk factors than whites. (Because these data were collected from patients presenting with indications for coronary angiography, it is necessary to place appropriate caveats on such data given their questionable representativeness for the population at actual risk for coronary atherosclerosis.)

In terms of survival following myocardial infarction, some studies have shown either slightly higher or no differences in in-hospital case-fatality rates of acute myocardial infarction in whites versus nonwhites [57, 59]. From data on patients hospitalized in 19 coronary care units in metropolitan Seattle between 1988 and 1990 and after a variety of characteristics, including demographics and prior medical history, were adjusted for, race was not shown to be independently related to hospital mortality following acute myocardial infarction [60]. Rates of out-of-hospital sudden cardiac death have been observed to be higher among blacks than whites [61,62], although a large community-based study in Baltimore found markedly lower incidence rates of sudden death in black males than in white males, with an opposite trend seen in black females [63].

Primary Risk Factors Associated with CHD

Cigarette Smoking

Tobacco is a custome lothesome to the Eye, hatefull to the Nose, harmful to the Brain, dangerous to the Lungs, and in the black stinking fume thereof, nearest resembling the horrible, stigian smoke of the pit that is bottomlesse.

King James I, 1604

A case control study that associated cigarette smoking with angina pectoris and myocardial infarction in middle-aged men was published in 1940 [64]. This investigation was followed approximately 15 years later by a large prospective study of almost 190,000 men aged 50 to 69 years that identified dose-responsive higher death rates from CHD in regular cigarette smokers compared to nonsmokers [65]. Thus, early supportive evidence for the adverse effects of smoking on morbid and mortal CHD events was provided. The discussants of the initial published observation had several interesting insights into the possible association of tobacco and coronary disease and pointed to the need for further systematic study of the possible health hazards associated with cigarette smoking.

One may conclude from laboratory and clinical investigations and statistical reports that smoking is not an innocent habit; it may even be a contributing etiologic factor in coronary disease. Observations convince me that smoking is a distinct menace to patients with hypertension and coronary disease and that it may provoke an attack of angina and auricular fibrillation. . . . It is only by impartial analyses of great masses of clinical material that is not available to many of us, of carefully studied patients, that we can hope to arrive at a fair-minded conclusion and an approximately true conception of the real effects of tobacco smoking [64].

Since these early observations and despite some unwarranted skepticism as to the etiological importance of cigarette smoking in CHD [66], cigarette smoking has been consistently related in a dose-responsive manner to the development of fatal and nonfatal CHD events. Despite the general strength and consistency of these observations, data from the Framingham Heart Study have shown a lack of association between cigarette smoking and angina pectoris in both men and women. The study does show, however, that the consumption of cigarettes is clearly related to the risk of myocardial infarction, sudden cardiac death, and CHD mortality in the two sexes (Figure 1-8) [67].

Cigarette smoking has not been shown to be a potent risk factor for CHD in those populations, such as the Japanese, that are characterized

by low levels of serum cholesterol [68]. These observations, taken in conjunction with the results of studies that have shown a markedly decreased risk of CHD in men and women after they have quit smoking [69, 70, 71] (with the excess risk of CHD declining substantially and relatively quickly after quitting), suggest that smoking may act as a triggering event, rather than as a necessary underlying substrate for CHD. Even among patients suffering acute myocardial infarction, the risk of subsequent mortality and reinfarction is dramatically lower among ex-smokers than among continuing smokers [72, 73]. Nicotine and the smoking of cigarettes have been shown to have adverse affects on the cardiovascular system, including undesirable effects on platelet adhesiveness and clotting factors; increased heart rate, catecholamine levels, and myocardial oxygen demand; and decreased oxygen-carrying capacity of the blood. Providing yet another link in the causal chain of evidence associating smoking with the risk of CHD, particularly in those populations with epidemic levels of coronary atherosclerosis, a recent study has shown a markedly increased occurrence of episodes of silent my-

Figure 1-8.   Risk of selected CHD manifestations by smoking status (Framingham Heart Study).

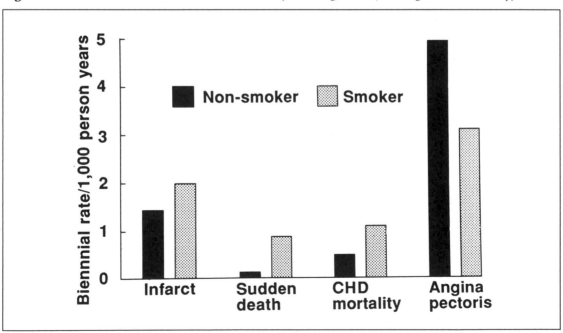

ocardial ischemia among smokers as compared to nonsmokers [74]. Pipe and cigar smokers appear to have only a slight, if any, increase in risk for CHD, with the observed absolute and relative risks considerably lower than those observed for cigarette smokers [70]. The lower risk for CHD among pipe and cigar smokers is thought to be related, in part, to the tendency for pipe and cigar smokers not to inhale the smoke.

Given the continued high prevalence of cigarette smoking and clearly documented evidence of the benefits of smoking cessation in both healthy persons and those with CHD, clinicians and other health care professionals should direct considerable attention to this potentially modifiable risk factor. Indeed, given the marked increase in tobacco use in China and other developing countries [75], attention also needs to be directed to the growing overseas "brown plague" [76] and to the societal and economic factors that contribute to these unacceptable trends.

Blood Pressure

Elevation of either systolic or diastolic blood pressure has been repeatedly shown to be predictive of the subsequent risk of CHD, with hypertension consistently and independently established as a major risk factor for CHD in national and international studies [2, 3, 4]. The role of excess dietary salt intake in the genesis of hypertension has also been clearly shown [76a]. The risk of morbid and mortal CHD events is related to increasing levels of blood pressure in a direct and continuous manner with no clear cutoff point below which risk becomes negligible. A meta-analysis recently examined data from nine large prospective observational studies and assessed the relation of baseline levels of diastolic blood pressure to the development of CHD. This analysis included a combined sample of approximately 420,000 persons and a total of over 4850 fatal and nonfatal CHD events [77]. As can be seen in Figure 1-9, there was a direct and continuous relationship between increasing levels of diastolic blood pressure and the risk of CHD events. From a clinical point of view, borderline as well as definite hypertension is highly correlated with the development of CHD, even within the so-called mild range. Actuarial studies published by insurance companies have also clearly shown higher all-cause mortality rates with increasing levels of either systolic or diastolic blood pressure.

Marked and favorable changes have come about in the United States in the management and control of hypertension [78]. Increasing attention is being paid to the promising results obtained from the modification of lifestyle factors (reduction in salt and alcohol intake, weight loss, increased physical activity, relaxation therapy) in the primary and secondary prevention of elevated blood pressure. Despite these favorable trends, however, the benefits of reductions in blood pressure through pharmacologic means in mildly hypertensive individuals in terms of reduced CHD morbidity and mortality remain unproved and controversial [79, 80]. In major national and international randomized trials that evaluated morbidity and mortality patterns in patients with diastolic pressures between 90 and 114 mm Hg, no beneficial effects of treatment were seen in terms of overall and cardiovascular mortality [79]; only slight differences in the risk of major nonfatal cardiovascular events were seen in treated individuals, with the magnitude of these differences differing in the various trials analyzed. Another pooled analysis of the data from nine controlled clinical trials suggested a slight decrease in the incidence rates of fatal and nonfatal coronary events among treated hypertensives, although a clear-cut benefit of antihypertensive treatment in these events was lacking [81]. Recently, however, two large studies (Swedish Trial in Old Patients with Hypertension; Systolic Hypertension in the Elderly Program) have shown important and significant reductions in morbidity and mortality from cardiovascular disease and stroke in elderly patients with hypertension, clearly establishing the value of antihypertensive treatment in this age group. Such definitive evidence is still lacking for younger age groups [81a, 81b].

These findings have called attention to the need to find the optimal therapeutic levels at

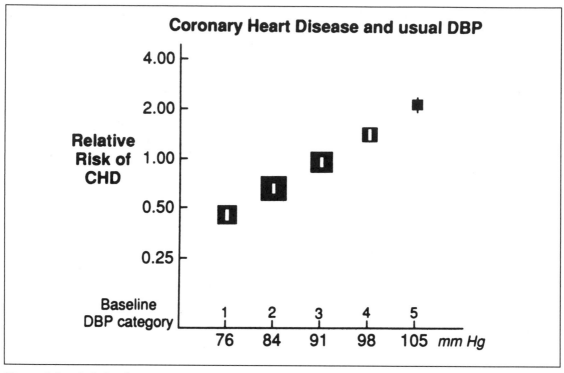

Figure 1-9. Relation between CHD and usual diastolic BP in nine major prospective observational studies. Solid squares represent disease risk in each category relative to risk in the whole study population; sizes of squares are proportional to number of events in each DBP category; 95 percent confidence intervals for estimates of relative risk are denoted by vertical lines.

which benefit is enhanced and risk minimized in treating hypertensives in terms of the future risk of acute myocardial infarction and/or coronary-related mortality [82, 83]. Two schools of thought have emerged on this topic. One school maintains that the lower the blood pressure the better in terms of subsequent CHD events. The other school has proposed that a J-shaped curve exists in relation to blood pressure and CHD morbidity and mortality and that if blood pressure is lowered below certain critical levels, not only may the benefits of treatment be lacking but deleterious effects may even be observed. These conflicting opinions were addressed recently by an examination of 13 prospective studies as well as randomized trials involving over 48,000 subjects [84]. In summarizing the findings of these studies, the authors found a consistent J-shaped relationship between the level of treated diastolic pressures and cardiac events. Based on these findings as

well as other observations in the literature, caution should be exercised in the aggressive lowering of diastolic blood pressure levels to levels below 85 mm Hg, particularly in patients with underlying coronary disease. The previously held belief that the lower the better needs to be reassessed in light of these recent findings, and further investigative work is needed in this area.

Cholesterol

Evidence accumulated from observational epidemiologic studies over the past several decades strongly supports the contention that total serum cholesterol is a major predictive factor in the development of CHD [2, 3, 4]. Data culled from observations between countries (as in the Seven Countries Study), from population-based investigations within the United States (as best illustrated by the Framingham Heart Study), and from additional prospective epidemiologic investigations summarized in the Pooling Project, in conjunction with the results of studies in migrant populations, have established in a clear, dose-related, and temporal manner the important role of total serum cholesterol in the development of CHD. Findings from the Multiple Risk Factor Intervention Trial (MRFIT) provide additional support for the relationship of increased total serum cholesterol levels to the risk of dying from CHD [85] (Figure 1-10). Among the approximately 356,000 males between the ages of 35 and 57 years who were screened for this trial, a continuous and graded relationship between the level of serum cholesterol at the time of initial screening and deaths from CHD over a six-year follow-up period was observed. These results reinforce previous findings that showed that a "safe" level of cholesterol below which the risk of CHD is negligible is much lower than previously thought. Evidence collected from prospective population-based studies in the United States, Finland, and England also suggests an

increased risk of dying from CHD among persons with preexisting coronary disease who have increased cholesterol levels [86, 87, 88].

Data obtained from the Pooling Project Research Group [21], the Framingham Heart Study [89], and other epidemiologic investigations have suggested that with advancing age the association between blood levels of cholesterol and mortality from CHD may diminish. Two recent studies of white male enrollees at the Kaiser Permanente Medical Care Program [90] and elderly cohort attendees of the Honolulu Heart Program [91] suggest, however, an independent role for serum cholesterol levels even in elderly men in relation to the incidence of coronary events as well as to mortality from CHD (see also the discussion of relative versus attributable risk, Chapter 4).

These epidemiologic observations of the atherogenicity of elevated levels of serum cholesterol are consistent with information obtained from randomized clinical trials that suggest a beneficial effect of lowering blood cholesterol

Figure 1-10.   Relation between screening total cholesterol level and CHD mortality (MRFIT).

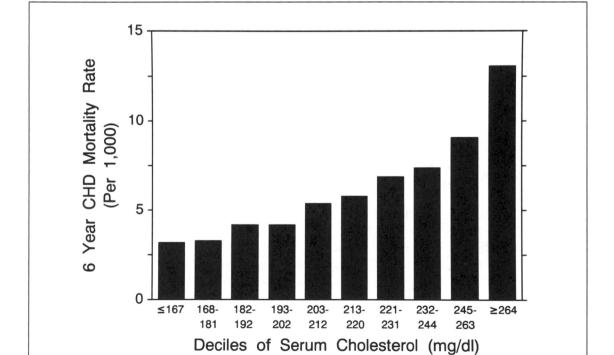

levels on the risk of developing clinical CHD [92, 93]. Data obtained from treatment studies in humans also suggest that, through the use of dietary and pharmacologic interventions, important effects on the rates of progression of the advanced underlying atherosclerotic process and/or actual regression can be achieved in treated individuals through favorable alterations in lipid and lipoprotein parameters [94, 95, 96]. Experimental and pathologic studies in humans and laboratory animals over the past 75 years have also demonstrated a key role for serum cholesterol in the pathogenesis of atherosclerosis [97]. Deposition of lipid, particularly cholesterol, and ingestion of modified low-density lipoproteins by macrophages with ultimate transformation to foam cells are hallmark events in the evolution of the atherosclerotic lesions, from the earliest fatty streaks to the clinically relevant fibrous plaques and complicated lesions.

Cholesterol, an essential component of cell membranes throughout the body, is insoluble in water and is transported in the blood via lipoproteins, which contain varying degrees of lipid and protein complexes. The five major classes of lipoproteins are characterized by their density as well by their mobility on electrophoretic assays. The lipoproteins consist of chylomicrons, very low-density lipoproteins (prebeta lipoprotein), intermediate-density lipoproteins, low-density lipoproteins (beta lipoprotein), and high-density lipoproteins (alpha lipoproteins). In addition, four major categories of apoproteins exist, namely, apoproteins A, B, C, and E. (Chapter 3 discusses these topics in more detail.)

Low-density lipoprotein (LDL) cholesterol and high-density lipoprotein (HDL) cholesterol have emerged as the most important lipoprotein complexes related to the onset of clinical events resulting from coronary atherosclerosis. LDL is the major carrier of cholesterol in the serum, having a lipid core composed almost entirely of cholesterol esters. Information obtained from a number of epidemiologic studies has shown the levels of LDL cholesterol to be positively related to the incidence rates of CHD [2, 3, 4, 89, 98]. The other important lipoprotein related to the development of CHD is HDL cholesterol, the smallest of the lipoproteins. Whereas high levels of LDL are positively associated with an increased risk for CHD, levels of HDL cholesterol are inversely related to the incidence rates of CHD; that is, high levels of HDL cholesterol have a protective effect and are associated with a reduced risk of CHD.

The inverse relationship between plasma levels of HDL cholesterol and the incidence of CHD has been observed in prospective epidemiologic investigations from several countries [2, 3, 4, 89, 98, 99, 100, 101, 102]. Data from the Framingham Study show a beneficial effect of increased levels of HDL cholesterol with decreased risk of CHD in both men and women [39] (Figure 1-11). In a review of the data from two prospective studies in the United States (the Framingham Heart Study and the Lipid Research Clinics Prevalence Mortality Follow-up Study) and from the control groups of two randomized, controlled intervention trials (the Multiple Risk Factor Intervention Trial and the Lipid Research Clinics Coronary Primary Prevention Trial), a pronounced effect of increases in HDL cholesterol on the risk of CHD and deaths from cardiovascular events was seen [103]. For each 1-mg/dl increase in HDL cholesterol observed in these studies, a 2-percent reduction in the risk of CHD events in men and an approximate 3-percent reduction in women were observed. Even more pronounced trends were seen for the association between increased levels of HDL cholesterol and reductions in death rates from cardiovascular disease. Based on the evidence linking levels of lipids and lipoproteins to the incidence rates of CHD, the use of total serum cholesterol level, ratio of LDL to HDL, or ratio of total cholesterol to HDL has been advocated as a useful methodology for judging an individual's future risk of CHD and as a gauge for the efficacy of dietary or pharmacologic interventions.

With regard to the apoproteins, CHD has been shown to be positively associated with apolipoprotein B, the principal protein moiety

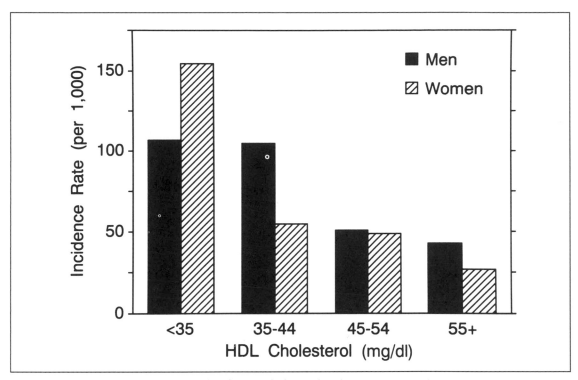

Figure 1-11.   Relation between levels of HDL cholesterol and CHD (Framingham Heart Study).

of LDL cholesterol, and inversely associated with apolipoprotein A, the principal apolipoprotein of HDL cholesterol [104, 105, 106].

Debate continues with regard to the role of triglycerides as an independent risk factor for CHD. Some studies have, whereas others have not, found triglycerides to correlate with the subsequent risk of CHD [107, 108, 109, 110, 111, 112, 113]. When multivariate analyses are carried out in which the other lipoprotein fractions and coronary risk factors are simultaneously controlled for, triglycerides appear to exert little, if any, independent influence on the risk of CHD [114, 115]. Questions concerning the independent role of triglycerides nonetheless remain, with more recent findings from the Framingham Study suggesting that higher levels of triglycerides are related to CHD, especially in women [116].

A twelfth-century Chinese work on the dietetic methods of treatment stated that "When food is in order, the body is also in order." The

relationship between elevated blood lipids and specific lipoprotein fractions and risk of CHD has been consistently demonstrated and is well established, but concerns continue to be expressed regarding the relationship of dietary habits to CHD. In the Seven Countries Study, a significant and independent association was seen among the population percentage of calories coming from saturated fat, the amount of cholesterol in the diet, and the occurrence of CHD (Figure 1-12)[117]; longitudinal studies published over the past decade have also suggested an independent association between selected dietary variables, primarily saturated fat and cholesterol, and risk of and mortality from CHD [118, 119, 120, 121]. International comparisons in varying population samples have shown similar associations (see Chapter 6) [121, 122]. Human metabolic studies and feeding experiments in animals have also implicated the habitual consumption of diets high in saturated fats and dietary cholesterol as causing increased

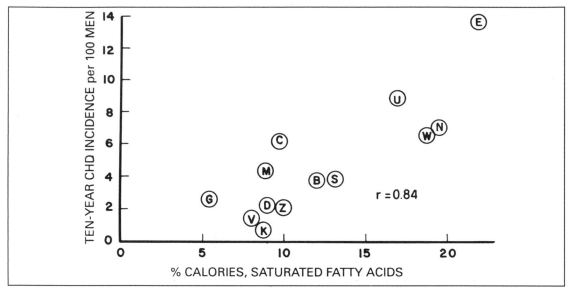

Figure 1-12.   Relation between percentage of calories from saturated fatty acids and CHD (Seven Countries Study). (B)-Belgrade Faculty, (C)-Crevalcore, (D)-Dalmatia, (E)-East Finland, (G)-Corfu, (K)-Crete, (N)-Zutphen, (M)-Montegiorgio, (S)-Slavonia, (U)-U.S. Railroad, (V)-Velika Krsna, (W)-West Finland, (Z)-Zrenjanin

levels of cholesterol in the blood [123, 124, 125, 126, 127]. On the other hand, within-country studies of dietary intake have not been persuasive in correlating diet to the level of serum cholesterol and CHD [128]. This is most likely a consequence of the limited variation within the atherogenic diet consumed among the populations studied and/or due to the inadequacy of the dietary assessment methodology utilized.

A definitive test of the diet-heart hypothesis has not been carried out, although a feasibility study of this issue was proposed over two decades ago [129]. A formal, nationally based, controlled dietary study examining the role of diet in the development of CHD has not been undertaken because of design, implementation, and cost considerations. Despite the fact that such a trial has not been conducted to resolve this ongoing controversy, dietary intervention for prevention and treatment is considered to be the cornerstone of therapy to reduce the population burden from CHD, and its use is reinforced in the goals and objectives of the National Cholesterol Education Project [130]. While controversy may still linger as to the beneficial effects to be obtained from directed lipid-intervention approaches, in many minds the controversy is over [131]. Future research activities should provide additional insights into the relationship between cholesterol and CHD and into those primary and secondary prevention approaches that may be efficacious and cost effective in the management of this enormous public health problem [132].

Secondary Risk Factors for CHD

Diabetes Mellitus

CHD is the most common underlying cause of death in diabetic adults in the United States, accounting for greater than one-third of all deaths in diabetic adults 40 years of age and older [133, 134]. Other macrovascular sequelae, including cerebrovascular disease, congestive heart failure, and peripheral vascular disease, occur more frequently in diabetics than in nondiabetics. Despite the consistency of these observations, questions remain as to the role of asymptomatic hyperglycemia in relation to the development of CHD. In addition, the majority of studies have failed to observe an association between the duration of diabetes and subsequent risk of CHD. Conversely, control of diabetes as reflected by the level of hyperglycemia has also not been shown to be related to the risk of CHD. These issues are explored in depth in Chapter 14.

Maturity-onset diabetics commonly have the risk factors of obesity, elevated serum lipids, and hypertension [135, 136]. Substantial evidence exists to show that diabetes exerts an independent influence on the risk of developing as well as dying from CHD irrespective of these concomitant risk factors [134]. As opposed to the usual disproportionate burden that CHD places on men, the effect of diabetes appears to be relatively stronger in women. Data from the Framingham Heart Study, for example, have shown an approximate threefold increased risk of selected coronary events in diabetic women relative to nondiabetic women, and an approximate twofold increase among diabetic men as compared to nondiabetic men [137, 138]. The impact of diabetes on cardiovascular disease was also seen to diminish with advancing age in women, with less apparent trends seen in men. Also shown by the Framingham Study is that adult-onset diabetes mellitus appears to exact its greatest relative toll on intermittent claudication and congestive heart failure. However, the greatest absolute increase in risk in diabetes is seen in coronary disease, because of its far higher incidence rates. Autopsy studies have also shown more extensive atherosclerosis in diabetics than in nondiabetics.

While controversy continues concerning the independent role of plasma insulin levels in the development of CHD [139, 140, 141, 142], several lines of evidence suggest that hyperinsulinemia is an important risk factor for coronary atherosclerosis and contributes directly to adverse effects on the arterial wall and to the development of hyperlipidemia. A recent investigation from the San Antonio Heart Study suggests that prediabetic individuals are characterized not only by hyperinsulinemia but by a more atherogenic pattern of CHD risk factors relative to those persons who subsequently do not go on to develop diabetes [143]. These findings suggest that the increased atherogenicity associated with the prediabetic state may make a significant contribution to the subsequent risk of CHD even before clinically apparent diabetes develops.

The results of this study indicate that a multifactorial risk-intervention program in diabetics, possibly even extended to those in the prediabetic state if an accurate characterization of such individuals can be achieved, might be of great value. Such a program should include efforts directed at increasing physical activity, reducing obesity, eliminating cigarette smoking, and making favorable dietary alterations.

Obesity

When more food than is proper has been taken, it occasions disease.

Hippocrates

Substantial evidence exists to confirm Hippocrates' observation — increased body weight for height, or obesity, is associated with various risk factors for CHD and may also more directly influence the risk of CHD, although the latter association remains less evident and inconsistent between studies.

Based on studies that utilize either comparison of weight relative to a desirable standard, as compiled by the Metropolitan Life Insurance Company, or body mass indexes as proxy measures for obesity, obesity has been shown to be positively related to levels of serum cholesterol and to blood pressure in a continuous and graded manner, as well as to categorical definitions of hypertension and hypercholesterolemia [144, 145, 146]. Prevalence rates of diabetes have also been shown to be higher in overweight as compared to normal-weight persons. While a consistent association of obesity with an unfavorable coronary risk factor profile has been observed repeatedly in cross-sectional and prospective epidemiologic studies, and weight change among adults studied in Framingham was associated with a corresponding change in CHD risk factors [147], an apparent paradox exists with regard to the independent association of obesity with CHD incidence.

Widely discrepant results have been reported from investigations in this area. Data from the

Pooling Project found that among the several cohorts studied, there was a lack of, a U-shaped, or a positive association of obesity with CHD [21, 146]. A review of the major longitudinal studies from North America, carried out primarily among men, that utilized multivariate analyses to control for other potentially confounding sociodemographic and coronary risk factors, found a significant independent relation between obesity and the incidence of CHD, primarily in the younger cohorts studied [145]. In contrast, in a review of data from cross-cultural and population-based studies, divergent results were observed in terms of the association of obesity with subsequent risk of CHD, as well as to the CHD endpoint examined [146]. For example, in the Framingham Study, a significant association was observed between excess body weight and risk of sudden death and angina pectoris, but not with myocardial infarction [147].

The few prospective studies of obesity and CHD in women have found either a lack of association [148, 149] or a strong positive association between relative weight and the incidence of CHD [150]. As with the results observed in the Framingham Study [150], the largest of the prospective epidemiologic studies carried out to date among women that examined the relation of obesity to risk of CHD found a strong and consistent relation between extent of overweight, as measured by the platelet index, and risk of fatal and nonfatal CHD events among over 115,000 middle-aged nurses [151]. Extending and refining work in this area, studies carried out in the past decade suggest that the distribution of adipose tissue ("pears" versus "apples"), i.e., central versus peripheral obesity, is an independent risk factor for the development of CHD [152].

Given that an estimated 20 percent of the adult United States population is overweight [144], and given the observed associations of overweight with coronary risk factors, CHD, total mortality, and possibly other chronic diseases of major public health importance, reduction of weight through either modification of caloric intake or changes in physical-activity patterns is highly desirable among obese persons.

Physical Activity

Parts of the body unused and left idle become liable to disease, defective in growth and age quickly.

Hippocrates

Beginning with such landmark studies as those of bus drivers and conductors in the London transport system [153] and of San Francisco longshoremen [154], which showed a protective effect of high-level energy expenditure, considerable evidence has accumulated for the independent role of increased physical activity in the primary prevention of CHD. Indeed, this subject has been the focus of a number of extensive reviews in the past decade, and the common conclusion has been that individuals engaged in regular physical activity are at reduced risk for CHD when compared to their more sedentary counterparts [155, 156, 157].

A meta-analysis of the available literature has recently assessed the role of physical activity in the prevention of CHD [158]. Such an analysis must deal with numerous methodologic considerations: varying definitions of physical activity used, measurement of activity levels either at work or during leisure time, and potential confounding of the apparent association between physical activity and CHD by the influence of changes in physical activity on the prevalence as well as the severity of accompanying coronary risk factors, including body weight, HDL cholesterol, blood pressure, cigarette smoking and possibly thrombogenic factors. Nonetheless, this exhaustive review of the findings from 27 cohort studies concluded that a beneficial effect of physical activity in terms of a decreased risk of CHD was observed; this association was strongest when highly physically active groups were compared with sedentary ones and in the more methodologically rigorous studies.

Despite the relative weight of supportive evidence in this area, few investigations have directly examined the relation between physical fitness, as assessed through objective quantifiable measures, and future risk of CHD morbidity and/or mortality. In the Lipid Research Clinics Prevalence Survey, data obtained from submaximal exercise treadmill testing among over 3000 men between the ages of 30 and 69 years showed that the risk of dying from CHD was significantly greater among men with low levels of physical fitness [159]. Consistent with prior work in this area, persons at the highest levels of fitness also tended to have a more favorable risk factor profile; however, the beneficial effect of fitness remained after multivariate adjustment for age and accompanying cardiovascular fisk factors. In another recent study, all-cause mortality, as well as deaths from cardiovascular disease, was shown to be highly inversely correlated with the level of physical fitness, as measured longitudinally in over 13,000 healthy men and women [160]. In reviewing previous studies of physical fitness and CHD, the authors found an approximate twofold increase of fatal and nonfatal CHD events in unfit men. This level of increased risk compares well with the average relative risk observed in studies of physical activity and CHD [155]. The topic of physical activity and CHD is more fully explored in Chapter 10.

Alcohol

Consumption of ethanol has not been shown to lead to an increased risk of CHD. The majority of studies examining the association of alcohol use with CHD have suggested either a negative or a U-shaped relationship between alcohol consumption and CHD [161, 162, 163, 164, 165, 166]. In the Framingham Study, a beneficial effect of moderate alcohol consumption on mortality from CHD as well as from all causes was seen, particularly in males, with inconsistent patterns seen for females [167]. Recent evidence from a large cohort of men enrolled originally in the American Cancer Society Prospective Study has also shown reduced overall death rates, as well as death rates from CHD, among persons consuming moderate amounts of alcohol (less than three drinks per day) [168].

While the majority of studies examining the association of alcohol consumption patterns and cardiovascular disease have been carried out among men, data from the Nurses Health Study, a large cohort study of over 87,000 female nurses, have shown essentially similar results: when compared with nondrinkers and after adjusting for additional coronary risk factors, an approximate 50-percent lower risk of nonfatal myocardial infarction or death due to coronary disease was observed among women consuming approximately one alcoholic drink per day [169]. The consensus of findings supports an association of moderate alcohol consumption with decreased mortality rates from cardiovascular disease, irrespective of the type of alcoholic beverage consumed. Alcohol may reduce the risk of CHD, in part, through mechanisms such as increases in HDL cholesterol levels, increased fibrinolysis, or its peripheral vasodilating effects. Although appropriate concerns have been expressed over public health recommendations for ethanol consumption, given the well-documented deleterious effects of excessive alcoholic intake (encouragement of family disruption and unhealthy lifestyle habits such as cigarette smoking, increased risk of hypertension, drunk driving, liver disease), the abundance of data in this area suggests, on balance, a protective benefit of small daily amounts of ethanol on morbidity and mortality from CHD [170].

Psychosocial Factors

The type A, or coronary-prone, behavior pattern described by Osler as a "keen and ambitious man, the indicator of whose engine is always set at full speed ahead" [171] and originally studied by Rosenman and Friedman [172], has been actively investigated over the past several decades in relation to CHD and summarized in detail [173, 174]. Type A behavior, which is the behavior shown by an individual when challenged or prevented from engaging in a particular activity (as opposed to being an actual personality trait), is characterized by any or all of the following: a sense of time urgency, impatience, competitiveness, drive, and intense desire to achieve [175]. A variety of measurement tools, including the Structured Interview, the Jenkins Activity Survey, and the Framingham Type A Scale, have been used to assess the type A behavior pattern.

Early case-control and prospective investigations of the relation between the type A behavior pattern and risk of CHD found a positive association independent of the major coronary risk factors [176, 177]. On the other hand, recent findings from the MRFIT trial, the Aspirin Myocardial Infarction Study, and the Western Collaborative Group Study have shown no association between the type A behavior pattern and CHD [178, 179, 180], findings that are consistent with studies carried out over the past decade [173].

Recent attention has been focused on the role of hostile and suspicious anger and aggressiveness in relation to elevated serum cholesterol levels as well as to risk of CHD and total mortality [181, 182, 183]. Consistent suppressed anger may be related to an overactive "fight or flight" response in predisposed individuals, which may have an adverse effect on catecholamines as well as on hemostasis. Recent findings among patients undergoing coronary angiography [184], however, failed to support earlier findings in this area and are consistent with several other recent studies that also failed to observe an association between hostility and the occurrence of CHD [185, 186]. Further research in this area may provide additional insights into those inborn or environmentally determined personality factors and traits that may be related to the risk of developing or dying from CHD and how behavioral interventions might modify these risk factors on a long-term basis. See Chapter 11 for a fuller development of this topic.

Family History and Genetics

Familial as well as environmental risk factors are intimately involved in the pathogenesis of coronary artery disease [187, 188]. Early studies assessing the role of genetic factors in the etiology of CHD demonstrated familial aggregation of this disease among the relatives of those with CHD when compared to relatives of those without CHD [189, 190]. Studies of separated monozygotic twins and dizygotic twins have also provided supportive evidence for the heritability of CHD through comparison of concordance rates of myocardial infarction and risk factors for CHD [187, 191]. Studies of the offspring of patients with premature myocardial infarction have reported higher serum cholesterol levels than the total serum cholesterol levels seen in children whose parents did not have CHD and significant clustering of the lipoprotein profile among siblings [192, 193, 194, 195]. The relative contributions of shared genes and environmental influences to the familial clustering of coronary disease remain incompletely understood [196] and are an active focus of ongoing research.

A limited number of studies have examined the predictive utility for CHD of a positive family history of coronary disease while simultaneously adjusting for the role of concomitant coronary risk factors. Among men followed longitudinally in the Western Collaborative Group Study, a parental history of CHD was shown to be predictive of CHD, primarily in younger men [197]; findings from the Framingham Study of an older brother's positive history for CHD [198] and from the Paris Prospective Study of a paternal history of CHD [199] also showed family history to be independently predictive of CHD. The Rancho Bernardo Study showed that among men, but not among women, a family history of myocardial infarction is related to deaths from cardiovascular and ischemic heart disease [200]. On the other hand, the Nurses Health Study showed that a parental history of premature myocardial infarction in women is independently predictive of CHD [201].

Taken as a whole, studies of the family history of CHD suggest that family history is an important predictor for the risk of subsequent CHD, particularly in men, with a risk approximately one and one-half to two times greater for those with a parental history of CHD. Finally, since familial aggregation of CHD and its predisposing factors do not necessarily discriminate between nature and nurture, since families share more than genes, limited evidence suggests a possible etiologic link between genetic polymorphisms and occurrence rates of CHD as well as to variations in lipoproteins [202].

Oral Contraceptives

Women who use oral contraceptives have been shown to be at increased risk for venous thromboembolic disease and cerebrovascular accidents [203]. Several case reports published in the British literature in the early to mid-1960s suggested that the use of oral contraceptives might be associated with an increased risk of myocardial infarction [204, 205, 206]. The following letter to the editor is an illustrative example of one of these insightful case reports that questioned the association of oral contraceptives and coronary thrombosis [206], an association subsequently corroborated in observational epidemiologic investigations.

Sir — Up until recently I have felt quite justified in prescribing oral contraceptives for my patients. However, on Boxing Day a patient of mine, a young woman aged 33, the mother of six children, died suddenly from coronary thrombosis (confirmed at necropsy). She had been taking oral contraceptives for three years and had no ill effects whatsoever. In fact according to her it was only since taking the pill that she had had any life at all. She was happy and contented, looking after her children well and no longer waiting in fear and trepidation in case her next period did not arrive. One cannot draw conclusions from a single case, but is there an increased risk of coronary thrombosis in those taking the pill, and if so are we justified in subjecting our patients to this risk?

Subsequent case-control and longitudinal studies confirmed that use of oral contraceptives was associated with an increased risk of fatal and nonfatal myocardial infarction, being approximately three to four times greater among current users than among women who had never used oral contraceptives [203, 207, 208, 209, 210]. The risk was shown to increase in a multiplicative fashion with age; in individuals with other risk factors for CHD, most particularly cigarette smoking and hypertension; and in those with underlying coronary atherosclerosis [211]. While current use of oral contraceptives has been shown to place women at

increased risk for CHD, this risk diminishes relatively soon after discontinuation of use [203]. Two studies have also examined the residual effects, if any, of the use of oral contraceptives in the past among ex-users [212, 213]. These data were collected from a large case-control study of incident cases of acute myocardial infarction among women 25 to 49 years of age hospitalized in coronary care units along the eastern seaboard [212] and from over 119,000 women between the ages of 30 and 55 years participating in the Nurses Health Study [213]. The Nurses Health Study, in accord with numerous smaller investigations, found a lack of association between past use of oral contraceptives and present risk of major coronary or cardiovascular disease events; there was also no increase in risk of CHD with increasing duration of use. On the other hand, the case-control study showed that the risk of myocardial infarction among long-term users of these agents in the past was elevated approximately twofold among a subgroup of premenopausal women 40 to 49 years of age when compared to women who had never used oral contraceptives [212].

Placing these findings in context, the absolute risk of myocardial infarction remains low even among current users of oral contraceptives. The relative risk of myocardial infarction and other thromboembolic events could be reduced if these agents are not provided to women who are considered to be at increased risk for coronary thrombosis based on their age and risk factor profile.

Hemostatic Factors

Given the recent rediscovery of the role of the thrombus in the onset of acute coronary disease and the significant benefit of clot-lysing agents in patients with evolving myocardial infarction, interest in the role of plasma fibrinogen in the pathogenesis of CHD has been rekindled and remains the subject of current inquiry. Data from the Northwick Park Heart Study and the Framingham Heart Study have identified raised fibrinogen levels with an increased risk for CHD [214, 215]. In addition, several case-control and cross-sectional studies have also demonstrated an association of increased fibrinogen levels with either clinical or angiographically confirmed coronary artery disease [216, 217]. Previous reports have shown varying degrees of correlation between fibrinogen and the primary risk factors for CHD, particularly smoking. When these and other potential covariates associated with the development of CHD were adjusted for in the prospective Gothenburg, Sweden, study, baseline fibrinogen level was shown to be predictive of subsequent myocardial infarction in univariate analyses, but the strength of this potential predictor diminished when the other well-established risk factors for CHD were adjusted for [218].

Vasectomy

Experimental studies in monkeys suggested a possible association between vasectomy and the severity of atherosclerosis [219, 220]. Given the millions of men throughout the world who have chosen vasectomy as a method of contraception, this issue is of some importance. Several observational studies have examined the association of vasectomy to the subsequent development of CHD. Data collected from studies carried out in populations with a high incidence of CHD, as well as from studies carried out in developing countries in which the occurrence rates of CHD are lower, have suggested a lack of association between vasectomy and increased risk of CHD [221, 222, 223, 224]. The current consensus provides reassurance as to the lack of adverse cardiovascular effects associated with this contraceptive method.

Other Risk Factors

Investigators have examined a number of other potential risk factors for CHD. While varying degrees of association or absence of association with either the risk of developing or dying from CHD have been observed with regard to these factors, they will only be mentioned here because of a relative lack of supportive data. These factors include the hardness of drinking water, environmental and air pollutants, sucrose consumption, body iron stores, serum uric acid levels, and gout.

Multifactorial Nature of CHD

It is clear that CHD is a multifactorial disease with its pathogenic roots in the first and second decades of life. The clinical manifestations of the atherosclerotic process reflect the interaction of host and environmental factors.

A variety of formulations using stratified and multivariate analytic techniques have been utilized to identify those persons at high risk for CHD through various combinations of the primary and secondary risk factors for coronary disease. These estimates not only have provided analytic rigor in showing the independence of the well-established risk factors associated with the development of CHD but have also shown how the risk factors interact in an additive as well as a multiplicative fashion. Data from the Framingham Heart Study convincingly demonstrate the relation between multiple coronary risk factors and the likelihood of developing CHD in both middle-aged men and women (Figure 1-13). These risk estimates have allowed for the characterization of those asymptomatic persons among whom approximately one-half of all incident cases of CHD will appear and in whom these risk factors may be readily assessed in a clinician's office (see Chapter 4 for further information on patient risk profiling).

While the risk factors for CHD relate to the different clinical manifestations of coronary ath-

Figure 1-13. Eight-year risk of CHD (per 1,000) according to number of coronary risk factors (Framingham Heart Study).

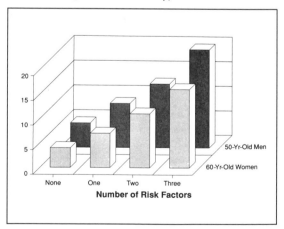

erosclerosis in slightly different ways and with varying degrees of predictive utility, depending on the endpoint examined and the interaction of other risk factors, practicing clinicians are armed with considerable information with which to assess an individual's future risk of CHD as well as with an array of pharmacologic and nonpharmacologic approaches that can be prescribed to delay or ultimately prevent the morbidity and disability associated with CHD. This task is formidable, however, given that multiple risk factors tend to cluster among individuals, that adverse lifestyle habits may have lifelong roots with complex biobehavioral determinants, and that regular and consistent reinforcement most likely will need to be provided to achieve targeted goals.

Summary and Future Directions

Despite favorable trends in declining mortality rates from CHD, heart disease remains the nation's leading cause of death. A constellation of risk factors as well as risk markers have been identified in association with the occurrence of CHD. Future research activities need to focus not only on those risk factors that have been shown to be related to CHD but also on those risk factors in which conflicting findings have been reported in the literature, in an attempt to resolve such discrepancies. Investigative work needs to be carried out at various levels to identify how these risk factors interact and set into motion the disease process at both the pathophysiologic and clinical levels. Future research also needs to focus on the efficacy and cost effectiveness of currently utilized intervention approaches for modifying the risk factors for CHD and on the development of novel approaches for modifying such risk factors, to enhance compliance to these measures and hopefully to lessen the associated disease burden. Epidemiologic as well as clinically based research should also identify those persons likely or not to respond to various intervention strategies and in whom additional and possibly tailored intervention approaches can be delivered. This chapter has provided an overview of the epidemiology of CHD. Later chapters will expand more fully each of the topics introduced here.

References

1. U.S. Department of Health and Human Services. Morbidity and mortality chartbook on cardiovascular, lung and blood diseases 1990. National Institutes of Health: National Heart, Lung and Blood Institute, 1990.
2. Inter-Society Commission for Heart Disease Resources: Atherosclerosis study group and epidemiology study group. Primary Prevention of the atherosclerotic diseases. Circulation 1970; 42:A55–A94.
3. WHO Expert Committee on the Prevention of Coronary Heart Disease. Prevention of coronary heart disease. World Health Organization technical report. Series no. 678. Geneva: World Health Organization, 1982.
4. AHA Committee Report. Risk factors and coronary disease. A statement for physicians. Circulation 1980; 62:449A–55A.
5. Dawber TR, Meadors GF, Moore FE, Jr. Epidemiological approaches to heart disease: The Framingham Study. Am J Publ Health 1951; 41:279–86.
6. Gordon T, Kannel WB. Premature mortality from coronary heart disease. The Framingham Study. JAMA 1971; 215:1617–25.
7. Stamler J, Lindberg HA, Berkson DM, et al. Prevalence and incidence of coronary heart disease in strata of the labor force of a Chicago industrial corporation. J Chron Dis 1960; 11:405–20.
8. Paul O, Lepper MH, Phelan WH, et al. A longitudinal study of heart disease. Circulation 1963; 28:20–31.
9. Epstein FH, Ostrander LD Jr, Johnson BC, et al. Epidemiological studies of cardiovascular disease in a total community — Tecumseh, Michigan. Ann Intern Med 1965; 62:1170–87.
10. Doyle JT, Heslin AS, Hilleboe HE, et al. A prospective study of degenerative cardiovascular disease in Albany: report of three years' experience. I. Ischemic heart disease. Am J Publ Health 1957; 47:25–32.
11. Chapman JM, Goerke LS, Dixon W, et al. The clinical status of a population group in Los Angeles under observation for two to three years. Am J Publ Health 1957; 47:33–42.
12. Keys A, Taylor HL, Blackburn H, et al. Coronary heart disease among Minnesota business and professional men followed 15 years. Circulation 1963; 28:381–95.
13. Rosenman RH, Friedman M, Straus R, et al. A

predictive study of coronary heart disease: The Western Collaborative Group Study. JAMA 1964; 189:15–22.

14. Feinleib M, Kannel WB, Garrison RJ, et al. The Framingham Offspring Study. Design and preliminary data. Prev Med 1975; 4:518–25.

15. Reid DD, Hamilton PJS, McCartney P, Rose G. Smoking and other risk factors for coronary heart disease in British civil servants. Lancet 1976; 2:979–83.

16. Kagan A, Gordon T, Rhoads GG, Schiffman JC. Some factors related to coronary heart disease incidence in Honolulu Japanese men: the Honolulu Heart Study. Int J Epidemiol 1975; 4:271–9.

17. Groen JJ, Medalie JH, Neufeld HN, et al. An epidemiologic investigation of hypertension and ischemic heart disease within a defined segment of the adult male population of Israel. Isr J Med Sci 1968; 4:177–94.

18. Johnson KG, Yano K, Kato H. Coronary heart disease in Hiroshima, Japan: a report of a six-year period of surveillance, 1958–1964. Am J Publ Health 1968; 58:1355–67.

19. Carlson LA, Bottiger LE. Ischemic heart disease in relation to fasting values of plasma triglycerides and cholesterol. Stockholm Prospective Study. Lancet 1972; 1:865–8.

20. Keys A, Aravanis C, Blackburn H, et al. Epidemiological studies related to coronary heart disease. Characteristics of men aged 40–59 in seven countries. Acta Med Scand 1967; 180: Suppl 460:1–392.

21. The Pooling Project Research Group. Relationship of blood pressure, serum cholesterol, smoking habit, relative weight and ECG abnormalities to incidence of major coronary events: final report of the Pooling Project. J Chron Dis 1978; 31:201–306.

22. Toor M, Katchalsky A, Agmon J, Allalouf D. Serum lipids and atherosclerosis among Yemenite immigrants in Israel. Lancet 1957; 1:1270–3.

23. Prior IAM. Cardiovascular epidemiology in New Zealand and the Pacific. N Z Med J 1974; 80:245–252.

24. Worth RM, Kato H, Rhoads GG, et al. Epidemiologic studies of coronary heart disease and stroke in Japanese men living in Japan, Hawaii and California: Mortality. Am J Epidemiol 1975; 102:481–90.

25. Yano K, MacLean CJ, Reed DM, et al. A comparison of the 12-year mortality and predictive factors of coronary heart disease among Japanese men in Japan and Hawaii. Am J Epidemiol 1988; 127:476–87.

26. Steinberg D, Witztum JL. Lipoproteins and atherogenesis. Current Concepts. JAMA 1990; 264:3047–52.

27. McGill HC, ed. The geographic pathology of atherosclerosis. Baltimore: Williams and Wilkins, 1968.

28. Ross R, Glomset JA. The pathogenesis of atherosclerosis. N Engl J Med 1976; 295:369–77; 420–5.

29. Ross R. The pathogenesis of atherosclerosis — an update. N Engl J Med 1986; 314:488–500.

30. Herrick JB. Clinical features of sudden obstruction of the coronary arteries. JAMA 1912; 59:2015–20.

31. Muller JE, Tofler GH, Stone PH. Circadian variation and triggers of onset of acute cardiovascular disease. Circulation 1989; 79:733–41.

32. Pell S, D'Alonzo CA. Acute myocardial infarction in a large industrial population: Report of a 6-year study of 1,356 cases. JAMA 1963; 185:831–8.

33. Pedoe HT, Clayton D, Morris JN, et al. Coronary heart attacks in East London. Lancet 1975; 2:833–8.

34. Muller JE, Stone PH, Turi ZG, et al. and the MILIS Study Group. Circadian variation in the frequency of onset of acute myocardial infarction. N Engl J Med 1985; 313:1315–22.

35. Hjalmarson A, Gilpin E, Nicod P, et al. Differing circadian patterns of symptom onset in subgroups of patients with acute myocardial infarction. Circulation 1989; 80:267–75.

36. Willich SN, Levy D, Rocco MB, et al. Circadian variation in the incidence of sudden cardiac death in the Framingham Heart Study population. Am J Cardiol 1987; 60:801–6.

37. Rocco MB, Barry J, Campbell S, et al. Circadian variation of transient myocardial ischemia in patients with coronary heart disease. Circulation 1987; 75:395–400.

38. Goldberg RJ, Brady P, Muller JE, et al. Time of onset of symptoms of acute myocardial infarction. Am J Cardiol 1990; 66:140–4.

39. Castelli W, Leaf A. Identification and assessment of cardiac risk — an overview. Cardiol Clin 1985; 3:171–8.

40. Peel AAF. Age and sex factors in coronary heart disease. Br Heart J 1955; 17:319–26.

41. Pell S, D'Alonzo CA. Immediate mortality and five-year survival of employed men with a first myocardial infarction. N Engl J Med 1964; 270:915–22.

42. Goldberg RJ, Gore JM, Gurwitz JH, et al. The impact of age on the incidence and prognosis of initial acute myocardial infarction: the Worcester Heart Attack Study. Am Heart J 1989; 117:543–9.

43. Kannel WB. Metabolic risk factors for coronary heart disease in women: perspective from the Framingham Study. Am Heart J 1987; 114: 413–9.

44. Eaker ED, Castelli WP. Coronary heart disease and risk factors among women in the Framingham Study. In: Eaker ED, Packard B, Wenger NK, et al., eds. Coronary heart disease in women: proceedings of an NIH workshop. New York: Haymarket Doyma, 1987: 22–8.

45. Kannel WB, Abbott RD. Incidence and prognosis of unrecognized myocardial infarction: an update on the Framingham Study. N Engl J Med 1984; 311:1144–7.

46. Fiebach NH, Viscoli CM, Horwitz RI. Differences between women and men in survival after myocardial infarction. Biology or methodology? JAMA 1990; 263:1092–6.

47. Robinson K, Conroy RM, Mulcahy R, Hickey N. Risk factors and in-hospital course of first episode of myocardial infarction or acute coronary insufficiency in women. JACC 1988; 11:932–6.

48. Tofler GH, Stone PH, Muller JE, et al. Effects of gender and race on prognosis after myocardial infarction. JACC 1987; 9:473–82.

49. Dittrich H, Gilpin E, Nicod P, et al. Acute myocardial infarction in women: influence of gender on mortality and prognostic variables. Am J Cardiol 1988; 62:1–7.

50. Kannel WB, Sorlie P, McNamara PM. Prognosis after myocardial infarction: the Framingham Study. Am J Cardiol 1979; 44:53–9.

51. Weinblatt E, Shapiro S, Frank CW. Prognosis of women with newly diagnosed coronary heart disease — comparison with course of disease among men. Am J Public Health 1973; 63:577–93.

52. Johansson S, Bergstrand R, Ulvenstam G, et al. Sex differences in pre-infarction characteristics and long-term survival among patients with myocardial infarction. Am J Epidemiol 1984; 119:610–23.

53. Gillum RF. Coronary heart disease in black populations. I. Mortality and morbidity. Am Heart J 1982; 104:839–50.

54. Report of National Heart Lung and Blood Institute Working Conference on coronary heart disease in black populations and proceedings of a symposium on coronary heart disease in black populations. Am Heart J 1984; 108:633–62.

55. Gillum RF, Grant CT. Coronary heart disease in black populations. II. Risk factors. Am Heart J 1982; 104:852–64.

56. Rowland ML, Fulwood R. Coronary heart disease risk factor trends in blacks between the first and second National Health and Nutrition Examination Surveys, United States, 1971–1980. Am Heart J 1984; 108:771–9.

57. Roig E, Castaner A, Simmons B, et al. In-hospital mortality rates from acute myocardial infarction by race in U.S. hospitals: findings from the National Hospital Discharge Survey. Circulation 1987; 76:280–8.

58. Maynard C, Fisher LD, Passamani ER, Pullum T. Blacks in the Coronary Artery Surgery Study: Risk factors and coronary artery disease. Circulation 1986; 74:64–71.

59. Goldberg RJ, Kennedy HL. The influence of race on prognosis after acute myocardial infarction: a community-wide perspective. J Cardiac Rehab 1983; 3:195–201.

60. Maynard C, Litwin PE, Martin JS, et al. Characteristics of black patients admitted to coronary care units in metropolitan Seattle: results from the Myocardial Infarction Triage and Intervention Registry (MITI). Am J Cardiol 1991; 67:18–23.

61. Keil JE, Saunders DE, Lackland DT, et al. Acute myocardial infarction: period prevalence, case fatality, and comparison of black and white cases in urban and rural areas of South Carolina. Am Heart J 1985; 109:776–84.

62. Hagstrom RM, Federspiel CF, Ho YC. Incidence of myocardial infarction and sudden death from coronary heart disease in Nashville, Tennessee. Circulation 1971; 44:884–90.

63. Kuller L. Sudden death in atherosclerotic heart disease. The case for preventive medicine. Am J Cardiol 1969; 24:617–28.

64. English JP, Willius FA, Berkson J. Tobacco and coronary disease. JAMA 1940; 115:1327–9.

65. Hammond EC, Horn D. Smoking and death rates — report on forty-four months of follow-up of 187,783 men. II. Death rates by cause. 1958; 166:1294–1308.

66. Seltzer CO. Smoking and coronary heart disease: what are we to believe? (editorial). Am Heart J 1980; 100:275–80.

67. Wilhelmsen L. Coronary heart disease: epidemiology of smoking and intervention studies of smoking. Am Heart J 1988; 115:242–9.

68. Robertson PL, Kato H, Gordon T, et al. Epidemiological studies of coronary heart disease and stroke in Japanese men living in Japan, Hawaii, and California: coronary heart disease risk factors in Japan and Hawaii. Am J Cardiol 1977; 39:244–9.

69. Kristein MM. 40 years of U.S. cigarette smoking and heart disease and cancer mortality rates. J Chron Dis 1984; 37:317–24.

70. U.S. Department of Health and Human Services. The health consequences of smoking. Cardiovascular disease. A report of the Surgeon General. USDHHS publ. no. (PHS) 84-50204, 1983.

71. Ockene JK, Kuller LH, Svendsen KH, Meilahn E. The relationship of smoking cessation to coronary heart disease and lung cancer in the Mul-

tiple Risk Factor Intervention Trial (MRFIT). Am J Publ Health 1990; 80:954–8.

72. Wilhelmsson C, Elmfeldt D, Vedin JA, et al. Smoking and myocardial infarction. Lancet 1975; 1:415–20.

73. Sparrow D, Dawber TR, Colton T. The influence of cigarette smoking on prognosis after a first myocardial infarction. J Chron Dis 1978; 31:425–32.

74. Barry J, Mead K, Nabel EG, et al. Effect of smoking on the activity of ischemic heart disease. JAMA 1989; 261:398–402.

75. Yu JJ, Mattson ME, Boyd GM, et al. A comparison of smoking patterns in the People's Republic of China with the United States. An impending health catastrophe in the Middle Kingdom. JAMA 1990; 264:1575–9.

76. Foege WH. The growing brown plague. JAMA 1990; 264:1580.

76a. Stamler J, Rose G, Stamler R, et al. INTERSALT study findings: Public health and medical care implications. Hypertension 1989; 14:570–7.

77. MacMahon S, Peto R, Cutler J, et al. Blood pressure, stroke, and coronary heart disease. I. Prolonged differences in blood pressure — prospective observational studies corrected for the regression dilution bias. Lancet 1990; 335:765–74.

78. Dannenberg AL, Drizd T, Horan MJ, et al. Progress in the battle against hypertension. Change in blood pressure levels in the United States from 1960 to 1980. Hypertension 1987; 10:226–33.

79. Sacks HS, Chalmers TC, Berk AA, Reitman D. Should mild hypertension be treated? An attempted meta-analysis of the clinical trials. Mt. Sinai J Med 1985; 52:265–70.

80. Chobanian AV. Antihypertensive therapy in evolution. N Engl J Med 1986; 314:1701.

81. MacMahon SW, Cutler JA, Furberg CD, Payne GH. The effects of drug treatment for hypertension on morbidity and mortality from cardiovascular disease: a review of randomized controlled trials. Prog Cardiovasc Dis 1986; 29: Suppl I:99–118.

81a. Dahlöf B, Lindholm LH, Hansson L, et al. Morbidity and mortality in the Swedish Trial in Old Patients with Hypertension (STOP-Hypertension). Lancet 1991; 338:1281–5.

81b. SHEP Cooperative Research Group. Prevention of stroke by antihypertensive drug treatment in older persons with isolated systolic hypertension; final results of the Systolic Hypertension in the Elderly Program (SHEP). JAMA 1991; 265:3255–64.

82. Cruickshank JM, Thorp JM, Zacharias FJ. Benefits and potential harm of lowering high blood pressure. Lancet 1987; 1:581–3.

83. Kaplan NM, Alderman MH, Flamenbaum DA, et al. Guidelines for the treatment of hypertension. Am J Hypertens 1989; 2:75–7.

84. Farnett L, Mulrow CD, Linn WD, et al. The J-curve phenomenon and the treatment of hypertension. Is there a point beyond which pressure reduction is dangerous? JAMA 1991; 265:489–95.

85. Stamler J, Wentworth D, Neaton JD for the MRFIT Research Group. Is relationship between serum cholesterol and risk of premature death from coronary heart disease continuous and graded? Findings in 356,222 primary screenees of the Multiple Risk Factor Intervention Trial (MRFIT). JAMA 1986; 256:2823–8.

86. Pekkanen J, Linn S, Heiss G, et al. Ten-year mortality from cardiovascular disease in relation to cholesterol level among men with and without pre-existing cardiovascular disease. N Engl J Med 1990; 322:1700–7.

87. Heliovaara M, Karvonen MJ, Punsar S, Haapakoski J. Importance of coronary risk factors in the presence or absence of myocardial ischemia. Am J Cardiol 1982; 50:1248–52.

88. Phillips AN, Shaper AG, Pocock SJ, et al. The role of risk factors in heart attacks occurring in men with pre-existing ischaemic heart disease. Br Heart J 1988; 60:404–10.

89. Kannel WB, Castelli WP, Gordon T. Cholesterol in the prediction of atherosclerosic disease: new perspectives based on the Framingham Study. Ann Intern Med 1979; 90:85–91.

90. Rubin SM, Sidney S, Black DM, et al. High blood cholesterol in elderly men and the excess risk for coronary heart disease. Ann Intern Med 1990; 113:916–20.

91. Benfante R, Reed D. Is elevated serum cholesterol level a risk factor for coronary heart disease in the elderly? JAMA 1990; 263:393–6.

92. The Lipid Research Clinics Program. The Lipid Research Clinics Coronary Primary Prevention Trial Results. I. Reduction in incidence of coronary heart disease. JAMA 1984; 251:351–64.

93. Frick MH, Elo O, Happa K, et al. Helsinki Heart Study: primary-prevention trial with gemfibrozil in middle-aged men with dyslipidemia: safety of treatment, changes in risk factors, and incidence of coronary heart disease. N Engl J Med 1987; 317:1237–45.

94. Brensike JF, Levy RI, Kelsey SF, et al. Effects of therapy with cholestyramine on progression of coronary atherosclerosis. Results of the NHLBI type II Coronary Intervention Study. Circulation 1984; 69:313–24.

95. Blankenhorn DH, Nessim SA, Johnson RL, et al. Beneficial effects of combined colestipol-niacin therapy on coronary atherosclerosis and cor-

onary venous bypass grafts. JAMA 1987; 257:3233–40.

96. Cashin-Hemphill L, Mack WJ, Pogoda JM, et al. Beneficial effects of colestipol-niacin on coronary atherosclerosis. A 4 year follow-up. JAMA 1990; 264:3013–7.

97. Anitschkow N. Über die Veränderungen der Kaninchenaorta bei experimenteller cholesterinsteatose. Bietr Path Anat Allg Path 1913; 56:379–404.

98. Conference on the Health Effects of Blood Lipids. Optimal distributions for populations. Workshop report: Epidemiological section. Prev Med 1979; 8:612–78.

99. Gordon T, Castelli WP, Hjortland MC, et al. High density lipoprotein as a protective factor against coronary heart disease: the Framingham Study. Am J Med 1977; 62:707–14.

100. Miller NE, Forde OH, Thelle DS, Mjos OD. The Tromso Heart Study: high-density lipoprotein and coronary heart disease: a prospective case-control study. Lancet 1977; 1:965–70.

101. Keys A. Alpha lipoprotein (HDL) cholesterol in the serum and the risk of coronary heart disease and death. Lancet 1980; 2:603–6.

102. Goldbourt U, Holtzman E, Neufeld HN. Total and high density lipoprotein cholesterol in the serum and risk of mortality: evidence of a threshold effect. Br Med J 1985; 290:1239–43.

103. Gordon DJ, Probstfield JL, Garrison RJ, et al. High density lipoprotein cholesterol and cardiovascular disease. Four prospective American studies. Circulation 1989; 79:8–15.

104. De Backer G, Rosseneu M, Deslypere JP. Discriminative value of lipids and apoproteins in coronary heart disease. Atherosclerosis 1982; 42:197–203.

105. Maciejko JJ, Holmes DR, Kottke BA, et al. Apolipoprotein A-I as a marker of angiographically assessed coronary heart disease. N Engl J Med 1983; 309:385–9.

106. Brunzell JD, Sniderman AD, Albers JJ, Kwiterovich PO Jr. Apoproteins B and A-I and coronary artery disease in humans. Arteriosclerosis 1984; 4:79–83.

107. Albrink MJ, Mann EB. Serum triglycerides in coronary artery disease. Arch Intern Med 1959; 103:4–8.

108. Carlson LA. Serum lipids in men with myocardial infarction. Acta Med Scand 1960; 167:399–413.

109. Rosenman RH, Brand RJ, Sholtz RI, Friedman M. Multivariate prediction of coronary heart disease during 8.5 year follow-up in the Western Collaborative Group Study. Am J Cardiol 1976; 37:903–10.

110. Tibblin G, Wilhelmsen L, Werko L. Risk factors for myocardial infarction and death due to ischemic heart disease and other causes. Am J Cardiol 1975; 35:514–22.

111. Brunzell JD, Austin MA. Plasma triglyceride levels and coronary disease. N Engl J Med 1989; 320:1273–5.

112. Calabresi L, Franceschini G, Sirtori M, et al. Influence of serum triglycerides on the HDL pattern in normal subjects and patients with coronary artery disease. Atherosclerosis 1990; 84:41–8.

113. Gotto AM. Interrelationship of triglycerides with lipoproteins and high-density lipoproteins. Am J Cardiol 1990; 66:A20–A23.

114. Hulley SB, Rosenman RH, Bawol RD, Brand RJ. Epidemiology as a guide to clinical decisions. The association between triglyceride and coronary heart disease. N Engl J Med 1980; 302:1383–9.

115. Rhoads GG, Feinleib M. Serum triglyceride and risk of coronary heart disease, stroke, and total mortality in Japanese-American men. Arteriosclerosis 1983; 3:316–22.

116. Castelli WP. The triglyceride issue: a view from Framingham. Am Heart J 1986; 112:432–7.

117. Keys A. *Seven Countries: A multivariate analysis of death and coronary heart disease.* Cambridge: Harvard University Press, 1980.

118. Shekelle RB, Shryock AM, Paul O, et al. Diet, serum cholesterol, and death from coronary heart disease. The Western Electric Study. N Engl J Med 1981; 304:65–70.

119. Kushi LH, Lew RA, Stare FJ, et al. Diet and 20-year mortality from coronary heart disease. The Ireland-Boston diet-heart study. N Engl J Med 1985; 312:811–8.

120. Lapidus L, Anderson H, Bengtsson C, Bosaeus I. Dietary habits in relation to incidence of cardiovascular disease and death in women: a 12-year followup of participants in the population study of women in Gothenburg, Sweden. Am J Clin Nutr 1986; 44:444–8.

121. McGee DL, Reed DM, Yano K, et al. Ten-year incidence of coronary heart disease in the Honolulu Heart Program. Am J Epidemiol 1984; 119:667–76.

122. Connor SL, Gustafson JR, Artaud-Wild SM, et al. The cholesterol-saturated fat index: an indication of the hypercholesterolemic and atherogenic potential of food. Lancet 1986; 1:1229–32.

123. Hegsted DM, McGandy RB, Meyers ML, Stare FJ. Quantitative effects of dietary fat on serum cholesterol in man. Am J Clin Nutr 1965; 17:281–95.

124. Mattson FH, Grundy SM. Comparisons of effects of dietary saturated, monounsaturated and

polyunsaturated fatty acids on plasma lipid and lipoproteins in man. J Lipid Res 1985; 26:194–202.

125. Nichaman MZ, Hamm P. Low-fat, high carbohydrate diets and plasma cholesterol. Am J Clin Nutr 1987; 45:1155–60.

126. Bonanome A, Grundy SM. Effect of dietary stearic acid on plasma cholesterol and lipoprotein levels. N Engl J Med 1988; 318:1244–8.

127. Kris-Etherton PM, Krummel D, Russell ME, et al. The effect of diet on plasma lipds, lipoproteins, and coronary heart disease. J Am Diet Assoc 1988; 88:1373–1400.

128. Stamler J, Shekelle R. Dietary cholesterol and human coronary heart disease. The epidemiologic evidence. Arch Path Lab Med 1988; 112:1032–40.

129. National Diet-Heart Study Research Group. National Diet-Heart Study Final Report. Circulation 1968; 37:Suppl I:I-260–I-274.

130. National Cholesterol Education Program Expert Panel. Report on detection, evaluation, and treatment of high blood cholesterol in adults. Arch Intern Med 1988; 148:36–69.

131. Steinberg D. The cholesterol controversy is over: why did it take so long? Circulation 1989; 80:1070–8.

132. Grundy SM. Cholesterol and coronary heart disease. Future directions. JAMA 1990; 264:3053–9.

133. Kleinman JC, Donahue RP, Harris MI, et al. Mortality among diabetics in a national sample. Am J Epidemiol 1988; 128:389–401.

134. Barrett-Connor E, Orchard T. Diabetes and heart disease. In: Diabetes in America: diabetes data compiled 1984. National Diabetes Data Group, U.S. Department of Health and Human Services. USDHHS pub. no. (NIH) 85-1468, 1985.

135. Mattock MB, Fuller JH, Maude PS, Keen H. Lipoproteins and plasma cholesterol esterification in normal and diabetic subjects. Atherosclerosis 1979; 34:437–49.

136. Wingard DL, Barrett-Connor E, Criqui MH, Suarez L. Clustering of heart disease risk factors in diabetic compared to nondiabetic adults. Am J Epidemiol 1983; 117:19–26.

137. Kannel WB, McGee DL. Diabetes and cardiovascular disease. The Framingham Study. JAMA 1979; 241:2035–8.

138. Kannel WB, Hjortland M, Castelli WP. Role of diabetes in congestive heart failure: the Framingham Study. Am J Cardiol 1974; 34:29–34.

139. Reaven GM. Role of insulin resistance in human disease. Diabetes 1988; 37:1595–1607.

140. Stout RW. Insulin and atheroma — an update. Lancet 1987; 1:1077–9.

141. Jarrett RJ. Is insulin atherogenic? Diabetologia 1988; 31:71–5.

142. Stern MP, Haffner SM. Body fat distribution and hyperinsulinemia as risk factors for diabetes and cardiovascular disease. Arteriosclerosis 1986; 6:123–30.

143. Haffner SM, Stern MP, Hazuda HP, et al. Cardiovascular risk factors in confirmed prediabetic individuals. Does the clock for coronary heart disease start ticking before the onset of clinical diabetes? JAMA 1990; 263:2893–8.

144. National Institutes of Health Consensus Development Panel on the Health Implications of Obesity. Health implications of obesity. Ann Intern Med 1985; 103:1073–7.

145. Hubert HB. The importance of obesity in the development of coronary risk factors and disease: the epidemiologic evidence. Ann Rev Public Health 1986; 7:493–502.

146. Barrett-Connor EL. Obesity, atherosclerosis, and coronary artery disease. Ann Intern Med 1985; 103:1010–9.

147. Ashley FW, Jr, Kannel WB. Relation of weight change to changes in atherogenic traits: the Framingham Study. J Chron Dis 1974; 27:103–14.

148. Noppa H, Bengtsson C, Wedel H, Wilhelmsen L. Obesity in relation to morbidity and mortality from cardiovascular disease. Am J Epidemiol 1980; 111:682–92.

149. Tuomilehto J, Salonen JT, Marti B, et al. Body weight and risk of myocardial infarction and death in the adult population of eastern Finland. Br Med J 1987; 295:623–7.

150. Hubert HB, Feinleib M, McNamara PM, Castelli WP. Obesity as an independent risk factor for cardiovascular disease: a 26-year follow-up of participants in the Framingham Heart Study. Circulation 1983; 67:968–77.

151. Manson JE, Colditz GA, Stampfer MJ, et al. A prospective study of obesity and risk of coronary heart disease in women. N Engl J Med 1990; 322:882–9.

152. Despres JP, Moorjani S, Lupien PJ, et al. Regional distribution of body fat, plasma lipoproteins, and cardiovascular disease. Arteriosclerosis 1990; 10:497–511.

153. Morris JN, Heady JA, Raffle PAB, et al. Coronary heart disease and physical activity of work. Lancet 1953; 2:1053–7; 1111–20.

154. Paffenbarger RS, Hale WE. Work activity and coronary heart mortality. N Engl J Med 1975; 292:545–50.

155. Powell KE, Thompson PD, Caspersen CJ, Kendrick JS. Physical activity and the incidence of coronary heart disease. Ann Rev Public Health 1987; 8:253–87.

156. Oberman A. Exercise and the primary prevention of cardiovascular disease. Am J Cardiol 1985; 55:10D–20D.

157. Shephard RJ. Exercise in coronary heart disease. Sports Med 1986; 3:26–49.

158. Berlin JA, Colditz GA. A meta-analysis of physical activity in the prevention of coronary heart disease. Am J Epidemiol 1990; 132:612–28.

159. Ekelund LG, Haskell WL, Johnson JL, et al. Physical fitness as a predictor of cardiovascular mortality in asymptomatic North American men. The Lipid Research Clinics Mortality Follow-up Study. N Engl J Med 1988; 319:1379–84.

160. Blair SN, Kohl HW, Paffenbarger RS, Jr, et al. Physical fitness and all-cause mortality. A prospective study of healthy men and women. JAMA 1989; 262:2395–401.

161. LaPorte RE, Cresanta JL, Kuller LH. The relationship of alcohol consumption to atherosclerotic heart disease. Prev Med 1980; 9:22–40.

162. Moore RD, Pearson TA. Moderate alcohol consumption and coronary heart disease. Medicine 1986; 65:242–67.

163. Klatsky A, Friedman GD, Siegelaub AB. Alcohol and mortality: a ten year Kaiser-Permanente experience. Ann Intern Med 1981; 95:139–45.

164. Blackwelder WC, Yano K, Rhoads GG, et al. Alcohol and mortality: the Honolulu Heart Study. Am J Med 1980; 68:164–9.

165. Marmot MG, Rose G, Shipley MJ, Thomas BJ. Alcohol and mortality: a U-shaped curve. Lancet 1981; 1:580–3.

166. Castelli WP, Doyle JT, Gordon T, et al. Alcohol and blood lipids: the Cooperative Lipoprotein Phenotyping Study. Lancet 1977; 2:153–5.

167. Friedman LA, Kimball AW. Coronary heart disease mortality and alcohol consumption in Framingham. Am J Epidemiol 1986; 124:481–9.

168. Boffetta P, Garfinkel L. Alcohol drinking and mortality among men enrolled in an American Cancer Society Prospective Study. Epidemiology 1990; 1:342–8.

169. Stampfer MJ, Colditz GA, Willett WC, et al. A prospective study of moderate alcohol consumption and the risk of coronary disease and stroke in women. N Engl J Med 1988; 319:267–73.

170. Ellison RC. Cheers! Epidemiology 1990; 1:337–9.

171. Osler W. Lecture on angina pectoris and allied states. NY Med J 1896; 64:177–183.

172. Friedman M, Rosenman RH. Association of a specific overt behavior pattern with increases in blood cholesterol, blood clotting time, incidence of arcus senilis and clinical coronary heart disease. JAMA 1959; 169:1286–96.

173. Krantz DS, Contrada RJ, Hill DR, Friedler E. Environmental stress and biobehavioral antecedents of coronary heart disease. J Consult Clin Psych 1988; 56:333–41.

174. Matthews KA, Haynes SG. Type A behavior pattern and coronary disease risk: update and critical evaluation. Am J Epidemiol 1986; 123:923–60.

175. Jenkins CD. The coronary-prone personality. In: W.D. Gentry & R.B. Williams, eds. Psychological aspects of myocardial infarction and coronary care. St. Louis, MO: Mosby, 1979.

176. Jenkins CD, Rosenman RH, Zyzanski SJ. Prediction of clinical coronary heart disease by a test for the coronary-prone behavior pattern. N Engl J Med 1974; 290:1271–5.

177. Haynes SG, Feinleib M, Kannel WB. The relationship of psychosocial factors to coronary heart disease in the Framingham Study. II. Eight-year incidence of coronary heart disease. Am J Epidemiol 1980; 111:37–58.

178. Shekelle RB, Gale M, Norusis M. Type A score (Jenkins Activity Survey) and risk of recurrent coronary heart disease in the Aspirin Myocardial Infarction Study. Am J Cardiol 1985; 56:221–5.

179. Shekelle RB, Hulley SB, Neaton JD, et al. The MRFIT Behavior Pattern Study. II. Type A behavior and incidence of coronary heart disease. Am J Epidemiol 1985; 122:559–70.

180. Ragland DR, Brand RJ. Type A behavior and mortality from coronary heart disease. N Engl J Med 1988; 318:65–9.

181. Williams RB Jr, Haney TL, Lee KL, et al. Type A behavior, hostility, and coronary atherosclerosis. Psychosom Med 1980; 42:539–49.

182. Shekelle RB, Gale M, Ostfeld AM, Paul O. Hostility, risk of coronary heart disease, and mortality. Psychosom Med 1983; 45:109–14.

183. Dembroski TM, MacDougall JM, Williams RB, et al. Components of type A, hostility, and anger-in: relationship to angiographic findings. Psychosom Med 1985; 47:219–33.

184. Helmer DC, Ragland DR, Syme SL. Hostility and coronary artery disease. Am J Epidemiol 1991; 133:112–22.

185. Leon GR, Finn SE, Murray D, Bailey JM. Inability to predict cardiovascular disease from hostility scores or MMPI items related to type A behavior. J Consult Clin Psychol 1988; 56:597–600.

186. Hearn MD, Murray DM, Luepker RV. Hostility, coronary heart disease, and total mortal-

ity: a 33-year follow-up study of university students. J Behav Med 1989; 12:105–21.

187. Goldbourt U, Neufeld HN. Genetic aspects of arteriosclerosis. Arteriosclerosis 1986; 6:357–77.

188. Robertson FW. The genetic component in coronary heart disease — a review. Genet Res 1981; 37:1–16.

189. Thomas CB, Cohen BH. The familial occurrence of hypertension and coronary artery disease, with observations concerning obesity and diabetes. Ann Intern Med 1955; 42:90–127.

190. Slack J, Evans KA. The increased risk of death from ischemic heart disease in the first degree relatives of 121 men and 96 women with ischemic heart disease. J Med Genet 1966; 3:239–57.

191. Feinleib M, Garrison RJ, Fabsitz R, et al. The NHLBI twin study of cardiovascular disease risk factors: methodology and summary of results. Am J Epidemiol 1977; 106:284–95.

192. Shear CL, Frerichs RR, Weinberg R, Berenson GS. Childhood sibling aggregation of coronary artery disease risk factor variables in a biracial community. Am J Epidemiol 1978; 107:522–8.

193. Morrison JA, Khoury P, Laskarzewski PM, et al. Familial associations of lipids and lipoproteins in families of hypercholesterolemic probands. Arteriosclerosis 1982; 2:151–9.

194. Hennekens CH, Jesse MJ, Klein BE, et al. Cholesterol among children of men with myocardial infarction. Pediatrics 1976; 58:211–7.

195. Glueck CJ, Fallat RW, Tsang R, Buncher CR. Hyperlipidemia in progeny of parents with myocardial infarction before age 50. Am J Dis Child 1974; 127:70–5.

196. King MC, Lee GM, Spinner NB, et al. Genetic epidemiology. Annu Rev Public Health 1984; 5:1–52.

197. Sholtz RI, Rosenman RH, Brand RJ. The relationship of reported parental history to the incidence of coronary heart disease in the Western Collaborative Group Study. Am J Epidemiol 1975; 102:350–6.

198. Snowden CB, McNamara PM, Garrison RJ, et al. Predicting coronary heart disease in siblings — a multivariate assessment. The Framingham Heart Study. Am J Epidemiol 1982; 115:217–22.

199. Cambien F, Richard JL, Ducimetiere P. Familial history of coronary heart diseases and high blood pressure in relation to the prevalence of risk factors, and the incidence of coronary heart disease. Rev Epidemiol Sante Publ 1980; 28:21–37.

200. Barrett-Connor E, Khaw KT. Family history of heart attack as an independent predictor of death due to cardiovascular disease. Circulation 1984; 69:1065–9.

201. Colditz GA, Stampfer M, Willett WC, et al. A prospective study of parental history of myocardial infarction and coronary heart disease in women. Am J Epidemiol 1986; 123:48–58.

202. Berg K. Inherited lipoprotein variation and atherosclerotic disease. In: Scanu AM, Wissler W, Getz GS, eds. The biochemistry of atherosclerosis. New York: Marcel Dekker, 1979:419–90.

203. Stadel BV. Oral contraceptives and cardiovascular disease. N Engl J Med 1981; 305:672–7.

204. Boyce J, Fawcett JW, Noall EWP. Coronary thrombosis and conovid. Lancet 1963; 1:111.

205. Hartveit F. Complications of oral contraception. Br Med J 1965; 1:160.

206. Naysmith JH. Oral contraceptives and coronary thrombosis. Br Med J 1965; 1:250.

207. Mann JI, Vessey MP, Thorogood M, Doll R. Myocardial infarction in young women with special reference to oral contraceptive practice. Br Med J 1975; 2:241–5.

208. Mann JI, Doll R, Thorogood M, et al. Risk factors for myocardial infarction in young women. Br J Prev Soc Med 1976; 30:94–100.

209. Jick H, Dinan B, Rothman KJ. Oral contraceptives and nonfatal myocardial infarction. JAMA 1978; 239:1403–6.

210. Rosenberg L, Hennekens CH, Rosner B, et al. Oral contraceptive use in relation to nonfatal myocardial infarction. Am J Epidemiol 1980; 111:59–66.

211. Dalen JE, Hickler RB. Oral contraceptives and cardiovascular disease. Am Heart J 1981; 101:626–39.

212. Slone D, Shapiro S, Kaufman DW, et al. Risk of myocardial infarction in relation to current and discontinued use of oral contraceptives. N Engl J Med 1981; 305:420–4.

213. Stampfer MJ, Willett WC, Colditz GA, et al. A prospective study of past use of oral contraceptive agents and risk of cardiovascular diseases. N Engl J Med 1988; 319:1313–7.

214. Meade TW, Mellows S, Brozovic M, et al. Haemostatic function and ischaemic heart disease: principal results of the Northwick Park Heart Study. Lancet 1986; 2:533–7.

215. Kannel WB, Wolf PA, Castelli WP, D'Agostino RB. Fibrinogen and risk of cardiovascular disease. The Framingham Study. JAMA 1987; 258:1183–6.

216. Yarnell JWG, Sweetnam PM, Elwood PC, et al. Haemostatic factors and ischaemic heart disease. The Caerphilly Study. Br Heart J 1985; 53:483–7.

217. Lowe GDO, Drummond MM, Lorimer AR, et al. Relation between extent of coronary artery disease and blood viscosity. Br Med J 1980; 1:673–4.
218. Wilhelmsen L, Svardsudd K. Korsan-Bengtsen K, et al. Fibrinogen as a risk factor for stroke and myocardial infarction. N Engl J Med 1984; 311:501–5.
219. Alexander NJ, Clarkson TB. Vasectomy increases the severity of diet-induced atherosclerosis in Macaca fascicularis. Science 1978; 201:538–41.
220. Clarkson TB, Alexander NJ. Long-term vasectomy: effects on the occurrence and extent of atherosclerosis in rhesus monkeys. J Clin Invest 1980; 65:15–25.
221. Massey FJ, Bernstein GS, O'Fallon WM, et al. Vasectomy and health: results from a cohort study. JAMA 1984; 252:1023–9.
222. Rosenberg L, Schwingl PJ, Kaufman DW, et al. The risk of myocardial infarction 10 or more years after vasectomy in men under 55 years of age. Am J Epidemiol 1986; 123:1049–56.
223. Guang-Hua T, Yu-Hui Z, Yue-Min M, et al. Vasectomy and health: cardiovascular and other diseases following vasectomy in Sichuan Province, People's Republic of China. Int J Epidemiol 1988; 17:608–17.
224. Petitti DB. Epidemiologic studies of vasectomy. In: Zatuchni GI, Goldsmith A, Spieler JM, Sciarra JJ, eds. Male contraception: advances and future prospects. New York: Harper and Row, 1985:24–33.

2

Temporal Trends and Declining Mortality Rates from Coronary Heart Disease in the United States

ROBERT J. GOLDBERG

EDITORS' INTRODUCTION

Over the last four decades heart disease mortality has fallen to 55 percent of the 1950 rate, and the pace at which CHD deaths have been declining has accelerated in recent years. Understanding the causes for this change is so important that it clearly deserves a separate chapter. Here Dr. Goldberg analyzes the phenomenon and looks at the evidence linking risk factor modification to the diminution of CHD risk. To a large extent the changes parallel those predicted from the outcome of clinical trials such as the Lipid Research Clinic's Coronary Primary Prevention Trial and vindicate our belief in CHD prevention through risk factor modification. Treatment factors such as the use of pharmacologic beta-blockade and interventions such as bypass surgery and coronary angioplasty are also discussed, and the relative contributions of prevention and treatment are evaluated. It may be that the encouraging implications of at least the primary prevention aspects of these findings are not necessarily limited to heart disease — it is reasonable to surmise that at least certain forms of cancer may eventually also respond to risk factor control, although the lag time is likely to be longer.

Beginning at the turn of the twentieth century, death rates from coronary heart disease (CHD) in the United States increased dramatically, reaching epidemic proportions by the mid-1960s [1, 2, 3, 4, 5, 6]. Since that time, the age-adjusted mortality atributed to CHD has leveled off and then turned markedly downward, declining by approximately 2 to 3 percent annually (Figure 2-1). All-cause mortality as well as mortality from cardiovascular disease and stroke have also declined over time. The observed declines in all causes of death, CHD, and stroke since 1968 are shown in Figure 2-2. The annual number of deaths and the crude death rate from CHD and acute myocardial infarction (MI) have exhibited consistent declines over the past two decades (Table 2-1); there were approximately 175,000 fewer deaths due to CHD and 120,000 fewer deaths due to acute MI in 1989 than at the beginning of the decline in CHD deaths in 1968. A particularly steep decline (4 percent) has been observed in the most recently published (1985 to 1989) annual age-adjusted mortality rates from CHD (1985: 126 per 100,000; 1989: 105 per 100,000) and acute MI (1985: 69 per

100,000; 1989: 56 per 100,000). While this significant and encouraging decline appears real, being seen in all age groups, both sexes, and the major race/ethnic groups examined and not due to artifactual changes in death certification or recording practices, the reasons for this decrease remain unknown. CHD remains the leading cause of death in the United States, accounting for nearly one-half million deaths, or approximately one-quarter of all deaths on an annual basis, and is responsible for over two million hospitalizations annually. The yearly direct and indirect costs associated with CHD are estimated to be approximately 140 billion dollars [7].

The decline in mortality rates attributed to CHD has been observed not only in the United States but also in certain other countries, namely, Australia, Belgium, Canada, Finland, Israel, Japan, and New Zealand [8]. The World Health Organization is collecting data on recent temporal trends (1984–1994) in the incidence rates of fatal and nonfatal coronary events and on the primary risk factors for cardiovascular disease from a uniform and standardized world-

Figure 2-1. Age-adjusted death rates for selected causes of death: United States.

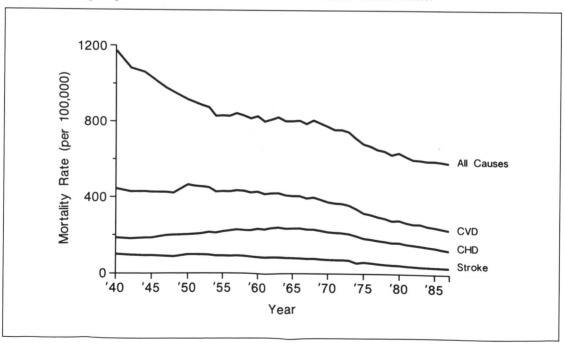

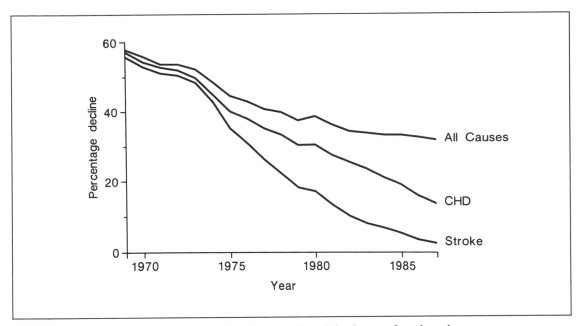

Figure 2-2. Cumulative percentage decline in age-adjusted death rates for selected causes: United States.

Table 2-1. Temporal trends in annual deaths and death rates from coronary heart disease and acute myocardial infarction in the United States

Year	Coronary heart disease[a]		Acute myocardial infarction[b]	
	Number of deaths	Crude death rate[c]	Number of deaths	Crude death rate
1968	674,747	338	369,610	185
1969	669,829	332	361,583	179
1971	674,292	332	357,714	173
1973	684,066	326	351,662	168
1975	642,719	302	324,652	152
1977	638,427	295	306,398	142
1979	551,365	251	300,462	137
1981	555,158	242	292,504	128
1983	555,492	236	286,300	122
1985	536,805	225	274,199	115
1987	512,138	210	253,542	104
1989	497,850	201	247,020	100

[a]International Classification of Diseases (ICD) Code 410–414.
[b]ICD Code 410.
[c]Per 100,000 population.

wide perspective among the 26 countries participating in the MONICA project [9,10]. Nonetheless, reasons for the dramatic decline in death rates remain uncertain, and a paucity of population-based data exists to ascertain whether the observed temporal trends are due to changes in the incidence rates of new coronary events, changes in survival after an acute coronary episode, or combinations thereof. These data are particularly needed to determine the relative contributions of primary and secondary preventive and therapeutic efforts to declining CHD death rates.

Declines in the incidence rates of CHD would suggest that the mortality decline may be due to a decrease in the occurrence rates of acute MI and sudden cardiac death (SCD) secondary to modification of lifestyle characteristics and changes in the prevalence and/or levels of the major coronary risk factors. If, however, the reported incidence rates of acute MI and out-of-hospital SCD have stabilized or even increased, a likely explanation for the observed downward trend in CHD mortality would be improvements in medical care. The following sections describe changes over time in the commonly accepted primary and secondary risk factors for CHD, from either a national or population-based perspective where such data are available. They also examine secular trends in the incidence and case-fatality rates of acute MI and SCD and in the therapeutic management of patients with CHD.

Temporal Trends in the Primary Risk Factors for CHD

Cigarette Smoking

Since the issuance of the Surgeon General's first report on smoking and health in 1964 and following repeated public warnings concerning the hazards of cigarette smoking, the prevalence of cigarette smoking has decreased over the past two decades in the United States [11, 12]. Based on data from the National Health Interview Survey of adults 20 years of age and older (Figure 2-3), while the two sexes have exhibited consistent decreases in the population prevalence

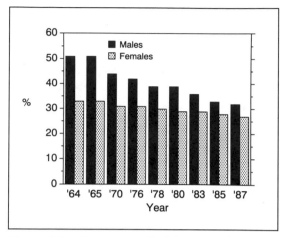

Figure 2-3. Percentage of adults currently smoking in the United States.

of cigarette smoking between 1964 and 1987, more marked declines have been observed among males. Slightly more than one-half of all males were smoking cigarettes in 1965; this percentage declined to 32 percent in 1987. Thirty-three percent of women smoked cigarettes in 1965, 31 percent approximately a decade later, and 27 percent in 1987.

Overall population rates of cigarette smoking have declined from 40 percent of the adult population being smokers in 1965 to 37 percent in 1970, 33 percent in 1980, 30 percent in 1985, and 29 percent in 1987, for a relative decline of 28 percent in the population prevalence of smoking between 1965 and 1987. More marked decreases in smoking rates have been observed among whites compared to blacks. In 1965 40 percent of whites were smoking cigarettes, with this proportion declining to 29 percent in 1987. Among black adults, approximately 43 percent were smokers in 1965; this percentage declined to 34 percent in 1987. Declines in estimates of cigarette smoking prevalence have also been reported recently from the Minnesota Heart Survey [13] and the Framingham Heart Study [14]. Between the two survey periods in the Minnesota Heart Survey of 1980–82 and 1985–87, the age-adjusted rate of current cigarette smoking declined to approximately 14 percent in men (34 percent to 30 percent) and 18 percent in women (34 percent to 28 percent) aged 25 to 74 years and surveyed in the Minneapolis–St. Paul metropolitan area. Among three middle-aged (50–59 years) male cohorts surveyed in the Framingham Heart Study during 1950, 1960, and 1970, the percentage of current smokers declined from 56 percent in 1950 to 52 percent in 1960 and to 34 percent in 1970.

Despite the encouraging decline in the national and selected population-sample prevalence estimates of current cigarette smoking, the proportion of heavy smokers has increased, particularly among women [11, 12] (Figure 2-4). Between 1965 and 1985 the percentage of heavy smokers among current smokers increased by approximately 29 percent in men and 77 percent in women. Similar national prevalence estimates of the extent of current and heavy smoking have been observed in the Health Promotion and Disease Prevention Survey of the National Health Interview Survey conducted in 1985 [15]. This survey showed that approximately 30 percent of persons 18 years of age and older currently smoked cigarettes, with higher rates of smoking observed among men (33 percent) than women (28 percent). Among current smokers, approximately 27 percent smoked 25 cigarettes or more per day, with a greater percentage of male (32 percent) than female (21 percent) heavy smokers. Because it is easier for lighter than for heavy smokers to quit smoking, we are being left with an increasingly "difficult"

Figure 2-4.   Percentage of adult smokers currently smoking 25 or more cigarettes per day.

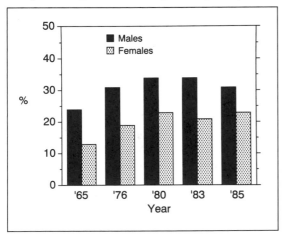

population of heavy smokers. National efforts continue to be made to decrease the overall prevalence of current cigarette smoking throughout the United States, with targeted efforts to enhance cessation among heavy smokers [16], increase the visibility and growth of tobacco use prevention and control coalitions [17], and place increasing emphasis on the role of health care providers in helping their patients stop smoking [18, 19, 20, 21]. It will therefore be important to continue to monitor population trends in cigarette smoking and progress in smoking prevention and cessation.

Elevated Blood Pressure and Hypertension

Several community-based studies carried out in the 1960s gave rise to the "rule of halves" concerning the awareness, management, and control of hypertension, suggesting neglect by the public as well as by health care providers of an important public health problem. These studies essentially showed that approximately one-half of all hypertensives were aware of their condition as reflected by having been told by a health professional that they were hypertensive; of those aware, approximately one-half were being treated with antihypertensive medication; and of those under treatment, approximately one-half had their blood pressure adequately managed and controlled. In 1967 the landmark Veterans Administration Study showed that lowering blood pressure could substantially improve morbidity and mortality associated with hypertension among treated patients with moderate to severe hypertension [22]. Following this study there was increased recognition of elevated blood pressure as a public health problem of national importance, with educational efforts begun by the National High Blood Pressure Education Program in the early 1970s [23] and then by publication and widespread dissemination of the first Joint National Committee Report on the Detection, Evaluation and Treatment of High Blood Pressure, which established guidelines for the treatment and stepped-care management of hypertension [24].

Data compiled from several nationally based representative population surveys have indeed shown marked increases in the population awareness and control of hypertension between the early 1960s and late 1970s. Utilizing data from the cross-sectional National Health Examination Survey carried out in 1960 to 1962 (NHES I), the initial National Health and Nutrition Examination Survey conducted during 1971 to 1974 (NHANES I), and its successor carried out in 1976–1980 (NHANES II), the proportion of adults with undiagnosed hypertension steadily declined from 1960 (52 percent) to 1980 (29 percent), the percentage of diagnosed hypertensives receiving antihypertensive medications increased over the same two decades (30 percent in 1960 to 45 percent in 1980), and the proportion of hypertensives receiving medication and whose condition was consistently controlled increased from 39 percent in 1960 to 1962 to 52 percent in 1976 to 1980 (Table 2-2).

While there have been significant improvements in the percentage of hypertensives whose blood pressure has been controlled, sizable black/white and male/female gaps continue to exist, and there has been a slight increase in the prevalence of adults with definite hypertension. Updating and extending these findings based on the results from other study samples, the household-based survey of the civilian noninstitutionalized population (Health Promotion and Disease Prevention) demonstrated that approximately 61 percent of men and 70 percent of women with elevated blood pressure readings were currently taking medication for this condition in 1985 [15]. Data collected from community-based studies of hypertension in Chicago (1967 to 1971) and Minneapolis (1980 to 81) showed marked increases in the proportion of hypertensives under treatment (25 to 69 percent) and of those with hypertension under control (11 to 61 percent)[25]. Recent findings from the Minnesota Heart Survey have shown a slight decline in the average age-adjusted systolic blood pressure in women surveyed between 1980 to 82 and 1985 to 87, whereas no change was observed in the average age-adjusted systolic pressure among men [13]. Among the three male cohorts assembled from different time periods in the Framingham Heart

Study, the percentage of men with definite hypertension declined between the 1950 and the 1970 cohorts (from 21 percent to 15 percent) while the percentage of hypertensive men receiving antihypertensive medication and having their blood pressure controlled approximately doubled between 1960 (11 percent taking medication; of these 30 percent had their hypertension controlled) and 1970 (22 percent taking medication; of these 60 percent had their hypertension controlled) [14]. Data from both males and females in the original cohort of the Framingham Heart Study have shown no apparent trends in the incidence rates of hypertension in the 1950s, 1960s, and 1970s, although the proportion of hypertensive persons receiving antihypertensive medication increased consistently from the mid-1950s to the late 1970s and early 1980s [26].

Given the recent introduction of new classes of agents to control elevated blood pressure (e.g., ACE inhibitors, beta-adrenergic blocking agents, calcium channel blockers) and interest in numerous nonpharmacologic approaches to the prevention and management of elevated blood pressure (including weight control, sodium and alcohol restriction, regular sustained aerobic exercise, and relaxation therapy), as well as provider awareness of the importance and need for intervention among persons with mild hypertension, improving trends in the prevention and management of hypertension are likely to continue into the 1990s. Hypertension remains a major public health problem, however, since it affects approximately 58 million Americans.

Serum Cholesterol Levels

Declines in the overall as well as the age-specific average population cholesterol levels have been observed over time in the United States (Figure 2-5). Based on data collected by the National Center for Health Statistics in nationally based health surveys of the noninstitutionalized population of the United States (Health and Examination Survey, or HES I, in 1960 to 1962, NHANES I carried out in 1971 to 1974, and NHANES II conducted in 1976 to 1980), the average age-adjusted race- and sex-specific serum cholesterol levels declined slightly over

Table 2-2. Results of national surveys of elevated blood pressure among adults 18–74 years of age

| | NHES (1960–62) | | | | |
| | | White | | Black | |
	Total	Males	Females	Males	Females
Percentage of adult population with definite hypertension	21	19	20	32	36
Percentage of definite hypertensives diagnosed	48	39	57	30	59
Percentage of diagnosed hypertensives under medication	30	21	38	18	44
Percentage of medicated hypertensives under control	39	39	41	15	38

| | NHANES I (1971–74) | | | | |
| | | White | | Black | |
	Total	Males	Females	Males	Females
Percentage of adult population with definite hypertension	21	21	19	32	33
Percentage of definite hypertensives diagnosed	40	31	47	41	53
Percentage of diagnosed hypertensives under medication	32	25	39	24	40
Percentage of medicated hypertensives under control	43	43	45	48	37

| | NHANES II (1976–80) | | | | |
| | | White | | Black | |
	Total	Males	Females	Males	Females
Percentage of adult population with definite hypertension	22	22	20	26	31
Percentage of definite hypertensives diagnosed	71	61	79	66	87
Percentage of diagnosed hypertensives under medication	45	34	56	35	63
Percentage of medicated hypertensives under control	52	44	57	36	60

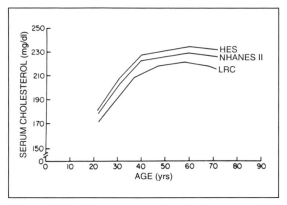

Figure 2-5. Changes over time in the age-specific total serum cholesterol levels in selected national studies.

the periods under study among each of the population groups examined (Table 2-3) [27]. On average these serum cholesterol levels decreased by 3 to 4 percent among the surveyed sample, with a significant decline observed in men (from 217 mg/dl to 211 mg/dl) and women (from 223 mg/dl to 215 mg/dl) from the time of the initial cross-sectional survey in 1960 to 1962 to that of the later survey in 1976 to 1980. While the average serum cholesterol levels declined in both whites and blacks, the trends were more apparent and statistically significant in whites.

In the mid-1980s the National Institutes of Health, as a result of the deliberations of the Consensus Development Conference on Lowering Blood Cholesterol to Prevent Heart Disease [28] and the Expert Panel on the Detection, Evaluation, and Treatment of High Blood Cholesterol in Adults [29], published guidelines and new cutpoints by which adults were to be considered at moderate or high risk for the development of CHD and in need for dietary or pharmacologic intervention. Based on these guidelines, individuals with serum total cholesterol levels less than 200 mg/dl were considered as having desirable cholesterol levels. Those with blood cholesterol levels of 200 to 239 mg/dl were considered at borderline-high risk for CHD, while those with levels 240 mg/dl and greater were considered at high risk for CHD.

Based on these recommendations and data derived from the Lipid Research Clinics Population Study to approximate the levels of serum cholesterol in the population, a large percentage of the adult U.S. population remains at moderate or high risk for the development of CHD [27] (Table 2-4). Despite this relatively large population burden, slight declines in the proportion of men (3 percent) and women (5 percent) considered at high risk for CHD were observed between 1960 to 1962 and 1976 to 1980. Slight decreases were also observed in the age-adjusted percentage of men and women consid-

Table 2-3. Secular trends in the age-adjusted mean serum cholesterol levels of adults aged 20–74 years, by race and sex

	Cholesterol levels (mg/dl)		
	HES I *(1960–1962)*	*NHANES I* *(1971–1974)*	*NHANES II* *(1976–1980)*
Sex			
Male	217	214	211
Female	223	216	215
Race/sex			
White			
Male	218	214	211
Female	224	216	215
Black			
Male	211	213	209
Female	216	218	214

Table 2-4. Age-adjusted percentage of adults aged 20–74 years at selected risk for CHD on the basis of serum cholesterol levels

	HES I (1960–1962)	NHANES I (1971–1974)	NHANES II (1976–1980)
	High-risk cholesterol levels (≥240 mg/dl) (%)		
Sex			
Male	18.1	16.4	15.5
Female	22.9	18.1	17.8
	Moderate-risk cholesterol levels (200–239 mg/dl) (%)		
Sex			
Male	15.0	12.8	12.8
Female	15.3	13.8	13.6

ered at moderate risk for CHD based on the observed cholesterol distribution. Based on data from the population-based Minnesota Heart Survey [13] and middle-aged cohorts from the Framingham Heart Study [14], between 1980 to 1982 and 1985 to 1987 average age-adjusted serum total cholesterol levels declined significantly in men (from 205 mg/dl to 200 mg/dl) and women (from 201 mg/dl to 195 mg/dl) residing in the Twin Cities metropolitan area, as well as among men studied in Framingham, Massachusetts between 1950 (228 mg/dl) and 1970 (221 mg/dl). Updated findings from the Minnesota Heart Survey also showed an increasing awareness of their condition among hypercholesterolemic individuals between 1980 to 1982 and 1985 to 1987 and an increasing likelihood for persons with elevated cholesterol levels to be treated with lipid-lowering agents and to have their condition controlled [30].

A recent national telephone survey of approximately 1600 physicians and 4000 adults showed positive and continuing changes in physician practices and public health behaviors as related to serum cholesterol [31]. Physicians reported treating considerably lower levels of serum cholesterol with diet and drug therapy in 1990 than had been reported in surveys carried out in 1986 and 1983. The percentage of adults who reported having had their cholesterol level checked increased from 35 percent in 1983 to 46 percent and 65 percent in 1986 and

1990, respectively. These and other findings from this survey suggest impressive gains in the treatment and awareness of high serum cholesterol levels by both providers and the general population and also provide insights into those areas in which future educational efforts remain needed.

Based on guidelines from the National Cholesterol Education Program that present schemata for the classification and treatment of individuals based on their cholesterol levels as well as accompanying risk factors for CHD [29], the population burden for receipt of medical advice and intervention due to elevated blood cholesterol levels among adults in the United States has been shown to be considerable [32]. According to these estimates, approximately 41 percent of adults would need a lipoprotein analysis based on their serum cholesterol distribution and accompanying CHD risk factor profile, with a greater percentage of men (45 percent) than women (36 percent) in need of such an analysis. Among persons needing a lipoprotein analysis, the great majority (88 percent) would be considered to be candidates for medical advice and intervention based on their low-density lipoprotein levels. Slightly over one-third (36 percent) of all adults in the United States would be candidates for counseling and intervention for their elevated blood cholesterol levels.

Given the positive results of recent primary prevention trials utilizing various pharmacologic agents (either alone or in conjunction with dietary measures) in terms of reduction in fatal and nonfatal CHD events [33, 34], the potential for regression of coronary artery disease through aggressive pharmacologic treatment (as evidenced by such studies as the Cholesterol-lowering Atherosclerosis Study [35], and increased awareness by the public and health care providers of serum cholesterol as a primary risk factor for CHD (through the efforts of the National Cholesterol Education Project), even more favorable trends in population cholesterol levels may become apparent over the next decade.

Dietary Changes

Since the beginning of the twentieth century and until the mid-1960s, data on national trends in per capita food availability have shown favorable shifts in the consumption of animal and vegetable fats, although total fat intake has increased. Appropriate qualifiers need be placed on the interpretation of these data, however, since all estimates are based on the extent to which food is available at the wholesale and retail levels as opposed to actual ingestion by individuals. These estimates do not allow for food waste or spoilage, factors that may have changed over time given changes in food-handling and preparation practices.

An examination of secular trends in dietary fats in the United States since the turn of the twentieth century shows that while total fat intake increased between 1910 and the mid-1960s the composition of available fats changed significantly. Between 1910 and 1965 per capita availability of animal fats slightly decreased, while there was a greater than twofold increase in the intake of vegetable or polyunsaturated fats [36]. More recent changes over time in the annual per capita availability of selected foods have been examined since the beginning of the decline in CHD mortality rates in the late 1960s (Figure 2-6) [37]. While the availability of red meat, poultry, and fish increased in the aggregate by approximately 4 percent over the periods examined (1968 to 1985), consumption of red meat slightly decreased, whereas consumption of fish, shellfish, and poultry markedly in-

creased. In terms of selected dairy products, the availability of eggs and whole milk declined by 17 percent and 43 percent, respectively, whereas use of low fat milk approximately doubled between the late 1960s and the mid-1980s (Table 2-5). The availability of animal fat and oils declined by 16 percent, while the use of vegetable fats and oils increased by 30 percent; the majority of the latter increase was accounted for by a large increase over time in the use of salad and cooking oils. Finally, the availability of fresh and processed fruits and vegetables increased by 7 percent and 12 percent, respectively, primarily due to increases in the availability of fresh produce.

An analysis of studies carried out in the United States since the 1920s that assessed actual individual dietary intake has shown relatively similar results [38]. When results were pooled across the more than 150 studies examined, several findings of note were observed. The percentage of fat, as a proportion of total energy, increased from the 1920s (36 percent) to the 1960s (40 percent), after which time a small decline (to 38 percent) was seen between 1970 to 1979 and 1980 to 1985. In addition, the percentage of saturated fat in relation to total energy declined over time with a concomitant increase in polyunsaturated fatty acids. Essentially similar trends over time in the percentage of energy consumed as either total or type of fat were seen for adult males and females.

With particular regard to the consumption of fruits and vegetables, data obtained from a single 24-hour dietary recall from the NHANES II Survey of the adult U.S. population carried out between 1976 and 1980 showed that less than 10 percent of the U.S. population met the recommended national guidelines for three or more servings of vegetables and two or more servings of fruit on a daily basis [39]. These data also showed that 11 percent of the survey sample ate neither fruit nor vegetables on the day of the dietary assessment, 45 percent had no fruit, and 22 percent no vegetables. These findings are similar to those obtained in the Nationwide Food Consumption Survey carried out by the United States Department of Agri-

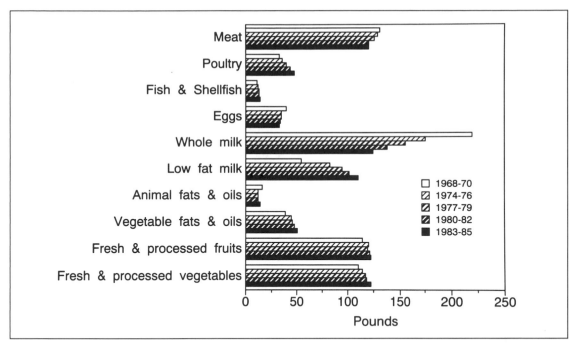

Figure 2-6. Secular trends in the annual per capita availability of selected commodities (pounds).

Table 2-5. Secular trends in the annual per capita availability of selected commodities (pounds)

	Meat	Poultry	Fish and shellfish	Eggs	Whole milk	Low fat milk	Animal fats and oils	Vegetable fats and oils	Fresh and processed fruits	Fresh and processed vegetables
1968–1970	131	33	11	40	220	55	16	39	115	111
1974–1976	129	36	12	35	176	83	12	45	121	115
1977–1979	126	40	13	35	156	95	12	46	120	118
1980–1982	121	44	13	34	138	102	13	48	122	119
1983–1985	121	48	14	33	125	111	14	51	123	123

culture in 1977 to 1978, in which between 8 and 10 percent of the study population aged 19–50 years reported eating no fruit or vegetables on the day of the dietary recall [40], as well as to the Continuing Survey of Food Intakes, in which there were no significant changes in the proportion of women or men consuming any vegetables or fruits between 1977 and 1985 [41].

Temporal Trends in Secondary Risk Factors for CHD

Obesity
The prevalence of obesity, as expressed in terms of body mass index (kg/m²), has increased over time, based on data obtained from selected National Health Examination Surveys [42].

Between 1960 to 1962 and 1976 to 1980, the frequency of obesity among white males slightly increased from 25 percent to 27 percent; essentially no changes were observed in the prevalence of obesity among white females (27 percent in 1960 to 1962; 28 percent in 1976 to 1980). The greatest temporal increases in the prevalence of obesity were observed among blacks, particularly black males. In black males the prevalence of overweight increased from 24 percent in 1960 to 1962 to 31 percent in 1976 to 1980; increases from 47 percent to 50 percent for black females were observed over similar survey periods.

Expressed from the perspective of changes in mean height and weight, both men and women were taller and heavier compared to earlier national cross-sectional samples. Among adult males 18 to 74 years of age, the average weight increased from 75.3 kg at the time of the NHES in 1960 to 1962 to 78.0 kg in both NHANES I (1971 to 1974) and NHANES II (1976 to 1980). Increases in average body weight from 63.5 kg to 64.9 kg to 65.3 kg, respectively, were seen among adult women over the times of the three surveys [43]. Based on the prevalence of obesity among respondents to the National Health Interview Survey in 1985 [15], approximately one-fourth of adults in the United States were 20 percent or more above desirable body weight for height, with marked racial differences observed, particularly among women. Data from the Minnesota Heart Survey (1980 to 1982, 1985 to 1987) also showed increases over time in the average body mass index in both men and women [13]. In accord with these observations, the average caloric intake of selected subgroups in the United States population has increased. The average energy intake of women between the ages of 19 and 50 years and among their offspring aged 1 to 5 years were assessed as part of the Survey of Food Intakes by Individuals carried out initially in 1977 to 1978 and again in 1985 [43]. The mean caloric intake of women increased over time from 1573 kilocalories per day in 1977 to 1661 kilocalories in 1985, with concomitant increases in the daily caloric intake of their children (from 1335 kcal/day to 1446 kcal/day). Data from adults in NHANES II

showed that the mean daily energy intake of white males was 2510 calories, of black males 2291 calories, of white females 1538 calories, and of black females 1471 calories [44]. Few differences, however, were observed among these four groups with regard to percentage of calories coming from total fat (36 percent) or from saturated fat (13 percent). The average daily cholesterol intakes for white and black males and for white and black females were 440 mg, 485 mg, 271 mg, and 302 mg, respectively.

Physical Activity

Despite interest in examining changes over time in the physical activity levels of the U.S. population and an apparent national obsession with physical fitness, only limited data exist to assess temporal trends in physical activity, and methodologic concerns limit extrapolation and comparability. The extent of and changes in adult leisure-time levels of physical activity as well as sedentariness have been examined in the NHANES surveys and National Health Interview Survey supplements in 1975 and 1985.

While appropriate caveats must be placed on the interpretation of temporal trends in physical activity given the lack of uniform questioning and definitions utilized, the age and sex-specific prevalence rates of vigorous leisure-time physical activity, as based on results of the Perrier Survey, the Centers for Disease Control Survey, and the National Health Interview Survey supplement, have all shown increases over time (1978 to 1985) [45]. Consistent with these observations, the proportion of the population engaged in little or no exercise has declined over time (1971 to 1985), based on the findings of the NHANES and the National Health Interview Surveys [45]. Among the adults surveyed, 41 percent were classified as sedentary in 1971, based on individual self reports; this percentage declined to 39 percent in 1975, to 34 percent in 1976 to 1980, and to 27 percent in 1985. As measured in the most recent (1985) segment of the Health Promotion and Disease Prevention portion of the National Health Interview Survey [15], 40 percent of persons 18 years of age and older in the United States exercised or played sports on a regular basis. Of the adults surveyed, about 28 percent reported being very physically active in the past two weeks, yet only 4 percent described attaining the extent of exercise considered desirable for cardiovascular fitness (three times per week for 20 minutes per session).

While isolated and anecdotal impressions suggest that work-related physical activity has declined in the United States, little to no information exists to systematically address changes over time in occupation-related energy expenditure.

Despite the methodologic and measurement concerns of these surveys, it nonetheless appears that leisure-time activity among adults in the United States has increased since the beginning of the decline in CHD mortality rates until the time of the most recent assessment in 1985 and that women have increased their activity levels to a greater degree than men over the periods surveyed. When available, the data from the 1990 National Health Interview Survey of Health Promotion and Disease Prevention will provide a more detailed and updated examination of national trends in physical activity and an assessment as to whether exercise objectives for the nation are being satisfactorily achieved [46].

Alcohol Consumption

Consumption of alcohol, as reported in the National Health Interview Surveys in 1964, 1979, and 1984, has shown little change over time based on rates of abstention for both men (23 percent in 1964; 24 percent in 1984) and women (40 percent in 1964; 36 percent in 1984) [47, 48]. In terms of the frequency of alcohol consumption, a similar absence of secular trends was seen in terms of daily (13 percent versus 12 percent) or weekly (35 percent versus 37 percent) consumption of alcohol by men in 1964 and 1984, respectively as well as in daily (5 percent in 1964; 4 percent in 1984) or weekly (18 percent in 1964; 21 percent in 1984) consumption of alcohol by women. From the perspective of per capita consumption of pure alcohol, there has been little change in the consumption of beer, wine, or spirits between the years 1968 and 1987, al-

though per capita consumption of alcohol exhibited consistent increases between 1968 and 1981, after which time there has been a consistent decline back to the levels seen in the late 1960s [49]. For example, among persons aged 14 years and older in 1968, per capita consumption of alcohol was 2.5 gallons; this amount increased to 2.8 gallons in 1980 with a continuing decline thereafter to 2.7 gallons in 1982, 2.6 gallons in 1985, and to 2.5 gallons in 1987 [49].

Diabetes

The incidence rates of noninsulin-dependent diabetes mellitus, as measured in the National Health Interview Surveys, showed declines among both males and females from 1968 up until the late 1970s but then increased [50]. Among males the incidence rate (per 1000 persons) declined by approximately 9 percent between 1968 (2.4) and 1979 to 1981 (2.2). A twofold greater decline of approximately 19 percent was observed among females from 1968 (2.9 per 1000 population) to 1979 to 1981 (2.3), although the consistency of these trends was less apparent. Taken for the two sexes collectively, the incidence rates of diabetes declined by approximately 14 percent between 1968 and 1979 to 1981, based on these national surveys of probability samples of the U.S. population. Since 1980, however, the overall age-adjusted incidence rates of diabetes mellitus have shown increases [51]. These rates have increased from 2.4 (per 1000) in 1980 to 2.9 in 1987. Females showed an increase in the incidence rates of diabetes between 1980 (2.4 per 1000) and 1987 (3.4), whereas the incidence rate among males was relatively stable.

Temporal Trends in the Secondary Prevention of CHD

Medical Management

Particularly striking changes have taken place in the medical management of patients with acute MI, with the most striking of these changes occurring within the past decade [52,

53]. The medical management of MI has evolved from a strategy of "wait and see" to a more active role of attempting to restore perfusion to the ischemic myocardium, thereby preventing or reducing the risk of complications associated with the extent of acute myocardial necrosis. The medical management of patients hospitalized with acute MI has recently evolved from the use of mainstay therapeutic interventions such as anticoagulants, selected antiarrhythmic agents, digoxin, and sublingual nitrates to the use of antiplatelet and beta adrenergic blocking agents, calcium channel blockers, intravenous nitroglycerin, and thrombolytic therapy. Based on the results of a number of recent promising secondary-prevention trials employing thrombolytic agents, the current management of acute MI focuses on the restoration and maintenance of the patency of the acutely occluded infarct-related artery with the use of thrombolytic agents, solely or in combination with coronary angioplasty or bypass surgery.

A meta-analysis that summarized the results of randomized trials evaluating treatments commonly utilized in the management of acute MI has shown anticoagulants, aspirin, beta blockers, nitrates, and thrombolytic agents to be of benefit in the acute management of patients hospitalized with recent-onset MI, with questionable benefit deriving from the use of prophylactic lidocaine and calcium channel blockers in the short-term management of these patients [54] (Table 2-6). Indeed, thrombolytic agents and beta blockers have been shown to be effective to the point where they are now considered to be the current standard of care for acute MI. From the community-wide viewpoint of the Worcester Heart Attack Study, significant changes over time have been observed in the therapeutic management of approximately 4750 patients hospitalized with validated acute MI between 1975 and 1988 [55] (Table 2-7). The use of anticoagulants, beta blockers, and nitrates increased dramatically over the periods under study, while utilization of aspirin in the short-term management of patients with acute MI increased more than twofold between 1986 and 1988. The use of digoxin and other anti-

arrhythmic agents has declined consistently over time, whereas the use of diuretics and lidocaine after 1975 has remained relatively stable. Calcium channel blockers are now routinely utilized in the management of patients with acute MI, while the use of thrombolytic agents has approximately doubled between 1986 and 1988.

The average length of hospital stay of patients admitted with acute MI in the community-wide Worcester Heart Attack Study declined significantly over the periods examined. Among patients hospitalized with acute MI in 16 hospitals in metropolitan Worcester, Massachusetts, in 1975, the average length of total hospital stay was 18.4 days; the average length of stay declined to 15.7 days in 1978 and 1981, to 12.9 days in 1984, to 11.9 days in 1986, and to 11.8 days in 1988. Data compiled from the National Health Survey series have also shown a progressive decline in the average length of stay for patients hospitalized with a first-listed diagnosis of acute MI from 18.8 days in 1968 to 12.6 days in 1980 and to 8.9 days in 1986 [56]. In relative concert with these findings, a survey of the management practices of more than one thousand randomly selected physicians involved in the care of patients with uncomplicated acute MI found significant trends in the length of stay and in management practices between 1970 and 1987 [57]. The median hospital stay for patients with uncomplicated acute MI declined from 21 days in 1970 to 14 days in 1979 and to 9 days in 1987. The routine use of beta blockers and nitrates during hospitalization increased progressively over the two periods surveyed, and aspirin and calcium antagonists were commonly used in the management of patients hospitalized with acute MI in 1987. Given the highly successful results of secondary-intervention trials employing thrombolytic agents and beta blockers and the association of benefit from these agents to the timing of administration soon after the onset of symptoms suggestive of acute coronary disease, increased health education efforts continue to be important in decreasing the time delay from patient perception of symptoms of acute MI to the receipt of definitive care.

Table 2-6.   Summary results of treatment approaches used in the in-hospital management of acute MI

Therapy	Number of clinical trials	Number of patients	Estimated risk reduction on in-hospital case fatality	95% confidence intervals on observed risk reduction
Aspirin	2	17,600	−21	−13, −28
Anticoagulants	6	4,500	−22	−8, −35
Beta blockers	27	27,000	−13	−2, −25
Calcium channel blockers	3	6,000	+10	−9, +35
Lidocaine	10	8,500	+11	−16, +46
Nitrates	10	2,000	−35	−18, −49
Streptokinase	9	1,000	−18	−44, +19
Tissue plasminogen activator	5	6,500	−26	−11, −39

Table 2-7.   Temporal trends in selected therapies: Worcester Heart Attack Study

Therapy	Percentage of patients treated with selected therapies*					
	1975	1978	1981	1984	1986	1988
Anticoagulants	36	61	72	75	77	72
Antiplatelets	15	20	14	20	22	49
Beta blockers	21	33	42	51	48	47
Calcium channel blockers	—	—	—	—	59	64
Digoxin	40	40	42	36	31	30
Diuretics	60	54	61	66	52	55
Lidocaine	32	52	44	47	44	47
Other antiarrhythmics	31	28	22	22	17	20
Nitrates	56	72	84	93	89	90
Thrombolytic agents	—	—	—	—	9	20

*Of 4750 patients hospitalized with validated acute MI.

Surgical Management and Invasive and Noninvasive Procedures

While controversy continues concerning the efficacy of coronary artery bypass surgery in prolonging the survival of patients with CHD, several studies have indicated that this surgical intervention prolongs life in patients with left main coronary artery disease and in those with extensive multivessel disease and left ventricular dysfunction. Coronary artery bypass surgery in comparison to medical therapy does not, however, appear to prolong life in patients with lesser degrees of coronary vessel involvement. Despite the inherent methodologic difficulties

in assessing the population-wide impact of bypass surgery on declining CHD death rates, the number of bypass operations and other mechanical interventions has increased dramatically [58, 59]. It has been estimated that in the late 1960s approximately 15,000 persons underwent coronary artery bypass surgery annually. Estimates of the number of individuals annually undergoing coronary bypass grafting increased to over 100,000 a little more than a decade later, to approximately 191,000 in 1983 and to 332,000 in 1987.

While there have been clear increases in the use of coronary artery bypass surgery and refined indications for its use, percutaneous transluminal coronary angioplasty (PTCA) is also being increasingly utilized in the management of patients with CHD since its introduction in the late 1970s, with a particularly recent increase in its use [60, 61]. Since being utilized in only a few cases between 1977 and 1980, PTCA was performed on an estimated 26,000 persons in 1983 and 184,000 in 1987. As opposed to projected estimates of coronary artery bypass surgery, with only a slight, if any, increase in volume expected over the next several years, marked increases are projected for PTCA; over 200,000 patients were expected to have undergone PTCA in 1988 and between 300,000 and 400,000 in 1990.

While more aggressive mechanical interventions, including PTCA and coronary artery bypass surgery, are being increasingly employed in the management of acute MI as a means of revascularizing the acutely ischemic myocardium, the role and proper timing of these therapies and their contribution to declining CHD death rates remain unclear. In the population-based Worcester Heart Attack Study, we have observed marked changes over time in the use of various invasive and noninvasive diagnostic tests and procedures, as well as in the use of mechanical interventions in patients hospitalized with acute MI between 1975 and 1988 [62, 63] (Figures 2-7, 2-8, 2-9). There was a dramatic increase in the use of noninvasive tests between 1975 and 1984; between 1984 and 1988, however, use of these tests declined, with the exception of echocardiography (Figure 2-7). On the other hand, in examining secular trends in the use of invasive diagnostic tests and mechanical interventions (Figures 2-8 and 2-9), the use of each of these procedures increased between 1975 and 1988, with the exception of cardiac pacing, which has remained essentially stable. The use of multiple invasive and noninvasive diagnostic tests and mechanical interventions has also increased over time, with attendant cost implications. An examination of the utilization of four invasive tests/interventions (cardiac catheterization, coronary artery bypass surgery, intra-aortic balloon counterpulsation, and pulmonary artery catheteriza-

tion) between 1975 and 1988 found that 91 percent of patients hospitalized with acute MI in participating Worcester, Massachusetts, area hospitals in 1975 received none of these procedures/interventions; this proportion declined to 81 percent in 1981 and to 58 percent in 1988, and corresponding increases were noted in the use of multiple (two or more) invasive intervention approaches between 1975 (2 percent), 1981 (3 percent), and 1988 (8 percent). More marked changes in the use of multiple noninvasive (echocardiography, exercise treadmill testing, Holter monitoring, radionuclide studies) diagnostic tests were observed over time; in 1975, 1 percent of patients with acute MI received any two of these tests, with this percentage increasing to 21 percent in 1981 and to 28 percent in 1988.

Emergency Medical Services

The modern management of patients suffering from out-of-hospital SCD was introduced by the work of Kouwenhoven and colleagues approximately three decades ago [64]. These investigators convincingly demonstrated that closed-chest cardiac massage combined with artificial ventilation could result in the significant salvage of patients found in cardiac arrest. These critically important observations led to the widespread deployment of cardiopulmonary resuscitation (CPR), with CPR training efforts extended to health care professionals and subsequently to the lay public.

Since the landmark conference on the setting of standards and guidelines for CPR and emergency cardiac care in 1973 [65], millions of Americans have been trained in this technique, and the importance of bystander-initiated CPR has been repeatedly demonstrated. Bystander-administered CPR followed by advanced cardiac life support has been consistently shown to be effective in enhancing the long-term survival as well as the neurologic outlook of patients experiencing out-of-hospital sudden cardiac arrest [66, 67]. Survival after out-of-hospital cardiac arrest has also been shown to be favorably affected by the institution of basic life support followed by the delivery of prehospital defibrillation by trained emergency medical tech-

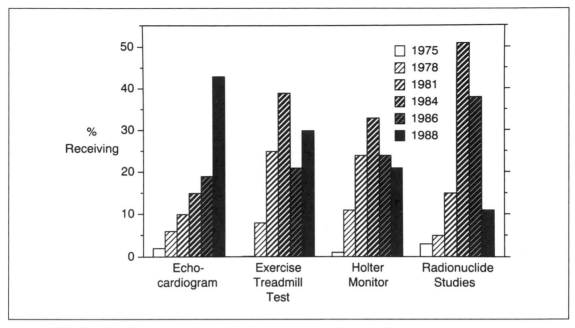

Figure 2-7.   Temporal trends in selected noninvasive diagnostic procedures (Worcester Heart Attack Study).

Figure 2-8.   Temporal trends in selected invasive diagnostic procedures (Worcester Heart Attack Study).

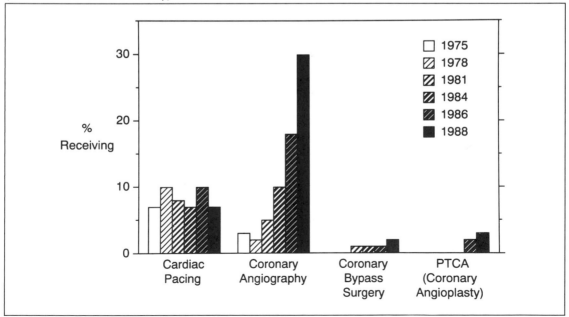

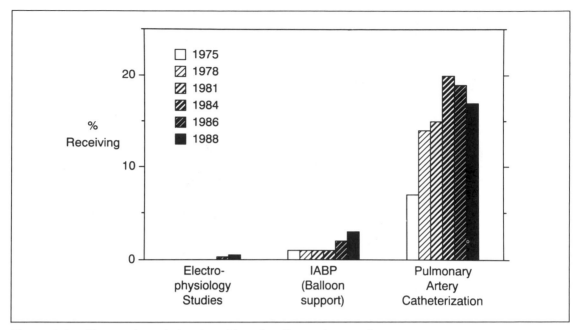

Figure 2-9.   Temporal trends in selected invasive diagnostic procedures
(Worcester Heart Attack Study).

nicians (EMTs) in outlying areas [68] as well as through the use of automatic external defibrillation in the hands of skilled firefighters [69].

While the millions of Americans trained in CPR and the several-fold larger pool of persons expressing interest in such training are encouraging and noteworthy, with the exception of findings reported from community-based emergency medical services systems in Seattle, Washington [70], and Charlottesville, Virginia [71], few published data exist to show a substantial impact of basic or advanced life support systems on the declining population rates of CHD. Reasons for an apparent absence of effect include the rapidity of the actual cardiac event and the severity of underlying CHD, lack of immediate access to and availability of prehospital support systems for many individuals and communities throughout the United States, prolonged paramedic response times and delayed defibrillation, and lack of effective utilization of EMTs in a tiered response system.

Given the continuing extent of SCD in the community, novel approaches to the prevention

and treatment of this problem continue to be needed, including dispatcher-assisted CPR instruction by telephone, which may provide a cost-effective means to increase the rates of bystander CPR in communities with low levels of training [72]. We [73] and others [74] have suggested that given limited and strained health care resources, CPR training should be more focused and directed at those subgroups of persons most likely to use such skills, namely, family members of patients who have suffered a recent acute MI or survived an episode of cardiac arrest and who are at increased risk for SCD. Given the extensive annual contact of physicians with these targeted high-risk family members, an opportunity exists for the consistent delivery of a simple yet directed message encouraging CPR training, with the expected dividend of increased survival rates when cardiac arrest occurs.

Coronary Care Units

Coronary care units (CCUs), with their specialized monitoring techniques and skilled nursing staff, were originally designed in the early to mid-1960s to detect serious cardiac rhythm disturbances promptly in hospitalized patients so that effective resuscitation might be delivered [75]. These units are now oriented toward the reduction of serious complications associated with acute myocardial necrosis, with the goal of favorably altering the in-hospital survival of acute MI. A variety of study designs have been utilized to examine the impact of CCUs on the short-term survival associated with acute MI. These designs have included before-and-after and sequential observational comparisons as well as experimental controlled trials [76]. A surfeit of literature exists that initially proselytized and subsequently questioned the effectiveness of these units from both a medical and an economic point of view. Two randomized clinical trials carried out in Great Britain by Mather et al. [77] and subsequently by Hill and colleagues [78] in the 1970s, utilizing observational nonexperimental study design approaches, failed to show an advantage in in-hospital survival for patients with mild to moderate acute MIs admitted to these units compared to those receiving home care. A recent analysis of the mortality experience of patients hospitalized with acute MI in 18 urban and rural hospitals in Great Britain failed to observe a significant difference in mortality rates for patients with acute MI treated in CCUs compared to those treated in general medical wards [79]. Thus, the precise effects of the CCU on declining CHD mortality trends remain controversial and difficult to assess. Certainly the majority of patients with acute MI currently admitted to hospitals in the United States continue to be admitted to these specialized-care units.

Temporal Trends in Incidence Rates of Acute Myocardial Infarction

In addition to examining secular trends in factors that may have affected the survival of patients with acute and chronic manifestations of CHD, a number of population-based studies have examined changes over time in the incidence and survival rates of acute MI and SCD,

providing further insights into the contribution of primary- and secondary-prevention efforts to declining CHD mortality rates. This section and the following sections summarize these studies.

Over the last two decades several community-based studies in Rochester [80] and Minneapolis-St. Paul, Minnesota [81], Worcester, Massachusetts [82, 83], the Pee Dee area of South Carolina [84], and one worksite-based study of DuPont Company employees [85] have examined temporal trends in the incidence rates of acute MI (Table 2-8). Appropriate caution should be exercised in the interpretation of these data, given that the sociodemographic characteristics of the populations under study and the diagnostic criteria for acute MI may have differed, that the size of the populations varied, and that the periods of investigation were limited, thus making estimates of temporal trends tenuous. Nonetheless, each of these population-based investigations showed a decline in the incidence rates of acute coronary events over the periods examined.

On the other hand, data from the National Hospital Discharge Survey, which utilized information based on patients discharged from short-term nonfederal hospitals, showed an increase in both the numbers of patients hospitalized with a first-listed diagnosis of acute MI and in the annual discharge rate of patients with the diagnosis between 1968 and 1986 [56, 86] (Table 2-9). Part of the large increase in the overall number of patients with a discharge diagnosis of acute MI and the rate of discharge observed between 1980 and 1982 among those with a primary diagnosis of acute MI may be explained by the coding decision to reclassify circulatory diagnoses involving acute MI, thus creating a possible artifact in the interpretation of trends thereafter. It should also be noted that, as opposed to the population-based studies examining secular trends in the incidence rates of acute MI in which actual medical records were reviewed and validated, data from the National Hospital Discharge Survey are based on the nonvalidated discharge summaries of patients hospitalized with acute MI and do not discriminate between initial and recurrent cases.

Table 2-8. Population-based studies of temporal trends in the incidence rates of acute MI

Study population	Periods under study	Incidence rates (per 100,000)
Charleston heart study Pee Dee area, South Carolina	1978[a] 1985[a]	1978:350 1985:347
Male employees of the DuPont Company	1957–1983	1957–1959:319[b] 1963–1965:292[b] 1969–1971:270[b] 1975–1977:270[b] 1981–83:229

Minneapolis–St. Paul, Minnesota, metropolitan area	1970, 1980	Males
		    1970:794
		    1980:727
		Females
		    1970:337
		    1980:249

Rochester, Minnesota	1950–1975	1950–1954:222[b] 1955–1959:294[b] 1960–1964:234[b] 1965–1969:278[b] 1970–1975:258[b]
Worcester, Massachusetts, standard metropolitan statistical area	1975 1978 1981 1984	1975:255[c] 1978:257[c] 1981:280[c] 1984:186[c]

[a]Period prevalence.
[b]Age-adjusted.
[c]Initial MIs, age-adjusted.

Temporal Trends in In-Hospital Case Fatality Rates of Acute MI

Several population-based studies have examined changes over time in the in-hospital case fatality rates associated with acute MI (Table 2-10) [80, 81, 82, 83, 84, 85, 87, 88]. As with the examination of hospital-based incidence data of acute MI, appropriate reservations should be exercised in the interpretation of the case fatality data. Factors such as the various sizes of the study samples, the diagnostic criteria for acute MI utilized, length of hospital stay, and differing characteristics of the populations compared, particularly with regard to those factors that might affect short-term prognosis (e.g., the extent and the severity of acute MI) as well as the therapeutic interventions employed make interpretation of the findings across studies difficult. Despite these caveats, an improvement in in-

hospital survival is seen in each of the studies examined, with the sole exception being the study of nonvalidated cases of acute MI admitted to acute care hospitals in the greater Boston, Massachusetts, area [87]. Declines in in-hospital case-fatality rates between 1970 and 1981, for both males and females, have also been seen in an analysis of data from the National Hospital Discharge Survey [86]. More recent estimates have shown declines in the in-hospital case fataility rates of patients discharged from short stay hospitals in the United States with a diagnosis of acute MI. For example, in 1982, 19.9 percent of patients with a discharge diagnosis of acute MI died; this percentage decreased to 16.1 percent in 1984 and to 15.6 percent in 1986. Data compiled from the Professional Activity Survey have also shown a decline in the in-hospital case fatality rates of patients with acute MI admitted to hospitals that reported data to this source between 1970 and 1977.

Table 2-9. Temporal trends in the annual discharge rates and number of patients discharged with a first-listed diagnosis of acute MI

Time period	Discharge rate (per 1000)	Number of discharged patients
1968	1.9	372,000
1970	1.7	342,000
1972	1.8	374,000
1974	1.8	382,000
1976	1.9	400,000
1978	2.0	425,000
1980	1.9	431,000
1982	3.0	681,000
1984	3.0	700,000
1986	3.2	758,000

Table 2-10. Selected studies examining secular trends in in-hospital case-fatality rates following acute MI

Population under study	Study year	Sample size	MI order (initial or recurrent)	In-hospital case fatality rates (%)
20 hospitals in metropolitan Baltimore, Maryland	1966–1967 1971	503 802	Initial and recurrent	28.9[c] 22.4[c]
63 hospitals in metropolitan Boston, Massachusetts	1973–1974 1978–1979	8524[a] 8572[a]	Initial and recurrent	22.0 23.0
DuPont Company male employees	1957–1983	6284	Initial	1957–1959:30.4[d] 1963–1965:33.0[d] 1969–1971:34.8[d] 1975–1977:29.1[d] 1981–1983:24.3[d]
35 hospitals in Minneapolis–St. Paul, Minnesota, area	1970	3842[b]	Initial and recurrent	Males:16.7 Females:16.6
30 hospitals in Minneapolis–St. Paul, Minnesota, area	1980	3736[b]	Initial and recurrent	Males:11.9 Females:12.2
7 hospitals in Pee Dee area, South Carolina	1978 1985	193 232	Initial and recurrent	14.0 9.9
Rochester, Minnesota, hospitals	1950–1975	1321	Initial	1950–1954:22.1 1955–1959:16.7 1960–1964:19.0 1965–1969:18.0 1970–1975:9.3
16 SMSA hospitals in Worcester, Massachusetts	1975 1978 1981 1984 1986 1988	780 845 999 714 765 659	Initial and recurrent	21.2 19.8 18.5 15.7 16.2 17.9

[a] Primary diagnosis of acute MI.
[b] Number of discharges.
[c] Multivariate adjusted.
[d] Died within 30 days.

Temporal Trends in Long-Term Survival of Acute Myocardial Infarction

A number of investigations in the United States (in metropolitan Baltimore, Maryland, between 1966 to 1967 and 1971 [88], in Rochester, Minnesota, between 1950 and 1975 [80], and among male enrollees of the Health Insurance Plan of New York surviving an initial MI in the 1960s and 1970s [89] have examined changes over time in the long-term prognosis of hospital survivors of acute MI. These studies failed to demonstrate an improvement over time in the long-term prognosis of discharged hospital survivors of acute MI. In concert with these findings, an analysis of the long-term survival patterns of over 3800 patients discharged from hospitals in metropolitan Worcester, Massachusetts, in 1975, 1978, 1981, 1984, 1986, and 1988 failed to observe secular improvements in the post-discharge survival experience of patients discharged from the hospital after acute MI between 1975 and 1988 (Figure 2-10). A similar lack of change in long-term prognosis was seen among patients discharged after either an initial or a recurrent acute MI. The sole study that has shown an improvement over time in the long-term survival of discharged hospital patients of acute MI is the Minnesota Heart Survey [90]. This population-based study showed, after adjustment for a variety of demographic and clinical factors that might affect long-term prognosis, a 35-percent improvement in the four-year survival rates of men discharged from Minnesota hospitals after a definite acute MI in 1980, compared to those discharged in 1970, and a 27-percent improvement in long-term survival among women.

Out-of-Hospital Deaths Due to CHD

Despite the use of different criteria to define out-of-hospital deaths due to CHD, each of the major population-based studies of CHD in the United States have shown consistent declines in the incidence rates of out-of-hospital deaths due to CHD, particular SCD. Declines in the incidence rates of out-of-hospital deaths attributed

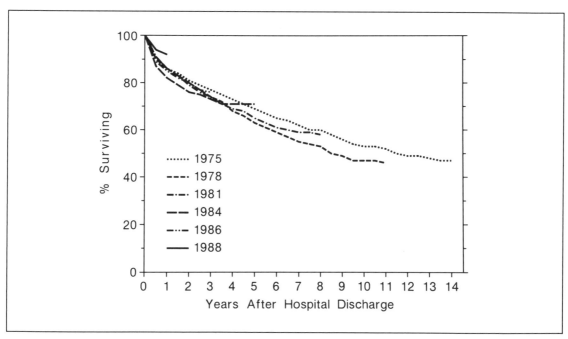

Figure 2-10.   Temporal trends in long-term survival after hospital discharge in patients with acute MI (Worcester Heart Attack Study).

to CHD have been observed in the Minneapolis-St. Paul metropolitan area (1970–1978), in Rochester, Minnesota (1950 to 1975), in young white males of Allegheny County, Pennsylvania (1970 to 1981), in the Pee Dee area of South Carolina (1978 to 1985), and in Worcester, Massachusetts (1975 to 1984) [80, 81, 82, 83, 84, 91]. A decline in the occurrence rates of SCD was also seen in the more select study of DuPont employees over the period 1972 to 1983 [85].

The occurrence of SCD from a demographically mixed, national perspective has been examined for the period 1980 to 1985 [92]. Routinely collected data compiled from the National Center for Health Statistics were analyzed to examine temporal trends in deaths due to heart disease occurring outside the hospital or in hospital emergency rooms as proxy representations for the occurrence of SCD. These death certificate data were collected from 40 states, representing approximately 70 percent of the U.S. population. In an examination of temporal trends in the incidence rates of SCD, encouraging and consistent declines were seen in out-of-hospital deaths between the study years of 1980 and 1985, although death rates in emergency rooms actually increased. Despite these differences in the setting of death, the age-adjusted out-of-hospital deaths plus emergency room deaths attributed to ischemic heart disease declined by 19 percent in white men, 16 percent in white women, 20 percent in black men, and 19 percent in black women.

Two community-based pathology studies examined temporal trends in the extent of coronary artery lesions in whites and blacks in New Orleans between 1960 to 1964 and 1969 to 1978 [93] and in the prevalence of MI scars among residents of Olmsted County, Minnesota, who died between 1950 and 1979 [94]. While variations in the pathologic techniques used, the coronary atherosclerotic vascular changes examined, the composition of the autopsied samples, and other characteristics may make comparability of these two studies difficult, differing temporal trends in the population burden of atherosclerosis were observed. The age-adjusted prevalence rates of MI scars found at autopsy among persons 30 years of age and older in Olmsted county exhibited little change over time (39 percent in 1950 to 1954, 41 percent in 1960 to 1964, 37 percent in 1975 to 1979). On the other hand, in an examination of secular trends in raised lesions of the coronary intimal surface, a decline over time (1960 to 1964 to 1969 to 1978) in the extent of coronary atherosclerosis was observed in New Orleans in young white males aged 25–44 without CHD but not among black males.

Contributions of Primary and Secondary Preventive and Therapeutic Efforts to Declining CHD Mortality Rates

Despite the lack of adequate and systematically collected sources of data to distinguish contributions of primary from those of secondary prevention to declining CHD mortality trends, two investigations have attempted to sort out the contributions of changes in lifestyle characteristics from those of secondary prevention during the period of declining CHD mortality rates from 1968 to 1976 [3, 5]. The most recent of these publications attempted to estimate the contribution of secular trends in the major coronary risk factors and medical care interventions to national declines in death rates due to ischemic heart disease [5]. The lifestyle factors examined in this latter study included reductions in serum cholesterol levels and cigarette smoking, while the medical care interventions included an assessment of the impact of prehospital resuscitation efforts, CCUs, coronary artery bypass surgery, medical treatment of CHD, and treatment of hypertension on declining CHD death rates (Table 2-11). Based on data from a multiplicity of published sources, the authors estimated that favorable reductions in the examined lifestyle factors may have accounted for slightly over one-half of the observed decline in CHD mortality rates between 1968 and 1976, whereas medical care interventions may have contributed approximately 40 percent of the decline.

Table 2-11.   Estimated benefit of interventions on ischemic heart-disease mortality rates, 1968–1976

	Estimated number of lives saved	Estimated decline in mortality (%)
Medical care interventions		
Coronary care units	85,000	13.5
Prehospital resuscitation	25,000	4
Coronary artery bypass surgery	23,000	3.5
Medical treatment of CHD	61,000	10
Treatment of hypertension	55,000	8.5
Subtotal	249,000	39.5
Lifestyle changes		
Reduction in serum cholesterol levels	190,000	30
Reduction in cigarette smoking	150,000	24
Subtotal	340,000	54
Not explained by examined factors	41,000	6.5
Total	630,000	—

Summary

A review of temporal trends in the major risk factors for CHD, incidence rates of acute MI and SCD, and in-hospital case-fatality rates from acute MI makes it obvious that favorable declines in these factors have occurred since the beginning of the decline in CHD death rates in 1968. It also becomes readily apparent that there have been dramatic and rapidly emerging changes in the therapeutic management of patients with CHD and a heightened public as well as provider awareness of the nation's number one health problem. While speculation will most likely continue concerning the reasons for the observed decline in CHD death rates, and considerable data will be generated by cardiovascular epidemiologists attempting to disentangle the various contributors to this dramatic and ongoing decline through community-based surveillance activities, the collective findings in this area provide encouragement for the apparent benefits of favorable lifestyle changes, for the development and use of medical care interventions, and just for "doing the right things" [95]. While a return to the hunter-gatherer lifestyle of our Cro-Magnon ancestors is not advocated, the rediscovery of the essential cultural and lifestyle elements of our Paleolithic ancestors may yet place our chronic and degenerative diseases of civilization into retreat [96].

References

1. Havlik RJ, Feinleib M, eds. Proceedings of the Conference on the Decline in Coronary Heart Disease Mortality. Washington, DC: Government Printing Office, 1979. Pub. no. USDHEW (NIH) 79-1610.
2. Higgins MW, Luepker RV, eds. Trends in coronary heart disease mortality. The influence of medical care. New York: Oxford University Press, 1988.
3. Stern M. The recent decline in ischemic heart disease mortality. Ann Intern Med 1979; 91:630–40.
4. Thom JJ, Kannel WB. Downward trend in cardiovascular mortality. Annu Rev Med 1981; 32:427–34.
5. Goldman L, Cook EF. The decline in ischemic heart disease mortality rates. An analysis of the comparative effects of medical interventions and changes in lifestyle. Ann Intern Med 1984; 101:825–36.
6. Kannel WB. Meaning of the downward trend in

cardiovascular mortality. JAMA 1982; 247:877–80.

7. U.S. Department of Health and Human Services. Morbidity and mortality chartbook on cardiovascular, lung and blood diseases 1990. National Institutes of Health, National Heart, Lung and Blood Institute, 1990.

8. Thom TJ. International mortality from heart disease: rates and trends. Int J Epidemiol 1989; 18:Suppl 1:S20–8.

9. WHO MONICA Project Principal Investigators. The World Health Organization MONICA Project (monitoring trends and determinants in cardiovascular disease): a major international collaboration. J Clin Epidemiol 1988; 2:105–14.

10. WHO MONICA Project. WHO MONICA Project: objectives and design. Int J Epidemiol 1989; 18:Suppl 1:S29–S37.

11. U.S. Department of Health and Human Services. Reducing the health consequences of smoking. Twenty-five years of progress. A report of the Surgeon General. USDHHS publ. no. (CDC) 89-8411, 1989.

12. McGinnis JM, Shopland D, Brown C. Tobacco and health: trends in smoking and smokeless tobacco consumption in the United States. Ann Rev Publ Health 1987; 8:441–67.

13. Sprafka JM, Burke GL, Folsom AR, et al. Continued decline in cardiovascular disease risk factors: results of the Minnesota Heart Survey, 1980–1982 and 1985–1987. Am J Epidemiol 1990; 132:489–500.

14. Sytkowski PA, Kannel WB, D'Agostino RB. Changes in risk factors and the decline in mortality from cardiovascular disease. The Framingham Heart Study. New Engl J Med 1990; 322:1635–41.

15. U.S. Department of Health and Human Services. Health promotion and disease prevention. United States, 1985. Data from the National Health Interview Survey. Series 10, #163. USDHHS publ. no. (PHS) 88-1591. Hyattsville, MD: National Center for Health Statistics, 1988.

16. Cummings KM, Sciandra R, Pechacek T, Lynn WR. For the community intervention trial for smoking cessation research group: smoker's beliefs about the health benefits of smoking cessation — 20 U.S. communities, 1989. Morbidity and Mortality Weekly Report 1990; 39:653–5.

17. Centers for Disease Control. State coalitions for prevention and control of tobacco use. Morbidity and Mortality Weekly Report 1990; 39:476; 483–5.

18. Orleans CT: Understanding and promoting smoking cessation: overview and guidelines for physician intervention. Annu Rev Med 1985; 36:51–61.

19. Health and Public Policy Committee, American College of Physicians. Methods for stopping cigarette smoking. Ann Intern Med 1986; 105:281–91.

20. Wilson DM, Taylor DW, Gilbert JR, et al. A randomized trial of a family physician intervention for smoking cessation. JAMA 1988; 260:1570–4.

21. Ockene JK, Quirk ME, Goldberg RJ, et al. A resident's training program for the development of smoking intervention skills. Arch Intern Med 1988; 148:1039–45.

22. Freis ED and the Veterans Administration Cooperative Study Group on Antihypertensive Agents. Effects of treatment on morbidity in hypertension. I. Results in patients with diastolic blood pressures averaging 115 through 129 mmHg. JAMA 1967; 202:1028–34.

23. National Conference on High Blood Pressure Education. Report on proceedings. Bethesda, MD: U.S. Department of Health, Education and Welfare, Public Health Service, National Institutes of Health. USDHEW publ. no. (NIH) 73-486, 1973.

24. Report of the Joint National Committee on Detection, Evaluation and Treatment of High Blood Pressure. A cooperative study. JAMA 1977; 237:255–61.

25. Moser M. A decade of progress in the management of hypertension. Hypertension 1983; 5:808–13.

26. Dannenberg AL, Garrison RJ, Kannel WB. Incidence of hypertension in the Framingham Study. Am J Public Health 1988; 78:676–9.

27. National Center for Health Statistics, National Heart, Lung and Blood Institute Collaborative Lipid Group. Trends in serum cholesterol levels among U.S. adults aged 20–74 years. Data from the National Health and Nutrition Examination Surveys, 1960 to 1980. JAMA 1987; 257:937–42.

28. Consensus Conference. Lowering blood cholesterol to prevent heart disease. JAMA 1985; 253:2080–6.

29. National Cholesterol Education Program Expert Panel. Report on detection, evaluation and treatment of high blood cholesterol in adults. Arch Intern Med 1988; 148:36–69.

30. Burke GL, Sprafka JM, Folsom AR, et al. Trends in serum cholesterol levels from 1980 to 1987. The Minnesota Heart Survey. N Engl J Med 1991; 324:941–6.

31. Schucker B, Wittes JT, Santanello NC, et al. Change in cholesterol awareness and action. Results from national physician and public surveys. Arch Intern Med 1991; 151:666–73.

32. Sempos C, Fulwood R, Haines C, et al. The prevalence of high blood cholesterol levels

among adults in the United States. JAMA 1989; 262:45–52.

33. Lipid Research Clinics Program. The Lipid Research Clinics Coronary Primary Prevention Trial results. Reduction in the incidence of coronary heart disease. JAMA 1984; 251:351–64.

34. Frick MH, Elo O, Haapa K, et al. Helsinki Heart Study: Primary-prevention trial with gemfibrozil in middle-aged men with dyslipidemia. N Engl J Med 1987; 317:1237–45.

35. Blankenhorn DH, Nessim SA, Johnson RL, et al. Beneficial effects of combined colestipol-niacin therapy on coronary atherosclerosis and coronary venous bypass grafts. JAMA 1987; 257:3233–40.

36. Stamler J. Primary prevention of coronary heart disease: the last 20 years. Am J Cardiol 1981; 47:722–35.

37. U.S. Department of Health and Human Services. Nutrition and health. A report of the Surgeon General. USDHHS publ. no. (PHS) 88-50210.

38. Stephen AM, Wald NJ. Trends in individual consumption of dietary fat in the United States, 1920–1984. Am J Clin Nutr 1990; 52:457–69.

39. Patterson BH, Block G, Rosenberger WF, et al. Fruit and vegetables in the American diet: data from the NHANES II Survey. Am J Public Health 1990; 80:1443–9.

40. U.S. Department of Agriculture, Science and Education Administration. Food and nutrient intakes of individuals in 1 day in the United States, Spring 1977. NFCS 1977–78 Preliminary Report no. 2, 1980.

41. U.S. Department of Agriculture, Human Nutrition Information Service. Nationwide Food Consumption Survey, continuing survey of food intakes by individuals, women 19–50 years and their children 1–5 years, 1 day, 1986. NFCS, CSFII Report no. 86-1. Washington, DC: USDA, 1987.

42. Higgins M, Thom T. Trends in CHD in the United States. Int J Epidemiol 1989; 18:Suppl 1:S58–S66.

43. Simopoulos AP. Characteristics of obesity: an overview. Ann NY Acad Sci 1987; 499:4–13.

44. Block G, Rosenberger WF, Patterson BH. Calories, fat and cholesterol: intake patterns in the U.S. population by race, sex and age. Am J Public Health 1988; 78:1150–5.

45. Stephens T. Secular trends in adult physical activity: exercise boom or bust? Res Quart Exerc Sport 1987; 58:94–105.

46. Caspersen CJ, Christenson GM, Pollard RA. Status of the 1990 physical fitness and exercise objectives — evidence from NHIS 1985. Public Health Reports 1986; 101:587–92.

47. Hilton ME. Trends in U.S. drinking patterns: further evidence from the past 20 years. Br J Addiction 1988; 83:269–78.

48. Hilton ME, Clark WB. Changes in American drinking patterns and problems. J Stud Alcohol 1987; 48:515–22.

49. U.S. Department of Health and Human Services. Alcohol and health. National Institute on Alcohol Abuse and Alcoholism. USDHHS publ. no. (ADM) 90-1656, 1990.

50. Everhart J, Knowler WC, Bennett PH. Incidence and risk factors for noninsulin-dependent diabetes. In: Diabetes in America. Diabetes data compiled 1984. U.S. Department of Health and Human Services, NIH pub. no. 85-1468.

51. Prevalence and Incidence of Diabetes Mellitus — United States, 1980–1987. Morbidity and Mortality Weekly Report 1990; 39:809–12.

52. Gore JM, Dalen JE. Cardiovascular disease. JAMA 1989; 261:2829–31.

53. Braunwald E. The aggressive treatment of acute myocardial infarction. Circulation 1985; 71:1087–92.

54. Yusuf S, Wittes J, Friedman L. Overview of results of randomized clinical trials in heart disease. I. Treatments following myocardial infarction. JAMA 1988; 260:2088–93.

55. Goldberg RJ, Gore JM, Alpert JS, Dalen JE. Therapeutic trends in the management of patients with acute myocardial infarction (1975–1984): the Worcester Heart Attack Study. Clin Cardiol 1987; 10:3–8.

56. National Center for Health Statistics. Detailed diagnoses and procedures for patients discharged from short-stay hospitals, United States. Vital and Health Statistics Series 13, selected annual issues. Public Health Service. Washington, DC: U.S. Government Printing Office.

57. Hlatky MA, Cotugno HE, Mark DB, et al. Trends in physician management of uncomplicated acute myocardial infarction, 1970 to 1987. Am J Cardiol 1988; 61:515–8.

58. McIntosh HD, Garcia JA. The first decade of aortocoronary bypass grafting, 1967–1977. A review. Circulation 1978; 57:405–31.

59. Feinleib M, Havlik RJ, Gillum RF, et al. Coronary heart disease and related procedures. National Hospital Discharge Survey data. Circulation 1989; 79:Suppl I: I-13-8.

60. Grüntzig AR, Senning A, Siegenthaler WE. Nonoperative dilatation of coronary-artery stenosis. Percutaneous transluminal coronary angioplasty. N Engl J Med 1979; 301:61–8.

61. King SB, Talley JD. Coronary arteriography and percutaneous transluminal coronary angioplasty. Changing patterns of use and results. Circulation 1989; 79:Suppl I:I-19-23.

62. Gore JM, Goldberg RJ, Alpert JS, Dalen JE. The

increased use of diagnostic procedures in patients with acute myocardial infarction: a community-wide perspective. Arch Intern Med 1987; 147:1729–32.

63. Gore JM, Goldberg RJ, Spodick DH, et al. A community-wide assessment of the use of pulmonary artery catheters in patients with acute myocardial infarction. Chest 1987; 92:721–7.

64. Kouwenhoven WB, Jude JR, Knickerbocker GG. Closed-chest cardiac massage. JAMA 1960; 173:1064–7.

65. Standards for cardiopulmonary resuscitation (CPR) and emergency cardiac care (ECC). JAMA 1974; 227:Suppl:833–68.

66. Cobb LA, Hallstrom AP, Thompson RG, et al. Community cardiopulmonary resuscitation. Annu Rev Med 1980; 31:453–62.

67. Eisenberg MS, Copass MK, Hallstrom AP, et al. Treatment of out-of-hospital cardiac arrests with rapid defibrillation by emergency medical technicians. N Engl J Med 1980; 302:1379–83.

68. Stults KR, Brown DD, Schug VL, Bean JA. Prehospital defibrillation performed by emergency medical technicians in rural communities. N Engl J Med 1984; 310:219–23.

69. Weaver WD, Copass MK, Hill DL, et al. Cardiac arrest treated with a new automatic external defibrillator by out-of-hospital first responders. Am J Cardiol 1986; 57:1017–21.

70. Eisenberg M, Bergner L, Hallstrom A. Paramedic programs and out-of-hospital cardiac arrest. II. Impact on community mortality. Am J Public Health 1979; 69:39–42.

71. Crampton RS, Aldrich RF, Gascho JA, et al. Reduction of prehospital, ambulance and community coronary death rates by the community-wide emergency cardiac care system. Am J Med 1978; 58:151–65.

72. Kellermann AL, Hackman BB, Somes G. Dispatcher-assisted cardiopulmonary resuscitation. Validation of efficacy. Circulation 1989; 80:1231–9.

73. Goldberg RJ. Physicians and CPR training in high-risk family members. Am J Public Health 1987; 77:671–2.

74. St. Louis P, Carter WB, Eisenberg MS. Prescribing CPR: a survey of physicians. Am J Public Health 1982; 72:1158–60.

75. Day HW. History of coronary care units. Am J Cardiol 1972; 30:405–7.

76. Gordis L, Naggan L, Tonascia J. Pitfalls in evaluating the impact of coronary care units on mortality from myocardial infarctions. Johns Hopkins Med J 1977; 141:287–95.

77. Mather HG, Morgan DC, Pearson NG, et al. Myocardial infarction: a comparison between home and hospital care for patients. Br Med J 1976; 1:925–9.

78. Hill JD, Hampton JR, Mitchell JRA. A randomized trial of home-versus-hospital management for patients with suspected myocardial infarction. Lancet 1978; 1:837–41.

79. Reznik R, Ring I, Fletcher P, Siskind V. Differences in mortality from acute myocardial infarction between coronary care unit and medical ward: treatment or bias? Br Med J 1987; 295:1437–40.

80. Elveback LR, Connolly DC, Kurland LT. Coronary heart disease in residents of Rochester, Minnesota. II. Mortality, incidence, and survivorship, 1950–1975. Mayo Clin Proc 1981; 56:665–72.

81. Gillum RF, Folsom A, Luepker RV, et al. Sudden death and acute myocardial infarction in a metropolitan area, 1970–1980. The Minnesota Heart Survey. N Engl J Med 1983; 309:1353–8.

82. Goldberg RJ, Gore JM, Alpert JS, Dalen JE. Recent changes in attack and survival rates of acute myocardial infarction (1975–1981): the Worcester Heart Attack Study. JAMA 1986; 255:2774–9.

83. Goldberg RJ, Gore JM, Alpert JS, Dalen JE. Incidence and case fatality rates of acute myocardial infarction (1975–1984): the Worcester Heart Attack Study. Am Heart J 1988; 115:761–7.

84. Keil JE, Gazes PC, Litaker MS, et al. Changing patterns of acute myocardial infarction: decline in period prevalence and delay in onset. Am Heart J 1989; 117:1022–9.

85. Pell S, Fayerweather WE. Trends in the incidence of myocardial infarction and in associated mortality and morbidity in a large employed population, 1957–1983. N Engl J Med 1985; 312:1005–11.

86. Gillum RF. Acute myocardial infarction in the United States, 1970–1983. Am Heart J 1987; 113:804–11.

87. Goldman L, Cook F, Hashimoto B, et al. Evidence that hospital care for acute myocardial infarction has not contributed to the decline in coronary mortality between 1973–1974 and 1978–1979. Circulation 1982; 65:936–42.

88. Goldberg R, Szklo M, Tonascia J, Kennedy H. The trends in prognosis of patients with myocardial infarction: a population-based study. Johns Hopkins Med J 1979; 144:73–80.

89. Weinblatt E, Goldberg JD, Ruberman W, et al. Mortality after first myocardial infarction. Search for a secular trend. JAMA 1982; 247:1576–81.

90. Gomez-Marin O, Folsom AR, Kottke TE, et al. Improvement in long-term survival among patients hospitalized with acute myocardial infarction, 1970 to 1980. The Minnesota Heart Survey. N Engl J Med 1987; 316:1353–9.

91. Kuller LH, Perper JA, Dai WS, et al. Sudden

death and the decline in coronary heart disease mortality. J Chron Dis 1986; 39:1001–19.

92. Gillum RF. Sudden coronary death in the United States. 1980–1985. Circulation 1989; 79:756–65.

93. Strong JP, Oalmann MC, Newman WP, et al. Coronary heart disease in young black and white males in New Orleans: community pathology study. Am Heart J 1984; 108:747–58.

94. Elveback L, Lie JT. Continued high incidence of coronary artery disease at autopsy in Olmsted County, Minnesota, 1950 to 1979. Circulation 1984; 70:345–9.

95. Stamler J. Coronary heart disease: doing the "right things" (editorial). N Engl J Med 1985; 312:1053–5.

96. Eaton SB, Konner MJ, Shostak M. Stone agers in the fast lane: chronic degenerative diseases in evolutionary perspective. Am J Med 1988; 84:739–49.

3

Pathobiology of Hypercholesterolemia and Atherosclerosis: Genetic and Environmental Determinants of Elevated Lipoprotein Levels

ROBERT J. NICOLOSI
ERNST J. SCHAEFER

EDITORS' INTRODUCTION

An abnormality of serum lipids is the key requirement for the development of CHD. Drs. Nicolosi and Schaefer describe the various lipids and lipoproteins, provide us with an overview of cholesterol and lipoprotein metabolism, and take us through the dyslipoproteinemias, both primary and secondary. They then help us understand the important interrelationship between genetic and environmental factors, particularly the exceedingly important role of diet. The relative roles played by dietary cholesterol and polyunsaturated, monounsaturated, and saturated fats are clarified, as is the role of marine oils.

It is now understood that the development of clinical CHD depends on a complex interplay of hyperlipidemia, altered hemostasis, and vessel wall factors. The central nature of the lipid abnormality, the pathophysiology of the atherosclerotic lesion, and the function of other risk factors as accelerators of the atherosclerotic process are all explained. Finally, the available measurement methodologies for lipids and lipoproteins are described, as well as their associated benefits and drawbacks, and recommendations are given for appropriate use and standardization.

Plasma Lipids, Lipoprotein Classes, and Apoproteins

The major circulating lipid classes in plasma are cholesterol, as either free cholesterol (FC) or cholesterol ester (CE), phospholipid (PL), triglycerides (TG), and unesterified or free fatty acids (FFA). The FFAs circulate in the blood stream in association with albumin. Because of their hydrophobic nature (i.e., insolubility in water), all other lipids are packaged into large molecular-weight molecules called lipoproteins. The densities of individual plasma lipoproteins are determined by their relative contents of protein and lipid. Differences in density, composition, and electrophoretic mobility have been used to divide lipoproteins into five major classes, which are described in Table 3-1. Chylomicrons are triglyceride-rich lipoproteins produced by the intestine and have a density (d) of approximately 0.95 g/ml. Triglyceride-rich very low density lipoprotein (VLDL)(d < 1.006 g/ml) is made by the liver and has prebeta mobility on electrophoresis. Intermediate-density lipoprotein (IDL)(d = 1.006 to 1.019 g/ml) is produced by the catabolism of VLDL and has electrophoretic mobility between prebeta and beta. Low-density lipoprotein (LDL)(d = 1.019 to 1.063 g/ml) is derived from the catabolism of both VLDL and IDL and has beta mobility on electrophoresis. LDLs are the major cholesterol-carrying lipoproteins of plasma in humans. LDL has been further subdivided by ultracentrifugation into LDL_1 (d = 1.019 to 1.035 g/ml) and LDL_2 (d = 1.035 to 1.065 g/ml), although these densities may vary. It is the larger LDL particle, LDL_1, that generally fluctuates in response to environmental factors such as diet or drug or hormonal intervention. High-density lipoprotein (HDL)(d = 1.063 to 1.21 g/ml) has alpha mobility and is derived from a variety of sources, including the liver, the intestine, other lipoproteins, and other tissue. HDL has been further subfractionated by ultracentrifugation into HDL_2 (d = 1.063 to 1.125 g/ml) and HDL_3 (d = 1.125 to 1.21 g/ml). Changes in HDL levels by environmental factors are usually associated with the larger HDL_2 fraction.

Lipoprotein(a) (Lp(a)), recently reviewed by several investigators [1, 2], was first described as early as 1963. It has recently received considerable attention because high circulating levels are significantly correlated with the incidence of coronary heart disease [3, 4] and predilection to vein graft occlusion following coronary bypass surgery [5]. Lp(a) resembles an LDL particle, in which the major apoprotein of LDL, apo B-100, is disulfide-linked to a specific apoprotein designated apo(a), which has a striking homology to plasminogen, a protein involved in the regulation of fibrinolysis [1]. Apo(a) is heterogeneous in size and density with a molecular weight of approximately 600,000 daltons. At least seven apo(a) isoforms have been

Table 3-1. Classification of plasma lipoproteins

Lipoprotein class	Density (g/ml)	Electrophoretic mobility	Sources	Composition (Wt%)				
				FC	CE	TG	PL	PROT
Chylomicrons	<0.95	Origin	Intestine	1	3	90	4	2
Very-low density lipoproteins (VLDL)	0.95–1.006	Prebeta	Liver	7	14	55	16	8
Intermediate-density lipoproteins (IDL)	1.006–1.019	Between beta and prebeta	Catabolism of VLDL	6	22	30	24	18
Low-density lipoproteins (LDL)	1.019–1.063	Beta	Catabolism of VLDL and IDL	7	48	5	20	20
High-density lipoproteins (HDL)	1.063–1.210	Alpha	Liver, intestine, other	4	15	4	27	50

FC = free cholesterol; CE = cholesterol ester; TG = triglycerides; PL = phospholipids; PROT = protein

described, and their size appears to be inversely correlated with Lp(a) concentration.

Lipoproteins can also be classified according to their apolipoprotein composition, whose major function is lipid transport (Table 3-2). The differences in the composition of apolipoproteins between and within lipoprotein classes oftentimes determines their metabolic fate. The apoproteins classified as the major apo Bs are B-48, synthesized in the intestine and carried by chylomicrons, and B-100, produced by the liver and carried on the surface of VLDL, IDL, and LDL. The apo As (A-I, A-II, and A-IV) are made by both the intestine and the liver and are transported in both chylomicron and HDL particles. The apo Cs (C-I, C-II, and C-III) are made by the liver and are found in chylomicrons, VLDL, IDL, and HDL. Apolipo-

Table 3-2.   Characteristics and functions of major apolipoproteins

Apolipo-protein	Lipoproteins	Approximate molecular weight (daltons)	Sources	Average plasma concentration (mg/dl)	Physiologic function
B-48	Chylomicrons	264,000	Intestine	Trace	Major structural apoprotein; secretion and clearance of chylomicrons
B-100	VLDL, LDL	550,000	Liver	100–125	Ligand for LDL receptor; structural apoprotein of VLDL and LDL
A-I	HDL, Chylomicrons	28,000	Intestine, liver	100–120	Structural apoprotein of HDL; cofactor for LCAT
A-II	HDL, Chylomicrons	17,000	Intestine, liver	35–45	Structural apoprotein of HDL; cofactor for hepatic lipase
A-IV	HDL, Chylomicrons	46,000	Intestine, liver	10–20	Unknown
Apo(a)	Lp(a)	600,000	Liver	1–10	Unknown
C-I	Chylomicrons, VLDL, HDL	5,800	Liver	6–8	Cofactor for LCAT
C-II	Chylomicrons, VLDL, HDL	9,100	Liver	3–5	Cofactor for LPL
C-III	Chylomicrons, VLDL, HDL	8,750	Liver	12–15	Inhibitor of LPL; involved in lipoprotein remnant uptake
E-2	Chylomicrons, VLDL, HDL	35,000	Liver, peripheral tissues	4–5	Ligand for cell receptor
E-3	Chylomicrons, VLDL, HDL	35,000	Liver, peripheral tissues	4–5	Ligand for cell receptor
E-4	Chylomicrons, VLDL, HDL	35,000	Liver, peripheral tissues	4–5	Ligand for cell receptor

protein E (apo E) is transported as a constituent of chylomicrons, VLDL, IDL, and HDL. It exists in several polymorphic forms due to the presence of multiple, genetically determined alleles at a single gene locus. Three homozygous (E4/4, E3/3, and E2/2) and three heterozygous (E4/3, E4/2, and E3/2) phenotypes have been detected, with E3/3, which is present in 60 percent of the population, being the most common [6].

Overview of Cholesterol Metabolism

Cholesterol is an essential steroid molecule in cell membranes and lipoproteins, having particularly important functions for permeability and enzyme activities in membranes. Cholesterol and/or its derivatives are precursors of adrenal steroids (hydrocortisone and aldosterone), sex hormones (estrogens and androgens), bile acids, which facilitate the absorption of intestinal fat, and vitamin D. Although all nucleated mammalian cells can produce cholesterol, the major organs of synthesis are the intestine and the liver (Figure 3-1). Since the liver is the major organ capable of metabolizing cholesterol, an elaborate system of cholesterol transport via lipoproteins from peripheral tissues back to the liver has evolved (Figures 3-2, 3-3, 3-4, and 3-5).

Figure 3-1.   Overview of cholesterol metabolism.

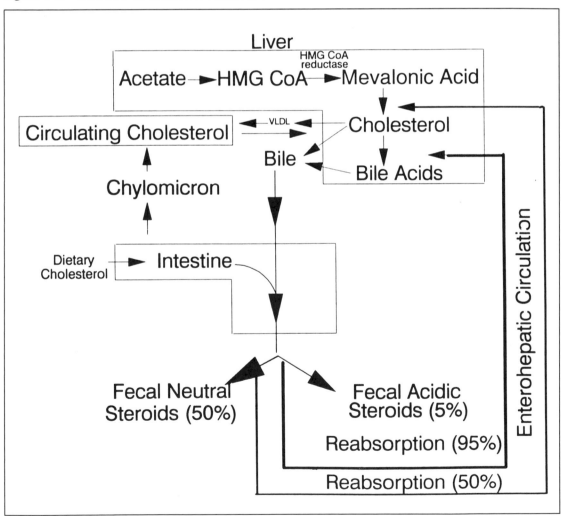

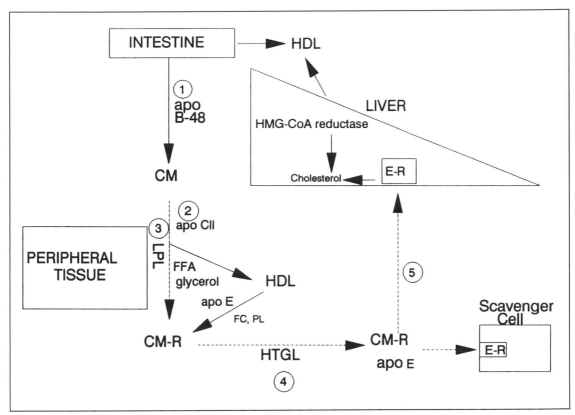

Figure 3-2. Chylomicron metabolism
CM = chylomicron, LPL = lipoprotein lipase, CM-R = chylomicron remnant, HGTL = hepatic triglyceride lipase, E-R = apoE receptor, FC = free cholesterol, PL = phospholipids. Numbers represent sites of regulation where metabolic defects can occur. Solid arrows = synthetic pathways; dashed arrows = catabolic pathways.

Sources of Cholesterol

Cholesterol in the intestinal lumen originates from two major sources, the diet and bile, although some cholesterol is also derived from the desquamation of intestinal mucosal cells.

In humans, the amount of dietary cholesterol can vary from virtually zero, as in the case of vegetarians, to 2000 mg/day in people consuming large quantities of animal fats. The average intake of adult men and women is 450 mg/day. All dietary cholesterol is from animal sources. Plants do not contain cholesterol but instead have other cell membrane sterols such as sitosterol.

Absorption of Cholesterol

As described in Figure 3-1, approximately 50 percent of the cholesterol entering the lumen of the intestine is absorbed, and the remainder is excreted in the feces. Because of the insoluble nature of cholesterol, it is first solubilized into micelles that contain bile acids and more polar lipids such as fatty acids, monoglycerides, and lecithin. In the intestinal lumen, the detergent nature of these more polar lipids facilitates the solubilization of cholesterol, which, upon incorporation into the intestinal mucosal cell, is packaged along with more nonpolar lipids (triglycerides and cholesterol ester) and protein into chylomicrons for secretion into the bloodstream.

Hepatic Synthesis and Catabolism of Cholesterol

As previously mentioned, the liver is the major site of cholesterol synthesis. Briefly, as de-

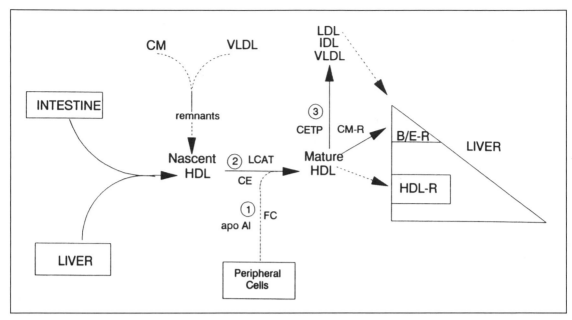

Figure 3-3. HDL metabolism.
HDL-R = HDL receptor, CETP = cholesterol-ester transfer protein, CE = cholesterol ester, LCAT = lecithin cholesterol acyl transferase, CM-R = chylomicron remnant. Numbers represent sites of regulation where metabolic defects can occur. Solid arrows = synthetic pathways; dashed arrows = catabolic pathways.

scribed in Figure 3-1, the synthesis of cholesterol is initiated from the conversion of the 2-carbon fragment, acetate to 3-hydroxy-3-methylglutaryl coenzyme A (HMG CoA). The conversion of HMG CoA to mevalonic acid is mediated via the enzyme HMG CoA reductase and is the rate-limiting step in cholesterol biosynthesis. Approximately 600–800 mg of cholesterol is synthesized per day. The cholesterol, which accumulates in the liver, may have three fates: (1) it may be repackaged as VLDL and enter the circulation; (2) it may be converted to the primary bile acids, cholate and chenodeoxycholate, by the regulatory enzyme 7 alpha hydroxylase; or (3) it may be secreted into the bile and, therefore, the intestine, as biliary cholesterol along with bile acids.

Enterohepatic Circulation

The process of continuous transport of cholesterol and bile acids between the liver and the intestine is referred to as the enterohepatic circulation. During this process, approximately one-half of the dietary cholesterol entering the intestine is reabsorbed and returns to the liver. The amount of cholesterol that returns to the liver can regulate the degree of hepatic synthesis of cholesterol by feedback inhibition of HMG CoA reductase. Thus, the more cholesterol reabsorbed by the liver, the greater the inhibition of cholesterol synthesis. The hepatic synthesis of bile acids is also regulated by feedback inhibition through their return to the liver via the enterohepatic circulation. Approximately 95 percent of the bile acids synthesized by the liver and secreted into the bile and eventually the intestine are returned to the liver in this process.

Overview of Lipoprotein Metabolism

Chylomicrons

The metabolism of lipoproteins has been reviewed by several investigators, including Schaefer and Levy [7]. In humans and most subhuman species, lipoproteins are produced by the intestine and the liver. As shown in Figure 3-1, the intestine secretes chylomicrons, which

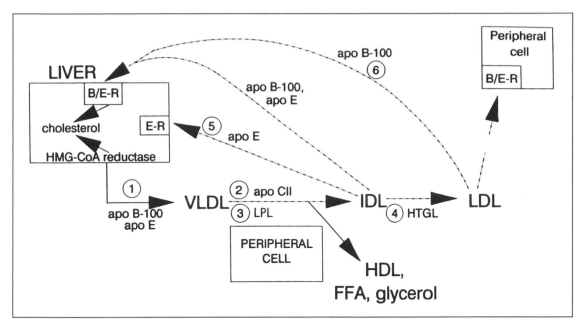

Figure 3-4. VLDL and LDL metabolism.
B/E-R = LDL receptor, E-R = apo E receptor, LPL = lipoprotein lipase, HTGL = hepatic triglyceride lipase. Numbers represent sites of regulation where metabolic defects can occur. Solid arrows = synthetic pathways; dashed arrows = catabolic pathways.

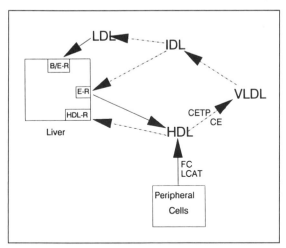

Figure 3-5. Reverse cholesterol transport.
FC = free cholesterol, CE = cholester ester,
CETP = cholesterol-ester transfer protein,
LCAT = lecithin cholesterol acyl transferase,
HDL-R = HDL receptor, E-R = apo E receptor,
B/E-R = LDL receptor. Solid arrows = synthetic
pathways; dashed arrows = catabolic pathways.

contain several apoproteins, the most essential one for chylomicron secretion being apo B-48, the intestinal form of apo B. This large, triglyceride-rich particle originates in the intestine in response to such dietary factors as fat. Once these chylomicrons are secreted from the intestine into the circulation, they are acted on by the enzyme lipoprotein lipase (LPL), which, after activation by apo C-II, results in the hydrolysis of triglycerides and the formation of chylomicron remnants. The enzyme hepatic triglyceride lipase (HTGL) is also active in the formation of chylomicron remnants from chylomicrons. During the process of lipolysis, triglycerides are catabolized to form FFAs and glycerol. As the core of chylomicrons is depleted of triglycerides, surface components such as apo A-I, apo A-II, apo Cs, and phospholipids are released to form nascent HDL, which goes on to form mature HDL (Figure 3-3). During the process of HDL metabolism, certain of its surface components, such as apo E, are transferred to chylomicron remnants. The TG-poor chylomicron remnants, enriched in apo E, are then taken up by the apo E receptor in the liver. The apo E receptor is not regulated by environmental factors.

VLDL

The liver also secretes VLDL and, in particular, apo B-100 (Figure 3-4). The secretion and synthesis of VLDL is increased in obese individuals and is also responsive to dietary variables, such as high carbohydrate intake and increases in dietary fatty acids. The catabolism of VLDL triglycerides is similar to chylomicron degradation, involving both lipoprotein lipase and hepatic triglyceride lipase. During the formation of VLDL remnants (IDL) from the catabolism of VLDL, certain constituents such as apo E and apo C are also transferred to HDL while apo B-100 remains with the IDL particle. The major product of VLDL and IDL catabolism is LDL, although some VLDL may be removed from plasma prior to LDL formation, especially in individuals with severe hypertriglyceridemia.

LDL

LDL, the major cholesterol-transporting lipoprotein in humans, is derived predominantly from the catabolism of VLDL and IDL, although in certain individuals with familial hypercholesterolemia [8, 9] and in some animal models, such as the pig [10, 11], there is some direct LDL synthesis. LDL can be catabolized by both hepatic and extrahepatic tissues with approximately 75 percent of LDL being catabolized by the liver and the remaining 25 percent by extrahepatic tissue [12,13]. The clearance of LDL by these tissues involves both receptor-mediated and non-receptor-mediated pathways (see Figure 3-4). The predominant pathway of clearance is receptor mediated via the B-E receptor (LDL receptor), accounting for nearly 75 percent of the clearance of LDL, while approximately 25 percent is cleared by non-receptor pathways [14, 15]. During catabolism of LDL via the B-E receptor, LDL binds to the receptor and becomes internalized in association with cytoplasmic lysosomes. Once internalized, the receptors disassociate themselves from LDL and return to the cell surface to be used again.

The cholesterol esters and apo B of LDL are hydrolyzed by enzymes within the lysosome to unesterified cholesterol and amino acids, respectively. The unesterified cholesterol can be used for cell membrane components, be reesterified as cholesterol ester for storage, or leave the cell, as in the case of the liver, where it can become incorporated into bile for final fecal excretion. The B-E receptor appears to be influenced by changes in the levels of dietary cholesterol [16, 17], the type of dietary fat [18, 19, 20], hormones [21], and increasing age [22, 23]. The amount of cholesterol entering the cell can regulate the synthesis of cholesterol and the rate of LDL receptor synthesis by influencing the activity of HMG CoA reductase [24], the major enzyme that controls cholesterol synthesis. Environmental factors that regulate LDL receptor synthesis and activity are discussed in a later section.

Lp(a)

Very little information is currently available on Lp(a) metabolism. The liver is the primary site of synthesis of Lp(a) and, although its catabolic site has not been determined with certainty, the LDL receptor pathway has emerged as a major route, although possibly not as effective as it is for LDL [25, 26]. Levels of Lp(a) seem to be regulated by rates of synthesis [25]. Its value as a predictor of coronary heart disease risk probably resides in its striking homology with plasminogen [27]. Plasminogen is converted to plasmin, which normally dissolves clots. Lp(a) at high concentrations competes with plasminogen, counteracting the fibrinolytic system and thereby increasing the risk of thrombosis.

HDL

HDLs are a heterogeneous group of particles that can be divided into several subfractions depending on the method of separation used. In general the mature HDL particle is spherical in shape, while the precursor or nascent HDL particles are usually viewed as disks consisting of phospholipid bilayers enriched with apo A-I and/or apo E molecules. As outlined in Figures 3-2 and 3-3, nascent HDL (sometimes referred

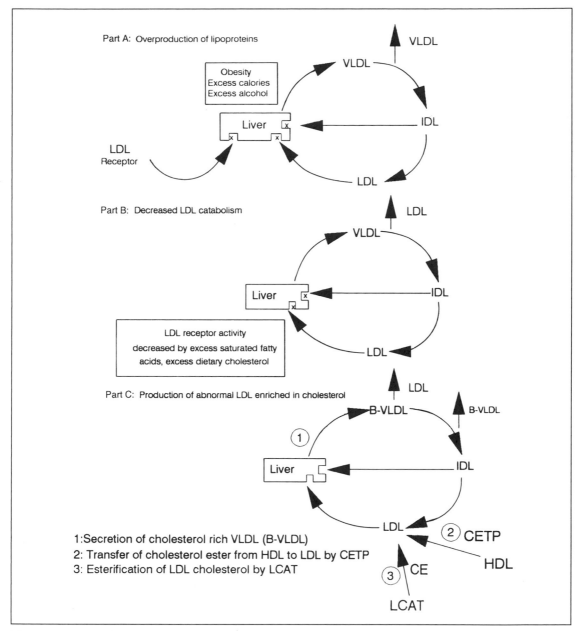

Figure 3-6.   Overview of dietary regulation of VLDL and LDL metabolism.

to as HDL₃) can originate from the catabolism of VLDL and chylomicrons. As outlined in Figure 3-3, nascent HDL can also be secreted directly by the liver and the intestine. These nascent forms of HDL may associate with cholesterol and phospholipid originating from the degradation of cell membranes. Nascent HDL particles also provide excellent substrates for lecithin-cholesterol acyl-transferase (LCAT), the major plasma-cholesterol-esterifying enzyme. By acquiring cholesterol esters generated during the LCAT reaction, these disc-shaped nascent HDLs (HDL₃) are converted to mature, spherical HDL (HDL₂ particles) in plasma upon movement of cholesterol ester into the hydrophobic core regions of HDL. The cholesterol esters from the core of HDL can be exchanged or transferred to chylomicrons or VLDL in exchange for triglyceride molecules by a cholesterol ester transfer protein (CETP). These cholesterol esters transferred to triglyceride-rich lipoproteins may then be cleared from circulation via the LDL receptor or remnant pathway. Some HDL particles may be directly cleared from plasma by the liver through a putative HDL receptor [28], although probably not as intact particles, since the rates of removal of HDL lipid and apoproteins differ [29].

Reverse Cholesterol Transport

Since cholesterol can be degraded and excreted only by the liver, any removal of excess cholesterol from peripheral tissues, such as blood vessel walls, must involve the transport of cholesterol back to the liver. Figure 3-5 outlines the mechanism of reverse cholesterol transport. In this scenario, unesterified cholesterol, a normal constituent of cellular membranes, but also found in atherosclerotic plaques, is transferred to HDL and through the action of the enzyme LCAT becomes esterified cholesterol. Some of the HDL cholesterol ester is transferred to VLDL by CETP. The cholesterol ester in VLDL can then be returned to the liver by direct incorporation of VLDL remnants (IDL) through the apo E receptor or can be taken up by the B/E receptor subsequent to conversion of VLDL to LDL.

Definition of Dyslipoproteinemias

Dyslipoproteinemias (DLPs) are disorders of plasma lipid transport that can be associated with deficiencies of apolipoproteins, enzymes, lipid transfer proteins, or cellular receptors. Because the end result includes alterations in the synthesis and/or removal of lipoproteins from the blood stream, the critical significance of the DLPs is therefore attributable to their involvement in enhanced risk of atherosclerosis and coronary heart disease.

It is important to understand that true familial hyperlipidemias account for only a minor portion of individuals with elevated serum cholesterol levels. For the majority of such individuals, their hyperlipidemia reflects both a genetic tendency to develop elevated lipid levels combined with environmental characteristics (e.g., high-fat diet or obesity) that allow the tendency to be expressed. Thus, an individual with a serum cholesterol of 230 mg/dl is not likely to have a clearly defined familial hyperlipidemia; nonetheless, a genetic influence must be present, since other individuals with similar diets will have lower lipid levels. The familial dyslipidemias are of importance because they include the most severe forms of lipid abnormalities, and also because the study of these disorders has proven invaluable in augmenting our understanding of lipid physiology and the consequent treatment of abnormal states.

A precise diagnosis of lipoprotein abnormalities must be based on age- and gender-specific norms. Such norms, based on the Lipid Research Clinic's population, are provided in Table 3-3, which is taken from the review article of Schaefer and Levy [7]. The major reasons to use such norms are the significant age-related increases in plasma cholesterol, plasma triglyceride, VLDL, and LDL cholesterol levels. In addition, there is a significant gender difference with regard to HDL cholesterol after the age of puberty, which persists throughout the rest of life. Therefore, while approximate cutpoints such as a total cholesterol of ≥ 240 mg/dl and LDL cholesterol ≥ 160 mg/dl as well as an HDL cholesterol <35 mg/dl are all associated with increased heart disease risk [30], age- and gender-specific percentile values are more accurate for clearly defining an abnormality, specifically values that are above the ninetieth or below the tenth percentile of normal [31].

Classification, Physiology, and Pathology of DLPs

It should be emphasized that the classification of DLPs is continually changing. We have arbitrarily separated the DLPs into 12 different phenotypes, as described in Table 3-4. These phenotypes have been further divided into those DLPs that result in either elevated or reduced

Table 3-3. Normal plasma lipid and lipoprotein-cholesterol concentrations

	Plasma cholesterol (mg/dl)			Plasma triglyceride (mg/dl)			VLDL cholesterol (mg/dl)			LDL cholesterol (mg/dl)			HDL cholesterol (mg/dl)		
Percentile →	10	50	90	10	50	90	10	50	90	10	50	90	10	50	90
Males															
0–4	125	151	186	33	51	84	—	*	—	—	—	—	—	—	—
5–9	130	159	191	33	51	85	2	7	15	69	90	117	42	54	70
10–14	127	155	190	37	59	102	2	9	18	72	94	122	40	55	71
15–19	120	146	183	43	69	120	3	12	23	68	93	123	34	46	59
20–24	130	165	204	50	86	165	5	12	24	73	101	138	32	45	57
25–29	143	178	227	54	95	199	6	15	31	75	116	157	32	44	58
30–34	148	190	239	58	104	213	8	18	36	88	124	166	32	45	59
35–39	157	197	249	62	113	251	7	19	46	92	131	176	31	43	58
40–44	163	203	250	64	122	248	8	21	43	98	135	173	31	43	60
45–49	169	210	258	68	124	253	8	20	40	106	141	186	33	45	60
50–54	169	210	261	68	124	250	10	23	49	102	143	185	31	44	58
55–59	167	212	262	67	119	235	6	19	39	103	145	191	31	46	64
60–64	171	210	259	68	119	235	4	16	35	106	143	188	34	49	69
65–69	170	210	258	64	112	208	3	16	40	104	146	199	33	48	70
>70	162	205	252	67	111	212	3	15	31	100	142	182	33	48	70
Females															
0–4	120	156	189	38	59	96	—	1	—	—	—	—	—	—	—
5–9	134	163	195	36	55	90	1	9	19	73	98	125	38	52	67
10–14	131	158	190	44	70	114	3	10	20	73	94	126	40	52	64
15–19	126	154	190	44	66	107	4	11	20	67	93	127	38	51	68
20–24	130	160	203	41	64	112	3	10	22	62	98	136	37	50	68
25–29	136	168	209	42	65	116	4	11	22	73	103	141	40	55	73
30–34	139	172	213	44	69	123	2	9	20	76	108	142	40	55	71
35–39	147	182	225	46	73	137	3	13	26	81	116	161	38	52	74
40–44	154	191	235	51	82	155	5	12	26	89	120	164	39	55	78
45–49	161	199	247	53	87	171	4	14	32	90	127	173	39	56	78
50–54	172	215	268	59	97	186	4	14	32	102	141	192	40	59	77
55–59	183	228	282	63	106	204	4	18	40	103	148	204	39	58	82
60–64	186	228	280	64	105	202	3	13	30	105	151	201	43	60	85
65–69	183	229	280	66	112	204	3	15	36	104	156	208	38	60	79
>70	180	226	278	69	111	204	0	13	34	107	146	189	37	60	82

Source: Lipid Research Clinic's population studies in the United States and Canada for white males and females (nonusers of sex hormone) [31].
Notes: All subjects were tested in the fasting state. Values in the lowest fifth percentile and highest fifth percentile for all age and sex groups (mg/dl) are: cholesterol, 112–303; triglyceride, 29–327; VLDL cholesterol, 0–62; LDL cholesterol, 60–234; and HDL cholesterol, 27–91. To convert cholesterol and triglyceride values to millimoles per liter, multiply by 0.02586 and 0.01129, respectively.
*Dashes indicate that no data are available because there were fewer than 100 subjects in a cell.

Table 3-4. Primary DLPs

Type	Plasma lipid changes	Plasma lipoprotein changes	Genetic disorder	Apparent biochemical defect	Clinical manifestations
I	↑ Triglycerides	↑ Chylomicrons	Familial lipoprotein-lipase (LPL) deficiency	Loss of LPL activity	Acute pancreatitis, eruptive xanthomas, hepatosplenomegaly, lipemia retinalis
			Familial apo CII deficiency	Abnormal CII structure or levels	Acute pancreatitis
IIA	↑ Cholesterol	↑ LDL	Familial hypercholesterolemia	Deficiency of LDL receptor number and/or activity	Premature atherosclerosis; tendon xanthomas and corneal arcus
IIB	↑ Cholesterol, triglycerides	↑ LDL and VLDL	Familial combined hyperlipidemia	Unknown	Increased risk of premature coronary artery disease
III	↑ Cholesterol, triglycerides	↑ beta-VLDL	Familial type III hyperlipoproteinemia Homozygous for apo E-2	Defective clearance of triglyceride-rich remnants; hepatic lipase deficiency	Premature coronary artery and peripheral vascular disease, tuberous xanthomas, hyperuricemia, glucose intolerance
IV	↑ Triglycerides	↑ VLDL	Familial hypertriglyceridemia	Increased synthesis and decreased catabolism of VLDL	Acute pancreatitis, glucose intolerance, hyperuricemia
V	↑ Triglycerides, cholesterol	↑ VLDL and chylomicrons	Familial type V hyperlipoproteinemia	Defective lipolysis of triglyceride-rich lipoproteins and overproduction of VLDL triglycerides	Acute pancreatitis, eruptive xanthomas, glucose intolerance, hyperuricemia, peripheral neuropathy

Hyper Lp(a)	↑ Cholesterol	↑ Lp(a)	Familial hyper apo (a)	Resemblance to plasminogen causes competitive inhibition, lowering fibrinolytic activity in plasma	Increased coronary artery disease, xanthomatosis
Hyperapobetalipoproteinemia	↑ Triglycerides	↑ VLDL and LDL	Familial hyperapo B; Familial type IV	Increased VLDL apo B synthesis	Predisposition to coronary, cerebral, and peripheral atherosclerosis
Hyperalphalipoproteinemia	↑ Cholesterol	↑ HDL	Familial hyperalpha lipoproteinemia	CETP deficiency	Decreased frequency of CHD; increased longevity
Abetalipoproteinemia	↓ Cholesterol, triglycerides	↓ Chylomicrons, VLDL, LDL	Unknown	apo B-100 and apo B-48 not secreted into plasma	Fat malabsorption, acanthocytosis, retinitis pigmentosa
Familial hypobetalipoproteinemia	↓ Cholesterol, triglycerides	↓ Chylomicrons, VLDL, LDL	Unknown	Inability to synthesize apo B-100 and apo B-48	Development of neurological or eye complications, abnormal clotting function
Hypoalphalipoproteinemia (Tangier disease, fish eye disease)	↓ Triglycerides, cholesterol	↓ HDL	Unknown	LCAT deficiency, combined apo A-I, CIII deficiency, apo A-I defects — all of which may lead to abnormal metabolism of apo A-I and apo A-II	Premature coronary artery disease

levels of plasma lipids and lipoproteins. It is important to note that these DLPs can also occur secondary to other diseases (Table 3-5).

TYPE I DYSLIPOPROTEINEMIA

This rare disorder, known as familial type I dyslipoproteinemia, is associated with elevated levels of plasma triglycerides (triglyceride values > 1000 mg/dl) and severe chylomicronemia in the fasting state, with normal VLDL levels. It is associated with the inheritance of a recessive gene that causes a deficiency in either apo C-II, the apoprotein that activates lipoprotein lipase (Figure 3-2, Site 2) or extrahepatic lipoprotein lipase (see Figure 3-2, Site 3). These deficiencies result in an inability to clear chylomicrons from the circulation and therefore cause their accumulation in plasma [32, 33]. Clinical manifestations appear in childhood, and the disorder usually is not associated with an increased risk of CHD. The severity of the condition is exacerbated by a high-fat diet; thus, it is not unusual for plasma triglyceride levels to range up to 5,000 mg/dl, resulting in such severe complications as acute pancreatitis due to triglyceride deposition in the pancreas.

To reduce the occurrence of recurrent pancreatitis and eruptive xanthoma formation, it is imperative to reduce dietary fat intake to less than 20 percent of calories. While drugs such as niacin and gemfibrozil are often ineffective in

these individuals, fish oil capsules may be helpful to keep triglyceride levels below 1000 mg/dl.

TYPE II FAMILIAL HYPERCHOLESTEROLEMIA

Familial hypercholesterolemia (FH) is an autosomal dominant disorder, with the most frequent type involving mutations within the LDL receptor gene on chromosome 19, resulting in lack of expression of receptors or defective receptors [34] (see Figure 3-4, Site 6). Occasionally patients may have a defect within apo B-100 resulting in defective binding of LDL to the LDL receptor [35, 36]. Patients with familial hypercholesterolemia, which in its homozygous form often results in clinical disease in childhood, usually have hypercholesterolemia associated with increased levels of LDL only (type IIa). Familial hypercholesterolemia accounts for up to 6 percent of myocardial infarctions occurring prior to age 60 years. In type IIb dyslipoproteinemia, the increased levels of VLDL and LDL are responsible for elevations in both plasma cholesterol and triglycerides. Approximately one in 500 individuals is heterozygous for familial hypercholesterolemia, with plasma cholesterol levels typically greater than 250 mg/dl. The homozygote condition is very rare, with individuals typically having plasma cholesterol levels in excess of 500 mg/dl and frequently

Table 3-5. Secondary DLPs

Type	Associated diseases	Lipoproteins elevated	Underlying defects
I	Lupus erythematosus	Chylomicrons	Circulating LPL inhibitor
II	Nephrotic syndrome Cushing's syndrome	VLDL and LDL	Overproduction of VLDL particles; defective lipolysis of VLDL triglycerides
III	Hypothyroidism Dysglobulinemia	VLDL and LDL	Suppression of LDL receptor activity; overproduction of VLDL triglycerides
IV	Renal failure Diabetes mellitus Acute hepatitis	VLDL	Defective lipolysis of triglyceride-rich VLDL due to inhibition of LPL and HL
V	Non-insulin-dependent diabetes	VLDL	Overproduction and defective lipolysis of VLDL triglycerides

having decreased HDL cholesterol values. Since the LDL receptor plays a major role in the catabolism of LDL, the deficiency of LDL receptors that characterizes the heterozygotes and, in particular, the near absence of LDL receptors in the homozygote condition result in striking hypercholesterolemia and increases in plasma LDL cholesterol (see Figure 3-4, Site 6). Coronary artery disease often develops in the heterozygotes between the ages of 30 and 50 years, with clinical features that include tendon xanthomas and corneal arcus. The very high levels of serum cholesterol seen in homozygotes are also associated with tendinous xanthomas and tuberous xanthomas over elbows, hands, and knees [37], and coronary artery disease often develops in childhood, with males developing disease earlier than females. In addition to a reduced fractional catabolic rate of LDL because of the deficiencies in LDL receptors, increases in LDL synthesis, especially hepatic apo B secretion (see Figure 3-4, Site 1), are also demonstrable.

The heterozygote FH can be treated by a combination of diet, consistent with NCEP step 2 (see Chapter 9), bile acid resins such as cholestyramine or colestipol, and nicotinic acid. When these treatments do not sufficiently lower LDL cholesterol levels, HMG CoA reductase inhibitors such as lovastatin, which inhibit hepatic cholesterol synthesis, are recommended. In FH heterozygotes who are prepubertal, resins are the only agents that should be used. After the age of puberty, the use of most lipid-lowering agents is justified in FH heterozygotes. The most effective combination in heterozygotes is an anion exchange resin and lovastatin [38, 39]. Probucol, which has been shown to regress tendinous xanthomas, may be used as a third-line drug in FH heterozygotes.

Control of plasma cholesterol levels in the homozygote FH is extremely difficult. Dietary modification alone usually produces insignificant reductions in LDL cholesterol levels, and even the use of HMG CoA reductase inhibitors often fails to lower cholesterol levels into the normal range. For those homozygote individuals who are unresponsive to drugs, plasmapheresis every one to two weeks is sometimes effective [40]. Recently a more specific form of this therapy, LDL-apheresis, has been developed and appears to offer considerable promise [40a, 40b]. Currently there are no reliable assays for LDL receptor activity that can be performed in a routine clinical chemistry laboratory. Therefore, the diagnosis rests on finding an elevated LDL cholesterol level and tendinous xanthomas.

TYPE III DYSBETALIPOPROTEINEMIA

This is a polygenic disorder that occurs in one in 10,000 individuals and is associated with elevations of both serum cholesterol and triglycerides due to a marked increase in chylomicron and VLDL remnants or IDL. These cholesterol-rich VLDL particles (cholesterol:triglycerides >.3) [41, 42] have been termed B-VLDL, and their plasma levels often correlate with the severity of atherosclerotic lesions, especially in susceptible animal species [43]. Individuals with type III dysbetalipoproteinemia have been reported to have an increased frequency of the homozygous phenotype E2/2 [44, 45]. In this phenotype lipoproteins have a low affinity for LDL receptors, so VLDL remnants, which carry the apo E2/2 phenotype, are not cleared from plasma efficiently (see Figure 3-4, Sites 2–5). The delayed clearance of these VLDL remnants results in the accumulation of cholesterol esters, thus inducing the production of abnormal B-VLDL particles (see Figure 3-4, Site 1). Patients with type III dysbetalipoproteinemia are prone to the development of premature coronary artery disease and peripheral vascular disease as well as tuberous xanthomas. Afflicted individuals, who are usually adults, are often obese, diabetic, hypertensive, and hyperuricemic. Effective treatment includes the NCEP step 2 diet, cessation of beta blockers, and a program of exercise. Niacin, gemfibrozil, and lovastatin will lower lipids in these patients, with niacin being the most effective in terms of reducing the levels of both cholesterol and triglycerides [46].

TYPE IV DYSLIPOPROTEINEMIA

The estimated frequency of type IV dyslipoproteinemia is approximately 0.3 percent of the adult population and 15 percent of patients with premature CHD. It is characterized by an increase in circulating VLDL levels associated with elevated triglyceride levels in the range of 300 to 500 mg/dl. Other lipoprotein values are usually normal, although HDL cholesterol values may be reduced [47]. These elevations may result from an increase in hepatic VLDL triglyceride synthesis with normal apo B production [48, 49, 50, 51, 52, 53, 54, 55] (see Figure 3-4, Site 1). Those patients with decreased HDL levels have enhanced fractional catabolism of apo A-I, the major protein of HDL [36]. Although the exact cause of type IV dyslipoproteinemia is not known, it is more prevalent in both the diabetic with elevated insulin levels and the obese patient with male pattern (truncal) obesity. Treatment of affected individuals may include the NCEP step 2 diet, avoidance of beta blockers and thiazides, and a program of regular exercise. Patients with established CHD or thought to be at high risk may be treated with gemfibrozil or niacin to optimize their lipids.

Type V Dyslipoproteinemia

The prevalence of type V dyslipoproteinemia is approximately .2 percent in adult males and even less in females. Individuals with this condition can have severe hypertriglyceridemia (triglyceride values > 1000 mg/dl) associated with high circulating levels of both VLDL and chylomicrons. These patients are readily distinguishable from those with familial postheparin lipoprotein lipase deficiency (type I), in which the age of onset of symptoms is earlier, only chylomicrons are elevated, and heparin administration has no effect on clearing the serum of chylomicrons. Individuals with type V dyslipoproteinemia may have delayed chylomicron and VLDL clearance but may also have excess production of VLDL apo B [57] (see Figure 3-2 and Figure 3-4, Sites 1-4). Type V dyslipoproteinemia occurs more frequently in adults who are obese, are diabetic, and consume excessive levels of alcohol or take exogenous estrogens. Pancreatitis due to triglyceride deposition in the pancreas and eruptive xanthomas [58] characterize those individuals with extremely high levels of chylomicrons. Treatment consists of a calorie-restricted NCEP step 2 diet.

Medications that lower triglycerides to less than 500 mg/dl in these patients include gemfibrozil or fish oil capsules (six to ten capsules per day) or a combination of both [59]. In nondiabetic patients, niacin can be used.

Hyper Lp(a)

Hyper Lp(a) is thought to occur through autosomal dominant inheritance. The true prevalence of individuals with high Lp(a) levels is not known, but approximately 20 percent of patients with premature CHD have elevated Lp(a) values [47]. Patients with hyper Lp(a) have an increased risk of developing CHD [60]. Some individuals with hyper Lp(a) will have normal plasma cholesterol levels, while others will be hypercholesterolemic and develop characteristic xanthomas. A value over the ninetieth percentile of normal is considered elevated (above 40 mg/dl using assays that assess the level of the entire particle). Plasma concentrations greater than 30 mg/dl are associated with a 1.75-fold higher risk of myocardial infarction [61]. Lp(a) appears to promote atherosclerosis and thrombosis by deposition in the arterial wall and inhibition of fibrinolysis [60, 62, 63]. Elevated levels of Lp(a) are also observed in patients with heterozygous familial hypercholesterolemia [64]. The treatment of individuals with hyper Lp(a) presents a real problem since the condition does not respond to conventional approaches that lower LDL levels, such as diet and most medications (resins, HMG CoA reductase inhibitors). Niacin administration, however, has been reported to decrease Lp(a) levels [65].

Hyperapobetalipoproteinemia

The term hyperapobetalipoproteinemia (Hyperapo B) describes the condition in which the concentration of LDL apo B is increased above the ninetieth percentile (approximately 130 mg/dl), although normal concentrations of LDL cholesterol may exist [66, 67, 68]. This disorder is present in approximately 5 percent of patients with premature CHD [47]. The apparent mechanism(s) involved in this increase of apo B are not known with certainty, but they may include elevated rates of VLDL apo B synthesis (see Figure 3-4, Site 1), which can result in an increase in the pool of LDL apo B. LDL catabolism is thought to be normal in this condition. Individuals with hyperapobetalipoproteinemia often have normal triglyceride values but elevated postprandial triglycerides compared to those of normal subjects [69] and have an increased risk of developing atherosclerosis in coronary, cerebral, and peripheral arteries. Treatment should include a diet consistent with NCEP step 2 guidelines, caloric restriction if the patient is overweight, and a program of exercise. The use of niacin or HMG CoA reductase inhibitors to optimize lipids should be considered in patients at high risk or with established CHD.

HYPERALPHALIPOPROTEINEMIA

Hyperalphalipoproteinemia is associated with HDL cholesterol levels above the ninetieth percentile (greater than 70 mg/dl for males and 75 mg/dl for females), with normal levels of LDL and VLDL cholesterol and normal triglycerides [70]. Studies by Glueck et al. [71] suggest that familial hyperalphalipoproteinemia is inherited by an autosomal dominant transmission, and although its frequency in the population is unknown, it is probably greater than one in 3000. The mechanism for the elevation in HDL is uncertain, but a deficiency of CETP (see Figure 3-3, Site 3) appears to inhibit the transfer of cholesterol esters from HDL to VLDL, IDL, and LDL, resulting in high levels of plasma HDL and often low levels of LDL. A recent study of a Japanese family with CETP deficiency, high HDL cholesterol levels, and increased longevity provides some support for this association [72]. Individuals with hyperalphalipoproteinemia may have a decreased incidence of CHD and increased longevity and thus may benefit from this "disease."

ABETALIPOPROTEINEMIA

Approximately 50 cases of abetalipoproteinemia have been reported to date. It usually presents in childhood and is associated with diarrhea, fat malabsorption, and failure to gain weight normally. Untreated, these patients will develop spinocerebellar ataxia and retinitis pigmentosa in their teens and twenties. Plasma cholesterol, triglycerides, and HDL cholesterol values are approximately 40, 20, and 40 mg/dl, respectively, with no detectable plasma apo B levels. The metabolic defect appears to be associated with an inability to secrete intestinal apo B-48 (see Figure 3-2, Site 1) or apo B-100 (see Figure 3-4, Site 1) [73]. Intestinal apo B mRNA levels are increased [74]. Supplementation of vitamins A and E is recommended to prevent the onset of neuropathy [75, 76, 77]. Obligate heterozygotes (parents) have normal lipoproteins.

FAMILIAL HYPOBETALIPOPROTEINEMIA

Both the clinical and laboratory settings of patients with hypobetalipoproteinemia are the same as in those with abetalipoproteinemia [78, 79, 80]. However, obligate heterozygotes in these kindreds have LDL cholesterol and apo B values that are 50 percent of normal. The defect is due to an inability to synthesize normal amounts of apo B (see Figures 3-2 and 3-4, Site 1). In contrast to abetalipoproteinemia, intestinal apo B mRNA levels are decreased [81]. Treatment is the same as in abetalipoproteinemia and is indicated only in homozygotes.

Another variant of this disorder is associated with abnormal apo B molecular weight (truncated apo B), and these patients have marked deficiencies of VLDL and LDL and very low plasma apo B levels [82, 83, 84, 85, 86]. Cholesterol levels are generally approximately 40 mg/dl, but triglyceride levels can be as high as 100 mg/dl.

HYPOALPHALIPOPROTEINEMIA

Familial Hypoalphalipoproteinemia. Individuals afflicted with familial hypoalphalipoproteinemia have HDL cholesterol levels below the tenth percentile (less than 30 mg/dl) of normal in affected family members. Approximately 4 percent of patients with premature CHD have this disorder. An autosomal dominant mode of inheritance has been reported [87, 88]. All other lipoprotein values and plasma lipids are normal in these patients. Although the molecular defect is not known, metabolic studies in these patients suggest that a decrease in the HDL apo A-I production rate (see Figure 3-3, Site 2) is demonstrable [89]. Treatment of affected individuals includes a diet consistent with NCEP step 2 guidelines, calorie restriction if the patient is overweight, avoidance of beta blockers, and a program of regular exercise. Patients at high risk or with established CHD can be treated with gemfibrozil, niacin, or HMG CoA reductase inhibitors to optimize their lipid profile.

Apolipoprotein A-I Deficiency States. Three major deficiency states, of apolipoprotein A-I/C-III/A-IV [90, 91, 92], apolipoprotein A-I/C-III [93, 94, 95], and apolipoprotein A-I [96], have been identified. All are extremely rare. They involve point mutation or deletions of gene complexes resulting in marked reductions or no detectable levels of plasma apo A-I and/or C-III or A-IV. Treatment in all cases includes optimization of other risk factors.

Tangier Disease. Homozygotes for Tangier disease have striking HDL deficiency, decreased LDL cholesterol levels, and mild hypertriglyceridemia [97, 98]. Apo A-I levels are 1 percent of normal, while apo C-III and A-IV values are within normal limits. Heterozygotes have HDL cholesterol and apo A-I values that are 50 percent of normal [98]. Patients with Tangier disease have abnormal apo A-I, resulting in increased catabolism of HDL components (see Figure 3-3, Site 3) and, therefore, reduced levels of HDL. Heterozygotes have HDL levels that are 50 percent of normal, while the homozygote condition produces strikingly decreased levels of HDL cholesterol and apo A-I. These abnormalities in apo A-I sometimes interfere with or prevent the activation of LCAT (see Figure 3-3, Site 2). The inability to activate LCAT can result in the accumulation of nascent HDL, which can lead to complications such as renal failure and anemia. In patients with Tangier disease, these abnormal HDL particles do not function normally, as in reverse cholesterol transport (see Figure 3-5), so cholesterol esters can deposit in reticuloendothelial cells of homozygotes, causing enlarged tonsils and hepatosplenomegaly. Homozygotes may develop premature CHD and peripheral neuropathy [98]. Treatment consists of optimization of CHD risk factors.

Fish Eye Disease. Fish eye disease has been associated with mild hypertriglyceridemia and significant HDL deficiency. Patients with this disorder develop striking corneal opacification but have not been reported to have premature CHD. These patients have a deficiency of alpha-LCAT, which differs from beta-LCAT in that it acts only on HDL, whereas beta-LCAT acts on VLDL and LDL. This disorder appears to be a milder variant of LCAT deficiency [99].

Familial LCAT Deficiency. Familial LCAT deficiency is due to a deficiency of the enzyme LCAT, which is responsible for cholesterol esterification in plasma. Patients with LCAT deficiency have a very high proportion of plasma cholesterol in the unesterified form, marked HDL cholesterol deficiency, hypertriglyceridemia, and increased amounts of free cholesterol-rich VLDL and LDL. They develop marked corneal opacification, anemia, proteinuria, renal insufficiency, and atherosclerosis. Treatment consists of dietary restriction of saturated fat and cholesterol and renal dialysis and transplantation if necessary [99].

Secondary Dyslipoproteinemias

It is important to realize that dyslipoproteinemias can be the secondary result of a number of diseases, such as diabetes mellitus, nephrotic syndrome, renal failure, and hepatic diseases such as obstructive jaundice (see Table 3-5). The mechanisms resulting in the hyperlipoproteinemias associated with these lipid abnormalities have been previously reviewed [100]. For example, patients with elevated chylomicrons, typical of type I dyslipoproteinemia, could be afflicted with lupus erythematosus, which can produce an inhibitor of lipoprotein lipase that circulates in plasma. Elevations in plasma cholesterol levels, as in type II hyperlipoproteinemia, are characteristic of nephrotic syndrome. The underlying cause of the hypercholesterolemia seen in nephrotic syndrome is thought to be both overproduction and defective catabolism of VLDL particles. These patients also have elevations in plasma triglycerides because of increased production of VLDL triglycerides. Individuals with hypothyroidism can often be classified as having type II or type III dyslipo-proteinemia because of the elevations in both cholesterol and triglycerides and the associated increase in VLDL and LDL particles. As in the type II dyslipoproteinemias, the elevations in LDL seen in the hypothyroid individual are thought to be the result of suppression of LDL receptor activity. As in the type III dyslipopro-teinemia, individuals with hypothyroidism can have delayed clearance of VLDL remnants due to impaired lipolysis of triglyceride-rich lipo-proteins.

It is not unusual for individuals with renal failure, diabetes mellitus, or acute hepatitis to develop a pattern of type IV hyperlipoprotein-emia, with hypertriglyceridemia and elevations in LDL due to defective lipolysis of triglyceride-rich VLDL. Patients with non–insulin-depend-ent diabetes can also demonstrate a pattern re-sembling type V dyslipoproteinemia, with increased levels of triglycerides and VLDL due to both the overproduction of and the defective lipolysis of VLDL triglycerides. Patients with obstructive jaundice can manifest lipoprotein abnormalities that resemble LCAT deficiency, which often results in the accumulation of nas-cent HDL particles.

Secondary dyslipoproteinemia can also result from the intake of certain drugs and hormones. Progestins and estrogen-containing contracep-tives can elevate VLDL levels by increasing the production of VLDL. Anabolic steroids, such as those commonly used by athletes, can raise LDL cholesterol levels and lower HDL levels, sometimes to a striking degree [101, 102]. Sim-ilarly alcohol consumption can increase VLDL triglycerides by stimulating triglyceride synthe-sis and secretion, mimicking type IV dyslipo-proteinemia.

Interrelationships Between the Genetic and Environmental Factors Regulating Hyperlipidemia

Since elevations in apo B–containing lipopro-teins (VLDL, IDL, and LDL) are highly cor-related with an increased risk of CHD, it is particularly germane that we understand the re-lationships between genetic and environmental factors that influence these lipoproteins.

Basic Mechanisms of Diet-Induced Hypercholesterolemia

The three basic mechanisms that lead to ele-vations in LDL cholesterol, especially in re-sponse to. dietary cholesterol and the type of dietary fat are: (1) reduced catabolism of LDL; (2) overproduction of LDL and/or its precur-sors, VLDL and IDL; and (3) production of ab-normal LDL enriched in cholesterol.

The previous section on genetic dyslipopro-teinemias described abnormalities in the LDL receptor gene (as in type IIa dyslipoproteinemia) that lead to decreases in LDL receptor number and/or activity. However, several environmen-tal factors can regulate LDL receptor synthesis and/or activity (see Figure 3-6).

DIETARY CHOLESTEROL

We previously mentioned that dietary choles-terol can influence LDL receptor activity and/or synthesis [16, 17]. For example, perturba-tions that increase a regulatory pool of hepatic cellular cholesterol can decrease LDL receptor synthesis. Thus, increases in absorption of di-etary cholesterol [103, 104, 105], inability to downregulate cholesterol synthesis [106], and decreases in cholesterol catabolism or conver-sion to bile acids or neutral sterols [107] could lead to the accumulation of cellular cholesterol, thereby decreasing LDL receptor synthesis and/or activity.

SATURATED FATTY ACIDS

LDL receptor activity is also influenced by the type of dietary fatty acids. There is considerable evidence that saturated fatty acids, in general, raise serum cholesterol and, in particular, LDL cholesterol levels. Several epidemiologic studies have shown that populations consuming large amounts of saturated fatty acids, particularly of animal fat origin, have elevated levels of cir-culating cholesterol. In contrast those popula-tions that consume lower levels of saturated fatty acids have lower serum cholesterol levels. Studies performed by Keys et al. [108] and Hegsted et al. [109] support the notion that saturated fatty acids are the major nutrient that influences cholesterol levels. These investigators developed predictive equations that relate the degree of serum cholesterol increase to saturated fatty acid intake. These equations indicate that for every 1 percent of calories consumed from saturated fatty acid there is an approximate increase of 2.7 mg/dl in serum cholesterol. In addition more recent studies indicate that saturated fatty acids also increase LDL cholesterol [110, 111, 112]. While the cholesterol-raising action of dietary saturated fatty acids, as a lipid class, is well established, the mechanisms whereby these saturated fatty acids raise LDL is not well understood. Though many mechanisms have been postulated, the most probable explanation is that saturated fatty acids interfere with normal LDL receptor-mediated clearance of LDL [12, 20] (see Figure 3-6, Part B). However, the precise mechanism of down-regulation of the LDL receptor is not known. One possibility is that increased saturated fatty acid intake enlarges a hepatic pool of cholesterol, which can suppress the expression (messenger RNA levels) of the LDL receptor protein, an explanation supported by recent studies in animals fed saturated fatty acids and cholesterol [113]. In a recent review by Grundy [113a], it was suggested that this hepatic pool of cholesterol may not be the regulatory sterol. Instead, an oxygenated derivative of cholesterol (oxysterol) may modify the conformation of proteins adjacent to the promoter region of the LDL receptor and suppress transcription of the LDL receptor gene [113b]. Another mechanism postulated from both in vivo [20] and in vitro studies [114, 115] suggests that enrichment of phospholipid membranes of various cells by saturated fatty acids interferes with the normal function of LDL receptors, possibly through alterations in the binding and/or internalization of circulating LDL. It is also possible that newly secreted lipoproteins from cholesterol-fed animals, abnormally enriched in cholesterol or having altered apoproteins [116, 117], may be less avidly bound to the LDL receptor (see Figure 3-6, Part C).

Although dietary saturated fatty acids, in general, can raise serum cholesterol and LDL cholesterol levels, earlier studies [108, 109], as well as more recent evidence [112], suggest that the various saturated fatty acids have different serum cholesterol–raising effects. Saturated fatty acids with chain lengths less than 10 carbons, i.e., medium-chain fatty acids, are thought to have little or no cholesterol-raising capabilities [118, 119]. To what extent lauric acid, a 12-carbon-chain fatty acid, raises serum cholesterol levels is not known at this time with certainty. There is substantial evidence that myristic acid, a 14-carbon-chain fatty acid, and palmitic acid, a 16-carbon-chain fatty acid, increase both total and LDL serum cholesterol levels. Earlier studies by Keys et al. [108] and Hegsted et al. [109] and the more recent investigations from the laboratory of Grundy et al. [110, 111, 112] have clearly shown that palmitic acid increases serum total and LDL cholesterol levels when it is substituted for carbohydrates or for monounsaturated fat in the diet. Another saturated fatty acid found in animal fats and cocoa butter is stearic acid, an 18-carbon-chain fatty acid. Previous studies by Keys et al. [108] and Hegsted et al. [109] and more recent studies by Bononome and Grundy [112], suggest that stearic acid may be neutral in its cholesterol-raising capabilities, thus leaving palmitic, myristic, and possibly lauric acid as the major cholesterol-raising saturated fatty acids in the diet.

The source of saturated fatty acids in the diet is typically animal fats, although certain vegetable oils such as coconut oil, palm oil, palm kernel oil, and cocoa butter are rich in saturated fatty acids. Coconut oil and palm kernel oil have similar compositions and are particularly rich in the medium-chain fatty acids 8 to 12 carbons in chain length. Animal fat is relatively rich in myristic acid, but it can also contain substantial quantities of the medium-chain fatty acids. Palm oil can contain almost 50 percent of its fatty acids in the form of saturates with the major one being palmitic acid. While cocoa butter also contains a percentage of total saturated fatty acid similar to that of palm oil, it is predominantly made up of stearic acid, which, as just mentioned, is thought to be neutral in its cholesterol-raising ability. Beef fat is high in total saturated fatty acids and rich in both palmitic acid and stearic acid. Fat from pork and chicken generally has relatively high amounts of palmitic acid and lesser amounts of stearic acid.

Thus, the type of saturated fat in various foods is of considerable importance in determining the atherogenic potential of such foods. It may be possible, as suggested by St. John et al. [120] to "engineer" various foods, e.g., beef, to contain greater amounts of stearic acid and lesser amounts of palmitic acid and thus make them more "heart healthy."

POLYUNSATURATED FATTY ACIDS (N-6) FROM VEGETABLE OILS

In contrast to saturated fatty acids, which in general raise cholesterol levels, unsaturated fatty acids, which include monounsaturated acids such as oleic acid and polyunsaturated fatty acids such as linoleic acid, have a cholesterol-lowering effect when they replace saturated fat in the diet. Two types of polyunsaturated fatty acids have been identified. The predominant n-6 fatty acid (first double bond starts at the sixth carbon from the methyl end) is linoleic acid derived from plant oils, while the n-3 fatty acids (first double bond starts at the third carbon from the methyl end) eicosapentanoic (EPA) and docosahexanoic (DHA) are derived largely from fish oils. The action of these fish oil fatty acids is discussed later. Very early studies of Kinsell et al. [121, 122] and Ahrens et al. [123] clearly demonstrated that vegetable oils enriched in linoleic acid lowered serum cholesterol levels when they were substituted for saturated fatty acids. These observations led Keys et al. [108] and Hegsted et al. [109] to establish equations that quantified the cholesterol-lowering activity of linoleic acid. The mechanism by which polyunsaturated fatty acids, such as linoleic acid, lower serum cholesterol and LDL cholesterol levels has been investigated for many years. These mechanisms include enhanced fecal excretion of cholesterol from the body and reduced synthesis of apo B–containing lipoproteins. More recent evidence from both human and animal studies suggests that the substitution of linoleic acid for saturated

fatty acids increases the fractional clearance of LDL from the blood stream by up-regulation of LDL receptor activity [19, 20]. Although the exact mechanism by which polyunsaturated fatty acids increase LDL receptor activity is not known, hypotheses put forth include (1) a reduction in hepatic pools of cholesterol, which would normally down-regulate the receptor [24], and (2) an increase in membrane fluidity associated with enhanced incorporation of polyunsaturated fatty acids into membrane phospholipids, resulting in up-regulation of the LDL receptor by increasing binding and internalization of the LDL particle by the LDL receptor [114, 115]. All of these proposed mechanisms remain to be further established.

MONOUNSATURATED FATTY ACIDS

More recently monounsaturated fatty acids, oleic acid in particular, have been shown to lower plasma total and LDL cholesterol levels when substituted for saturated fatty acids [110, 124, 125]. Although the mechanism is not known with certainty, there are reports indicating that monounsaturates may decrease the suppression of LDL receptor activity that is produced by saturated fatty acids [126].

While recent investigations have indicated that monounsaturated fatty acids can lower serum LDL levels, these studies have focused on oleic acid, a monounsaturate with the cis configuration (the carbon moieties on the two sides of a double bond lie on the same side) as occurs in most natural fats and oils. However, during the process of hydrogenation of polyunsaturated vegetable and fish oils to produce fats that have more firmness and resist rancidity, trans fatty acids are formed (unsaturated fatty acids in which the carbon atoms on the two sides of the double bond point in opposite directions). The estimated daily intake of trans fatty acids in the United States is 8 to 10 grams, or 6 to 8 percent of total fat calories. The most abundant trans fatty acids are elaidic acid and its isomers, which are 18-carbon fatty acids with one double bond. Studies to determine whether serum cholesterol levels are influenced by the trans form of oleic acid (elaidic) have been inconsistent. One early study demonstrated that trans-unsaturated fatty acids elevated serum cholesterol levels [127], while several others [128, 129, 130, 131, 132] did not demonstrate an effect. However, a more recent study [133] demonstrated that a diet rich in trans fatty acids (11 percent of total fat calories) was associated with increased serum LDL and decreased HDL levels. Additional studies utilizing more reasonable intakes of trans fatty acid will need to be conducted before any conclusions can be drawn.

POLYUNSATURATED FATTY ACIDS (N-3) FROM FISH OIL

Animal studies of dietary fish oil have been inconsistent, with increases and decreases in receptor clearance of LDL (see Figure 3-4, Site 6) being reported. Dietary fish oils enriched in omega-3 fatty acids can influence lipoprotein metabolism by altering key lipolytic and transfer enzymes. The activity of LCAT, the enzyme largely responsible for the formation of plasma cholesterol ester, is significantly increased in rats [134] and cardiac patients [135] who are fed fish oil (see Figure 3-3, Site 2). In contrast, consumption of fish oil by monkeys [136] and normolipidemic patients [135] reduced LCAT activity.

The effect of fish oil consumption on lipoprotein lipase (LPL) activity, the enzyme that catabolizes TG-rich lipoproteins such as intestinal chylomicrons and hepatic VLDL, (see Figures 3-2 and 3-4, Site 3) has been equivocal, with reports of no effect [134] or of striking decreases in activity in rats [137]. A decrease in VLDL-TG and apo B production and secretion seems to be the predominant mechanism explaining the striking hypotriglyceridemic effect seen with fish oil consumption (see Figure 3-4, Site 1). While the hypotriglyceridemic action of fish oils has been consistently observed, their effect on serum cholesterol levels is less reproducible, for reasons that may include variability in the populations studied, the dosages and composition of fish oil, and the durations of study.

Human studies of the effect of dietary fish oils rich in EPA and DHA on total plasma and LDL cholesterol levels have also been equivocal. While early studies using pharmacologic doses of fish oil lowered total plasma and LDL cholesterol levels, more recent studies of fish oil consumption have shown small but significant increases in LDL cholesterol [138].

HIGH-CARBOHYDRATE DIETS

High-carbohydrate diets rich in monosaccharides, disaccharides, and polysaccharides can lower LDL cholesterol levels when replacing dietary fat, although the mechanism(s) are not well-established. A recent review article by Grundy and Denke [126] suggests that there may be a reduction in the suppression of LDL receptor activity by saturated fat.

OVERPRODUCTION OF LIPOPROTEINS

Increases in apo B–containing lipoproteins, and LDL cholesterol in particular, may result from the overproduction of lipoproteins. For example, in obesity associated with excessive caloric intake, an increased production of both VLDL and LDL apo B has been reported [139, 140, 141] (see Figure 3-6, Part A). This overproduction of lipoproteins is further augmented if the excessive caloric intake is in the form of saturated fatty acids, which would, in addition, suppress LDL receptor activity [142] (see Figure 3-6, Part B). Excessive alcohol consumption can also enhance VLDL production [143, 144, 145, 146]. Plasma LDL cholesterol can also be increased if a disproportionate increase in the cholesterol moiety occurs relative to LDL apo B. For example, VLDL rich in cholesterol, as occurs in animals fed excess cholesterol [116, 117], can lead to LDL particles also enriched in cholesterol. In humans, LDL can also be enriched in cholesterol by the action of CETP, which can transfer cholesterol from HDL to LDL, and by the enzyme LCAT, which can enrich the LDL particle in cholesterol ester (see Figure 3-6, Part C).

The Regulation of HDL

The regulation of HDL levels by environmental factors is only beginning to be understood. Dietary factors that have been demonstrated to influence HDL levels include the type of dietary fat and the level of dietary cholesterol and carbohydrates consumed. Human studies have demonstrated that a high-carbohydrate diet decreases levels of HDL by increasing the rate of catabolism of HDL with no effect on HDL synthesis [147]. Changing the polyunsaturated/saturated (P/S) fatty acid ratio in the diet from 0.25 to 4.0 in male subjects resulted in significant decreases in HDL cholesterol, which were associated with a decreased production rate in apo A-I with no effect on fractional catabolic rate [148]. Similarly studies in humans demonstrated that changing the diet from a high saturated fat level to a low fat intake caused significant reductions in both HDL cholesterol and apo A-I levels, which were significantly correlated with a decrease in apo A-I production rate [149]. Animal studies in which the P/S ratio of dietary fat was increased severalfold have also shown reductions in HDL cholesterol and apo A-I that were associated with increases in apo A-I fractional catabolic rate [150, 151] and decreases in apo A-I production rate, the latter also associated with a decrease in hepatic mRNA levels of apo A-I [152]. It should be mentioned that more modest increases in P/S ratios are not accompanied by decreases in HDL. It is also worth noting that, in most cases, LDL levels fall to a greater extent than HDL levels, giving rise to a favorable LDL/HDL ratio. Finally there are no intervention studies that have shown that diet or drug-induced reduction of HDL levels increases the risk of CHD.

Other environmental factors that influence HDL levels include certain hormones, increased alcohol consumption, and aerobic exercise. HDL cholesterol and apo A-I levels in women are generally higher than in men, and this observation has been associated with increased apo A-I synthesis in females as compared to males. Estrogen treatment raises HDL levels by prolonging the residence time of apo A-I in women [101]. The increase in HDL cholesterol seen with aerobic exercise is associated with enhanced catabolism of certain components of VLDL remnants and transfer to HDL, as well as prolonged residence time of HDL [153]. Alcohol-induced increases in HDL have been reported to result from both decreased HDL catabolism [154] and increased HDL production [155].

Diet and Hemostasis

The mechanisms that explain the effects of diet, and unsaturated fatty acids in particular, on the parameters of hemostasis, such as platelet function, are not well established. However, a considerable body of knowledge indicates that unsaturated fatty acids derived from vegetable oils, e.g., omega-6 fatty acids such as linoleic acid (C18:2) and arachidonic acid (C20:4), induce alterations in platelet function and in endothelial cells distinct from those observed with the omega-3 fatty acids of fish oil (Figure 3-7). Platelets function in hemostasis by aggregating on the exposed surface of collagen of a blood vessel wall in response to injury. The degree of platelet aggregation and vasoconstriction is modulated by the release of prostanoids, whose properties and function can be influenced by the source of unsaturated fatty acids. The prostanoid thromboxane A_2 (TXA_2), produced by platelets in response to the consumption of omega-6 fatty acids, especially linoleic (C18:2) and arachidonic acid (C20:4) derived from vegetable oils, has vasoconstrictor and proaggregatory effects, thereby increasing platelet aggregation (see Figure 3-7). The proaggregatory effects of TXA_2 are normally balanced by the vasodilator, antiaggregatory properties of PGI_2, a prostanoid secreted by endothelial cells of blood vessel walls. However, if the effects of TXA_2 released by the platelet exceed those of PGI_2 released by the endothelium, a shift in favor of thrombus formation results. In response to fish oil consumption, the omega-3 fatty acids (EPA and DHA) are incorporated into platelet phospholipids, reducing the synthesis of the proaggregatory TXA_2 in favor of TXA_3, which has little biologic activity. In addition consumption of fish oil enhances the antithrombotic environment by inducing endothelial cells to produce PGI_3, which acts in concert with PGI_2 to maintain the antiaggregatory property of the latter. (See Chapter 5 for further discussion of platelet-vessel wall interactions.)

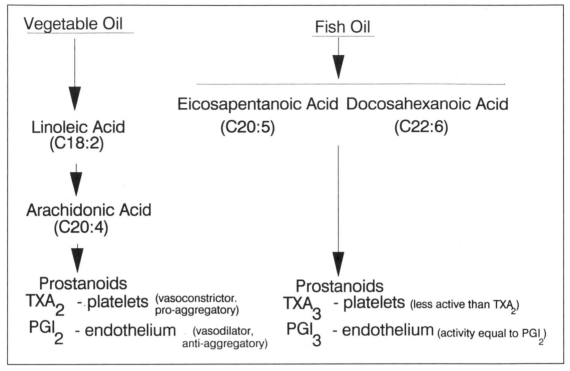

Figure 3-7.   Abbreviated flow chart of prostanoid formation.

Pathobiology of Atherosclerosis: The Role of Hypercholesterolemia and Altered Hemostasis

The role of hypercholesterolemia and hemostasis in the development of atherosclerosis as described here represents a synthesis of information derived from the reviews by Ross [156], Steinberg et al. [157], and Nicolosi and Stucchi [158]. Elevated serum cholesterol levels associated with the uptake by arteries of atherogenic lipoproteins such as LDL, VLDL remnants, and/or beta VLDL appear to be a necessary prerequisite for initiating atherogenesis (Figure 3-8). The enhanced uptake of these atherogenic lipoproteins may be associated with nonspecific endothelial dysfunction or endothelial injury resulting from risk factors such as hypertension, smoking, or diabetes. If endothelial dysfunction exists, once these lipoproteins move into the subintimal space, their residence time may be extended by their interaction with proteoglycans, substances that make up the connective tissue matrix of the blood vessel wall and that bind avidly to apo B–containing lipoproteins such as LDL and VLDL remnants. The increase in the residence time of these lipoproteins provides a greater opportunity for oxidative modification of LDL. Oxidized LDL acts as a chemoattractant, causing more monocytes to adhere to and penetrate the endothelium. In the presence of endothelial dysfunction, the increased adhesion of monocytes to the endothelial surface results in their release of growth factors and chemoattractants. As more monocytes penetrate the endothelium and move into the subendothelial space, they are converted to macrophages. Macrophages, having receptors for modified LDL, can take up more of the modified LDL, forming many intracellular lipid droplets laden with cholesterol esters, ultimately resulting in conversion of the macrophages into foam cells. These foam cells, engorged with oxidized lipid and apoproteins, may lyse, releasing their content into the extra-

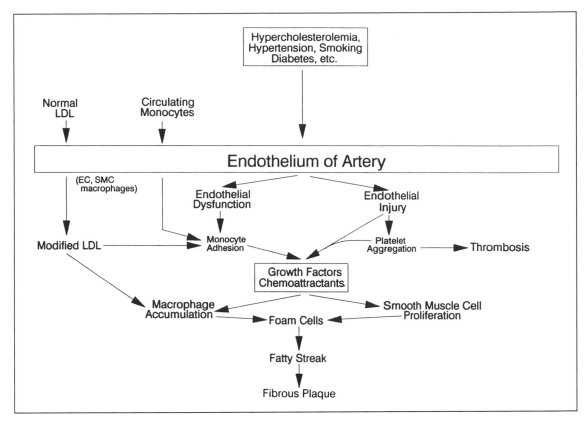

Figure 3-8.   Steps in atherosclerosis.

cellular space. This oxidized material is cyto-toxic and causes further endothelial injury. Thus, a vicious cycle develops, in which progressive endothelial injury and foam-cell production occur, accelerated by the presence of other risk factors. Ultimately, in response to progressive endothelial injury, platelets begin to adhere to the exposed underlying connective tissue and become activated, leading to the release of TXA$_2$, a vasoconstrictor that further enhances platelet aggregation. In response to increased platelet aggregation, platelet-derived growth factor (PDGF), and other similar growth factors released by monocytes, smooth muscle cells and altered endothelial cells stimulate smooth muscle cell migration and proliferation at the site of injury. These steps initiate the conversion of smooth muscle cell–derived foam cells to fatty streaks. With the concomitant increase in connective tissue formation and adhering thrombi, these fatty streaks can be converted to fibrous plaques, and further narrowing of the lumen of the artery results, eventually leading to thrombosis, luminal occlusion, and myocardial infarction.

The exact mechanisms by which risk factors directly affect the development of atherosclerosis are not well understood, but some general principles are operative. As already mentioned, it is likely that hypercholesterolemia, associated in particular with elevations of atherogenic lipoproteins, increases the infiltration of lipoproteins into the arterial wall, thereby enhancing the accumulation of intramural cholesterol. In response to the uptake of cholesterol by macrophages and smooth muscle cells, foam cells are formed leading to a cascade of events that ultimately transforms the fatty streak into the advanced lesion and the fibrous plaque. Hypertension contributes to the increased risk of atherosclerosis by enhancing the uptake of lipoproteins into the blood vessel wall and also by causing subsequent endothelial damage from the increased shear forces that result from the increase in blood pressure. Cigarette smoking probably increases the risk of atherosclerosis by multiple mechanisms, but many of the toxic products of cigarette smoke can induce hypoxia of the arterial wall, which can reduce circulating antioxidant levels so that more oxidized LDL is produced, leading to increased formation of macrophage-derived foam cells and the development of subsequent fatty streaks and fibrous plaques. Diabetes may promote the development of atherosclerosis by a combination of increases in serum lipid levels, modification of lipoproteins, and enhanced production of growth factors and chemoattractants, which may act together to accelerate the development of atherosclerosis.

Measurement Methodologies for Detecting Hypercholesterolemia

The importance given to the association between hyperlipidemia and the risk of CHD by various government and private health agencies, individual medical professionals, and the general public has made the development of accurate, precise, and reliable methods of measuring plasma lipids a top priority. In the United States efforts of the Department of Health and Human Services, the Public Health Service, and the National Institutes of Health, coordinated through the Laboratory Standardization Panel of the National Cholesterol Education Program, led to the development and subsequent publication (NIH pub. no. 90-2964) of guidelines for the measurement of plasma lipids by routine clinical laboratories. These same agencies also developed recommendations for the use of desk-top analyzers for cholesterol-screening programs, which were also subsequently published (NIH pub. no. 89-3045). Inappropriate standardization and inadequate quality control of measurements of plasma cholesterol, triglycerides, and lipoproteins by clinical laboratories and especially by users of desk-top analyzers can produce significant analytic error leading to misclassification of an individual's CHD risk. The consequences of these incorrect diagnoses can be major, leading to unnecessary

lifestyle changes, concerns, and possible pharmaceutical intervention. Brief descriptions of the recommendations given in both NIH publications follow. Those aspects of the recommendations for the measurement of plasma lipids and lipoprotein cholesterol by the routine laboratory (venipuncture sample) and the desktop analyzer (finger-prick sample) which are similar are discussed together.

VENOUS AND FINGER-PRICK SAMPLES FOR PLASMA LIPID AND LIPOPROTEIN MEASUREMENTS

Recommendations for Preanalytic Factors. It is well established that several biological factors that contribute to a patient's usual cholesterol level should be considered when preparing the patient for cholesterol measurements. Certainly both age and gender influence cholesterol level. Younger males generally have higher cholesterol levels than females, although in old age this relationship is reversed. Independent of sex, cholesterol levels tend to rise with age. Diurnal variation can influence cholesterol levels from 2 to 3 percent, such that serum cholesterols measured in the morning are often slightly higher than those determined at night. Seasonal variation can influence plasma cholesterol levels by as much as 5 percent. Cholesterol levels taken in the summer are usually lower than those taken in the winter, possibly due to seasonal changes in diet and physical activity, but in large part this difference is not well understood. Intraindividual variation, which reflects the daily biological variation that occurs within individuals independent of environmental influences, can be as high as 10 percent. Dietary fat and alcohol, as mentioned in previous sections, can influence serum cholesterol and triglyceride levels, and exercise can raise HDL levels. Certain drugs, such as hypertensive medications, including beta blockers and thiazides, and some oral contraceptives, can raise cholesterol levels. All of these phenomena are further described in the appropriate sections of this book.

In addition to these biologic factors, the Lipid Standardization Panel has made the following recommendations to control other preclinical factors that influence the cholesterol levels of all individuals:

- Individuals should be on their usual diet and their weight should be stable for at least 2 weeks before their lipids or lipoproteins are measured.
- Cholesterol measurements should be taken no sooner than 8 weeks after a myocardial infarction or any form of trauma (including surgery) or bacterial or viral infection.
- Patient preparation and blood collection procedures should be standardized in the following manner:
  — The patient should fast for at least 12 hours and not engage in any vigorous activity for 24 hours for any analyses other than total cholesterol.
  — Total cholesterol can be measured in either the fasting or the nonfasting state; however, if triglycerides and LDL cholesterol are to be measured, the patient should be instructed to take nothing by mouth, other than water, for at least 12 hours prior to sampling.
  — The patient should be in a sitting position for about 5 minutes prior to venipuncture. If a tourniquet is used, the sample should be obtained within 1 minute of tourniquet application.
  — Total cholesterol, triglycerides, and HDL can be measured in either serum or plasma. If EDTA is used as the anticoagulant, plasma cholesterol levels should be multiplied by 1.03 to obtain the true serum cholesterol measurement.

When complete lipoprotein fractionation or certain apolipoprotein measurements are to be performed, plasma should be prepared and immediately cooled to 2°C to 4°C to prevent compositional changes. When serum is used, the blood should stand for 45 minutes in a glass tube at room temperature to allow complete clotting. The serum then should be separated and ideally cooled to 2°C to 4°C before it is transported to the laboratory. For total cholesterol measurements, serum or plasma can be transported either at 4°C or frozen. Samples that are not going to be analyzed immediately should be stored frozen, preferably at −70°C or lower. All blood samples should be considered potentially infectious and should be handled accordingly. Care should be taken that the sample is not ingested or inhaled by or otherwise brought into contact with laboratory personnel. All laboratory personnel handling blood samples should use gloves and avoid leaving samples open to the atmosphere any longer than necessary.

Recommendations of the Lipid Standardization Panel for Analytic Factors. Enzymatic methods have generally replaced the strong acid methods of earlier years for routine analyses. The use of enzymes has improved specificity, permitting direct measurements without extraction or other pretreatment. Enzymatic reagents are less corrosive and thus better suited to the complex and expensive equipment in current use. Approximately 98 percent of all laboratories participating in standardized lipid measurement programs use enzymatic procedures. Because the choice of reagents can be a source of analytic error, it is important to realize that deterioration of the enzymatic reagent or variation in the source of the reagent can be a major problem. The enzymatic reagent should be (1) specific for cholesterol, (2) free from interference by other circulating substances, (3) stable, and (4) consistent from batch to batch. With regard to the instrument itself, the type of chemical analyzers, the consistency of temperature control, and the duration of sample incubation are all important factors in the reproducibility of the system. It is important to realize that every analytical system has an inherent level of reproducibility, which is a function of the instrument components. Therefore, some analytic systems, especially older or less sophisticated instruments, may not be capable of meeting some of the Lipid Standardization Panel's recommendations for both precision and accuracy. Concerning calibration, it is known that variation in calibration of an instrument is a major factor in influencing the run-to-run component of overall analytic variability and accuracy. Calibration material similar in nature to the fresh patient specimen is less likely to produce errors. The Lipid Standardization Panel recommends that calibrators and quality control materials be used with accurately assigned target values traceable to the National Resources for Cholesterol Standardization. Concerning the issues of internal quality assurance, clinical laboratories should have initial goals for analytic variation (precision) and bias (accuracy) of 5 percent or less for coefficient of variation and 5 percent or less for deviation from true value, respectively. An ideal goal of 3 percent or less for intralaboratory coefficient of variation and 3 percent or less for bias from target value should be achieved no later than 1992. Quality control materials for cholesterol should have concentrations near the two medical-decision levels for the test (i.e., 200 and 240 mg/dl). Concerning external quality control, the Lipid Standardization Panel recommends that laboratories participate in at least one external proficiency testing program. These external surveillance programs are provided by the Council for National Reference System for the Clinical Laboratory (NRSCL), the Centers for Disease Control (CDC), and the National Institute for Standards and Technology (NIST). It is recommended that any physician or health care worker who utilizes a laboratory for lipid determinations become familiar with the quality control procedures of that laboratory, the results achieved, and the laboratory's participation in an external standardization problem.

Recommendations for the Use of Desk-Top Analyzers. The precautions given concerning the standardization of plasma lipid and lipoprotein cholesterol measurement by routine clinical laboratories on venipuncture samples are even more necessary with the use of desk-top analyzers. Desk-top analyzers are particularly sensitive to physical differences between standards and biological samples. For example, lipid standards or calibrators that are dissolved in organic solvents or lyophilized may not be appropriate for estimating plasma lipids in biological samples, depending on the particular desk-top analyzer used. Some desk-top analyzers do not give reliable results on frozen serum samples. In general, most of these analyzers err on the high

side, highlighting the potential for misclassification of individuals. The need for laboratory quality control utilizing control samples that are traceable to the National Reference System for Cholesterol Measurements (NRSCM) established by the CDC and the National Bureau of Standards that are near the decision levels of 200 mg/dl and 240 mg/dl is even more critical with desk-top analyzers. The same stringent internal and external quality programs established for routine laboratory measurements of plasma lipids and lipoprotein cholesterol are also important for these machines. The same goals of acceptability of precision ($\pm 3\%$) and accuracy ($\pm 3\%$) are objectives that desk-top analyzers should attain by the year 1992. While appropriate staff training is necessary for both routine laboratory measurements of venipuncture samples and desk-top analysis of finger-prick samples, it is especially important for the latter, where environmental variables have a greater effect solely by virtue of the smaller sample volume.

Perhaps the greatest problem inherent in the use of desk-top analyzers is the setting in which they are used. Removed from the usual clinical laboratory and its system of quality control and professional supervision, these machines are used in low-volume offices, shopping malls, supermarkets, and mass screenings, where both training and quality control may be poor. Thus, results from desk-top machines, while theoretically quite reliable, must be viewed with a measure of skepticism unless one knows that operator training and quality control are optimal.

While appropriate referral and follow-up of patients is important for results obtained from both the laboratory and the screening site, it is especially critical for the latter, where convenience, ease, and rapid turnaround can often result in more people being screened than can be adequately counseled.

It should be emphasized that results from desk-top analyzers are to be used for screening, not for diagnosis. The final diagnosis should be determined by routine laboratory measurement. Although in the future it may be possible to use desk-top equipment for follow-up determination, at present the success of any diet or drug intervention should be evaluated on plasma lipids and lipoprotein cholesterol measurements performed by a clinical laboratory, not a desk-top analyzer.

References

1. Utermann G. Lipoprotein(a): a genetic risk factor for premature coronary heart disease. Current Opinion in Lipidology 1990; 1:404–10.

2. Loscalzo J. Lipoprotein(a): a unique risk factor for atherothrombotic disease. Arteriosclerosis 1990; 10:672–9.

3. Armstrong VW, Cremer P, Eberle E, et al. The association between Lp(a) concentrations and angiographically assessed coronary atherosclerosis — dependence on serum LDL levels. Atherosclerosis 1986; 62:249–57.

4. Rath M, Niendorf A, Reblin T, et al. Detection and quantification of lipoprotein(a) in the arterial wall of 107 coronary bypass patients. Arteriosclerosis 1989; 9:579–92.

5. Cushing GL, Ganbatz JW, Nava ML, et al. Quantitation and localization of apolipoprotein(a) and B in coronary artery bypass vein grafts resected at re-operation. Arteriosclerosis 1989; 9:593–603.

6. Utermann G, Steinmetz A, Weber W. Genetic control of human apolipoprotein e polymorphism: comparison of one- and two-dimensional techniques of isoprotein analysis. Hum Genet 1982; 60:344–51.

7. Schaefer EJ, Levy RI. Pathogenesis and management of lipoprotein disorders. N Engl J Med 1985; 312:1300–10.

8. Reardon MD, Poapst ME, Steiner G. The independent synthesis of intermediate density lipoproteins in Type III hyperlipoproteinemia. Metabolism 1982; 31:421–7.

9. Soutar AK, Myant NB, Thompson GR. Simultaneous measurement of apolipoprotein B turnover in very low and low density lipoproteins in familial hypercholesterolemia. Atherosclerosis 1977; 28:247–56.

10. Naraya N, Chung BH, Tauntin OD. Synthesis of plasma lipoproteins by the isolated perfused liver from the fasted and fed pig. J Biol Chem 1977; 252:5258–61.

11. Huff MW, Telford DE. Direct synthesis of low density lipoprotein apoprotein B in the miniature pig. Metabolism 1985; 34:36–42.

12. Spady DK, Dietschy JM. Interaction of dietary cholesterol and triglycerides in the regulation of hepatic low density lipoprotein transport in the hamster. J Clin Invest 1988; 81:300–9.

13. Spady DK, Turley SD, Dietschy JM. Rates of low density lipoprotein uptake and cholesterol synthesis are regulated independently in the liver. J Lipid Res 1985; 26:465–72.

14. Kesaniemi YA, Witzum JL, Steinbrecher UP. Receptor mediated catabolism of low density lipoprotein in man. Quantitation using glycosolated low density lipoprotein. J Clin Invest 1983; 71:950–9.

15. Bilheimer DW, Watanabe Y, Kita T. Impaired receptor-mediated catabolism of low density lipoprotein in the WHHL rabbit, an animal model of familial hypercholesterolemia. Proc Natl Acad Sci USA 1982; 79:3305–9.

16. Kovanen PT, Brown MS, Basu SK, et al. Saturation and suppression of hepatic lipoprotein receptors: a mechanism for the hypercholesterolemia of cholesterol-fed rabbits. Proc Natl Acad Sci USA 1981; 78:1396–1400.

17. Packard CJ, McKinney L, Carr K, Shepherd J. Cholesterol feeding increases low density lipoprotein synthesis. J Clin Invest 1983; 72:45–51.

18. Shepherd J, Packard CJ, Grundy SM, et al. Effects of saturated and polyunsaturated fat diets on the chemical composition and metabolism of low density lipoproteins in man. J Lipid Res 1980; 21:91–9.

19. Spady DK, Dietschy JM. Dietary saturated triacylglycerols suppress hepatic low density lipoprotein receptors in the hamster. Proc Soc Natl Acad Sci USA. 1985; 82:4526–30.

20. Nicolosi RJ, Stucchi AF, Kowala MC, et al. Effect of dietary fat saturation and cholesterol on LDL composition and metabolism. Arteriosclerosis 1990; 10:119–28.

21. Windler EE, Kovanen PT, Chao YS, et al. The estradiol-stimulated lipoprotein receptor of rat liver: a binding site that membrane mediates the uptake of rat lipoproteins containing apoproteins B and E. J Biol Chem 1980; 255:10464–71.

22. Miller NE. Why does plasma low density lipoprotein concentration in adults increase with age? Lancet 1984; 1:263–6.

23. Grundy SM, Vega GL, Bilheimer DW. Kinetic mechanisms determining variability in low density lipoprotein levels and their rise with age. Arteriosclerosis 1985; 5:623–30.

24. Brown MS, Goldstein JL. A receptor-mediated pathway for cholesterol homeostasis. Science 1986; 232:34–47.

25. Krempler F, Kostner GM, Rascher A, et al. Studies on the role of specific cell surface receptors in the removal of lipoprotein (a) in man. J Clin Invest 1983; 71:1431–41.

26. Hackes L, Jurgens G, Holasek A, van Berkel TJC. In vivo studies on the binding sites for lipoprotein (a) in parenchymal and nonparenchymal rat liver cells. FEBS Lett 1988; 227:27–31.

27. Karadi I, Kostner GM, Gries A, et al. Lipoprotein (a) and plasminogen are immunochemically related. Biochim Biophys Acta 1988; 960:91–7.

28. Oram JF. Cholesterol trafficking in cells. Current Opinion in Lipidology: Atherosclerosis-cell Biology and Lipoproteins 1990; 1:416–21.

29. Rifai N. Lipoproteins and apolipoproteins–composition, metabolism and association with coronary heart disease. Arch Pathol Lab Med 1986; 110:694–701.

30. National Cholesterol Education Program Expert Panel. Report on detection, evaluation, and treatment of high blood cholesterol in adults. Arch Intern Med 1988; 148:36–69.

31. The Lipid Research Clinics Population Studies Data Book. Vol. 1. The Prevalence Study. U.S. Department of Health and Human Services, Public Health Service. USDHHS publ. no. (NIH) 80-1527, 1980; 28–81.

32. Krauss RM, Levy RI, Fredrickson DS. Selective measurement of two lipase activities in postheparin plasma from normal subjects and patients with hyperlipoproteinemia. J Clin Invest 1974; 54:1107–12.

33. Breckenridge WC, Little JA, Steiner G, et al. Hypertriglyceridemia associated with a deficiency of apolipoprotein C-II. N Engl J Med 1978; 298:1265–73.

34. Goldstein JL, Brown MS. Familial hypercholesterolemia. In: Scriver CR, Beaudet AL, Sly WS, Valle D, eds. The metabolic basis of inherited disease. New York: McGraw Hill, 1989; 1215.

35. Vega GL, Grundy SM. In vivo evidence for reduced binding of low density lipoproteins to receptors as a cause of primary moderate hypercholesterolemia. J Clin Invest 1986; 78:1410–8.

36. Innerarity TL, Weisgraber KH, Arnold KS, et al. Familial defective apolipoprotein B-100: low density lipoproteins with abnormal receptor binding. Proc Natl Acad Sci USA 1987; 84:6919–25.

37. Sprecher DS, Schaefer EJ, Kent KM, et al. Cardiovascular features of homozygous familial hypercholesterolemia. Am J Cardiol 1984; 54:20–30.

38. Mabuchi H, Sakari T, Sakai Y, et al. Reduction of serum cholesterol in heterozygous patients with familial hypercholesterolemia: additive effects of compactin and cholestyramine. N Engl J Med 1983; 308:609–14.

39. Illingworth DR. Mevinolin plus colestipol in therapy for severe heterozygous familial hypercholesterolemia. Ann Intern Med 1984; 101:598–604.

40. Thompson GR, Miller JP, Breslow JL. Improved survival of patients with homozygous familial hypercholesterolemia treated with plasma exchange. Br Med J 1985; 291:1671–8.

40a. Keller C. LDL-apheresis — Results of long-term treatment and vascular outcome. Atherosclerosis 1991; 86:1–8.

40b. Kim SS, Kutsumi Y, Nakai T, et al. In vitro characterization of two types of LDL apheresis module and effect of repetitive LDL apheresis on plasma cholesterol levels and aortic atherosclerosis in heterozygous WHHL rabbits. Japanese Circ J (English Edition) 1991; 55:68–80.

41. Morganroth J, Levy RI, Fredrickson DS. The biochemical, clinical and genetic features of type III hyperlipoproteinemia. Ann Intern Med 1975; 82:158–63.

42. Hazzard WR, O'Donnell TF, Lee YL. Broad-beta disease (type III hyperlipoproteinemia) in a large kindred. Evidence for monogenic mechanism. Ann Intern Med 1975; 92:141.

43. Kris-Etherton PM, Cooper AD. Studies on the etiology of the hyperlipidemia in rats fed an atherogenic diet. J Lipid Res 1980; 21:435–42.

44. Utermann G, Pruin N, Steinmetz A. Polymorphism of apolipoprotein E and occurrence of dysbetalipoproteinemia in man. Nature 1977; 269:604–8.

45. Rall SC JR, Weisgraber KH, Innerarity TL, et al. Identical structural and receptor binding defects in apolipoprotein E2 in hypo-, normo-, and hypercholesterolemic dysbetalipoproteinemia. J Clin Invest 1983; 71:1023–30.

46. Schaefer EJ (discussant). Dietary and drug treatment, in type III hyperlipoproteinemia: diagnosis, molecular defects, pathology, and treatment. HB Brewer Jr (moderator). Ann Intern Med 1983; 98:part 1:633–7.

47. Genest JJ Jr, Martin-Munley S, McNamara JR, et al. Frequency of genetic dyslipidemia in patients with premature coronary artery disease. Circulation 1989; 9:701A.

48. Brunzell JD, Schrott HG, Motulsky AG, Bierman EL. Myocardial infarction in the familial forms of hypertriglyceridemia. Metabolism 1976; 25:313–8.

49. Janus ED, Nicoll AM, Turner PR, et al. Kinetic bases of the primary hyperlipidemias: studies of apolipoprotein B turnover in genetically defined subjects. Eur J Clin Invest 1980; 10:161–72.

50. Chait A, Albers JJ, Brunzell JD. Very low density lipoprotein overproduction in genetic forms of hypertriglyceridemia. Eur J Clin Invest 1980; 10:17–22.

51. Chait A, Foster D, Albers JJ, Brunzell JD. Familial hypercholesterolemia vs. familial combined hyperlipidemia: low density lipoprotein apolipoprotein-B kinetics. Arteriosclerosis 1981; 1:82a.

52. Kissebah AH, Alfarsi S, Adams PW. Integrated regulation of very low density lipoprotein triglyceride and apolipoprotein B kinetics in man: normolipidemic subjects, familial hypertriglyceridemia, and familial combined hyperlipidemia. Metabolism 1982; 30:856–68.

53. Beil V, Grundy SM, Crouse JR, Zech L. Triglyceride and cholesterol metabolism in primary hypertriglyceridemia. Arteriosclerosis 1982; 2:44–57.

54. Kesaniemi YA, Grundy SM. Overproduction of low density lipoproteins associated with coronary heart disease. Arteriosclerosis 1983; 3:40–6.

55. Brunzell JD, Albers JJ, Chait A, et al. Plasma lipoproteins in familial combined hyperlipidemia and monogenic familial hypertriglyceridemia. J Lipid Res 1983; 24:147–55.

56. Schaefer EJ, Ordovas JM. Metabolism of the apolipoproteins A-I, A-II, and A-IV. In: J. Segrest, J. Albers, eds. Methods in enzymology, plasma lipoproteins. Part B: characterization, cell biology and metabolism. New York: Academic Press 1985; 129:420–42.

57. Sigurdsson G, Nicoll A, Lewis B. The metabolism of very low density lipoproteins in hyperlipidemia: studies of apolipoprotein B kinetics in man. Eur J Clin Invest 1970; 6:167–77.

58. Greenberg BH, Blackwelder WC, Levy RI. Primary type V hyperlipoproteinemia. A descriptive study in 32 families. Ann Intern Med 1977; 87:526–34.

59. Saku K, Gartside PS, Hynd BA, Kashyap ML. Mechanism of action of gemfibrozil on lipoprotein metabolism. J Clin Invest 1985; 75:1702–12.

60. Dahlen GH, Guyton JR, Attar M, et al. Association of levels of lipoprotein Lp(a), plasma lipids, and other lipoproteins with coronary artery disease documented by angiography. Circulation 1986; 74:758–65.

61. Kostner GM, Avogaro P, Cazzolato G, et al. Lipoprotein Lp(a) and the risk for myocardial infarction. Atherosclerosis 1981; 38:51–61.

62. Hajjar KA, Gavish D, Breslow JL, Nachman RL. Lipoprotein (a) modulation of endothelial cell surface fibrinolysis and its potential role in atherosclerosis. Nature 1989; 339:303–5.

63. Loscalzo J, Weinfeld M, Gless GM, Scanu AM. Lipoprotein (a), fibrin binding and plasminogen activation. Arteriosclerosis 1990; 10:240–5.

64. Seed M, Hoppicher F, Reaveley D, et al. Relation of serum lipoprotein (a) concentration and apolipoprotein (a) phenotype to coronary heart disease in patients with familial hypercholesterolemia. N Engl J Med 1990; 322: 1494–9.

65. Gurakar A, Hoeg JM, Kostner G, et al. Levels of lipoprotein Lp(a) decline with neomycin and niacin treatment. Atherosclerosis 1985; 57:293–301.

66. Sniderman AD, Wolfson C, Teng B, et al. Association of hyperapobetalipoproteinemia with endogenous hypertriglyceridemia and atherosclerosis. Ann Intern Med 1982; 97:833–9.

67. Teng B, Thompson GR, Sniderman AD, et al. Composition and distribution of low density lipoprotein fractions in hyperapobetalipoproteinemia, normolipidemia, and familial hypercholesterolemia. Proc Natl Acad Sci USA 1983; 80:6662–6.

68. Sniderman AD, Teng B, Genest J, et al. Familial aggregation and early expression of hyperapobetalipoproteinemia. Am J Cardiol 1985; 55:291–5.

69. Genest J, Sniderman A, Cianflone K, et al. Hyperapobetalipoproteinemia. Plasma lipoprotein response to oral fat load. Arteriosclerosis 1986; 6:297–304.

70. Glueck CJ, Fallat RW, Millett F, et al. Familial hyperalphalipoproteinemia: studies in eighteen kindreds. Metabolism 1975; 24:1243–65.

71. Glueck CJ, Gartside PM, Tsang RC, et al. Neonatal familial hyperalphalipoproteinemia. Metabolism 1977; 26:469–74.

72. Inazu A, Brown ML, Hesler CB, et al. Increased lipoprotein levels caused by a common cholesteryl-ester transfer protein gene mutation. N Engl J Med 1990; 323:1234–8.

73. Gotto AM, Levy RI, John K, Fredrickson DS. On the nature of the protein defect in abetalipoproteinemia. N Engl J Med 1971; 284:813–8.

74. Lackner KJ, Monge JC, Gregg RE, et al. Analysis of the apolipoprotein B gene and messenger ribonucleic acid in abetalipoproteinemia. J Clin Invest 1986; 78:1701–12.

75. Muller DPR, Lloyd JK, Bird AC. Long-term management of abetalipoproteinemia. Arch Dis Child 1977; 52:209–14.

76. Muller DPR, Lloyd JK, Wolff OH. Vitamin E and neurological function. Lancet 1983; 1:225–7.

77. Hegele RA, Angel A. Arrest of neuropathy and myopathy in abetalipoproteinemia with high dose vitamin E therapy. Can Med Assoc J 1985; 12:41–5.

78. Levy RI, Langer T, Gotto AM, Fredrickson DS. Familial hypobetalipoproteinemia, a defect in lipoprotein synthesis. Clin Res 1970; 18:539–49.

79. Cottrill C, Glueck CJ, Leuba V, et al. Familial homozygous hypobetalipoproteinemia. Metabolism 1974; 23:779–91.

80. Berger GMB, Brown G, Henderson HE, Bon-

nici F. Apolipoprotein B detected in the plasma of a patient with homozygous hypobetalipoproteinemia: implications for aetiology. J Med Genet 1983; 20:189–97.

81. Ross RS, Gregg RE, Law SW, et al. Homozygous hypobetalipoproteinemia: a disease distinct from abetalipoproteinemia at the molecular level. J Clin Invest 1988; 81:590–601.

82. Steinberg D, Grundy SM, Mok HI, et al. Metabolic studies in an unusual case of asymptomatic familial hypobetalipoproteinemia and fasting chylomicronemia. J Clin Invest 1979; 64:292–301.

83. Young SG, Northey ST, McCarthy BJ. Low plasma cholesterol levels caused by a short deletion in the apo B gene. Science 1988; 241: 591–3.

84. Collins DR, Knott TJ, Pease RJ, et al. Truncated variants of apolipoprotein B cause hypobetalipoproteinemia. Nucleic Acids Res 1988; 16:8361–75.

85. Young SG, Peralta FP, Dubois BW, et al. Lipoprotein B37, a naturally occuring lipoprotein containing the amino-terminal portion of apolipoprotein B-100, does not bind to the apolipoprotein B,E (low density lipoprotein) receptor. J Biol Chem 1987; 262:16604–12.

86. Young SG, Bertics SJ, Curtis LK, et al. Genetic analysis of a kindred with familial hypobetalipoproteinemia; evidence for two separate gene defects: one associated with an abnormal apolipoprotein B species, apo B-37, and a second associated with low plasma concentrations of apo B-100. J Clin Invest 1987; 79:1842–51.

87. Vergani C, Bettale A. Familial hypoalphalipoproteinemia. Clin Chem Acta 1981; 114:45–52.

88. Third JLHC, Montag J, Flynn M, et al. Primary and familial hypoalphalipoproteinemia. Metabolism 1984; 33:136–46.

89. Le AN, Ginzberg HN. Heterogeneity of apolipoprotein A-I turnover with reduced concentrations of plasma high density lipoprotein cholesterol. Metabolism 1988; 37:614–7.

90. Schaefer EJ, Heaton, WH, Wetzel MG, Brewer HB Jr. Plasma apolipoprotein A-I absence associated with a marked reduction of high density lipoproteins and premature coronary artery disease. Arteriosclerosis 1982; 2:16–26.

91. Schaefer EJ, Ordovas JM, Law S, et al. Familial apolipoprotein A-I and C-III deficiency, variant II. J Lipid Res 1985; 26:1089–1101.

92. Ordovas JM, Cassidy DK, Civeira F, et al. Familial apolipoprotein A-I, C-III, and A-IV deficiency with marked high density lipoprotein deficiency and premature atherosclerosis due to a deletion of the apolipoprotein A-I, C-III, and A-IV gene complex. J Biol Chem 1989; 264:16339–42.

93. Norum RA, Lakier JB, Goldstein S, et al. Familial deficiency of apolipoproteins A-I and C-III and precocious coronary artery disease. N Engl J Med 1982; 306:1513–9.

94. Norum RA, Forte TM, Alaupovic P, Ginsberg HN. Clinical syndrome and lipid metabolism in hereditary deficiency of apolipoproteins A-I and C-III, variant I. Adv Exp Med Biol 1986; 201:137–49.

95. Karathanasis SK, Haddad I. DNA inversion within the apolipoprotein A-I/C-III/A-IV encoding gene cluster of certain patients with premature atherosclerosis. Proc Natl Acad Sci USA 1987; 84:7198–202.

96. Schmitz G, Lackner K. High density lipoprotein deficiency with xanthomas: a defect in apo A-I synthesis. Crepaldi G, Gotto AM, Manzato E, Baggio G., eds. Atherosclerosis VIII. Excerpta Medica Amsterdam 1989; 399.

97. Fredrickson DS, Altrocchi PH, Avioli LV, et al. Tangier disease — combined clinical staff conference at the National Institutes of Health. Ann Intern Med 1961; 55:1016.

98. Schaefer EJ, Zech LA, Schwartz DE, Brewer HB Jr. Coronary heart disease prevalence and other clinical features in familial high density lipoprotein deficiency (Tangier disease). Ann Intern Med 1980; 93:261.

99. Norum KR, Gjone E, Glomset JA. Familial lecithin: cholesterol acyltransferase deficiency including fish eye disease. In: Scriver CR, Beaudet AL, Sly WS, Valle D eds. Metabolic basis of inherited disease. New York: McGraw Hill, 1989; 1181–94.

100. Havel RJ, Goldstein JL, Brown MS. Lipoproteins and lipid transport. In: Bondy P. Rosenberg LE, eds. Metabolic control and disease. Philadelphia: W. B. Saunders, 1980; 393–494.

101. Hazzard WR, Haffner SM, Kushwaha RS, et al. Preliminary report: Kinetic studies on the modulation of high density lipoprotein, apolipoprotein, and subfraction metabolism by sex steroids in a post-menopausal woman. Metabolism 1984; 33:779–84.

102. Haffner WR, Kushwaha RS, Foster DM, et al. Studies on the metabolic mechanism of reduced high density lipoproteins during anabolic steroid therapy. Metab Clin Exp 1983; 32: 413–20.

103. Kesaniemi YA, Miettinen TA. Cholesterol absorption efficiency regulates plasma cholesterol level in the Finnish population. Eur J Clin Invest 1987; 17:391–5.

104. Kesaniemi YA, Ehnholm C, Miettinen TA. Intestinal cholesterol absorption efficiency in man is related to apoprotein E phenotype. J Clin Invest 1987; 80:578–81.

105. Miettinen TA, Kesaniemi YA. Cholesterol ab-

sorption: regulation of cholesterol synthesis and elimination and within population variations of serum cholesterol levels. Am J Clin Nutr 1989; 49:629–35.

106. McNamara DJ, Kolb R, Parker TS, et al. Heterogeneity of cholesterol homeostasis in man. J Clin Invest 1987; 79:1729–39.

107. Miettenen TA. Fecal fat bile acid excretion, and body height in familial hypercholesterolemia and hypertriglyceridemia. Scand J Clin Lab Invest 1972; 30: 85–8.

108. Keys A, Anderson JT, Frande F. Serum cholesterol response to changes in the diet. IV. Particular saturated fatty acids in the diet. Metabolism 1965; 14:776–87.

109. Hegsted DM, McGandy RB, Myers ML, Stare FJ. Quantitative effects of dietary fat on serum cholesterol in man. Am J Clin Nutr 1965; 17:281–95.

110. Mattson FH, Grundy SM. Comparison of effects of dietary saturated, monounsaturated and polyunsaturated fatty acids on plasma lipids and lipoproteins in man. J Lipid Res 1985; 26:194–202.

111. Grundy SM, Vega GL. Plasma cholesterol responsiveness to saturated fatty acids. Am J Clin Nutr 1988; 47:822–4.

112. Bonanome A, Grundy SM. Effect of dietary stearic acid on plasma cholesterol and lipoprotein levels. N Eng J Med 1988; 318:1244–8.

113. Fox JC, McGill Jr. HC, Carey KD, Getz GS. In vivo regulation of hepatic LDL receptor mRNA in the baboon: differential effects of saturated and unsaturated fat. J Biol Chem 1987; 262:7014–20.

113a. Grundy SM. Multifactorial etiology of hypercholesterolemia: implications for prevention of coronary heart disease. Arteriosclerosis and Thrombosis 1991; 11:1619–35.

113b. Dawson PA, Hofmann SL, van der Westhuyzen et al. Sterol-dependent depression of low density lipoprotein receptor promoter mediated by 16 base pair sequence adjacent to binding site for transcription factor Sp1. J Biol Chem 1988; 263:3372–9.

114. Kuo PC, Rudd MA, Nicolosi RJ, Loscalzo J. L. Effect of dietary fat saturation and cholesterol on low density lipoprotein degradation by mononuclear cells of cebus monkeys. Arteriosclerosis 1989; 9:919–27.

115. Loscalzo JL, Freedman J, Rudd MA, et al. Unsaturated fatty acids enhance low density lipoprotein uptake and degradation by peripheral blood mononuclear cells. Arteriosclerosis 1987; 7:450–5.

116. Noel S-P, Wong L, Dolphin PJ, et al. Secretion of cholesterol-rich lipoproteins by perfused livers of hypercholesterolemic rats. J Clin Invest 1979; 64:674–83.

117. Swift LL, Manowitz NR, Dun GD, et al. Cholesterol and saturated fat diet induces hepatic synthesis of cholesterol-rich lipoproteins. Clin Res 1979; 27:378A.

118. Grande F. Dog serum lipid responses to dietary fats differing in the chain length of the saturated fatty acids. J Nutr 1962; 76:255–64.

119. Hashim SA, Arteaga A, van Itallie TB. Effect of a saturated medium-chain triglyceride on serum lipids in man. Lancet 1960; 1:1105–8.

120. St. John LC, Young CR, Knabe DA, et al. Fatty acid profiles and sensory and carcass traits of tissues from steers and swine fed an elevated monounsaturated fat diet. J Anim Sci 1987; 64:1441–7.

121. Kinsell LW, Partridge WJ, Boling L, et al. Dietary modification of serum cholesterol and phospholipid levels. J Clin Endocrinol 1952; 12:909–13.

122. Kinsell LW, Michaels GD, Partridge JW, et al. Effect upon serum cholesterol and phospholipids of diets containing large amounts of vegetable fat. J Clin Nutr 1953; 1:231–44.

123. Ahrens EH, Hirsch J, Insull W, et al. The influence of dietary fats on serum-lipid levels in man. Lancet 1957; 1:943–53.

124. Mensink RP, Katan MB. Effect of a diet enriched with monounsaturated or polyunsaturated fatty acids on levels of low density and high density lipoprotein cholesterol in healthy women and men. N Engl J Med 1989; 321:436–41.

125. Dreon DM, Vranizan KM, Krauss RM, et al. The effects of polyunsaturated fat vs. monounsaturated fat on plasma lipoproteins. JAMA 1990; 263:2462–6.

126. Grundy SM, Denke MA. Dietary influences on serum lipids and lipoproteins. J Lipid Res 1990; 31:1149–72.

127. Vergroesen AJ. Dietary fat and cardiovascular disease: possible modes of action of linoleic acid. Proc Nutr Soc 1972; 31:323–9.

128. Grasso S, Gunning B, Imaichi K, et al. Effects of natural and hydrogenated fats of approximately equal dienoic acid content upon plasma lipids. Metabolism 1962; 11:920–4.

129. McOsker DE, Mattson FH, Swerningen HB, Kligman AM. The influence of partially hydrogenated dietary fats on serum cholesterol levels. JAMA 1962; 180:380–5.

130. Erickson BA, Coots RH, Mattson FH, Kligman AM. The effect of partial hydrogenation of dietary fats, of the ratio of polyunsaturated to saturated fatty acids and of dietary cholesterol upon plasma lipids in man. J Clin Invest 1964; 43:2017–25.

131. Mattson FH, Hollenback EJ, Kligman AM. Effect of hydrogenated fat on plasma cholesterol

and triglyceride levels of man. Am J Clin Nutr 1975; 28:726–31.

132. Laine DC, Snodgrass CM, Dawson EA, et al. Lightly hydrogenated soy oil versus other vegetable oils as a lipid lowering dietary constituent. Am J Clin Nutr 1982; 35:583–90.

133. Mensink RP, Katan MB. Effect of dietary trans fatty acids on high density and low density lipoprotein cholesterol levels in healthy subjects. N Eng J Med 1990; 323:439–45.

134. David JSK, Bazzan A, Weaver J, et al. Cholesterol lowering mechanism by omega 3 fatty acids in rat models. Arteriosclerosis 1987; 7:535a.

135. Davis JSK, de Pace N, Noval J, Reichle FA. Cholesterol-lowering mechanism of fish oil rich in omega 3 fatty acids in cardiac patients. Arteriosclerosis 1987; 7:512b.

136. Parks JS, Bullock BC, Rudel LL. The reactivity of plasma phospholipids with lecithin: cholesterol acyl transferase is decreased in fish oil-fed monkeys. J Biol Chem 1989; 264:2545–51.

137. Haug A, Hostmark AT. Lipoprotein lipases, lipoproteins and tissue lipids in rats fed fish oil or coconut oil. J Nutr 1987; 117:1011–6.

138. Failor RA, Childs MT, Bierman E. The effects of ω-3 and ω-6 fatty acid-enriched diets on plasma lipoprotein and apoproteins in familial combined hyperlipidemia. Metabolism 1988; 37:1021–7.

139. Kesaniemi YA, Grundy SM. Increased low density lipoprotein production associated with obesity. Arteriosclerosis 1983; 3:170–7.

140. Kesaniemi YA, Beltz WF, Grundy SM. Comparisons of metabolism of apolipoprotein B in normal subjects, obese patients and patients with coronary heart disease. J Clin Invest 1985; 76:586–95.

141. Egusa G, Beltz WF, Grundy SM, Howard BV. The influence of obesity on the metabolism of apolipoprotein B in man. J Clin Invest 1985; 76:596–603.

142. Cagguila AW, Christakis G, Ferrand M, et al. The multiple risk factor intervention trial (MRFIT) IV: Intervention on blood lipids. Prevent Med 1981; 10:443–75.

143. Nestel PJ, Hirsch EZ. Mechanism of alcohol-induced hypertriglyceridemia. J Lab Clin Med 1965; 66:357–65.

144. Baraona E, Lieber CS. Effects of ethanol on lipid metabolism. J Lipid Res 1975; 20:289–315.

145. Nikkila EA. Influence of dietary fructose and sucrose on serum triglycerides in hypertriglyceridemia and diabetes. In: Sipple H, McNutt KW, eds. Sugars in nutrition. New York: Academic Press, 1974; 439–48.

146. Wolfe BM, Havel RJ, Marlis EB, et al. Effects of a 3-day fast and ethanol on splanchnic metabolism of FFA, amino acids, and carbohydrates in healthy young men. J Clin Invest 1976; 57:329–40.

147. Blum CB, Levy RI, Eisenberg S, et al. High density lipoprotein metabolism in man. J Clin Invest 1977; 60:795–807.

148. Shepherd J, Packard CJ, Patsch JR, et al. Effects of dietary polyunsaturated and saturated fat on the properties of high density lipoprotein and metabolism of apolipoprotein A-I. J Clin Invest 1978; 61:1582–92.

149. Brinton EA, Eisenberg S, Breslow JL. Elevated high density lipoprotein cholesterol levels correlate with decreased apolipoprotein A-I and A-II fractional catabolism rate in women. J Clin Invest 1989; 84:262–9.

150. Chong KS. Nicolosi RJ, Rodger RF, et al. Effect of dietary fat saturation on plasma lipoproteins and high density lipoprotein metabolism of the rhesus monkey. J Clin Invest 1987; 79:675–83.

151. Parks JS, Rudel LL. Different kinetic fates of apolipoprotein A-I and A-II from lymph chylomicra of nonhuman primates. Effect of saturated vs. polyunsaturated dietary fat. J Lipid Res 1982; 23:410–21.

152. Sorci-Thomas M, Prack MM, Dashti N, et al. Differential effects of dietary fat on the tissue-specific expression of the apolipoprotein A-I gene: relationship to plasma concentration of high density lipoproteins. J Lipid Res 1989; 30:1397–1403.

153. Herbert PN, Bernier DN, Cullinane EM, et al. High density lipoprotein metabolism in runners and sedentary men. JAMA 1984; 252:1034–7.

154. Cluett-Brown J, Mullitan J, Igoe F, et al. Ethanol induced alterations in low and high density lipoproteins. Proc Soc Exp Biol Med 1985; 178:495–500.

155. Baraona E, Lieber CS. Effects of chronic ethanol feeding on serum lipoprotein metabolism in the rat. J Clin Invest 1970; 49:769–77.

156. Ross R. The pathogenesis of atherosclerosis — an update. N Engl J Med 1986; 314:488–500.

157. Steinberg D, Parthasarathy S, Carew TE, et al. Modifications of low-density lipoprotein that increase its atherogenicity. N Engl J Med 1989; 320:915–24.

158. Nicolosi RJ and Stucchi AF. n-3 fatty acids and atherosclerosis. Current Opinion in Lipidology 1990; 1:442–8.

4

The Rationale for Intervention

IRA S. OCKENE

EDITORS' INTRODUCTION

In this chapter we build upon the epidemiologic and lipid data already presented to derive the rationale for intervention for the prevention of CHD. We discuss the animal studies that clarified the pathophysiology of atherosclerosis and then examine the clinical trials that ultimately led to the present-day recommendations for risk-factor change. The particular problem of intervention in the elderly is then addressed, and two areas that generate more controversy than they should are clarified: the population approach versus the "high-risk" approach, and the "diet-heart" controversy. The chapter concludes with a discussion of relative risk versus attributable risk, a statistical concept that seems to cause much confusion, and a suggested methodology for the assessment of individual risk derived from the Framingham Heart Study.

Previous chapters have emphasized the great contribution that the epidemiologic method has made to our understanding of the atherosclerotic disorders. But epidemiologic investigation forms only one aspect of the many-faceted base of information that underlies the rationale for a forceful approach to the prevention of the atherosclerotic disorders. At the same time as large-scale population-based investigations were being undertaken, laboratory investigators were carrying out a series of animal experiments that gave us a truer picture of the pathophysiology of atherosclerosis. In this chapter we discuss these studies and then present the clinical intervention studies that grew out of the knowledge gained from epidemiologic and animal investigations and that provided the capstone in our understanding of the rationale for intervention. Finally we present an updated tool for assessing an individual's risk for coronary heart disease (CHD).

Animal Studies

Chapter 3 described the physiologic basis for the formation of the atherosclerotic plaque and Chapter 1 delineated the interrelationship between risk factors for CHD and the development of clinical disease. These discussions emphasized the primacy of the lipid abnormality in the development of CHD. In experimental animal models all of these observations are borne out, and we have the opportunity to observe the development of atherosclerotic lesions over a relatively short period of time, to observe in a controlled situation the manner in which the atherosclerotic plaque develops and those factors that affect its development and progression, and, ultimately, to gain an understanding of the manner in which the course of the atherosclerotic process can be slowed, arrested, and even reversed.

Atherosclerosis in animal models, especially in monkeys and swine, closely resembles that seen in humans [1, 2, 3, 4, 5]. Although developing over a much shorter period of time, the nature of the observed plaques — necrotic core, cholesterol clefts, and fibrous cap — is the same (Figure 4-1). In 1962 Taylor et al. reported

in a summary article the results of their early studies on the Rhesus monkey [2]. They utilized an atherogenic diet composed of normal monkey chow (175 g) to which had been added butterfat (30 g) and cholesterol (3 g). The mean serum cholesterol level, which had been 154 mg/dl on the control diet, rose to 382 mg/dl on the atherogenic diet, with 14 of 15 experimental animals having cholesterol levels greater than 250 mg/dl. Atherosclerosis developed in all but the one animal that was resistant to the atherosclerotic diet (her cholesterol level rose to only 192 mg/dl). Taylor and his colleagues made the following observations:

- The level of serum cholesterol required for the development of atherosclerosis in the Rhesus monkey seemed very similar to that of humans. No deposition of lipids in the arterial intima was seen when serum cholesterol levels were under 200 mg/dl. Lesions were always seen with cholesterol levels over 250 mg/dl; vascular injury reduced this to the 225-mg/dl level [6].
- The distribution of the atherosclerosis seen was strikingly similar to that seen in humans. Furthermore, the pattern of development was similar to that seen in humans, with the earliest lesions occurring in the aortic arch, the thoracic and abdominal aorta, the iliac arteries, the proximal coronary arteries (especially at branch points), and the coronary sinuses. Later on the coronary arteries became more heavily involved.
- Fatal myocardial infarction and gangrene of a lower extremity associated with atherosclerosis and thrombosis of the femoral and popliteal arteries was seen in monkeys with diet-induced atherosclerosis [7, 8].

In many ways the animal model, with atherosclerosis forced over a short period of time by a diet leading to very high serum cholesterol levels, is similar to the situation seen in humans with homozygous type II familial hyperlipidemia, where lesions develop in childhood as a consequence of markedly elevated blood cholesterol levels, but the lesions are pathologically no different than those seen in older patients

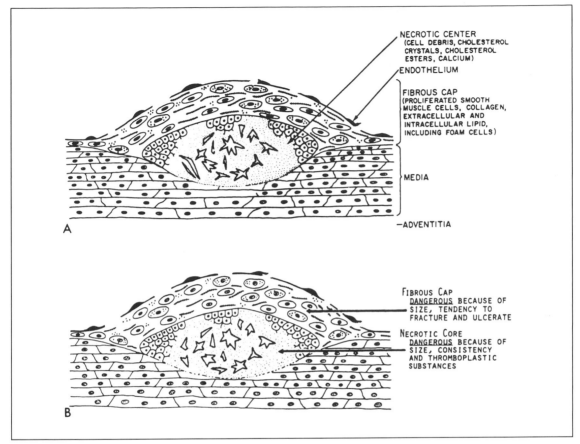

Figure 4-1. The nature of the atherosclerotic plaque. (Source: Wissler et al. Prev Med 12:84–99, 1983.)

with nonfamilial CHD [9]. These early studies and their favorable comparison with human atherosclerosis established the value of the animal model [10].

Later experiments looked at both the induction of atherosclerosis and its subsequent possible regression upon return of the animals to their normal low-saturated-fat, low-cholesterol diet. In a typical experiment carried out by Armstrong and colleagues involving the Rhesus monkey, a high-saturated-fat, high-cholesterol diet produced significant coronary atherosclerosis at the end of 17 months [11]. In this study the monkeys were divided into four groups. A control group was fed a low-fat, cholesterol-free diet throughout the 40-month study. The other monkeys were fed a high-saturated-fat, high-cholesterol diet for the first 17 months,

after which time they were divided into three groups: a group examined at autopsy for baseline atherosclerosis (group 1); a group fed a cholesterol-free, low-fat diet (group 2); and a group fed a cholesterol-free but relatively high-fat diet whose fat was provided by corn oil, an oil rich in polyunsaturated linoleate (group 3) (Table 4-1).

The high-saturated-fat, high-cholesterol diet produced a rapid rise in serum cholesterol from a control level of approximately 140 mg/dl (a level similar to that seen in humans eating a vegetarian diet) to a level of 700 mg/dl (similar to that seen in homozygous type II familial hyperlipidemia) (Table 4-2).

The diet-induced changes in serum cholesterol were associated with striking differences in the degree of atherosclerosis found at autopsy. The overall luminal narrowing found at

Table 4-1.   Rhesus monkey regression study — components of the diets

| | *Percentage of calories* | | |
	Group I *Atherogenic diet*	*Group II* *Low-fat diet*	*Group III* *Corn oil diet*
Protein	16	19	15
Carbohydrate	43	77	45
Fat	41	4	40
Cholesterol	1.2*	0*	0*

*Percentage by weight.

Table 4–2.   Rhesus monkey regression study — cholesterol levels

| | *Serum cholesterol levels (mg/dl)* | | |
Group	*At start of study*	*At 17 months*	*At 40 months*
Control	143±7	140±10	135±8
1	138±4	701±47	
2	142±9	712±68	136±11
3	140±5	703±37	138±7

all sites in the baseline animals sacrificed at 17 months (group 1) was 58 percent. In groups 2 and 3, which had been returned to cholesterol-free, low-saturated-fat diets, presumed regression of coronary artery disease was seen, with luminal narrowing markedly and significantly reduced to 18 percent in the group fed the low-fat diet (group 2) and to 22 percent in the corn-oil group (group 3).

Photomicrographic studies of the coronary arteries of the animals showed that in the regression specimens remarkable changes had occurred in the lesions, with a dramatic decrease in the lipid–rich necrotic core, including a decrease in both intra- and extracellular lipid and of foam cells.

Other studies have demonstrated that regression of lesions is associated with a marked reduction in the total-body cholesterol burden [12]. Studies by Wissler et al [13] indicate that reversal of the atherosclerotic process occurs rapidly, with almost half of the decrease in lesion area occurring during the first four months of the regression period. Furthermore, the addition of a cholesterol-lowering drug such as cholestyramine to the regression regimen resulted in even more rapid removal of lipid and lesion regression [14].

These and many similar studies are of great importance. They provide a firm pathophysiologic basis for the phenomena seen in epidemiologic studies. They strongly support the lipid hypothesis: the animals do not smoke, are not hypertensive, and in fact have no other risk factors for CHD, yet the disease develops rapidly. These studies also demonstrate that it is not only the amount of fat in the diet that is of importance; it is also the type of fat, with saturated fat being necessary to induce atherosclerosis. Nor is it necessary for the fat to be of animal origin. In the early studies of Taylor et al. butter was used as the source of saturated fat [1]; in many later studies saturated oils of vegetable origin, such as coconut and palm oil, were shown to be potent inducers of atherosclerosis [10].

Animal studies have also been used to examine the interrelationship of differing risk factors. In a particularly interesting study, Kaplan et al. investigated the effect of social environment and social status on coronary artery and aortic atherosclerosis in male cynomolgus monkeys (*Macaca fascicularis*) [15]. The study is worth looking at in detail as a particularly good example of the manner in which a useful animal model can be developed of a complex human situation combining dietary and social risk factors.

Kaplan et al. divided 30 experimental animals into six groups, and fed all animals a moderately atherogenic diet for 22 months, with 43 percent of calories as fat and .34 mg cholesterol/cal. On this diet mean serum cholesterol was 471 ± 83 mg/dl, and high-density lipoprotein (HDL) cholesterol was 41 ± 10 mg/dl. Fifteen monkeys (three groups of five each) were each assigned to either a stable or an unstable social housing condition; the animals in the unstable condition were rotated among the three groups, whereas the animals in the stable condition were allowed to remain with their group for the duration of the study. In addition, all of the monkeys were classified as having a dominant or a subordinate social status, based on patterns of aggressive and submissive behavior as carefully observed by the investigators. At the end of the study the coronary arteries and the aorta of each animal were carefully examined for evidence of atherosclerosis (Table 4-3).

Dominant monkeys in the unstable social condition had significantly greater levels of coronary atherosclerosis than did either dominant monkeys housed in stable social conditions or all of the subordinate monkeys. This was true when measured either by luminal involvement or by the degree of luminal stenosis. The behavioral effects were not explained by differences in serum lipids, blood pressure, or obesity. The authors concluded that social dominance is associated with increased coronary artery atherosclerosis when combined with a moderately atherogenic diet, but only when the animal is faced with the additional stress of having to deal with recurrent threats to its dominance.

Interestingly in a follow-up study in which

similar groups of monkeys were fed a diet patterned after the American Heart Association's "prudent diet," monkeys in the socially unstable condition still developed significantly more coronary artery atherosclerosis than did those in the socially stable state [16].

These investigations exemplify the contribution made by animal studies to our understanding of the mechanisms of atherosclerosis and the complex manner in which various risk factors may interact.

Clinical Intervention Studies

Epidemiologic investigation and animal studies provided a firm basis for the lipid hypothesis: the view that lipid abnormalities, in particular elevated levels of low-density lipoprotein cholesterol, are intimately involved in the atherogenic process. However, the last link in the chain remained to be forged. Still missing into the 1980s was the most critical bit of evidence: a clinical trial showing conclusively that lowering cholesterol would result in a reduction in coronary events. This gap was closed with the publication in 1984 of the results of the Lipid Research Clinics Coronary Primary Prevention Trial (LRC-CPPT) [17, 18].

The LRC-CPPT is often misunderstood. It was never intended to provide, in and of itself, the rationale for the important recommendations that have since been made to the public. It was intended, rather, to round out the large body of evidence that had accumulated to that time and to demonstrate what had to be shown before public health recommendations could be made with confidence — that intervention in adult human beings could influence the course of the atherosclerotic process.

In preparation for this trial, other alternatives

Table 4-3. Mean coronary artery intimal area measurements ($\pm$ sem) among dominant and subordinate monkeys in stable and unstable social conditions

Social condition	Mean coronary artery intimal area measurements (mm^2)	
	In dominant monkeys	In subordinate monkeys
Stable	0.32 ± 0.13	0.45 ± 0.12
Unstable	0.74 ± 0.12	0.38 ± 0.10

were considered. It was recognized that the ideal study of the efficacy of cholesterol lowering would in fact be a dietary trial, since both epidemiologic and animal studies had clearly established the link between a high-saturated-fat, high-cholesterol diet and the development of CHD. In 1971, however, the National Heart and Lung Institute Task Force on Arteriosclerosis recommended against conducting a large-scale, national diet-heart trial [19]. They reasoned that the sample size required would be enormous, the cost prohibitive, and the problems of maintaining a blinded trial design insurmountable. The LRC-CPPT was, therefore, designed as a feasible alternative that would prove the point in a much more manageable fashion. The study population was restricted to hypercholesterolemic men, an at-risk population with an anticipated relatively high incidence of clinical events, and a drug treatment was used, permitting a blinded design. It is important to bear in mind that it was intended from the beginning that the results of this trial should be interpreted in the light of all the other studies that had already been carried out and that the implications of those results would be extrapolated to populations other than the middle-aged hypercholesterolemic males directly involved in the study.

The study design was as follows: in 12 participating Lipid Research Centers 3,806 men aged 35 to 59 with plasma cholesterol levels at or above the ninety-fifth percentile (265 mg/dl or greater) and LDL cholesterol levels of 190 mg/dl or greater were randomized to receive the bile acid sequestrant cholestyramine resin at a dose of 24 gm/day (two to four equal doses,

six packets per day), or a placebo. (See Chapter 12 for more information about cholestyramine.) Men with triglyceride levels above 300 mg/dl were excluded, because cholestyramine is known to elevate triglyceride levels. All were also placed on a cholesterol-lowering diet. The primary end point of the trial was the combination of definite CHD death and/or definite myocardial infarction (MI). Numerous other clinical end points were also evaluated. All men were followed up for a period of time varying between seven and ten years.

Adherence to the study drug, an agent that causes frequent gastrointestinal side effects, was less than hoped for. In the first year the mean daily packet count was 4.2 in the cholestyramine group and 4.9 in the placebo group, falling to 3.8 and 4.6, respectively, by the seventh year. Perhaps as a consequence, the cholesterol-lowering effect seen was less than that predicted for this agent. During treatment the cholestyramine group experienced average plasma total cholesterol and LDL cholesterol reductions of 13.4 percent and 20.3 percent, respectively, levels that were 8.5 percent and 12.6 percent greater than those seen in the placebo group (p<.001) (Table 4-4).

The cholestyramine group experienced 155 definite CHD deaths and/or definite nonfatal MIs compared to 187 such events in the placebo group, an incidence rate of CHD estimated to be 19 percent lower in the active treatment group (p < .05) (Table 4-5).

The frequency with which other cardiovascular events occurred further confirmed the benefit provided by the cholesterol-lowering therapy. Positive exercise tests, the incidence of

Table 4-4. Mean plasma lipid and lipoprotein cholesterol concentrations in LRC-CPPT

	Placebo group				Cholestyramine resin group			
	Preentry		Postentry		Preentry		Postentry	
Lipid	Prediet	On-diet	1st year	7th year	Prediet	On-diet	1st year	7th year
Chol, mg/dl	291.8	279.2	275.4	277.3	291.5	280.4	238.6	257.1
LDL, mg/dl	216.2	204.5	198.8	197.6	215.6	205.3	159.4	174.9
HDL, mg/dl	45.1	44.4	44.5	45.5	45.0	44.4	45.6	46.6
HDL/Chol	0.16	0.16	0.16	0.17	0.16	0.16	0.20	0.19
TG, mg/dl	158.4	153.2	162.0	173.5	159.8	156.3	172.2	182.9

Table 4-5. Definite or suspected primary end points and all-cause mortality in LRC-CPPT

End point	Placebo group (n=1900)		Cholestyramine group (n=1906)		
	Number	Percent	Number	Percent	Percent reduction in risk
Definite CHD death and/or definite nonfatal MI	187	9.8	155	8.1	19*
Definite or suspected CHD death or nonfatal MI	256	13.5	222	11.6	15
All-cause mortality	71	3.7	68	3.6	7

*Significant at the .05 level.

Table 4-6. Other cardiovascular events in LRC-CPPT

End point	Placebo group (n=1900)		Cholestyramine group (n=1906)			p
	Number	Percent	Number	Percent	Percent reduction in risk	
Positive exercise test	345	19.8	260	14.9	25	<.001
Angina (Rose questionnaire)	287	15.1	235	12.4	20	<.01
Coronary bypass surgery	112	5.9	93	4.9	21	=.06
Congestive heart failure	11	0.6	8	0.4	28	NS*

*NS = nonsignificant.

angina as measured by the Rose questionnaire, and the frequency with which the subjects went on to coronary bypass surgery were all reduced in the cholestyramine group (Table 4-6).

Of particular interest is the life-table cumulative incidence of primary end points, shown in Figure 4-2, which demonstrated a shape that conformed to the theoretical expectation for a lipid-lowering intervention. For the first two years there was essentially no visible effect, a not-surprising occurrence for an intervention whose sole consequence is a slowing down of the steady rain of lipids into the arterial wall. From the two-year mark onward, however, there is a progressive separation between the placebo curve and the cholestyramine curve, with an even more dramatic separation toward the end of the study. This, too, is in accord with the recognized effect of such an intervention. Although at any given time the intervention effect is small, it is always present; as time continues to pass, a cumulative, snowballing effect

is seen. Thus, the greater the time interval, the more marked the intervention effect. This is in sharp contrast to the life-table curves seen with a potent but one-shot intervention, such as coronary artery bypass surgery, in which an initial benefit tends to disappear by the tenth year of follow-up [20].

In a companion article [18], the investigators analyzed the relation between change in plasma cholesterol and LDL cholesterol levels and the reduction in CHD events. They concluded that the relationship is continuous and graded, with an approximate 2-percent decline in events for each 1-percent drop in plasma cholesterol.

All-cause mortality was not significantly different in the two groups, reflecting an increase in deaths not related to CHD. The most striking difference was seen in deaths due to accidents and violence, a difference the authors attributed to chance (Table 4-7).

As pointed out earlier, the LRC-CPPT was intended to close out a chain of evidence. Al-

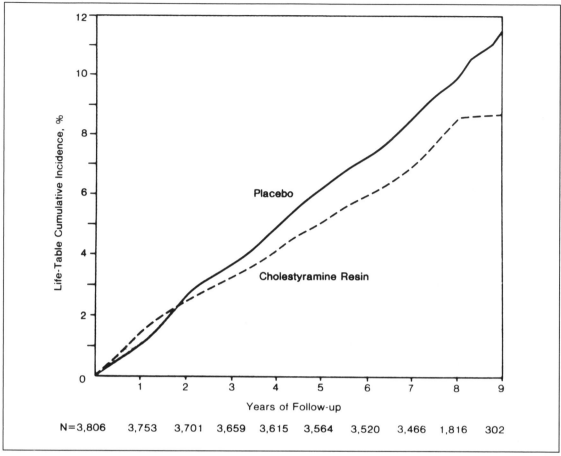

Figure 4-2. Life table event curves in the Lipid Research Clinics Trial: N = number of participants. (Source: The Lipid Research Clinics Program. JAMA 251:351–64, 1984.)

Table 4-7.   Causes of mortality in LRC-CPPT

	Number of deaths	
Cause of death	*Placebo group*	*Cholestyramine group*
CHD	44	32
Other vascular causes	3	5
Malignant neoplasm	15	16
Other medical causes	5	4
Accidents and violence	4	11
Total, all causes other than CHD	27	36
Total, all causes	71	68

though the investigators warned against incautious extrapolation of the results to population groups other than the one studied, they did go on to discuss the implications of the results.

The LRC-CPPT was not designed to assess directly whether cholesterol lowering by diet prevents CHD. Nevertheless, its findings, taken in conjunction with the large volume of evidence relating diet, plasma cholesterol levels, and CHD, support the view that cholesterol lowering by diet also would be beneficial. The findings of the LRC-CPPT take on additional significance if it is acknowledged that it is unlikely that a conclusive study of dietary-induced cholesterol lowering for the prevention of CHD can be designed or implemented [17]. . . . The trial's implications, however, could and should be extended to other age groups and women and, since cholesterol levels and CHD risk are continuous variables, to others with more modest elevations of cholesterol levels.

In late 1985 the National Institutes of Health (NIH) sponsored a Consensus Development Conference on "Lowering blood cholesterol to prevent heart disease." [21] The conference concluded that *"lowering definitely elevated blood cholesterol levels will reduce the risk of heart disease"* and noted that while this position had been established most convincingly for men with elevated blood cholesterol levels *"much evidence justifies the conclusion that similar protection will be afforded in women with elevated levels."*

Three years later a second study essentially replicated the major findings of the LRC-CPPT, using an entirely different population and a drug having a different pharmacologic mechanism. The Helsinki Heart Study took 4081 asymptomatic middle-aged men (aged 40 to 55) who were defined as being at increased risk for CHD by virtue of a non–HDL cholesterol (total cholesterol minus HDL) of 200 mg / dl or more, and randomized them to receive either a placebo or 600 mg of gemfibrozil twice daily for a five-year period [22]. Gemfibrozil is a fibric acid derivative that has a modest cholesterol-lowering effect, but it also raises HDL cholesterol and markedly lowers triglycerides (see Chapter 12). In the Helsinki Heart Study gemfibrozil produced an 8 percent reduction in cholesterol, an 8 percent reduction in LDL cho-

lesterol, a 35 percent reduction in triglycerides, and a 10 percent increase in HDL cholesterol. This combination of a modest reduction in total and LDL cholesterol and a modest elevation in HDL cholesterol produced a favorable shift in the cholesterol/HDL ratio; associated with these changes were significant favorable clinical effects. Overall there was a 34 percent reduction in coronary events in the gemfibrozil group ($p < .02$) with most of this difference occurring in the incidence of nonfatal MI. There was no difference in overall mortality between the treatment group and the placebo group, but as in the LRC-CPPT, the study was not designed to use overall mortality as an end point and thus lacked sufficient power for such an analysis.

There are striking parallels between the Helsinki Heart Study and the LRC-CPPT. Both studies involved drug intervention in asymptomatic hyperlipidemic men, the LRC trial using cholestyramine and the Helsinki Heart Study gemfibrozil. Despite the different mechanisms of these two agents, the outcomes were similar, with significant declines in nonfatal coronary end points. Interestingly the Helsinki Heart Study showed a life-table pattern remarkably similar to that seen in the LRC-CPPT (Figure 4-3), again showing an approximate two-year lag phase between the initiation of therapy and the appearance of a favorable effect. Also seen again in this study was an unexplained increase in accidental deaths. There is no a priori reason to expect that a cholesterol-lowering effect should be associated with personality change, but a recent review of the subject suggests that it is also unreasonable to dismiss these findings as pure coincidence and indicates the need for further study [23].

Within the last few years there has been a remarkable additional outpouring of data demonstrating the value of lipid modification for the prevention of CHD. The similarity of end-point results, despite differing methodologies, strongly suggests that the necessary and common element is favorable lipid modification, whether by major reduction in LDL, such as achieved in the LRC study with cholestyramine, by favorable change in the LDL/HDL ratio, as in the Helsinki Heart Study, or by both, as in

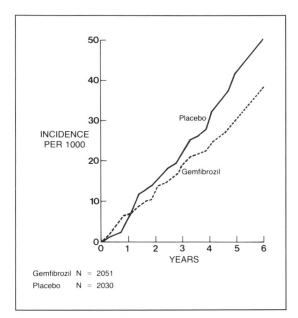

Figure 4-3. Life table event curves in the Helsinki Heart Study. (Source: Frick et al. NEJM 317:1237–45, 1987.)

the postbypass study carried out by Blankenhorn's group using cholestyramine and nicotinic acid in the Cholesterol-Lowering Atherosclerosis Study (CLAS) and the Familial Atherosclerosis Treatment Study (FATS) study carried out by Brown et al. [24, 25]. In both of the latter studies evidence of regression of coronary artery disease was seen. In an even more remarkable study carried out by Ornish et al., evidence of atherosclerosis regression was seen on serial quantitative angiographic examinations in a group of individuals treated with only intense life-style changes: a near-vegetarian diet resulting in marked reduction in LDL cholesterol levels, exercise, meditation, and smoking cessation. All of these regression studies are more fully discussed in Chapter 15.

Intervention in the Elderly

Although the rationale for a vigorous approach to risk factor modification has been established for young and middle-aged individuals, that the same approach is appropriate in the elderly has not yet been demonstrated [26]. The recommendations of the Adult Treatment Panel did not

distinguish between young and middle-aged adults and the elderly [27]. Applying to the elderly the same diet and pharmacologic intervention standards recommended for younger individuals would result in a large increase in health care costs; it is necessary, therefore, to ask if the data exist to justify such a level of treatment.

The traditional risk factors retain their predictive value in the older population. In a review of the Framingham Study experience in persons aged 60 to 70 years, Castelli and colleagues [28] noted that hyperlipidemia, hypertension, diabetes, and elevated fibrinogen levels retain their predictive power for CHD in the elderly. In particular, they emphasized the importance of total cholesterol concentration as a risk factor for CHD and the importance of high LDL and low HDL levels as markers for high risk. Also noteworthy is the disappearance of the female advantage with regard to CHD mortality with advancing age; by age 75 the male-female differential essentially disappears [29].

In the Framingham Study smoking lost its predictive power for CHD after age 65, although deaths due to smoking-related cancers accelerated rapidly [28]. This finding has not been universally accepted. In a report from the Honolulu Heart Study, Benfante and colleagues noted that in a population of men aged 65 to 74 incidence rates of CHD increased progressively in individuals classified at baseline as never, former, or current smokers [30]. The absolute excess risk associated with cigarette smoking in this study was nearly twice as high in elderly as compared to middle-aged men. (See Relative Risk vs. Attributable Risk, later in this chapter. The same relative risk in an older population with higher rates of disease results in a higher attributable risk; thus, treatment may lead to a greater absolute benefit).

In another recent study of 7178 men and women over age 65 and free of CHD at entry, LaCroix and colleagues found rates of total mortality among current smokers to be twice that of never-smoking participants [31]. Current smokers also had higher rates of cardiovascular mortality than never-smokers (relative risk 2.0, with a 95 percent confidence interval of 1.4 to 2.9 in men and 1.6, with a 95 percent confidence interval of 1.1 to 2.3, in women). Former smokers had cardiovascular mortality rates similar to those of never-smokers.

In a prospective study of a very old population (mean age 82±8years), Aronow and colleagues looked at risk factors for coronary events over a mean follow-up period of 41±6 months [32]. Using multivariate analysis, cigarette smoking, hypertension, diabetes, and serum cholesterol were predictive of CHD events in both men and women, and serum HDL and serum triglycerides were additionally predictive in women. For men and women with antecedent CHD, significant risk factors were cigarette smoking, diabetes, a serum cholesterol level of 250 mg/dl or greater, and a serum cholesterol-HDL ratio of 6.5 or more.

The Honolulu Heart Study also evaluated the contribution of serum cholesterol levels to CHD risk in men over the age of 65 years [33]. In a population of 1480 men followed up for an average of 12 years, the upper-quartile relative risk for serum cholesterol level was 1.64 (95 percent confidence interval of 1.14 to 2.36), identical to the relative risk for middle-aged men. Again, because of the greater incidence of CHD in the elderly, absolute risk was actually higher in this group. Data from the Kaiser Permanente Coronary Heart Disease in the Elderly Study also support the findings of excess risk of CHD in elderly men with elevated cholesterol levels [34].

Although the Framingham Heart Study and others such as that of Aronow and colleagues have found elevated cholesterol to be as predictive of risk in the elderly female population as in males, others have come to different conclusions [35]. In a study of 92 women (mean age 82) living in a nursing home in Paris, a five-year follow-up (during which time 53 of the women died) demonstrated a J-shaped mortality curve, with the lowest overall mortality at a cholesterol level of 270 mg/dl. Low cholesterol levels were associated with increased mortality, which was independent of cancer. Studies such as this, however, are liable to selection bias; nursing home inhabitants may not be reflective of the population at large. In another study of an elderly population in Glostrup, Denmark,

however, a J-shaped mortality curve for the elderly was also seen, with the highest-quartile cholesterol values associated with CHD and the lowest-quartile levels with an excess risk of cancer death [36].

Although it is true that risk factors retain their predictive power in the elderly, few studies exist to show that intervention in this age group is of value. Intervention studies such as the Lipid Research Clinics and Helsinki trials [17, 22] excluded older individuals. A diet–intervention trial in the elderly was reported in 1969, in which the effect of a high-polyunsaturated-fat, low-saturated-fat diet was compared with a control diet in 846 institutionalized men aged 50 to 89 [37]. The experimental diet lowered blood cholesterol levels from a mean of 233 mg/dl to 187 mg/dl. A significant reduction in deaths from CHD and stroke was seen, but the beneficial effect was restricted to those men who initially had higher cholesterol levels (> 233 mg/dl); this beneficial effect was present in both younger and older age groups. The National Heart, Lung, and Blood Institute is currently sponsoring a placebo-controlled, double-blind study of the value of lowering blood LDL levels in the elderly, using a hydroxymethylglutaryl coenzyme A reductase inhibitor as the intervention agent. This study should provide some of the answers now lacking.

In the absence of more definitive data that support intervention for modification of CHD risk in the elderly, an appropriate approach would be as follows:

• Smoking cessation and control of hypertension should be vigorously encouraged; smoking cessation for CHD prevention probably retains its importance even at advanced ages. In addition smoking contributes to mortality and morbidity from many diseases, including chronic obstructive lung disease and many forms of cancer. Control of hypertension is of value even in elderly patients with isolated elevation of systolic blood pressure [38].

• Although definitive clinical trials demonstrating the value of lipid modification in the elderly are not yet available, substantial evidence exists that elevated levels of cholesterol and

LDL and low levels of HDL remain risk factors for CHD, with levels of absolute risk that may actually increase because of the increasing frequency of CHD with advancing age. Furthermore, there is no sound physiologic reason to postulate a difference between younger and older individuals with regard to responsiveness to lipid-modifying therapy.

- The approach should be tempered by the realization that the lag time seen in cholesterol-intervention studies represents an increasingly larger proportion of remaining life expectancy as individuals age; this fact and the lack of definitive evidence of the effectiveness of intervention in the elderly should lead to an increase in our threshold for intervention.

- An increased-fiber, low-fat diet has many advantages for the elderly apart from CHD prevention, including improved digestibility, prevention of constipation and other gastrointestinal disorders, amelioration of diabetes, and prevention of cancer [39, 40, 41]. Furthermore, many older individuals are quite health conscious and feel neglected when a physician fails to give dietary advice. It is therefore appropriate to recommend a reduced-fat, low-cholesterol diet as recommended by the National Cholesterol Education Project guidelines (see Chapter 9).

- Pharmacologic therapy should be reserved for carefully selected individuals with a reasonable life expectancy and a high risk of CHD. (This topic is discussed in Chapter 12).

The Population Approach versus the High-risk Approach

In an attempt to control the epidemic of atherosclerotic disease, two general approaches are advocated. The first, which is much more comfortable for physicians because it is their usual *modus operandi*, is the high-risk approach, in which patients who are in the upper end of the risk spectrum are specifically sought, either by screening on an individual level in physicians' offices or by community screening programs. They are then treated on a one-to-one basis to reduce their risk. The second approach, which aims to lower the mean level of a risk factor in the entire population, is usually referred to as the population approach. Here, the goal is to shift the entire risk curve to the left (Figure 4-4), by altering risk factors on a population level, without necessarily dealing with individuals. Such interventions, familiar to epidemiologists and public health workers, might include antismoking campaigns, efforts to reduce the use of saturated fat and salt by fast-food restaurants, and education campaigns directed at reducing meat intake and increasing fruit and vegetable consumption across the entire country.

Geoffrey Rose has pointed out that these two approaches relate to two different etiological questions [42]. The individual-centered approach seeks the causes of cases and asks, "Why does this *person* have an elevated cholesterol level?" The population-centered approach seeks the causes of incidence and asks, "Why does this *population* have a higher mean cholesterol level and many individuals with elevated levels, when in other populations elevated cholesterol levels are rare?"

These two approaches are often discussed on an either-or basis, but they should not be viewed in this manner. Each approach has advantages and disadvantages, and both should be seen as complementary methodologies. Their relative advantages and disadvantages are summarized in Tables 4-8 and 4-9 (modified from Rose) [42].

Figure 4-4. Theoretical effect of a shift in the population distribution for blood cholesterol levels. A: Mean cholesterol 190 mg/dl; B: Mean cholesterol 220 mg/dl.

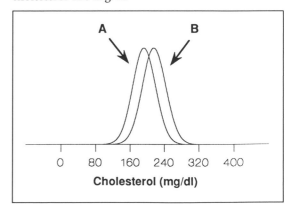

Table 4-8.   The high-risk strategy

Advantages	Disadvantages
Intervention appropriate to the individual	Difficulties and cost of screening
Subject motivation	Failure to deal with the root causes of the disease
Physician motivation	Limited potential for both the individual and the population
Cost-effective use of resources	Imposition of behavioral difficulties
Favorable risk-benefit ratio	Labeling of asymptomatic individuals as "sick"

Table 4-9.   The population approach

Advantages	Disadvantages
Potential to alter the root causes of the disease	Small benefit to the individual (the prevention paradox)
Larger potential for reducing disease incidence	Poor motivation of subject
Behavioral appropriateness	Poor motivation of physician
	Problematic risk-benefit ratio if intervention may not be entirely benign

The high-risk strategy appeals to physicians, who understand that detecting and treating an asymptomatic risk situation such as hypertension can lead to decreased morbidity and mortality. This triage approach — culling for special attention those at the high end of a risk distribution — is used in many other medical situations, ranging from high-risk pregnancies to prophylactic antibiotics for recurrent urinary tract infections. In taking this approach, the physician is treating an individual who understands the need to be treated ("I have high cholesterol and high blood pressure, so I need to change my diet"); both feel comfortable and are appropriately motivated. The high-risk approach also husbands scarce resources that can be applied to individuals who will have a higher payoff in terms of diminished risk. If the intervention has a down side, be it risk or cost, the risk-benefit ratio will be more favorable in the high-risk setting.

Despite the appeal of the high-risk approach, a number of problems are associated with it, one of the most important of which is the difficulty of screening a population. It is often the case in such situations that the people at highest risk are those least likely to be reached; it is commonplace at cholesterol-screening programs for the majority of participants to be relatively health-conscious older individuals who frequently already know their cholesterol levels, although the level of compliance with recommended follow-up is often suboptimal [43, 44]. The younger, hyperlipidemic, smoking, doctor-avoiding individual is far less likely to appear at a screening site. For an easily understandable comparison, imagine applying the same approach to the use of seat belts. The person taking the high-risk approach to this problem would say, "Why make everyone wear an uncomfortable seat belt? Surely the accident risk of the 60-year-old woman going shopping on a Wednesday morning at 10:00 must be very low, and asking her to wear a seat belt is of little utility. We need to target only the high-risk groups, such as alcoholic teenage drivers out on Saturday nights." Here, clearly, is a situation where the difficulty of the high-risk approach is apparent. The same logic applies to many other risk-altering situations: the population at highest risk is least likely to participate voluntarily in risk-modifying behaviors.

In addition to the difficulty of reaching high-risk individuals, there is an even more important disadvantage to this strategy: by seeking to protect only those most liable to be affected by a population-based condition, such as a diet high in saturated fat, the high-risk approach fails to alter the root cause of the problem and thus does not have the potential to eliminate the problem altogether. There will need to be a never-ending search for individuals at risk. Furthermore, our ability to predict risk for a given individual will never be more than mediocre except for those few individuals who fall into the highest risk category [45, 46]. Because so many more individuals are in the moderate- to low-risk categories, the number of cases in these groups far exceeds those that arise from the smaller group of individuals in the high-risk categories.

The high-risk strategy also requires individuals to make changes that put them at odds with peer groups or family. Quitting smoking when all your friends smoke, telling your spouse that the foods she loves to cook for you and that you love to eat are no good — these are difficult changes to make.

The population-based strategy, on the other hand, has many advantages. Shifting the entire risk curve of a population has the potential to truly alter the pattern of disease within a society. In fact, the decline in mortality in the United States from CHD, as described in Chapter 2, is entirely consistent with the pattern of risk-factor change that has occurred over the past 20 years [47]. Furthermore, changes occurring in an entire population support individual change — it is easier to quit smoking when your workplace is smoke-free and certainly easier to follow a low-fat diet when such choices are available in the company or school cafeteria and fast-food restaurants.

Because the population-based strategy is inherently designed to affect many individuals who are at low risk, it leads to a phenomenon that Rose has called the *prevention paradox*: preventive measures that greatly benefit the society as a whole bring little benefit to each individual [48]. This pattern is common in public health, however, and is equally true of immunization and seat-belt strategies. Because the gain for a given individual is small, motivating that person to make lifestyle changes may be difficult. Health-beneficial change is much easier when it becomes socially desirable, as when such phenomena as jogging are no longer seen as the preoccupation of a few "exercise nuts," but rather as a socially approved action with positive reinforcement from peers.

Because both approaches are of value, they should be combined into an overall national strategy. Several studies have looked at the likely relative contributions of the high-risk and population-based approaches. Kottke et al. [49,

50] used Monte Carlo simulations to assess the effects of several intervention strategies on CHD mortality rates in both Finnish and North American cohorts. They projected that lowering serum cholesterol by 4 percent, smoking by 15 percent, and diastolic blood pressure by 3 percent for the entire population — goals easily achievable and in the case of cholesterol and smoking already surpassed in the United States — would be expected to reduce the incidence of nonfatal MI by at least 13 percent and CHD deaths by at least 18 percent. By contrast, lowering serum cholesterol by 34 percent, smoking by 20 percent, and diastolic blood pressure to 90 mm Hg in the subset of the population with all three risk factors in the highest quartile would result in only a 6 to 8 percent reduction in nonfatal MI and a 2 to 9 percent reduction in deaths from CHD. More recently Goldman et al. [51] used Framingham Heart Study coefficients in a computer simulation (the Coronary Heart Disease Policy Model) to analyze the effect of targeting individuals with serum cholesterol levels greater than 250 mg/dl as opposed to a population-wide program to reduce everyone's cholesterol level. Their model suggests that a targeted program would reduce CHD incidence by 8 to 10 percent in men 35 to 54 years of age and by 1 to 4 percent in men aged 55 to 74. Such a reduction in CHD incidence could also be achieved by a 10-mg/dl population-wide reduction in serum cholesterol. As already pointed out, such a decline in cholesterol has already been seen in the United States and has been associated with an unprecedented decline in CHD mortality.

Goldman et al. point out that in women a targeted program would yield greater relative and absolute benefits and would be equivalent to an approximately 23-mg/dl population-wide reduction in serum cholesterol. The relatively greater impact of the targeted program in women is related to the greater tendency among women for CHD events to be concentrated among those persons with elevated cholesterol levels (but see Relative Risk versus Attributable Risk, below). The authors conclude that "relatively modest population-wide cholesterol reductions that are likely to be achievable . . . would be equivalent to very ambitious targeted programs."

The Diet–Heart Controversy

Although the discussion of the relative merits of the population-based and high-risk approaches to the control of CHD properly involves all of the major risk factors, the principal discussion has revolved around the control of hyperlipidemia, in particular the role of diet, frequently referred to as the diet-heart controversy [52]. Cigarette smoking is now clearly accepted as the cause of diseases of many organ systems other than the cardiovascular system, and the utility of population-based smoking cessation initiatives is clear [53]. Likewise the value of treating even relatively minor degrees of blood pressure elevation is now established [54]. The value of treating moderately elevated cholesterol levels, however, and especially the concept of large-scale dietary change, continues to provoke argument [55, 56], and articles in the lay press have contributed to public confusion [57].

Blackburn and Jacobs [52] point out that one important source of confusion about the relation between diet and heart disease is the inappropriate extrapolation of evidence derived from group data to the individual and vice versa. Factors that determine the usual population levels of risk characteristics are likely to be the determinants of mass disease, but they may not be the same as those factors that determine individual disease susceptibility within a given population. Rejecting important causal relationships in populations when relationships appear weak or absent in individual patients is an example of what has been termed the ecological fallacy [58, 59]. It is likely that widespread environmental factors, such as the saturated-fat content of the American diet, acting on a common inherent susceptibility, are responsible for strong population correlations, such as are seen between serum cholesterol levels and CHD risk. Genetic factors determine individual susceptibility and account for variation in levels of a risk factor and risk of the disease within a population, but they have relatively little to do with

large differences in disease rates between populations.

Large-scale studies that attempt to show a mortality difference from intervention with a risk factor such as serum cholesterol are likely to continue to meet with difficulty [52]. When an entire population has a very high exposure level, as with dietary fat and cholesterol, and the intervention effect is only modest, genetic variation in response may be the predominant factor that determines risk. It is difficult to accurately characterize individual behavior (for example, diet), and truly controlled trials in free-living communities are near impossible. Diet-disease relationships are much clearer when one has the opportunity to examine populations with very different dietary intakes [60]; this is true of cancer as well as CHD. There is no country in the world with a low average serum cholesterol level in which CHD is prevalent.

Relative Risk versus Attributable Risk

Considerable confusion over the value of intervention for risk factor modification has been caused by a lack of understanding of the difference between relative risk and attributable risk. Most studies of the relationship between risk factors and the incidence of CHD, whether observational or interventional, have reported results in terms of such relative measures as the risk ratio or the odds ratio [61]. Thus, the Multiple Risk Factor Intervention Trial (MRFIT) [62] showed that the six-year CHD death rate was four times as great in the top 10 percent of the cholesterol distribution as compared to the bottom 10 percent. Certainly it is important to know that one individual's risk is four times that of another, but it is equally important to ask, "Four times what?" If the risk for an individual in the low-risk group is very low, for example, one death per 1000 over the follow-up period, then a risk quadruple that is still very small and perhaps not worth intervention. On the other hand, if the low-risk figure is 50 per 1000, then a quadrupling of risk is serious indeed. Although the relative risk in both situations is 4.0, the *attributable risk*, or the difference between the high and low probabilities, is greatly different. In the first case it is .3 percent (.004 − .001); in the second case it is much higher, at 15 percent (.200 − .050). Attributable risk is often the more useful figure for a clinician, as it gives a truer picture of risk and benefit.

The difference between relative and attributable risk leads to some anomalous conditions. It is usually thought that the benefit of risk-factor change decreases with age, since the relative risk for such risk factors as cigarette smoking and hypercholesterolemia lessens with increasing years. In their insightful examination of this topic, Malenka and Baron [61] point out in an analysis of the MRFIT data that as relative risk of hypercholesterolemia decreases with age, attributable risk actually increases (Figure 4-5). This results because the smaller relative risk is superimposed on a much greater disease-incidence rate in the older population. Thus, intervention in the elderly for risk-factor control may be of value, even though analyses of relative risk show diminishing benefit.

Malenka and Baron [61] suggest that clinicians should use a variation of attributable risk they call *practical attributable risk*. This statistic is defined by the difference in disease incidence between a patient's current risk and that level of risk reduction that is practicably achievable, as opposed to that which is theoretically possible. The use of such a figure requires an assessment of the degree to which a given patient can reduce risk. Thus, it may be more reasonable to assume that a patient may reduce risk from the fifth quintile to the third, rather than to a level below the population mean. The perceived value of an intervention would then be correspondingly reduced.

Assessment of Individual Risk

Given that there is sufficient evidence to warrant intervention on both the individual and the population levels, it is desirable to develop predictive equations based on an individual's total risk factor pattern that would allow prediction of CHD risk. The best known of these equations have come from the Framingham Heart Study [63]. These equations were updated in 1991 to include additional data, particularly on older individuals. The database now includes individuals from the Framingham Offspring Cohort as well as from the original study population [64,

Figure 4-5.   Relative risk versus attributable risk. (Source: Malenka and Baron. Arch Int Med 149:1981–85, 1989.)
RR = relative risk, AR = attributable risk

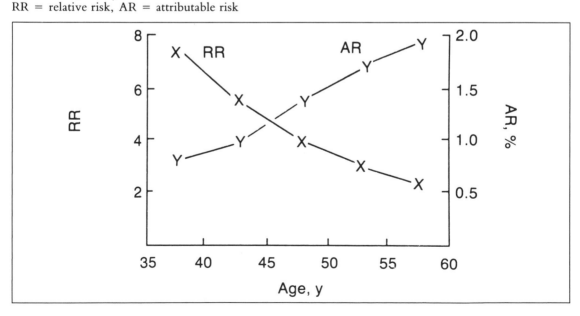

65]. The updated equations also reflect the influence of HDL cholesterol. The predictive chart from the Framingham Heart Study is reproduced in Figure 4-6.

CHD risk as predicted from the chart in Figure 4-6 includes all clinical CHD events: CHD death (sudden or nonsudden), MI, angina pectoris, and coronary insufficiency. For example, a 45-year-old man with an HDL level of 40, a cholesterol level of 245, and systolic blood pressure of 145 and who is a smoker but does not have either diabetes or electrocardiographic evi-

Figure 4-6. The Framingham Heart Study predictive chart for coronary heart disease. (Source: Anderson et al. Circulation. 83:356–62, 1991.)

1. Find points for each risk factor

Age (if female) (yr)				Age (if male) (yr)				HDL cholesterol			
Age	Points	Age	Points	Age	Points	Age	Points	HDL	Points	HDL	Points
30	−12	41	1	30	−2	48–49	9	25–26	7	67–73	−4
31	−11	42–43	2	31	−1	50–51	10	27–29	6	74–80	−5
32	−9	44	3	32–33	0	52–54	11	30–32	5	81–87	−6
33	−8	45–46	4	34	1	55–56	12	33–35	4	88–96	−7
34	−6	47–48	5	35–36	2	57–59	13	36–38	3		
35	−5	49–50	6	37–38	3	60–61	14	39–42	2		
36	−4	51–52	7	39	4	62–64	15	43–46	1		
37	−3	53–55	8	40–41	5	65–67	16	47–50	0		
38	−2	56–60	9	42–43	6	68–70	17	51–55	−1		
39	−1	61–67	10	44–45	7	71–73	18	56–60	−2		
40	0	68–74	11	46–47	8	74	19	61–66	−3		

Total cholesterol (mg/dl)				Systolic blood pressure (mm Hg)						Points	
Chol	Points	Chol	Points	SBP	Points	SBP	Points	Other factors		Yes	No
139–151	−3	220–239	2	98–104	−2	150–160	4	Cigarette smoking		4	0
152–166	−2	240–262	3	105–112	−1	161–172	5	Diabetes			
167–182	−1	263–288	4	113–120	0	173–185	6	Male		3	0
183–199	0	289–315	5	121–129	1			Female		6	0
200–219	1	316–330	6	130–139	2			ECG-LVH		9	0
				140–149	3						

2. Add points for all risk factors

+		+		+		+		+		+		=	
(Age)		(Total chol)		(HDL)		(SBP)		(Smoking)		(Diabetes)		(ECG-LVH)	(Total)

Note: *Minus points subtract from total.*

3. Look up risk corresponding to point total

	Probability (%)			Probability (%)			Probability (%)			Probability (%)	
Points	5 yr	10 yr	Points	5 yr	10 yr	Points	5 yr	10 yr	Points	5 yr	10 yr
≤1	<1	<2	9	2	5	17	6	13	25	14	27
2	1	2	10	2	6	18	7	14	26	16	29
3	1	2	11	3	6	19	8	16	27	17	31
4	1	2	12	3	7	20	8	18	28	19	33
5	1	3	13	3	8	21	9	19	29	20	36
6	1	3	14	4	9	22	11	21	30	22	38
7	1	4	15	5	10	23	12	23	31	24	40
8	2	4	16	5	12	24	13	25	32	25	42

4. Compare with average 10-year risk

Age (yr)	Probability (%)		Age (yr)	Probability (%)		Age (yr)	Probability (%)	
	Women	Men		Women	Men		Women	Men
30–34	<1	3	45–49	5	10	60–64	13	21
35–39	<1	5	50–54	8	14	65–69	9	30
40–44	2	6	55–59	12	16	70–74	12	24

HDL, high density lipoprotein; SBP, systolic blood pressure; ECG-LVH, left ventricular hypertrophy by electrocardiography.

dence of left ventricular hypertrophy (ECG-LVH) would have a point total of 19 and a five-year probability of developing CHD of 8 percent, with a ten-year probability of 16 percent.

Several important points need to be kept in mind when one uses the Framingham risk chart. The calculations are based on the Framingham population, and generalization to other populations should always be made with caution. The less similar the population from which the individual in question is drawn, the greater the level of caution that must be applied to the use of the chart. Thus, the equations may not be appropriate for use with populations or ethnic groups that have very low rates of CHD. Second, heredity is not factored into the chart, but because it does modify risk, assessment of this element should be used to alter appropriately the level of concern gained from the Framingham prediction. Third, the equations are probably not appropriate for individuals with markedly abnormal levels of a single risk factor, such as severe diabetes, familial hyperlipidemia, or malignant hypertension.

Summary

The evidence overwhelmingly demonstrates that CHD is not an inevitable consequence of aging but rather a disease process based on physiologic mechanisms related to abnormal concentrations of blood lipids, and is accelerated by a number of other risk factors, most of which are related to the diet and lifestyle associated with an industrialized, urban society. It is also clear that the pace of the atherosclerotic process can be modified by alteration of risk factors, even when significant arterial disease is already present. Future chapters address the various risk factors individually and explore methodologies that can be used to alter risk in real-world settings, where time, money, compliance, and patience all have their limits.

References

1. Taylor CB. Experimentally induced arteriosclerosis in non-human primates. In: Roberts JC, Straus R, eds. Comparative atherosclerosis. New York: Harper & Row, 1965; 215.

2. Taylor CB, Cox GE, Manalo-Estrella P, et al. Atherosclerosis in rhesus monkeys. II. Arterial lesions associated with hypercholesterolemia induced by dietary fat and cholesterol. Arch Pathol 1962; 74:16–34.

3. Wissler RW, Vesselinovitch D. Differences between human and animal atherosclerosis. In: Schettler G, Weizel A, eds. Atherosclerosis III. Proceedings of the 3rd International Symposium. New York: Springer-Verlag, 1974; 319–25.

4. Wissler RW, Vesselinovitch D. Atherosclerosis in non-human primates. In: Brandly CA, Cornelius CE, Simpson, CF, eds. Advances in veterinary science and comparative medicine. Vol. 21. New York: Academic, 1977; 351–420.

5. Weiner BH, Ockene IS, Jarmolych J, et al. Comparison of pathology and angiography in swine model of coronary atherosclerosis. Circulation 1985; 72:1081–6.

6. Taylor CB, Cox GE, Hall-Taylor BJ, et al. Atherosclerosis in areas of vascular injury in monkeys with mild hypercholesterolemia. Circulation 1954; 10:613.

7. Taylor CB, Cox GE, Counts M, et al. Fatal myocardial infarction in Rhesus monkey with diet-induced hypercholesterolemia. Amer J. Pathol 1959; 35:674.

8. Taylor CB, Cox GE, Counts M, et al. Fatal myocardial infarction in Rhesus monkey with diet-induced hypercholesterolemia. Circulation 1959; 20:975.

9. Buja LM, Kovanen PT, Bilheimer DW. Cellular pathology of homozygous familial hypercholesterolemia. Amer J Pathol 1979; 97:327.

10. Wissler RW, Vesselinovitch D. Special lecture: the complementary interaction of epidemiological and experimental animal studies: a key foundation of the preventive effort. Prev Med 1983; 12:84–99.

11. Armstrong ML, Warner ED, Connor WE. Regression of coronary atheromatosis in rhesus monkeys. Circ Res 1970; 27:59–67.

12. Wissler RW, Vesselinovitch D., Schaffner TJ, et al. Quantitating rhesus monkey atherosclerosis progression and regression with time. In: Gotto AM, Smith LC, Allen B, eds. Atherosclerosis V. Proceedings of the 5th International Symposium. New York: Springer, 1980; 757–61.

13. Wissler RW, Vesselinovitch D. Can atherosclerotic plaques regress — anatomic and biochemical evidence from nonhuman animal models. Am J Cardiol 1990; 65:F33-F40.

14. Wissler RW, Vesselinovitch D. Interaction of therapeutic diets and cholesterol-lowering drugs in regression studies in animals. In: Malinow MR, Blaton VH, eds. Regression of atherosclerotic lesions. New York: Plenum, 1984; 21–41.

15. Kaplan JR, Manuck SB, Clarkson TB, et al. Social status, environment, and atherosclerosis in cynomolgus monkeys. Arteriosclerosis 1982; 2:359–68.

16. Kaplan JR, Manuck SB, Clarkson TB, et al. Social stress and atherosclerosis in normocholesterolemic monkeys. Science 1983; 733–5.

17. The Lipid Research Clinics Program. The lipid research clinics coronary primary prevention trial results. I. Reduction in incidence of coronary heart disease. JAMA 1984; 251:351–64.

18. The Lipid Research Clinics Program. The lipid research clinics coronary primary prevention trial results. II. The relationship of reduction in incidence of coronary heart disease to cholesterol lowering. JAMA 1984; 251:365–74.

19. National Heart and Lung Institute Task Force on Arteriosclerosis. Arteriosclerosis: a report. U.S. Department of Health, Education, and Welfare, National Institutes of Health. USDHEW publ. no. (NIH) 72-137, vol. 1, 1971.

20. The Veterans Administration Coronary Artery Bypass Surgery Cooperative Study Group. Eleven-year survival in the Veterans Administration randomized trial of coronary bypass surgery for stable angina. N Engl J Med 1984; 311:1333–9.

21. NIH Consensus. Lowering blood cholesterol to prevent heart disease. Arteriosclerosis 1985; 5:404–12.

22. Frick MH, Elo O, Haapa K, et al. Helsinki Heart Study: Primary-prevention trial with gemfibrozil in middle-aged men with dyslipidemia: safety of treatment, changes in risk factors, and incidence of coronary heart disease. N Engl J Med 1987; 317:1237–45.

23. Wysowski DK, Gross TP. Deaths due to accidents and violence in two recent trials of cholesterol-lowering drugs. Arch Int Med 1990; 150:2169–72.

24. Blankenhorn DH, Nessim SA, Johnson RL, et al. Beneficial effects of combined colestipol-niacin therapy on coronary atherosclerosis and coronary venous bypass grafts. JAMA 1987; 257:3233–40.

25. Brown G, Albers JJ, Fisher LD, et al. Regression of coronary artery disease as a result of intensive lipid-lowering therapy in men with high levels of apolipoprotein-B. N Engl J Med 1990; 323:1289–98.

26. Denke MA, Grundy SM. Hypercholesterolemia in elderly persons: resolving the treatment dilemma. Ann Int Med 1990; 112:780–92.

27. National Cholesterol Education Program Expert Panel. Report on detection, evaluation, and treatment of high blood cholesterol in adults. Arch Intern Med 1988; 148:36–69.

28. Castelli WP, Wilson PWF, Levy D, et al. Cardiovascular risk factors in the elderly. Am J Cardiol 1989; 63:12H–19H.

29. Lerner DJ, Kannel WB. Patterns of coronary heart disease morbidity and mortality in the sexes: a 26-year follow-up of the Framingham population. Am Heart J 1986; 111:383–90.

30. Benfante R, Reed D, Frank J. Does cigarette smoking have an independent effect on coronary heart disease in the elderly? Am J Public Health 1991; 81:897–9.

31. Lacroix AZ, Lang J, Scherr P, et al. Smoking and mortality among older men and women in three communities. N Engl J Med 1991; 324:1619–25.

32. Aronow WS, Herzig AH, Etienne F, et al. 41-month follow-up of risk factors correlated with new coronary events in 708 elderly patients. J Am Geriatr Soc 1989; 37:501–6.

33. Benfante R, Reed D. Is elevated serum cholesterol level a risk factor for coronary heart disease in the elderly? JAMA 1990; 263:393–6.

34. Rubin SM, Sidney S, Black DM, et al. High blood cholesterol in elderly men and the excess risk for coronary heart disease. Ann Int Med 1990; 113:916–20.

35. Forette B, Tortrat D, Wolmark Y. Cholesterol as risk factor for mortality in elderly women. Lancet 1989; 1:868–70.

36. Agner E, Hansen PF. Fasting serum cholesterol and triglycerides in a ten year prospective study in old age. Acta Med Scand 1983; 214:33–41.

37. Dayton S, Pearce ML, Hoshimoto S, et al. A controlled trial of a diet high in unsaturated fat in preventing complications of atherosclerosis. Circulation 1969; 60:Suppl 2:1–63.

38. SHEP Cooperative Research Group. Prevention of stroke by antihypertensive drug treatment in older persons with isolated systolic hypertension: final results of the systolic hypertension in the elderly program (SHEP). JAMA 1991; 265:3255–64.

39. Burkitt DP, Walker AR, Painter NS. Dietary fiber and disease. JAMA 1974; 229:1068–74.

40. Steiner G. From an excess of fat, diabetics die (editorial). JAMA 1989; 262:398–9.

41. Doll R. An overview of the epidemiological evidence linking diet and cancer. Proc Nutr Soc 1990; 49:119–131.

42. Rose G. Sick individuals and sick populations. Internat J Epidem 1985; 14:32–8.

43. Wynder EL, Field F, Haley NJ. Population screening for cholesterol determination: a pilot study. JAMA 1986; 256:2839–42.

44. Fischer PM, Guinan KH, Burke JJ, et al. Impact of a public cholesterol screening program. Arch Int Med 1990; 150:2567–72.

45. Kannel WB, Garcia MJ, McNamara PM, et al.

Serum lipid precursors of coronary heart disease. Human Pathol 1971; 2:129–51.

46. Keys A. Coronary heart disease in seven countries. Circulation 1970; 41:1–211.

47. Goldman L, Cook EF. The decline in ischemic heart disease mortality rates. Ann Intern Med 1984; 101:825–36.

48. Rose G. Strategy of prevention: lessons from cardiovascular disease. Brit Med J 1981; 282:1847–51.

49. Kottke TE, Puska P, Salonen JT, et al. Projected effects of high-risk versus population-based prevention strategies in coronary heart disease. Am J Epidemiol 1985; 121:697–704.

50. Kottke TE, Gatewood LC, Wu SC, et al. Preventing heart disease: is treating the high risk sufficient? J Clin Epidemiol 1988; 41:1083–93.

51. Goldman L, Weinstein MC, Williams LW. Relative impact of targeted versus populationwide cholesterol interventions on the incidence of coronary heart disease: projections of the coronary heart disease policy model. Circulation 1989; 80:254–60.

52. Blackburn H, Jacobs D. Sources of the diet-heart controversy: confusion over population versus individual correlations. Circulation 1984; 70:775–80.

53. U.S. Department of Health and Human Services. Reducing the health consequences of smoking: 25 years of progress. A report of the surgeon general. Public Health Service, Centers for Disease Control, Center for Chronic Disease Prevention and Health Promotion, Office on Smoking and Health. USDHHS publ. no. (CDC) 89-8411, 1989.

54. Joint National Committee. The 1988 report of the Joint National Committee on detection, evaluation and treatment of high blood pressure. Arch Int Med 1988; 148:1023–38.

55. McCormick J, Skrabanek P. Coronary heart disease is not preventable by population intervention. Lancet 1988; 2:839–41.

56. Oliver MF. Prevention of coronary heart disease — propaganda, promises, problems, and prospects. Circulation 1986; 73:1–9.

57. Moore TJ. The cholesterol myth. Atlantic 1989; 37–70.

58. Morgenstern H. Uses of ecological analysis in epidemiological research. Am J Public Health 1982; 72:1336.

59. Robinson WS. Ecological correlations and the behavior of individuals. Am Sociol Rev 1950; 15:351.

60. Armstrong B, Doll R. Environmental factors and cancer incidence and mortality in different countries, with special reference to dietary practices. Int J Cancer 1975; 15:617–31.

61. Malenka DJ, Baron JA. Cholesterol and coronary heart disease: the attributable risk reduction of diet and drugs. Arch Int Med 1989; 149:1981–5.

62. Multiple Risk Factor Intervention Trial Research Group. Multiple Risk Factor Intervention Trial: risk factor changes and mortality results. JAMA 1982; 248:1465–77.

63. Kannel WB, McGee D, Gordon T. A general cardiovascular risk profile: the Framingham Study. Amer J Cardiol 1976; 38:46–51.

64. Anderson KM, Odell PM, Wilson PWF, et al. Cardiovascular disease risk profiles. Am Heart J 1990; 121:293–8.

65. Anderson KM, Wilson PWF, Odell PM, et al. An updated coronary risk profile: a statement for health professionals. Circulation 1991; 83:356–62.

5

Platelet–Vessel Wall Interactions in Coronary Heart Disease

RICHARD C. BECKER

EDITORS' INTRODUCTION

Chapter 3 introduced the concept of altered hemostasis as a determinant of CHD. In this chapter Dr. Becker brings us up to date on all of the current developments in this rapidly expanding field. It is now clear that platelet-coagulation protein–vessel wall interactions play a key role in the initiation of clinical coronary events and are probably also active in the progression of the atherosclerotic plaque. The deleterious effects of risk factors such as smoking, diabetes, and hypertension may be at least in part mediated through such a mechanism, and the connection between stress and CHD may also be through this pathway. Thus, to understand CHD, it is essential to understand the entire thrombotic-fibrinolytic system. Dr. Becker also looks at the pharmacology of platelet-inhibiting agents and discusses their use in both the primary and secondary prevention of CHD.

For over a century scientists have recognized platelets as a major component of normal physiological hemostasis, providing a first line of defense following vascular trauma. However, their pivotal role in coagulation protein interactions, fibrinolytic processes, and vascular endothelial cell function has been appreciated only more recently.

Under normal circumstances, platelets circulate freely through the vascular system. In pathological conditions, however, platelet–vessel wall interactions can initiate local thrombus formation, either causing an immediate impedance to physiological blood flow or serving as a stimulus for subsequent vascular events.

This chapter examines the important roles of platelet activity and platelet–vessel wall interactions in cardiovascular disease.

The Vascular Endothelium

The vascular endothelium is a structurally simple but functionally complex tissue. Its integrity is essential for normal vessel responsiveness and thromboresistance. Until recently the vascular endothelium was thought to represent no more than a protective barrier, separating platelets and the contact-activated coagulation factors from thrombogenic subendothelial connective tissues. It is now known that the endothelial lining is, in fact, a multifunctional organ system composed of metabolically active and physiologically responsive component cells that meticulously regulate blood flow. Moreover, we now appreciate that vascular endothelial cells are susceptible to injury (biochemical or mechanical), which may be relevant to certain disease processes such as coronary atherosclerosis.

Structural Anatomy

In most vertebrates vascular endothelial cells form a single layer of simple squamous lining cells (.1 to .5μ in thickness) joined by intercellular junctions. The cells themselves are polygonal, varying between 10 and 50μ, and elongated in the long axis of the vessel, thus orienting the cellular longitudinal dimension in the direction of blood flow.

The endothelial cell has three surfaces: nonthrombogenic (luminal), adhesive (subluminal), and cohesive. The luminal surface is nonthrombogenic and devoid of any electron-dense connective tissue. It does, however, possess an exterior coat, or glycocalyx, which consists primarily of starches and proteins secreted by the endothelial cells: oligosaccharides, glycoproteins, glycolipids, and sialoconjugates. Plasma proteins, including lipoprotein lipase, α_2 macroglobulin, antithrombin III, heparin cofactor II, albumin, and small amounts of fibrinogen and fibrin are adsorbed to the luminal surface. The luminal membrane itself adds significantly to the thromboresistant properties, carrying a negative charge that repels similarly charged circulating blood cells.

The subluminal, or abluminal, surface adheres to the connective tissue of the subendothelial zone. Small processes penetrate through a series of internal layers to form myoendothelial junctions with subjacent smooth muscle cells.

The third surface of the vascular endothelium is cohesive, joining endothelial cells to one another by cell junctions of two basic types: occluding (tight) junctions and communicating (gap) junctions. Occluding junctions represent a physical link between two adjoining cells, sealing the intercellular space. The communicating junctions provide the structural substrate for direct two-way communication between cells. They are instrumental in the electronic coupling and intracellular exchange of ions and small metabolites.

Normal Function

As an active site of protein synthesis, the vascular endothelium may be considered the largest and most productive organ system in the human body. Endothelial cells synthesize, secrete, modify, and regulate connective tissue components, vasodilators, vasoconstrictors, anticoagulants, procoagulants, fibrinolytic compounds, and prostanoids, each contributing to the maintenance of normal vasomotion, thromboresistance, and physiologic hemostasis (Figures 5-1 and 5-2).

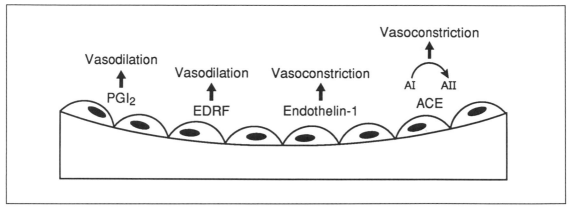

Figure 5-1. Vasoactive properties of the vascular endothelium.
PGI$_2$ = prostacyclin; EDRF-endothelium-derived relaxing factor; ACE = angiotensin-converting enzyme; AI = angiotensin I; AII = angiotensin II

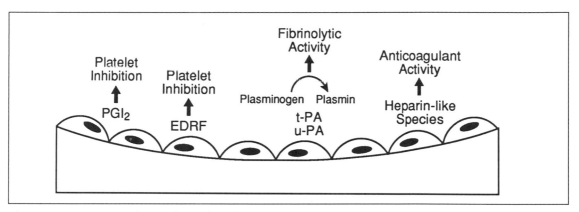

Figure 5-2. Anticoagulant and platelet-inhibiting properties of the vascular endothelium.
PGI$_2$ = prostacyclin; EDRF = endothelium-derived relaxing factor; t-PA = tissue plasminogen activator; u-PA = urokinase-type plasminogen activator

PROSTACYCLIN

Prostacyclin (PGI$_2$) is a potent vasodilating substance released locally in response to biochemical and mechanical mediators, including thromboxane A$_2$, thrombin, bradykinin, histamine, high-density lipoprotein, platelet-derived growth factor, tissue hypoxia, and hemodynamic stress [1]. PGI$_2$, by increasing intracellular cyclic adenosine monophosphate (cAMP), also inhibits platelet aggregation. Furthermore, there is evidence that PGI$_2$ increases the rate of smooth-muscle-cell cholesterol ester metabolism, suppresses lipid metabolism within macrophages, and inhibits the release of growth factors, which mediate proliferative responses to intravascular shear stress [2].

ENDOTHELIUM-DERIVED RELAXING FACTOR

Utilizing strips of arteries in organ baths (isolated system), Furchgott and Zawadski [4] discovered that acetylcholine-mediated vasodilation requires an intact vascular endothelium (i.e., it is endothelium dependent) (Table 5-1). Endothelium-derived relaxing factor (EDRF), recently identified as nitric oxide [5], is an L-arginine derivative that relaxes smooth muscles by increasing intracellular cyclic guanosine monophosphate (cGMP) (Figure 5-3). It is released locally in response to a number of mediators, including thrombin, bradykinin, thromboxane A$_2$, histamine, adenine nucleotides, and aggregating platelets. In addition to vasoactive properties, EDRF is also a potent inhibitor of platelet adhesion [6] and aggregation [7]. Moreover, EDRF and PGI$_2$ appear to have synergistic antiaggregatory properties [7].

ANGIOTENSIN II

Studied extensively over the past two decades, angiotensin II is a potent vasoconstrictor that exerts an important effect on vascular tone [8]. Although the systemic properties of angiotensin II have been known for some time, local synthesis, release, and vascular activity have just recently been appreciated. Angiotensin-converting enzyme (ACE), required for the conversion of angiotensin I to the active peptide angiotensin II, has been isolated from mammalian arteries and veins. While there has been some debate, most studies suggest that ACE is, indeed, synthesized within vascular endothelial cells. Moreover, there is mounting evidence that endothelial cells are also capable of producing enzymes, other than or in addition to ACE, capable of angiotensin II generation [9].

ENDOTHELIN

The vascular endothelium, in addition to synthesizing vasodilating substances such as PGI$_2$ and EDRF, also produces vasoconstrictors essential for maintaining vessel tone and responsiveness. Endothelin, a small peptide, has vasoconstricting properties ten times those of angiotensin II [10]. Although three structurally and pharmacologically distinct isopeptides have been isolated and characterized, only endothe-

lin-1 is synthesized by vascular endothelial cells [11]. While a majority of vasoactive mediators are released in surges following local mechanical or biochemical stimulation, endothelin-1 is released slowly and, via specific receptor-mediated mechanisms, activates intracellular protein C [12], leading to smooth muscle contraction (vessel constriction).

PLASMINOGEN ACTIVATORS

Vascular endothelial cells synthesize and release activators that are capable of converting plasminogen to the serine protease plasmin, an enzyme that proteolytically degrades fibrin (and fibrinogen). Tissue plasminogen activator and urokinase-type plasminogen activator generate plasmin locally; therefore, fibrinolysis is limited to the immediate environment. Stimuli for the release of vascular plasminogen activators include epinephrine, thrombin, heparin, interleukin-1, venous occlusion, aggregating platelets, and desamino-8-D-Arginine vasopressin (DDAVP).

HEPARIN-LIKE SPECIES

In the past, mast cells were thought to be the only cells capable of synthesizing anticoagulant-active heparin. Investigations performed by Teien et al. [13], Thomas et al. [14], and Rosenberg [15] have shown, however, that endothelial cells are, in fact, capable of synthesizing heparin-like molecules (heparin sulfate) with anticoagulant properties. As a result, it is currently accepted that thromboresistance is mediated, at least in part, through the

Table 5-1.   Endothelium-independent and -dependent vasodilators

Independent vasodilators	Dependent vasodilators
PGE$_1$, PGE$_2$, PGI$_2$	Acetylcholine
Adenosine	Serotonin
Atrial natriuretic polypeptide	Histamine
Bradykinin	Epinephrine, norepinephrine
Nitroglycerin	Thrombin
Sodium nitroprusside	Arachidonic acid
Nitric oxide	Leukotrienes (LTC$_4$, LTD$_4$)
Glucagon	Substance P
Insulin	

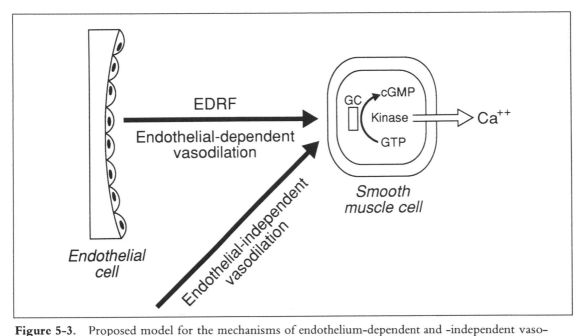

Figure 5-3. Proposed model for the mechanisms of endothelium-dependent and -independent vaso-dilation. A mediator may (a) trigger the release of endothelium-derived relaxing factor from the vascular endothelium, activating guanylate cyclase (endothelium-dependent) or (b) activate guanylate cyclase directly (endothelium-independent).
GC = guanylate cyclase; cGMP = cyclic guanosine monophosphate; GTP = guanosine triphosphate; Ca++ = calcium.

interaction of heparin-like substances with antithrombin III and heparin cofactor II (both located on the endothelial surface), accelerating the neutralization of hemostatic (procoagulant) proteins.

PLATELET–ACTIVATING FACTOR
A lipid capable of inducing platelet aggregation and secretion in a concentration-dependent fashion, platelet-activating factor (PAF) mobilizes platelet surface membrane arachidonic acid, which stimulates thromboxane A_2 synthesis.

TISSUE FACTOR
Tissue factor, also known as tissue thromboplastin, is a lipoprotein present in large quantities in a number of organ systems, including the brain and lung parenchyma. Although tissue factor is, under normal conditions, produced by endothelial cells in small amounts, synthesis can be increased markedly after mechanical or biochemical stimulation, accelerating the activation of factor X by factor VIIa [16, 17].

VON WILLEBRAND FACTOR
Circulating in plasma as a series of self-aggregated structures composed of a single glycoprotein subunit, von Willebrand factor is a vital component of normal hemostasis that mediates both platelet–vessel wall interactions and platelet-platelet interactions [18].

PLASMINOGEN–ACTIVATOR INHIBITOR
Plasminogen-activator inhibitor-1 (PAI-1) is a single-chain glycoprotein that forms stable complexes with tissue plasminogen activator and urokinase-type plasminogen activator, inhibiting their fibrinolytic activity [19]. Endothelial cells are able to increase PAI-1 production and do so following administration of exogenous t-PA or direct exposure to platelet lysates or compounds released from activated platelets (epidermal growth factor, transforming growth factor β [20, 21, 22].

Endothelial Dysfunction

The vascular endothelium can be structurally or functionally altered by a wide variety of chemical, mechanical, biological, and toxic substances (Table 5-2). The primary focus of the following discussion, however, is the effect(s) of coronary atherosclerosis on vascular responsiveness and thromboresistance.

Although described frequently as a focal process, coronary atherosclerosis is diffuse in nature, primarily involving the vessel intima (composed of the endothelium, the underlying basement membrane, and a layer of myointimal cells). A structurally and functionally normal coronary artery dilates in response to acetylcholine, physical exercise, or provocation. In contrast, an atherosclerotic coronary artery undergoes paradoxical vasoconstriction when exposed to acetylcholine [23] and a progressive decrease in cross-sectional luminal area follows rapid ventricular pacing [24]. The failure to dilate prevents an increase in physiological blood flow and, in addition, subjects the endothelial surface to excessive shear stress [25, 26, 27, 28, 29, 30].

Recently it has become apparent that hypercholesterolemia in and of itself may adversely affect endothelial-cell function. Despite being morphologically intact, the vascular endothelium in areas of intimal atherosclerosis fails to release EDRF [31, 32]. Of additional clinical importance, hypercholesterolemia has been shown to impair endothelium-dependent vascular relaxation in coronary resistance vessels, which are predominantly responsible for regulating myocardial perfusion [33].

Vascular endothelial cells are strategically positioned to play an important role in the regulation of local vascular clotting processes. These cells are also ideally positioned to promote thrombosis following vascular injury. However, damaged or "perturbed" endothelial cells can lose their ability to maintain thromboresistance and may promote pathologic thrombosis. Indeed, assembly of a complete coagulation pathway can take place on the endothelial surface of atherosclerotic vessels; in addition, impaired local fibrinolytic activity can prevent clot dissolution [34, 35, 36] (Figure 5-4).

Platelets

Despite being simple in appearance, platelets are complex cellular elements with complicated structural and functional characteristics (Figure 5-5).

Structural Anatomy
PERIPHERAL ZONE

The peripheral zone consists of membranes and closely associated structures that provide surfaces for the platelet itself and the tortuous channels of the open canalicular system. The peripheral zone consists of three distinct structural domains: the exterior coat, the unit membrane, and the submembrane region.

The exterior coat, or glycocalyx, is rich in glycoproteins (GPs). Recent biochemical studies have identified nine distinct glycoproteins: Ia, Ib, Ic, IIa, IIb, IIIa, IV, V, and IX. Many glycoproteins act as receptors for platelet–platelet and platelet–vessel wall interactions.

The unit membrane provides a physicochemical separation between intracellular and extracellular constituents and processes. Important components of the unit membrane include Na/K

Table 5-2. Disorders associated with endothelial cell dysfunction

Hereditary disorders
  Fabry's disease
  Protein S deficiency
  Plasminogen activator deficiency
  Homocysteinuria

Acquired disorders
  Trauma: mechanical, biochemical, toxic, infectious
  Diabetes mellitus
  Atherosclerosis

Immune mediated disorders
  Collagen vascular diseases
  Thrombotic thrombocytopenic purpura
  Behçet's disease
  Heparin-mediated endothelial antibodies
  Transplant rejection

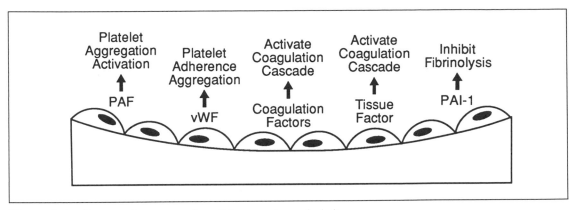

Figure 5-4. Procoagulant properties of the vascular endothelium.
PAF = platelet–activating factor; vWF = von Willebrand factor; PAI-1 = plasminogen–activator inhibitor.

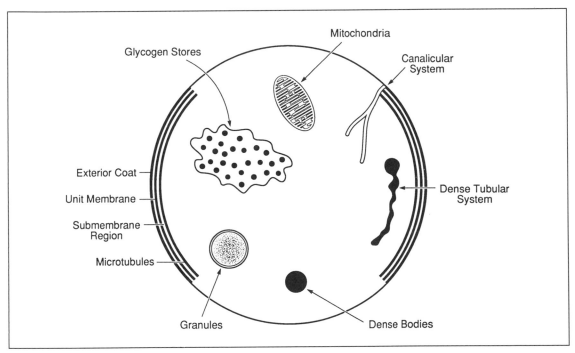

Figure 5-5. Normal discoid platelet (schematic representation), with a number of vital ultrastructural features depicted.

ATPASE and other anion or cation pumps that maintain transmembrane ionic gradients.

The submembrane region contains a specialized filamentous system similar to actin microfilaments. Functionally submembrane filaments assist circumferential microtubules, maintaining platelet discoid shape, controlling pseudo-pod extrusion, and interacting with other elements of the platelet contractile mechanism.

SOL-GEL ZONE

The sol-gel zone is the matrix of the platelet cytoplasm. It contains several fiber systems in various states of polymerization, maintaining the discoid shape of non-stimulated platelets and providing the intricate contractile system required to initiate shape change, pseudopod extension, internal contraction, and secretion.

ORGANELLE ZONE

The organelle zone consists of granules, electron-dense bodies, peroxisomes, lysosomes, and mitochondria randomly dispersed in the platelet cytoplasm. It is centrally involved with metabolic processes and also acts as a storage site for enzymes, adenine nucleotides, serotonin, calcium, and a variety of protein constituents.

MEMBRANE SYSTEMS

The platelet membrane systems include a surface-connected canalicular system, which provides access for plasma-borne substances to the platelet interior and an exit route for products of the release reaction, and a dense tubular system, which acts as a site for calcium sequestration and for storing prostaglandin precursors.

Normal Platelet Physiology
PLATELET ADHESION

Under normal conditions, platelets do not adhere to intact endothelial surfaces. However, they avidly adhere to damaged, disrupted, or dysfunctional vascular endothelium, particularly in areas of exposed subendothelial collagen fibers, such as those found in ulcerated atherosclerotic plaques.

Platelet surface membrane receptors are essential for adhesion (Figure 5-6). Glycoprotein Ia (GPIa) binds with collagen at low shear rates and may also contribute to platelet adherence in areas of vascular damage. Glycoprotein Ib (GPIb) serves as a binding site for von Willebrand factor, particularly at high shear rates. Glycoprotein IIb/IIIa (GPIIb/IIIa) may also participate in platelet adhesion within areas of high shear rates.

PLATELET AGGREGATION

Activated platelets undergo a progressive change in shape and release calcium from the dense tubular system. Adenosine diphosphate (ADP), serotonin, and thromboxane A_2 are subsequently released, exposing platelet receptors for fibrinogen, the molecular "glue" for platelet aggregation.

PLATELET–COAGULATION PROTEIN INTERACTIONS

Beyond their ability to provide coagulation proteins, including factors II, V, VII, IX, X, XI, and XIII, high-molecular-weight kininogen, and fibrinogen, platelets contain specific receptors for a number of circulating hemostatic proteases and can also trigger contact-activated coagulation. Moreover, platelets provide a protective nidus for activated clotting factors from circulating plasma inhibitors.

PLATELET–LIPID INTERACTIONS

Hypercholesterolemia has been shown to influence platelet activity. Increased adhesion, aggregation, and serotonin release have been reported [37], as have increased circulating levels of the potent platelet agonist thromboxane A_2 [38] and decreased sensitivity to the platelet-inhibiting properties of PGI_2 [39]. Cholesterol feeding is associated with increased platelet activatability [40, 41]; however, a reduction of cholesterol through either dietary or pharmacologic means returns platelet activity to its normal state [42].

Although the mechanism(s) underlying the relation between serum cholesterol concentration and platelet activity are not fully understood, it has been shown that changes in the cholesterol content of the platelet surface membrane profoundly affect overall membrane fluidity. In turn, fluidity, or the cells' lipid-water interface, influences lipase activity. Therefore, it has been proposed that hypercholesterolemia-mediated increases in the cholesterol content of the platelet surface membrane enhance diglyceride lipase or phospholipase A_2 activity (or both), which increases the release of arachidonic acid, the substrate for thromboxane A_2 synthesis [43, 44].

Hypercholesterolemia and atherosclerosis impair endothelium-dependent relaxation of major epicardial coronary arteries. Although marked intimal atherosclerosis is frequently observed in these vessels, the endothelium is mor-

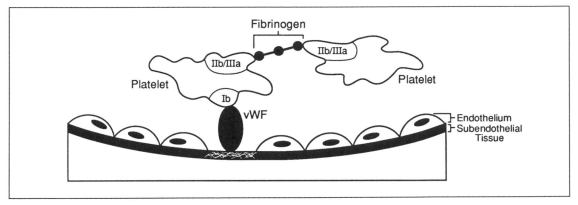

Figure 5-6. Schematic representation of platelet adhesion and aggregation. Following vascular injury, platelets adhere to subendothelial tissue (primarily collagen) via specific surface membrane receptors and von Willebrand factor. Aggregation is mediated primarily by fibrinogen, which binds with a specific GP receptor, GPIIb/IIIa complex.

phologically intact; however, it fails to release EDRF, which is a potent vasodilator and inhibitor of platelet aggregation [45, 46]. It is widely believed, therefore, that hypercholesterolemia in and of itself may directly impair vascular endothelial cell function and enhance platelet–vessel wall interactions prior to the development of overt atherosclerosis [47, 48, 49].

ATHEROGENESIS

Athough it is well known that platelets adhere readily to sites of endothelial disruption, their role in the overall atherogenic process has not been fully defined. Indeed, a series of complex pathologic events are required for the metamorphosis from platelet adhesion to plaque formation. Emerging evidence suggests that a unique platelet product known as platelet-derived growth factor (PDGF) may be a key factor.

PDGF is a polypeptide stored in platelet alpha granules. It is released during degranulation and is considered a major growth factor of human serum [50, 51]. In cell culture, smooth-muscle cells exposed to PDGF proliferate and increase their receptors for low-density lipoprotein, leading to increased lipid accumulation. Protein synthesis, including collagen and proteoglycan production, is also increased [52].

Beyond its mitogenic properties, PDGF is a potent vasoconstrictor and exhibits potent chemotactic properties for both smoothmuscle cells and neutrophils (Figure 5-7). Overall, PDGF may represent a critical link between initial platelet adherence, smooth muscle cell proliferation, and atherosclerotic plaque formation.

CORONARY ARTERIAL THROMBOGENESIS

Pathological, experimental, and clinical evidence supports the role of coronary mural thrombosis in the pathogenesis of acute coronary syndromes, including myocardial infarction (MI) and unstable angina.

Coronary artery thrombi consist of both platelet- and erythrocyte-rich zones, with the former predominating in most instances. A platelet-rich zone typically exists in an area of atherosclerotic plaque fissuring or rupture, while erythrocyte-rich zones extend proximally and distally (Figure 5-8). Careful examination of coronary artery thrombi using light microscopy, conventional staining techniques, or electron microscopy reveals an extensive network of platelets immersed in fibrin. Platelet masses and columns, consisting of tightly packed aggregates with varying degrees of cellular swelling, degranulation, and pseudopod extension along the vascular luminal surface, are also evident [53].

In addition to being directly involved in coronary thrombogenesis, activated platelets can

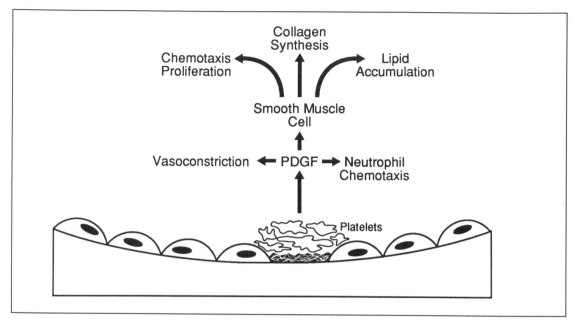

Figure 5-7.   Platelet activity in coronary atherosclerosis. Following adherence and activation, platelets release a potent growth factor, PDGF. In turn, PDGF stimulates smooth-muscle-cell migration, proliferation, and protein synthesis.

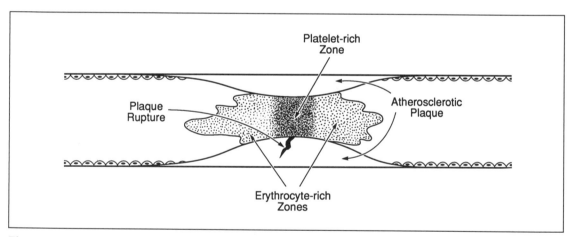

Figure 5-8.   Schematic representation of an atherosclerotic coronary artery containing an occlusive thrombus. A platelet-rich zone exists at the site of plaque rupture, while erythrocyte-rich zones extend both proximally and distally.

trigger intense vasoconstriction through the release of thromboxane A_2 and serotonin [54]. Indeed, coronary vasoplasm occurs proximal and distal to sites of endothelial disruption and has been shown to be proportional to the degree of platelet deposition [55].

PHARMACOLOGY OF PLATELET-INHIBITING AGENTS

The participation of platelets in the thrombotic process depends on their ability to adhere to an abnormal surface, aggregate to form an initial platelet plug, and activate, thus stimulating further aggregation and triggering the coagulation cascade. Therefore, pharmacologic strategies designed to inhibit platelet activity have focused on these three fundamental mechanisms of action. In addition, the recognition that growth factors released from platelets may influence cellular proliferation and atheroma formation has provided yet another potential target for newer agents [56, 57] (Table 5-3).

AGENTS THAT INHIBIT PLATELET ADHESION

In areas of severe coronary arterial narrowing caused by underlying atheroma, plaque rupture, or hemorrhage, platelet adhesion and aggregation are mediated by von Willebrand factor and the platelet receptors GPIb and GPIIb/IIIa. Monoclonal antibodies to von Willebrand factor [58], and aurintricarboxylic acid [59], a triphenylmethyl dye compound, inhibit platelets in regions of high shear stress through their binding to von Willebrand factor, preventing its interaction with platelet receptors and damaged or dysfunctional vessel walls. These agents may be useful for short-term therapy. Long-term ther-

Table 5-3. Pharmacology of platelet-inhibiting agents

Agents that inhibit platelet adhesion
   von Willebrand factor monoclonal antibodies
   Aurintricarboxylic acid

Agents that inhibit platelet aggregation
   Aspirin
   Glycoprotein IIb/IIIa receptor blockers
      Monoclonal antibodies
      RGD-containing peptides
   Ticlopidine
   Thromboxane synthetase inhibitors
   Thromboxane/endoperoxide receptor inhibitors
   Dextran
   Omega-3 fatty acids

Agents that inhibit platelet activation
   Dipyridamole
   Prostaglandin E_1
   Prostacyclin (PGI_2)
   Calcium-channel antagonists

Agent that inhibits platelet growth factors
   Trapidil

apy, however, may be associated with a significant risk of bleeding.

AGENTS THAT INHIBIT PLATELET AGGREGATION

Aspirin. Following oral ingestion, aspirin is rapidly absorbed in the stomach and the duodenum, achieving peak serum levels within 20 to 30 minutes. Enteric-coated preparations are less well absorbed (unless they are chewed), resulting in a delay in peak serum levels to approximately 60 minutes.

Aspirin irreversibly acetylates cyclooxygenase, impairing prostaglandin metabolism and thromboxane A_2 synthesis. As a result, platelet aggregation in response to collagen, ADP, and thrombin (in low concentrations) is inhibited [60]. Adherence and platelet release, however, are not affected. Because, unlike vascular endothelial cells, platelets lack the synthetic capacity to regenerate cyclooxygenase, aspirin's inhibitory effect persists for the lifespan of the platelet (7 ± 2 days). The antithrombotic effect of aspirin can be achieved with doses ranging from 160 to 325 mg per day; therefore, the toxic side effects seen with higher doses can be avoided [61].

Although nonsteroidal anti-inflammatory drugs also inhibit platelet cyclooxygenase, they do so in a reversible manner. In addition, these compounds have not been adequately tested in large randomized clinical trials. Therefore, their use in the prevention or treatment of cardiovascular disease cannot be recommended at this time [62].

GPIIb/IIIa Receptor Blockers. The platelet GP IIb/IIIa receptor is unique in two ways. First, normal platelets have an extremely large number of receptors ($\approx 50,000$) on their surface. Second, platelet activation exposes the GPIIb/IIIa receptor, leading to platelet aggregation. In essence, all physiologic platelet agonists act by exposing the GPIIb/IIIa receptor.

Monoclonal antibodies to the GPIIb/IIIa receptor have been developed recently. The $F(AB')_2$ fragment of this antibody can completely block in-vitro platelet aggregation induced by agonists thought to function in vivo, even in high concentrations or in combinations [63].

The ability of GPIIb/IIIa to bind a number of naturally occurring substances has been explained, at least in part, by the fact that it contains a binding site for the tripeptide arginine-glycine-aspartic acid (Arg-Gly-Asp). All substances that bind to the GPIIb/IIIa receptor contain this amino acid sequence; therefore, synthetic compounds containing the sequence can inhibit the binding of fibrinogen to GPIIb/IIIa. RGD (Arg-Gly-Asp), *RGDS* (Arg-Gly-Asp-Ser), and *RGDF* (Arg-Gly-Asp-Phe) peptides represent a new class of proteins that inhibit platelet aggregation [64].

Ticlopidine. Ticlopidine is structurally distinct from all other antiplatelet agents. It is a potent inhibitor of platelet aggregation induced by ADP and variably inhibits aggregation provoked by collagen, epinephrine, arachidonic acid, thrombin, and platelet-activating factor. Ticlopidine also inhibits the platelet release action and may impair platelet adhesion as well [65].

Thromboxane Synthetase Inhibitors. Thromboxane synthetase inhibitors (Dazoxiben, pirmagrel) have been developed to suppress platelet thromboxane A_2 synthesis, thereby preventing platelet aggregation [66, 67]. Despite their potential beneficial effects, currently available agents have been limited by two factors: incomplete thromboxane A_2 inhibition and the aggregating potential of endoperoxide intermediates.

Inhibitors of Thromboxane and Endoperoxide Receptors. The potential limitations of thromboxane synthetase inhibitors can, at least theoretically, be managed by inhibiting the receptors for both thromboxane A_2 and the active endoperoxide intermediates. In addition to inhibiting platelet aggregation, the vasoactive effects of thromboxane A_2 can also be blocked [68].

Dextran. Dextran is a polysaccharide that ranges in molecular weight from 65,000 to 80,000 daltons. It has been shown to prolong bleeding time in humans; however, its mechanism of action is unclear. There is evidence suggesting that dextran binds to the platelet surface, altering membrane receptor function and inhibiting platelet aggregation [69]. Decreased levels of the factor VIII:vWF (von Willebrand factor) complex have also been reported [70].

Omega-3 Fatty Acids. The n-3 class of polyunsaturated fatty acids, particularly eicosapentaenoic acid, may be valuable in preventing the thrombotic complications of cardiovascular disease [71]. Omega-3 fatty acid supplementation decreases the platelet membrane concentration of arachidonic acid, thus preventing thromboxane A_2 synthesis. In addition, eicosapentaenoic and docosahexaenoic acids compete with arachidonic acid for cyclooxygenase, leading to the formation of three biologically inactive prostanoids: PGG_3, PGH_3, and TXA_3. Within vascular endothelial cells, however, n-3 fatty acids are responsible for the synthesis of PGI_3, a potent platelet inhibitor [72, 73].

AGENTS THAT INHIBIT PLATELET ACTIVATION

Cyclic adenosine monophosphate (cAMP) is a major modulator of platelet activation and release. The platelet response to stimulation is inhibited when intracellular cAMP levels are elevated by agents that activate adenylate cyclase (the enzyme that converts ATP to cAMP), or that inhibit phosphodiesterase (the enzyme responsible for cAMP degradation).

Dipyridamole. Dipyridamole (Persantine) is a pyrimidopyrimidine derivative first used as an antianginal agent because of its vasodilating properties. It was subsequently shown to inhibit platelet activation and has been postulated to do so through one or more mechanisms, including inhibition of phosphodiesterase, stimulation and release of endothelial prostacyclin, or inhibiting cellular uptake and metabolism of adenosine, which increases its concentration at the platelet-vessel interface [74]. High concentrations of dipyridamole are required to influence platelet aggregation in vitro. It is not surprising, therefore, that the observed effects in vivo have been both modest and inconsistent.

Prostaglandin E_1. Prostaglandin E_1 (PGE_1) inhibits platelet activation and aggregation primarily by increasing intracellular cAMP. It may also have the capacity to deaggregate aggregated platelets [75]. The clinical usefulness of PGE_1 is limited by the extensive first-pass metabolism, which takes place in the lungs. Indeed, 70 percent of the activated compound is eliminated, resulting in extremely low plasma levels. Therefore, direct intravascular infusions are required to achieve therapeutic concentrations [76].

PGI₂. Prostacyclin (PGI_2) is a potent, naturally occurring platelet inhibitor. Its role in the treatment of cardiovascular disease has been limited by its instability in plasma and its propensity to cause systemic hypotension when given in doses required to inhibit platelet activation [77]. In contrast, the prostacyclin analogues Iloprost and ciprostene are chemically stable compounds. Because they are both platelet inhibitors, further investigation is in progress [78].

Calcium-Channel Antagonists. Because calcium plays a vital role in platelet activation and aggregation, the potential platelet-inhibiting properties of the calcium-channel antagonists nifedipine, diltiazem, and verapamil have been investigated. Indeed, each has been shown to inhibit platelet release and aggregation [79, 80, 81]. In addition, diltiazem appears to potentiate the inhibitory effects of aspirin [82] and prevent platelet-activating factor binding [83].

AGENT THAT INHIBITS GROWTH FACTORS

PDGF is a potent mitogen and chemoattractant capable of stimulating proliferation of smooth-muscle cells and fibroblasts in tissue culture [84]. The in vitro and in vivo stimulatory effect of PDGF is significantly reduced by Trapidil, a triazolopyrimidine derivative that also has vasodilatory and cholesterol-lowering properties [85]. Trapidil is currently undergoing clinical evaluation.

Abnormal Platelet–Vessel Wall Interactions in Systemic Disorders

DIABETES MELLITUS

There is a well-established association of diabetes mellitus with the development of ather-

osclerosis, microvascular disorders, and thromboembolic complications. Since platelets are known to release a number of potent mitogens and to contribute directly to physiologic and pathologic coagulative processes, their involvement in the accelerated vascular disease and thrombosis seen in persons with diabetes mellitus has been investigated.

Studies performed in experimental animal models, coupled with those in humans, suggest that diabetes mellitus is associated with a number of platelet abnormalities, including increased adhesion [86, 87], increased aggregation [88, 89], increased activation and release [90, 91], and increased thromboxane A_2 synthetic capacity [92, 93]. Moreover, an abnormality in vascular endothelium PGI_2 synthesis and release has also been observed [94], providing a nidus for thrombotic events.

The mechanisms responsible for these abnormalities are currently under investigation. However, the available evidence suggests that hyperglycemia itself [95], associated hyperlipidemic states, and chronic endothelial cell injury [96] may each contribute.

SMOKING

The first disease linked directly to smoking was lung cancer. In time, however, it was recognized that smoking was also strongly associated with heart disease [97]. With the link firmly established, large-scale epidemiologic studies were able to show that smoking caused more cardiovascular deaths than any of the other known risk factors, representing the largest preventable cause of heart disease in the United States [98]. More recently additional troubling facts have emerged, identifying an association between exposure to environmental tobacco smoke (passive smoking) and the development of heart disease in nonsmokers [99].

The risk of MI increases with the number of cigarettes smoked per day. Within a few years of complete cessation, however, the risk decreases markedly to a level similar to that of a person who has never smoked [100]. Smoking among patients with documented coronary artery disease is associated with an increased risk of MI and death. Smoking cessation decreases the risk, even among the elderly and patients with previous coronary artery bypass grafting [101]. Despite early optimism, low-yield cigarettes (decreased nicotine and carbon monoxide content) have not been shown to decrease the risk of MI [102].

Cigarette smoke has been shown to affect platelet activity. Platelet aggregability is increased, even among persons exposed only to passive smoke [103]. Moreover, platelet sensitivity to the antiaggregatory prostaglandins PGE_1 and PGI_2 is decreased in both smokers and nonsmokers exposed to tobacco smoke [104]. Similar abnormalities have been observed by other investigators, suggesting that exposure to tobacco smoke is associated with a prompt increase in platelet activity and activatability [105]. Although chronic exposure may cause a compensatory increase in the production of vascular PGI_2, heightened platelet activity persists, even among persons receiving aspirin [106].

In addition to increasing platelet activity, smoking has also been shown to adversely affect the vascular endothelium. Indeed, tobacco smoke is linked to the development of both atherosclerosis and endothelial cell dysfunction [107, 108].

Coupled with the procoagulant potential of increased circulating fibrinogen, the platelet and vessel-wall abnormalities associated with smoking provide a strong stimulus and an ideal environment for acute vascular events.

SYSTEMIC HYPERTENSION

Systemic hypertension is a major risk factor for the development of atherosclerosis, particularly ischemic heart disease and cerebrovascular disease. The hemodynamic theory of vessel-wall injury in hypertension has considerable support. In experimental animal models, hypertension produced by supravalvular aortic banding causes coronary arterial endothelial denudation with areas of platelet adherence and smooth-muscle-cell intimal proliferation [109]. Other studies have shown a tendency toward throm-

bus formation in areas of endothelial damage [110].

ISCHEMIC HEART DISEASE

A clear relation between platelet activity and vascular disease has been established. Subsequently attention has focused on thrombotic mechanisms and the role of platelets in acute thrombosis. As discussed later in this chapter, the significant reduction in coronary events yielded by aspirin use constitutes the most convincing indirect evidence that platelets play a central role in patients with ischemic heart disease. Until recently, however, there was no direct evidence that platelet reactivity was relevant to ischemic heart disease in the general population. Meade et al. [111] demonstrated increased platelet sensitivity to ADP agonists in subjects with ischemic heart disease. A subsequent study, the Caerphilly Collaborative Heart Study [112], based on a cohort of 2398 men aged 49 to 66 years, identified significant correlations between previous MI and electrocardiographic (ECG) evidence of ischemia and ADP-induced platelet aggregation, and between ECG evidence of ischemia and thrombin-induced aggregation. Overall, patients with the greatest degree of ADP-induced platelet aggregation were twice as likely to have experienced a previous MI compared with patients with minimal aggregability.

Recent evidence suggests that patients surviving an acute MI can be risk-stratified based on platelet activity. Patients with spontaneous in vitro platelet aggregation appear to be at increased risk for coronary events, including recurrent infarction and death [113].

STRESS

Although a difficult entity to quantitate, stress has received considerable attention, and much speculation has been generated regarding its role in the development of atherosclerotic disease and thrombotic complications [114]. In experimental animals, stressful stimuli have been shown to cause both structural changes in the arterial intima [115] and overt atherosclerosis, which developed despite cholesterol levels within the normal human range [116].

Epinephrine (adrenaline) is an endogenous catecholamine synthesized and released in response to stressful stimuli. It is capable of inhibiting adenylate cyclase, thus reducing intracellular cAMP concentration. In vitro, however, epinephrine is required in supraphysiologic concentrations to induce platelet aggregation. Therefore, it has been hypothesized that cooperative or synergistic effects are required in vivo. Indeed, epinephrine and ADP act synergistically, exposing latent fibrinogen receptors on the platelet surface.

Small-vessel platelet aggregation and myocardial necrosis have been produced in animals given an intravenous infusion of epinephrine. Since the degree of necrosis can be reduced with aspirin or dipyridamole pretreatment, it has been hypothesized that myocardial injury results from intravascular platelet aggregation [117].

Recent epidemiologic studies have demonstrated a circadian morning peak in the onset of disorders associated with intravascular thrombosis, in particular acute MI [118]. Furthermore, clinical studies have demonstrated a morning increase in platelet aggregability that appears to be related to assuming an upright posture [119]. As a surge in sympathetic tone due primarily to epinephrine release occurs in the morning hours as well, heightened platelet activity may reflect a response to physiological stress. An ability to modify the observed morning increase in MI with low-dose aspirin (325 mg every other day) lends additional support to the potential role of platelets in stress-related cardiac events [120].

Primary Prevention of Cardiac Events

The Physicians Health Study [121] was the first randomized, double-blind, placebo-controlled trial examining whether low-dose aspirin (325 mg every other day) could influence cardiovascular mortality in the general population. Overall, 22,071 male physicians between 40 and 84 years of age were followed for an average of 60.2 months. A 44-percent relative reduction in the incidence of MI was observed in the aspirin group (254.8 per 100,000 per year compared with 439.7 in the placebo group); however, cardiovascular mortality did not differ between groups. In addition, an increased rate of hemorrhagic stroke was seen in the aspirin group (relative risk 2.14; 95 percent CI, .96 to 4.77; p = .06).

A second primary prevention trial, the British Male Doctor Study [122], failed to reveal significant differences between men taking aspirin and those asked to avoid aspirin. The lack of a beneficial effect may reflect the large aspirin dose (500 mg per day), lack of placebo control, low compliance rate in the aspirin group, or the advanced age of physicians agreeing to participate in the study. Collectively, however, the Physicians Health Study and the British Male Doctor Study demonstrate a significant (p < .0001) reduction in nonfatal MI of about one-third among individuals taking aspirin. Of concern, a trend toward an increased incidence of disabling stroke was also evident.

Further analysis of the data compiled in the Physicians Health Study has revealed two interesting and clinically relevant findings [123]. First, the rate of nonfatal MI among aspirin users decreased solely in persons 50 years of age or older. Second, the benefits derived from aspirin were most pronounced in persons with coronary risk factors, i.e., those at greatest risk of experiencing a cardiac event (Table 5-4).

Based on the available information, patients more than 50 years of age with two or more risk factors (one of which can be male sex) for atherosclerotic coronary artery disease should be encouraged to take one aspirin (325 mg) every other day. Younger patients with two or more risk factors, including a family history of sudden death before age 50, should also be strongly considered for this therapy. Although the studies to date have not included women, similar benefits would be anticipated in high-risk individuals. Routine aspirin administration among individuals with long-standing, poorly controlled systemic hypertension should be undertaken with caution.

Table 5-4. Aspirin in the primary prevention of cardiac events

End point	Reduction (%±SD) (↑ = increase)			
	British Doctors Study	US Physicians Study	Combined	P value (combined)
Nonfatal MI	23±19	39±9	32±8	<0.0001
Nonfatal stroke	↑ 13±24	↑ 19±15	↑ 18±13	NS
Cardiovascular mortality (total)	7±14	2±15	5±10	NS
Any vascular event	4±12	18±7	13±6	<0.05

Secondary Prevention of Cardiac Events

Aortocoronary Bypass Graft Disease

Currently approximately 280,000 aortocoronary bypass graft procedures are performed yearly in the United States; over 5 percent are repeat (redo) operations. Saphenous vein graft occlusion rates per distal anastomosis are 8 to 18 percent in the first postoperative month and 16 to 26 percent at one year [124]. After eight to ten years, greater than 50 percent of saphenous vein grafts are either occluded or significantly diseased.

Saphenous vein graft disease can be divided into two major phases, an early phase and a late phase. In the early phase, endothelial damage to the saphenous vein occurs during surgical harvesting and upon its exposure to the high-pressure arterial system. Additional damage follows surgical handling and suturing. Upon the establishment of blood flow, platelets, which are activated within the extracorporeal system, adhere to areas of endothelial damage and initiate coagulation. Poor surgical technique and severe native vessel coronary disease may also compromise blood flow, enhancing focal procoagulant tendencies.

In a majority of cases, early saphenous vein graft occlusion is thrombotic in origin. As platelet activation begins intraoperatively, platelet-inhibitor therapy should be initiated before surgery. Preoperative treatment with dipyridamole has been shown in an animal model to

decrease extracorporeal platelet activation [125]. A subsequent study in patients undergoing bypass surgery [126] confirmed the clinical efficacy of initiating platelet-inhibitor therapy with dipyridamole preoperatively, followed postoperatively by the combination of aspirin and dipyridamole. In contrast, preoperative aspirin administration, while maintaining graft patency, has been associated with an excess of bleeding complications, transfusion requirements, and surgical reexploration [127]. A number of studies have demonstrated the benefit of platelet-inhibitor therapy in preventing early saphenous vein graft occlusion (see Table 5-5).

Current recommendations include the routine use of dipyridamole (100 mg qid) in the 48 hours preceding surgery, followed by aspirin (325 mg) initiated within the first 12 postoperative hours (typically 8 to 10 hours postop) and continued daily.

Late saphenous vein graft disease is characterized by smooth-muscle (intimal) hyperplasia with varying amounts of subocclusive or occlusive thrombus. The process itself is initiated by early platelet activation, followed by the release of potent mitogenic factors that stimulate the proliferation of smooth-muscle cells. In time, however, intimal fibrosis, containing smooth-muscle cells, collagen, foam cells (lipid-laden macrophages), and focal calcification develops, indistinguishable from native coronary atherosclerosis.

Platelet-inhibitor therapy has been shown to reduce the incidence of saphenous vein graft oc-

Table 5-5. **Antiplatelet therapy in early saphenous vein bypass graft disease**

Investigator	Number of patients	Treatment regimen	Time of angiography (days)	Graft patency		P
				Treatment	Control	
Chesebro [126]	407	DIP 100 mg qid for two days preoperatively, then ASA 325 mg tid plus DIP 75 mg tid	8	97	90	<.0001
Goldman [127]	772	ASA 325 mg qd or ASA 325 mg tid or ASA 325 mg qd plus DIP 75 mg tid or sulfinpyrazone, 267 mg tid	9	94	85	<.05
				90		NS
Limet [128]	173	Ticlopidine 250 mg bid		93	87	<.05
Sanz [129]	1112	DIP 100 mg qid for two days preoperatively, then ASA 50 mg tid; or ASA 50 mg tid plus DIP 75 mg tid	10	86	82	.058
				87.1		.01

ASA = aspirin; DIP = dipyridamole; NS = not significant.

clusion at least through the first postoperative year (Table 5-6), primarily by preventing thrombus formation. However, the agents currently in use do not prevent the release of platelet-derived growth factors, nor have they been shown to reduce the development of late saphenous vein atherosclerosis.

Current recommendations include the daily use of aspirin (325 mg) for the first postoperative year. Although the benefits beyond one year have not been established, continuation to prevent native vessel and bypass graft thrombosis would seem prudent.

Survivors of Acute MI

In a majority of cases, acute MI is caused by thrombotic occlusion of a major epicardial coronary artery, occurring typically at a site of atherosclerotic plaque rupture. Patients surviving an acute MI are at risk for recurrent cardiac events, including reinfarction and sudden death.

The thrombotic nature of many of these events has prompted several large randomized trials investigating the role of platelet-inhibitor therapy in secondary prevention (Table 5-7). Despite the large number of patients studied, beneficial effects have not been observed in any individual study. A pooled analysis of these trials, however, has revealed that platelet-inhibitor therapy given to survivors of MI reduces mortality, nonfatal recurrent infarction, and stroke by 13, 31, and 42 percent, respectively [141].

Current recommendations for MI survivors include 325 mg of aspirin daily. Larger doses have not been shown to provide additional benefit, and they are frequently associated with an increased rate of adverse effects. In addition, combined regimens do not appear to be superior to aspirin alone. Although the duration of aspirin's beneficial effects has not been established, continued use beyond the first postinfarction year, which is the period of greatest risk, is recommended.

Table 5-6. Antiplatelet therapy in late (≤1 year) saphenous vein bypass graft disease

Investigator	Number of patients	Treatment regimen	Time of angiography	Graft patency		P
				Treatment	Control	
Chesebro [130]	84	DIP 100 mg qid for two days preoperatively, then ASA 325 mg tid plus DIP 75 mg tid	1 year	89	75	<.0001
Mayer [131]	174	ASA 650 mg plus DIP 50 mg bid	3–6 months	92	77	<.02
Goldman [132]	53	ASA plus sulfin-pyrazone 267 mg tid	1 year	84	77	<.03
				82		NS
Limet [128]	173	Ticlopidine 250 mg bid	6 months	85	76	<.02
			1 year	84	74	<.01
Brown [133]	147	ASA 325 mg tid *or*	1 year	67	59	.04
		ASA 325 mg tid plus DIP 75 mg tid		74		.04

ASA = aspirin; DIP = dipyridamole.

Table 5-7. Secondary prevention of cardiac events in survivors of acute MI

Investigator	Number of patients	Treatment regimen	Event rate reduction (%)		
			Cardiac events	Cardiac mortality	Total mortality
Elwood [134]	1239	ASA 300 mg qd	NA	NA	25
CDP [135]	1529	ASA 324 mg tid	21	27	30
GAM [136]	946	ASA 1500 mg qd	36	42	NA
AMIS [137]	4524	ASA 500 mg bid	5	8	10
PARIS-I [138]	2206	ASA 234 mg tid *or*	21	24	18
		ASA 325 mg tid plus DIP 75 mg tid	25	24	16
PARIS-II [139]	3128	ASA 330 mg tid plus DIP 75 mg tid	24	6	3
ART [140]	1558	Sulfinpyrazone 267 mg tid	NA	24	28

CDP = Coronary Drug Project; GAM = German-Austrian Multicenter; AMIS = Aspirin Myocardial Infarction Study; PARIS-I = Persantine-Aspirin Reinfarction Study, Phase 1; ART = Anturane Reinfarction Trial; ASA = aspirin; DIP = dipyridamole; NA = not available.

Summary

Platelets have long been recognized as a major component of normal hemostasis. More recently we have come to recognize their importance in coagulation, fibrinolysis, and vascular endothelial function as well.

Under normal circumstances, platelets circulate freely within the vascular system. In pathologic conditions, however, platelet–vessel wall interactions occur, initiating nonphysiologic thrombus formation, which may impair normal blood flow.

The importance of platelet-inhibitor therapy among individuals with atherosclerotic coronary heart disease has been established. Future investigations must address the use of more potent platelet inhibitors and agents designed to inhibit either the release or the binding of PDGFs.

References

1. Piper P, Vane JR. The release of prostaglandins from the vascular endothelium and other tissues. Ann NY Acad Science 1971; 180:363–85.
2. Willis AL, Smith DL, Vigo C, Kluge AF. Effects of prostacyclin and orally active stable mimetic agent RS-93427-007 on bovine mechanisms of atherogenosis. Lancet 1986; 2:682–3.
3. Dadak CH, Leithner C, Sinzinger H, Silberbaver K. Diminished prostacyclin formation in umbilical arteries of babies born to women who smoke. Lancet 1981; 1:94.
4. Furchgott RF, Zawadski JV. The obligatory role of endothelial cells in the relaxation of arterial smooth muscle cells by acetylcholine. Nature 1980; 288:373–6.
5. Palmer RMJ, Ferige AG, Moncada S. Nitric oxide release accounts for the biologic activity of endothelium-derived relaxing factor. Nature 1987; 327:524–6.
6. Radomski MW, Palmer RM, Moncada S. Endogenous nitric oxide inhibits human platelet adhesion to vascular endothelium. Lancet 1987; 1:1057–8.
7. Radomski MW, Palmer RM, Moncada S. The antiaggregatory properties of vascular endothelium: interactions between prostacyclin and nitric oxide. Br J Pharmacol 1987; 92:639–46.
8. Heeg E, Meng K. Die wirkung des bradykinins, angiotensins und vasopressins auf verhof papillarmusckel, und isoliert durstromte herzpraparate des meerschweinchens. Navnyn schiedebergs. Arch Pharmacol 1965; 250:35–41.
9. Unger TH, Gohlke P, Ganten D, Lang RE. Converting enzyme inhibitors and their effects on the renin-angiotensin system of the blood vessel wall. J Cardiovasc Pharmacol 1988; 13:Suppl 3:S8–S16.
10. Simonson MS, Wann S, Mene P, et al. Endothelin-1 activates the phosphoinositide cascade in cultured glomerular mesangial cells. J Cardiovasc Pharmacol 1989; 13:Suppl 5:S80–S83.
11. Yanagisawa M, Kurihara H, Kimsura S, et al. A novel potent vasoconstrictor peptide produced by vascular endothelial cells. Nature 1988; 332:411–5.
12. Miyanchi T, Tomobe Y, Shiba R, et al. Involvement of endothelin in the regulation of human vascular tonus: potent vasoconstrictor effect and existence in endothelial cells. Circulation 1990; 81:1874–80.
13. Teien AN, Abildgaard U, Hook M, Lindahl U. The anticoagulant effect of heparin sulfate and dermatan sulfate. Thromb Res 1977; 11:107.
14. Thomas DP, Merton RE, Barrowcliffe TW, et al. Antifactor Xa activity of heparin sulfate. Thromb Res 1979; 14:501.
15. Marcum JA, Rosenberg RD. Heparin–like molecules with anticoagulant activity are synthesized by cultured endothelial cells. Biochem Biophys Res Commun 1985; 126:365.
16. Maynard JR, Dreyer BE, Stemerman MB, Pitlick FA. Tissue factor coagulant activity of cultured human endothelial and smooth muscle cells and fibroblasts. Blood 1977; 50:387–96.
17. Stern OM, Bank I, Naworth PP, et al. Self regulation of procoagulant events on the endothelial cell surface. J Exp Med 1985; 162:1223–35.
18. Giddings JC. von Willebrand factor–physiology. In: Gimbrone MA Jr., ed. Vascular endothelium in hemostasis and thrombosis. New York: Churchill-Livingstone, 1986; 142–68.
19. Erickson LA, Ginsberg MH, Loskutoff DJ. Detection and partial characterization of an inhibitor of plasminogen activator in human platelets. J Clin Invest 1984; 74:1465–72.
20. Lucore CL, Sobel BE. Interactions of tissue-type plasminogen activator with plasma inhibitors and their pharmacologic implications. Circulation 1988; 77:660–9.
21. Loskutoff DJ. Type 1 plasminogen activator inhibitor and its potential influence on thrombolytic therapy. Sem Thromb Hem 1988; 14:100–9.
22. Fujii S, Sobel BE. Induction of plasminogen activator inhibitor by products released from platelets. Circulation 1990; 82:1485–93.

23. Ludmer PL, Selwyn AP, Shook TL, et al. Paradoxical vasoconstriction induced by acetylcholine in atherosclerotic coronary arteries. N Engl J Med 1986; 315:1046–51.

24. Nabel EG, Selwyn AP, Ganz P. Paradoxical narrowing of atherosclerotic coronary arteries induced by increases in heart rate. Circulation 1990; 81:850–9.

25. Vita JA, Treasure CB, Ganz P, et al. Control of shear stress in the epicardial coronary arteries of humans: impairment by atherosclerosis. J Am Coll Cardiol 1989; 14:1193–9.

26. Coupe MO, Mak JCW, Yacoub M, et al. Autoradiographic mapping of calcitonin gene-related polypeptide receptors in human and guinea pig hearts. Circulation 1990; 81:741–7.

27. Yatani A, Yokoyama M, Akita H, Fakuzak H. Endothelium-dependent vasodilating effect of substance P during flow-reducing coronary stenosis in the dog. J Am Coll Cardiol 1990; 15:1374–84.

28. Schwartz JS, Carlyle PF, Cohn JN. Effect of dilation of the distal coronary bed on flow and resistance in severely stenotic coronary arteries in the dog. Am J Cardiol 1979; 43:219–24.

29. Jellke FW, Quillen JE, Brooks LA, Harrison DG. Endothelial modulation of the coronary vasculature in the vessels perfused via mature collaterals. Circulation 1990; 81:1938–47.

30. Peters KG, Marcus ML, Harrison DG. Vasopressin and the mature coronary collateral circulation. Circulation 1989; 79:1324–31.

31. Yamamoto H, Bossaller C, Cartwright J Jr, Henry PD. Videomicroscopic demonstration of defective cholinergic arteriolar vasodilation in atherosclerotic rabbit. J Clin Invest 1988; 81:1752–8.

32. Harrison DG, Armstrong ML, Freiman PC, Heistad DD. Restoration of endothelium dependent relaxation by dietary treatment of atherosclerosis. J Clin Invest 1987; 80:1808–11.

33. Sellke FW, Armstrong ML, Harrison DG. Endothelium-dependent vascular relaxation is abnormal in the coronary microcirculation of atherosclerotic primates. Circulation 1990; 81:1586–93.

34. Kwaan HC. Possible effects of risk factors on fibrinolysis. In: Chandler AB, ed. Thrombotic processes in atherosclerosis. New York: Plenum, 1978; 235–300.

35. Walker ID, Davidson JF, Hutton I, et al. Disordered fibrinolytic potential in coronary heart disease. Thromb Res 1977; 10:509–20.

36. Chakrabarti R, Hocking ED. Fibrinolytic activity and coronary heart disease. Lancet 1968; 1:987–90.

37. Zahavi J, Bitteridge JD, Jones NAG, et al. Enhanced in vivo platelet-release reaction and malondialdehyde formation in patients with hyperlipidemia. Am J Med 1981; 70:59–64.

38. Joist JH, Baker RK, Schonfeld G. Increased in vivo and in vitro platelet function in type II and type IV hyperlipoproteinemia. Thromb Res 1974; 15:95–108.

39. Strano A, Davi G, Averna M, et al. Platelet sensitivity to prostacyclin and thromboxane production in hyperlipidemic patients. Thromb Haemost 1982; 48:18–20.

40. Joist JH, Dolezel G, Kinlough-Rathbone RL, Mustard JF. Effect of diet-induced hyperlipidemia on in vitro function of rabbit platelets. Thromb Res 1976; 9:435–9.

41. Tremoli E, Folco G, Agradi E, Gall C. Platelet thromboxanes and serum cholesterol. Lancet 1979; 1:107–8.

42. Harker LA, Hazzare W. Platelet kinetic studies in patients with hyperlipoproteinemia: effect of clofibrate therapy. Circulation 1979; 60: 492–6.

43. Worner P, Patscheke H. Hyperreactivity by an enhancement of the arachidonate pathway of platelets treated with cholesterol-rich phospholipid-dispersions. Thromb Res 1980; 18:439–51.

44. Shattil SJ, Cooper RA. Role of membrane lipid composition, organization and fluidity in human platelet function. Prog Hemost Thromb 1978; 4:59–86.

45. Nabel EG, Ganz P, Selwyn AP. Atherosclerosis impairs flow-mediated dilation in human coronary arteries. Circulation 1988; 78:Suppl II:II-474.

46. Jayakody L, Sernaratne M, Thompson A, Kappagoda T. Endothelium-dependent relaxation in experimental atherosclerosis in the rabbit. Circ Res 1987; 60:251–64.

47. Cohen RA, Zitnay KM, Haudenschild CC, Cunningham LD. Loss of selective endothelial cell vasoactive functions caused by hypercholesterolemia in pig coronary arteries. Circ Res 1988; 63:903–7.

48. Yasue H, Matsuyama K, Matsuyama K, et al. Responses of angiographically normal human coronary arteries to intracoronary injection of acetylcholine by age and segment. Circulation 1990; 81:482–90.

49. Vita JA, Treasure CB, Nabel EG, et al. Coronary vasomotor response to acetylcholine relates to risk factors for coronary artery disease. Circulation 1990; 81:491–7.

50. Ross R, Glomset J, Kariya B, et al. A platelet-dependent serum factor that stimulates the proliferation of arterial smooth muscle cells in vitro. Proc Natl Acad Sci USA 1974; 71:1207.

51. Antoniades HN, Hunkapiller MW. Human platelet derived growth factor (PDGF) amino-

terminal amino acid sequence. Science 1983; 220:963–5.

52. Grotendorst GR, Seppa EJ, Kleinman HK, et al. Attachment of smooth muscle cells to collagen and their migration toward platelet-derived growth factor. Proc Natl Acad Sci USA 1981; 78:3669.

53. Friedman M, Van den Bovenkamp EJ. The pathogenesis of a coronary thrombus. Am J Path 1966; 48:19–44.

54. Rasmanis G, Vastergvist O, Green K, et al. Effects of intermittent treatment with aspirin on thromboxane and prostaglandin formation in patients with acute myocardial infarction. Lancet 1988; I:245–7.

55. Lam JYT, Chesebro JH, Steele PM, et al. Is vasospasm related to platelet deposition? Relationship in a porcine preparation of arterial injury in vivo. Circulation 1987; 75:243–8.

56. Libby P, Warner SJC, Salomon RN, Birinyi LK. Production of platelet-derived growth factor-like mitogen by smooth-muscle cells from human atheroma. N Engl J Med 1988; 318:1493–8.

57. Williams LT. Signal transduction by the platelet-derived growth factor receptor. Science 1989; 243:1564–5.

58. Badimon L, Badimon JJ, Chesebro JH, Fuster V. Inhibition of thrombus formation: blockage of adhesive glycoprotein mechanisms versus blockage of the cyclooxygenase pathway. J Am Coll Cardiol 1988; 11:Suppl A:30A (abstract).

59. Strony J, Phillips M, Brands D, et al. Aurintricarboxylic acid in a canine model of coronary artery thrombosis. Circulation 1990; 81:1106–14.

60. Cattaneo M, Chahil A, Somers D, et al. Effect of aspirin and sodium salicylate on thrombosis, fibrinolysis, prothrombin time, and platelet survival in rabbits with indwelling aortic catheters. Blood 1983; 61:353–61.

61. Hirsh J. Progress review: the relationship between dose of aspirin, side-effects and antithrombotic effectiveness. Stroke 1985; 16:1–4.

62. Neri Serneri GG, Castellani S. Platelet and vascular prostaglandins: Pharmacological and clinical implications. In Born GVR, Neri Serneri GG, eds. Antiplatelet therapy: twenty years experience. Proceedings of a European conference. Amsterdam: Elsevier Excerpta Medica, 1987:37–51.

63. Yasuda T, Gold HK, Leinbach RC, et al. Lysis of plasminogen activator-resistant platelet-rich coronary artery thrombus with combined bolus injection of recombinant tissue-type plasminogen activator and antiplatelet GPIIb/IIIa antibody. J Am Coll Cardiol 1990; 16:1728–35.

64. Musial J, Niewiarowski S, Rucinski B, et al.

Inhibition of platelet adhesion to surfaces of extracorporeal circuits by disintegrins. RGD-containing peptides from viper venoms. Circulation 1990; 82:261–73.

65. Saltiel R, Ward A. Ticlopidine: a review of its pharmacodynamics and pharmacokinetic properties and therapeutic efficacy in platelet-dependent disease states. Drugs 1987; 34:222–62.

66. Fitzgerald GA, Reilly LA, Pederson AK. The biochemical pharmacology of thromboxane synthase inhibition in man. Circulation 1985; 72:1194–1201.

67. Mullane KM, Foinabaio D. Thromboxane synthetase inhibitors reduce infarct size by a platelet dependent, aspirin-sensitive mechanism. Circ Res 1988; 62:668–78.

68. Saussy DL Jr, Mais DE, Knapp DR, Halushka PV. Thromboxane A_2 and prostaglandin endoperoxide receptors in platelets and vascular smooth muscle. Circulation 1985; 72:1202–7.

69. Evans RJ, Gordon JD. Mechanisms of the antithrombotic actions of dextran. N Engl J Med 1974; 290:748–56.

70. Weiss HJ. The effect of clinical dextran on platelet aggregation, adhesion, and ADP release in man: in vivo and in vitro studies. J Lab Clin Med 1967; 69:37–46.

71. Clubb FJ, Schmitz JM, Butler MM, et al. Effect of dietary omega-3 fatty acid on serum lipids, platelet function, and atherosclerosis in Watanabe heritable hyperlipidemic rabbits. Arteriosclerosis 1989; 9:529–37.

72. Spector AA, Kaduce TL, Figard PH, et al. Eicosapentaenoic acid and prostacyclin production by cultured human endothelial cells. J Lipid Res 1983; 24:1595–1604.

73. Needleman P, Sprecher H, Whitaker MO, Wyche A. Mechanism underlying the inhibition of platelet aggregation by eicosapentaenoic acid and its metabolites. In: Samuelsson B, Ramwell PW, Paoletti R, eds. Advances in prostaglandin and thromboxane research. New York: Raven, 1980.

74. Fitzgerald GA. Dipyridamole. N Engl J Med 1987; 316:1247–56.

75. Emmons PR, Hampton JR, Harrison MJG, et al. Effect of prostaglandin E_1 on platelet behavior in vitro and in vivo. Br Med J 1967; 2:468–72.

76. Terres W, Beythien C, Kupper W, Bleifeld W. Effects of aspirin and prostaglandin E_1 on in vitro thrombolysis with urokinase. Circulation 1989; 79:1309–14.

77. Weksler BB. Prostaglandins and vascular function. Circulation 1984; 70:Suppl III:III-63–71.

78. Fisher CA, Kappa JR, Sinha AK, et al. Comparison of equimolar concentrations of iloprost, prostacyclin, and prostaglandin E_1 on human

platelet function. J Lab Clin Med 1987; 109:184–90.

79. Kiyomoto A, Sasaki Y, Odawara A, Morita T. Inhibition of platelet aggregation by diltiazem. Comparison with verapamil and nifedipine and inhibitory potencies of diltiazem metabolites. Circ Res 1983; 52:Suppl I:115–9.

80. Mehta P, Mehta J, Ostrowski N, Brigmon L. Inhibitory effects of diltiazem on platelet activation caused by ionophore A23187 plus ADP or epinephrine in subthreshold concentrations. J Lab Clin Med 1983; 102:332–9.

81. Addonizio VP, Fisher CA, Strauss JF, et al. Effects of verapamil and diltiazem on human platelet function. Am J Physiol 1986; 250:H366–71.

82. Altman R, Scazziota A, Dujovne C. Diltiazem potentiates the inhibitory effect of aspirin on platelet aggregation. Clin Pharmacol Ther 1988; 44:320–5.

83. Wade PJ, Lunt DO, Lad N, et al. Effect of calcium and calcium antagonists on [³H]-PAF-Acether binding to washed human platelets. Thrombosis Res 1986; 41:251–62.

84. Fischer-Dzoga K, Kuo YF, Wissler RW. The proliferative effect of platelets and hyperlipidemic serum on stationary primary cultures. Atherosclerosis 1983; 47:35–45.

85. Tiell ML, Sussman II, Gordon PB. Suppression of fibroblast proliferation in vitro and of myointimal hyperplasia in vivo by the triazolopyrimidine, trapidil. Artery 1983; 12:33–50.

86. Jones RL, Peterson CM. Hematologic alterations in diabetes mellitus. Am J Med 1981; 70:339–52.

87. Shaw S, Pegrum GD, Wolff S, Ashtono WL. Platelet adhesiveness in diabetes mellitus. J Clin Path 1967; 20:845–7.

88. Kwaan HC, Colwell JA, Cruz S, Suwanela N, Dobbie JG. Increased platelet aggregation in diabetes mellitus. J Lab Clin Med 1972; 80:236–46.

89. Sagel J, Colwell JA, Crook L, Laimens M. Increased platelet aggregation in early diabetes mellitus. Ann Int Med 1975; 82:733–8.

90. Burrows AW, Chavin SI, Hockaday TDR. Plasma thromboglobulin concentrations in diabetes mellitus. Lancet 1978; 1:235–7.

91. Preston FE, Ward JD, Marrola BH, et al. Elevated β-thromboglobulin levels and circulating platelet aggregates in diabetic microangiopathy. Lancet 1978; 1:238–9.

92. McDonald JWD, Dupre J, Rodger NW, et al. Comparison of platelet thromboxane synthesis in diabetic patients on conventional insulin therapy and continuous insulin infusions. Thromb Res 1982; 28:705–12.

93. Halushka PV, Rogers RC, Lisadholt CB, Colwell JA. Increased thromboxane synthesis in diabetes mellitus. J Lab Clin Med 1981; 97:87–96.

94. Silberhaur K, Schernthaner G, Sinzinger H, Piza-Katzer H, Winter M. Decreased vascular prostacyclin in juvenile-onset diabetes. N Engl J Med 1979; 300:366–7.

95. Landgraf-Leurs MMC, Landgraf R, Loy A, Weber PC, Herberg LL. Aggregation and thromboxane formation by platelets and vascular prostacyclin production from BB rats. An animal model for type I diabetes. Prostaglandins 1982; 24:35–46.

96. Lepape A, Gutman N, Guitton JD, Legrand Y, Muh JP. Nonenzymatic glycosylation increases platelet aggregating potency of collagen from placenta of diabetic human beings. Biochem Biophys Res Commun 1983; 111:602–10.

97. U.S. Department of Health and Human Services. The health consequences of smoking. A report of the Surgeon General. USDHHS publ. no. (PHS) 84-50204, 1983.

98. Cigarette smoking in the United States, 1986. MMWR 1987; 36:581–5.

99. Wells A. An estimate of adult mortality in the United States from passive smoking. Environ Int 1988; 14:249–65.

100. Hennekens CH, Buring JE. Smoking and coronary heart disease in women. JAMA 1985; 253:3003–4.

101. Hermanson B, Omenn GS, Kronmal RA, Gersh BJ. Beneficial six-year outcome of smoking cessation in older men and women with coronary artery disease. Results from the CASS registry. N Engl J Med 1988; 319:1365–9.

102. Palmer JR, Rosenberg L, Shapiro S. "Low yield" cigarettes and the risk of nonfatal myocardial infarction in women. N Engl J Med 1989; 320:1569–73.

103. Davis J, Shelton L, Eigenberg D, et al. Effects of tobacco and non-tobacco cigarette smoking on endothelium and platelets. Clin Pharmacol Ther 1985; 37:529–33.

104. Sinzinger H, Kefalides A. Passive smoking severely decreses platelet sensitivity to antiaggregatory prostaglandins. Lancet 1982; 2:392–3.

105. Burghuber O, Punzengruber C, Sinzinger H, Haber P, Silberbauer K. Platelet sensitivity to prostacyclin in smokers and non-smokers. Chest 1986; 90:34–8.

106. Davis J, Shelton L, Eigenberg D, Hignite C. Lack of effect of aspirin on cigarette smoke-induced increase in circulating endothelial cells. Haemostasis 1987; 7:66–9.

107. Ross R. The pathology of atherosclerosis — an update. N Engl J Med 1986; 314:488–500.

108. Albert R, Vanderlaan F, Nishizumi M. Effect

of carcinogens on chicken atherosclerosis. Cancer Res 1977; 37:2232–5.

109. Meairs S, Weihe E, Mittmann U, et al. Morphologic investigation of coronary arteries subjected to hypertension by experimental supravalvular aortic stenosis in dogs. Lab Invest. 1984; 50:469.

110. Downing SE, Vidone RA, Brandt HM, Liebow AA. The pathogenesis of vascular lesions in experimental hyperkinetic pulmonary hypertension. Am J Pathol 1963; 43:739.

111. Meade TW, Vickers MV, Thompson SG, et al. Epidemiological characteristics of platelet aggregability. Br Med J 1985; 290:428–31.

112. Elwood PC, Renaud S, Sharp DS, et al. Ischemic heart disease and platelet aggregation. The Caerphilly Collaborative Heart Disease Study. Circulation 1991; 83:38–44.

113. Trip MD, Cats VM, vanCapelle FJL, Vreeken J. Platelet hyperactivity and prognosis in survivors of myocardial infarction. N Engl J Med 1990; 322:1549–54.

114. Kannel WB, Schatzkin A. Risk factor analysis. Prog Cardiovasc Dis 1983; 26:309–32.

115. Gordon D, Guyton JR, Kaarnovsky MJ. Intimal alterations in rat aorta induced by stressful stimuli. Lab Invest 1981; 45:14–27.

116. Kaplan JR, Manuck SB, Clarkson TB, et al. Social stress and atherosclerosis in normocholesterolemic monkeys. Science 1983; 220:733–5.

117. Haft JI, Gershengorn K, Kranz PD, Oestreicher R. Protection against epinephrine-induced myocardial necrosis by drugs that inhibit platelet aggregation. Am J Cardiol 1972; 30:838–43.

118. Muller JE, Stone PH, Turi ZG, et al. Circadian variation in the frequency of onset of acute myocardial infarction. N Engl J Med 1985; 313:1315–22.

119. Brezinski DA, Tofler GH, Muller JE, et al. Morning increase in platelet aggregability: association with assumption of the upright posture. Circulation 1988; 78:35–40.

120. Ridker PM, Manson JE, Buring JE, et al. Circadian variation of acute myocardial infarction and the effect of low-dose aspirin in a randomized trial of physicians. Circulation 1990; 82:897–902.

121. Steering Committee of the Physicians Health Study Research Group. Final report on the aspirin component of the ongoing Physicians Health Study. N Engl J Med 1989; 321:129–35.

122. Peto R, Gray R, Collins R, et al. Randomized trial of prophylactic daily aspirin in British male doctors. Br Med J 1988; 296:313–6.

123. Fuster V, Cohen J, Halperin J. Aspirin in the prevention of coronary disease. N Engl J Med 1989; 321:183–5.

124. Fuster V, Chesebro JH. Role of platelets and platelet inhibitors in aortocoronary artery vein-graft disease. Circulation 1986; 2:227–32.

125. Josa M, Lie JT, Bianco RL, Kaye MP. Reduction of thrombosis in canine coronary bypass grafts with dipyridamole and aspirin. Am J Cardiol 1981; 47:1248–54.

126. Chesebro JH, Clements IP, Fuster V, et al. A platelet inhibitor drug trial in coronary artery bypass operations: benefits of perioperative dipyridamole and aspirin therapy on early postoperative vein graft patency. N Engl J Med 1982; 307:73–8.

127. Goldman S, Copeland J, Moritz T, et al. Improvement in early saphenous vein graft patency after coronary artery bypass surgery with antiplatelet therapy: results of a Veterans Administration Cooperative Study. Circulation 1988; 77:1324–33.

128. Limet R, David JL, Magotteaux P, et al. Prevention of aortocoronary bypass graft occlusion. Beneficial effect of ticlopidine on early and late patency rates of venous coronary bypass grafts: a double-blind study. J Thorac Cardiovasc Surg 1987; 94:773–83.

129. Sanz G, Pajaron A, Alegria E, et al. Prevention of early aortocoronary bypass occlusion by low-dose aspirin and dipyridamole. Circulation 1990; 82:765–73.

130. Chesebro JH, Fuster V, Elveback LR, et al. Effect of dipyridamole and aspirin on late vein graft patency. N Engl J Med 1984; 310:209–14.

131. Mayer JE Jr, Lindsay WG, Castaneda W, et al. Influence of aspirin and dipyridamole on patency of coronary artery bypass grafts. Ann Thorac Surg 1981; 31:204–10.

132. Goldman S, Copeland JG, Moritz T, et al. Saphenous vein graft patency 1 year after coronary artery bypass surgery and effects of antiplatelet therapy. Results of a Veterans Administration Cooperative Study. Circulation 1989; 80:1190–7.

133. Brown BG, Cuckingnan RA, DeRouen T, et al. Improved graft patency in patients treated with platelet-inhibiting therapy after coronary bypass surgery. Circulation 1985; 72:138–46.

134. Elwood PC, Cochrane AL, Burr ML, et al. A randomized controlled trial of acetylsalicylic acid in the secondary prevention of mortality from myocardial infarction. Brit Med J 1974; 1:436–40.

135. The Coronary Drug Project Research Group. Aspirin in coronary heart disease. J Chron Dis 1976; 29:625–42.

136. Breddin K, Loew D, Lechner K, et al. Secondary prevention of myocardial infarction: comparison of acetylsalicylic acid, phenprocoumon and placebo. Hemostasis 1980; 9:325–44.

137. Aspirin Myocardial Infarction Study Research Group. A randomized, controlled trial of aspirin in persons recovered from myocardial infarction. JAMA 1980; 243:661–9.
138. The Persantine-Aspirin Reinfarction Study Research Group. Persantine and aspirin in coronary heart disease. Circulation 1980; 62: 449–61.
139. Klimt CR, Knatterud GL, Stamler J, Meier P. Persantine-Aspirin Reinfarction Study. Part II.

Secondary coronary prevention with persantine and aspirin. J Am Coll Cardiol 1986; 7:251–69.
140. The Anturane Reinfarction Trial Research Group. Sulfinpyrazone in the prevention of sudden death after myocardial infarction. N Engl J Med 1980; 302:250–6.
141. Antiplatelet Trialists Collaboration. Secondary prevention of vascular disease by prolonged antiplatelet treatment. Brit Med J 1988; 296:320–31.

6

An International Perspective on Coronary Heart Disease and Related Risk Factors

JUAN CARLOS ZEVALLOS
DAVID CHIRIBOGA
JAMES R. HEBERT

EDITORS' INTRODUCTION

We often make decisions based on our own limited experience, without realizing that the situation elsewhere may be very different. Nowhere is this more true than in the area of risk factors for CHD. A serum cholesterol level that is low for the United States may be in the highest decile of the population cholesterol distribution in China; our low-fat diet with 30 percent of calories from fat would be a high-fat diet for a rural villager in Ecuador. A consequence of the wide spread of risk factor levels among the various populations of the world is that we are able to see relationships between risk factors and disease that are masked when the risk factor distribution is within a relatively narrow range, such as occurs for dietary fat in the United States. It is for this reason that interpopulation studies such as the Seven Countries Study were so productive. There is still much to be learned from a broadening of our horizon. This chapter presents the international perspective, with emphasis on both the value and the limitations of such analyses. International aspects of specific risk factors are discussed, and the cultural, sociologic, and economic forces that determine the distribution of such risk factors as tobacco consumption and the types of food fats eaten are analyzed. A particularly close look is taken at Japan, where changing economic and social conditions are resulting in dramatic shifts in risk factor prevalence. The material in this chapter will provide the reader with the broader perspective that is needed to understand some of the problems of risk factor modification in different environments and also to better understand the meaning of such terms as "normal" and "desirable" as they apply to the entire world.

This chapter reviews the available data on international morbidity and mortality for coronary heart disease (CHD) and the distribution of CHD risk factors in different countries. Analysis of the international distribution of CHD morbidity, mortality, and risk factors, though complicated by limitations of the available data, can provide insights into the complex interrelationships among the different factors and help in identifying those risk factors that can and should be targets of intervention.

The Limitations of International Data

In the analysis of worldwide rates of change in CHD morbidity, mortality, and relevant risk factors, incomplete reporting, poor quality of the available information, and lack of data standardization continue to be important problems.

With regard to morbidity data, in most countries the lack of adequate and standardized diagnostic criteria for the different clinical manifestations of CHD (e.g., angina pectoris, ischemic cardiomyopathy) make it difficult to evaluate the incidence and prevalence of CHD. Most of the available studies use only diagnostic criteria for myocardial infarction (MI) to address the problem of CHD morbidity, since standardization of this diagnosis is clearest. Even for this relatively straightforward diagnosis, however, it is not an easy task to monitor the incidence of acute MI over time using standardized methods, even within one community [1, 2, 3]. For example, in the United States in 1986 there were two million hospital discharges with CHD as the first-listed diagnosis [4]. Approximately 35 percent of these were for acute MI. Estimates of incidence cannot be inferred from hospital discharges, because first events are not differentiated from recurrent events. There were over ten million office visits for CHD [5], and the prevalence of CHD was estimated to be approximately 7 million, or 29 per 1000 [6].

Mortality data in many countries of the world show striking deficiencies. In approximately 30 percent of nonindustrialized countries, more than 15 percent of all deaths are certified as having occurred because of senility or other ill-defined causes [7]. The convention in ecological studies (i.e., cross-national studies that rely on aggregate estimates of risk factors and disease rates) is to exclude these countries from analysis [8, 9], the assumption being that the data are of poor quality. Even in countries with excellent overall death registration, mortality data can demonstrate a bias resulting from nonrepresentative sampling and low quality of the data from specific subpopulations. Many countries comprise several distinct populations with marked ethnic and cultural differences, which may make mortality data even more difficult to interpret.

In addition to the difficulties involved in assessing morbidity and mortality in various countries, there are also numerous problems in the assessment of risk factors for CHD. Cigarette or food consumption data are often based on economic or trade surveys and reports that do not necessarily target the population on which incidence rates are based [10]. Such data also do not differentiate at-risk subgroups, whose data often demonstrate the most severe skewing of either disease incidence or risk factor levels present in the least developed countries [11].

As an example of the type of information used in international nutrition studies, data on types and percentage composition of food usually come from the United Nations' Food and Agriculture Organization (FAO) data sheets, which list the average amount of food consumed by each person from a country in a particular year, based on the amount of food disposed of in that country (total grown + imports − exports, with adjustments for wastage and nonfood usage) divided by the total population. Although this method may appear artificial, the Seven Countries Study [12] has shown patterns of food consumption similar to those published by the FAO. In the absence of a superior database, it seems reasonable to use this information, bearing in mind its inherent limitations.

At times ecological correlations from different countries do not depict as strong a relationship as expected between risk factors for CHD and disease levels. Several explanations are possible: (1) high measurement variability may obscure the relationship; (2) the relationship may not exist; (3) the analyses do not reflect the structure of the relationship between the two trends (e.g., there is a lag period between changes in risk factor levels and changes in clinical event rates) [13]; or (4) a risk factor may act as an accelerator of CHD, as opposed to having a causal relationship, and in the absence of the necessary causal factor no correlation with CHD will be seen.

Despite these problems international data represent a much broader range of distribution of important risk factors than can be observed within individual countries [14, 15]. Such broad distributions can make risk factor–disease relationships easier to discern amid the noise of measurement variability and are essential for the analysis of causes of CHD.

Morbidity and Mortality

Cardiovascular diseases (CVD), which include hypertension, rheumatic heart disease, and such parasitic disorders as Chagas' disease, cause approximately one-quarter of all deaths worldwide (Figure 6-1). In industrialized countries one-half of all deaths are due to CVD. Although in nonindustrialized countries the proportion of deaths caused by CVD is approximately 16 percent (after respiratory and infectious diseases), the absolute number of deaths caused by CVD is greater in the nonindustrialized part of the world, since 78 percent of all deaths in the world occur in nonindustrialized countries [16].

The rapid increase in CVD seen in the industrialized nations after World War II prompted large-scale epidemiologic research beginning in the 1950s. Longitudinal studies, conducted both within and between countries, were initiated [17, 18, 19]. In the early 1950s a retrospective study comparing autopsy records from southern Japan and Minnesota [20] showed a striking differential in atherosclerotic coronary disease between the two populations, with atherosclerosis much less evident in the specimens from Japan.

Changes in CHD mortality rates for selected industrialized countries in two periods of time (1952 to 1967 and 1970 to 1985) are shown in Table 6-1. In the first time period, the majority of countries show an increase in mortality rates from CHD, whereas from 1970 to 1985 there is a decline in CHD mortality rates in many of the same countries. Men living in the United States, Australia, and Israel showed the greatest decline in mortality rates from CHD (− 49 percent, − 46 percent, and − 45 percent, respectively). Women in Israel (− 62 percent), Japan (− 53 percent), Australia (− 51 percent), and the United States (− 48 percent) also demonstrated large mortality rate declines. From 1970 to 1985, however, Poland, Hungary, and Spain experienced increased mortality rates for both sexes [21].

The U.S. decline in CHD mortality rates began in the mid-1960s and accelerated through the 1970s and early 1980s, so that age-standardized rates have decreased 2 to 3 percent per year for the last 15 years [22]. (See Chapter 2 for further discussion of this topic.) Subsequent to the development of these trends, the World Health Organization (WHO) Working Group developed an international collaborative study, the WHO MONICA Project, to monitor the trends and determinants of CVD over time in countries around the world [23].

The primary objectives of the MONICA Project (1985 to 1995) are the measurement of trends of cardiovascular mortality, CHD, and cerebrovascular disease morbidity and the assessment of the extent to which these trends are related to changes in known risk factors, daily living habits, health care, and major socioeconomic features in defined communities in 27 different countries. Each participating MONICA Collaborating Center collects annual population demographic and mortality data and continuous registration of coronary events over a ten-year period. At least 500 consecutive acute coronary care cases are monitored at the beginning and at the end of the event registration period, or, if feasible, all registered cases are closely monitored. In approximately one-half of the centers there is also registration of stroke events. Risk factor surveys are conducted at the beginning and at the end of the ten-year period

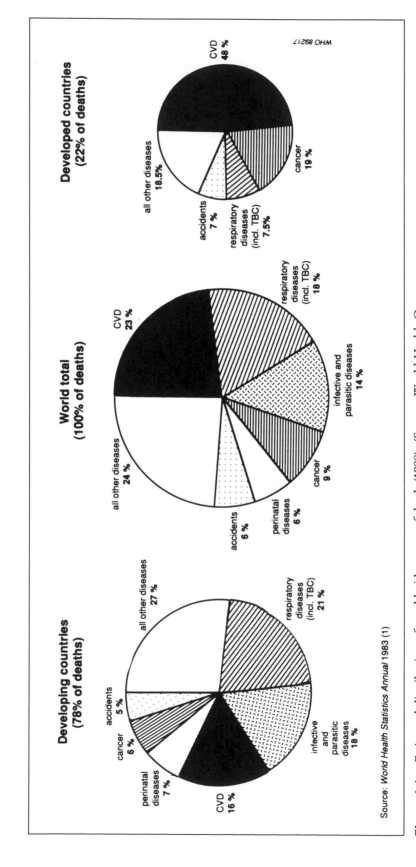

Figure 6-1. Estimated distribution of worldwide causes of death (1980). (Source: World Health Organization. World health statistics annual 1983. Geneva: WHO, 1983.)

Table 6-1. Percentage change in age-standardized death rates from ischemic heart disease in selected industrialized countries

Region/country	Males* 1952–1967	Males* 1970–1985	Females* 1952–1967	Females* 1970–1985
North America				
Canada	+7.0	−40.9	−12.4	−43.0
United States	+4.1	−48.6	−9.3	−48.1
Asia and the Middle East				
Israel	—	−45.0	—	−62.4
Japan	−.07	−38.8	−30.3	−52.7
Eastern Europe				
Czechoslovakia	+9.6	+10.2	−40.9	−2.3
Hungary	+63.9	+38.6	+17.1	+15.2
Poland	—	+72.0	—	+59.1
Northern Europe				
Finland	+23.8	−23.0	−7.5	−31.1
Norway	+98.6	−13.6	+27.2	−23.3
UK (England and Wales)	+23.7	−10.9	−6.3	−2.1
Southern Europe				
Italy	+24.2	−12.6	−36.1	−33.9
Portugal	91.4	−14.2	+44.1	−31.9
Spain	−10.7	+49.2	−49.4	+24.9
Western Europe				
Belgium	77.1	−36.6	+6.9	−40.8
France	60.3	−8.5	+21.0	−28.4
Oceania				
Australia	19.3	−46.1	+9.8	−50.5
New Zealand	39.0	−31.8	+14.6	−31.2

*Age 30 to 69.
— = Data not available.
Source: WHO data bank. Data based on the 7th (pp. 420–22) 8th (pp. 410–14) and 9th (pp. 410–14) revisions of the International Classification of Diseases (ICD). (Ischemic heart disease codes are not exactly equivalent.)

and preferably also at the mid point of the study.

The final results of the MONICA Project will provide valuable information in the ongoing collaborative international effort to solve the epidemiologic puzzle of CHD. Some of the already published data are presented here.

Figure 6-2 shows a comparison of CHD and cardiovascular mortality rates from selected industrialized countries for both sexes. Scotland has one of the highest CHD mortality rates in the world, whereas Japan has the lowest rate of any of the nations in this graph. Figure 6-3 shows a comparison of CHD mortality rates for five countries: two countries with low CHD mortality rates (Japan and France), one with an average CHD mortality rate (the United States), and two with high CHD mortality rates (Scotland and the Soviet Union), utilizing data from the WHO 1990 statistics report [24]. This figure demonstrates the remarkably wide spread of CHD mortality rates and the consistent female advantage. Table 6-2 compares overall mortality data for the five countries for men and women, ranked by CHD mortality rate. Interestingly there is a similar gradient in mortality rates for all causes in both sexes.

Baseline risk factor measurements obtained at the WHO MONICA centers [25] for these countries are the source for comparison, although it is important to bear in mind the limitations of these data. In each center measurements were obtained from a population

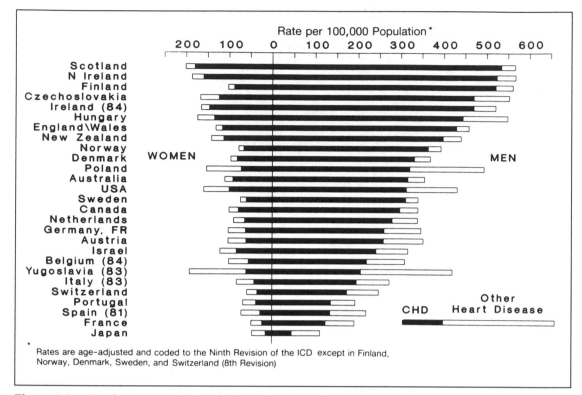

Figure 6-2. Death rates per 100,000 for heart disease and CHD by sex, ages 45 to 64, in 27 countries, 1985. (Source: Thom TJ. International mortality from heart disease: rates and trends. Int J Epidemiol 1989; 18:Suppl 1:S20–S28, with permission.)

Figure 6-3. CHD age-adjusted mortality rates for both sexes in selected industrialized countries, 1988 (France, United States, Soviet Union) and 1989 (Japan, Scotland). (Source: World Health Organization. World health statistics annual 1990. Geneva: WHO, 1991.)

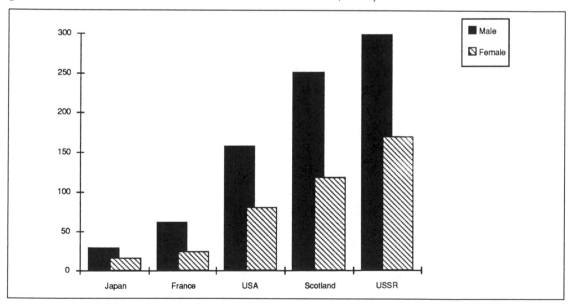

Table 6-2.   Mortality rates for men and women in selected industrialized countries, 1988

	Mortality rate, per 100				
Cause: men	Japan[a,b]	France[c]	United States[d]	Scotland[a,e]	Soviet Union[f]
All causes	518.5	654.0	715.2	831.3	1099.2
Infectious diseases	8.2	7.6	9.7	4.4	29.2
Cancer, all sites	151.1	202.2	162.6	199.5	196.4
Lung, bronchia, and trachea cancer only	30.2	46.8	56.7	73.6	62.7
Circulatory diseases	166.1	177.1	283.3	376.0	513.2
IHD only	29.9	63.0	158.8	250.6	297.5
Cerebrovascular only	65.0	43.9	34.3	75.9	155.4
All respiratory diseases	59.5	37.9	57.8	99.1	104.9
Chronic bronchitis, emphysema, and asthma only	10.4	9.5	8.0	11.5	41.1
All digestive diseases	26.4	37.8	26.3	24.2	33.4
Cirrhosis only	13.7	21.1	12.4	7.9	—
All injuries and poisonings	51.8	83.5	81.4	54.1	148.3

	Mortality rate, per 100				
Cause: women	Japan[a,b]	France[c]	United States[d]	Scotland[a,e]	Soviet Union[f]
All causes	295.2	330.3	423.9	524.9	621.9
Infectious diseases	4.0	4.4	6.8	3.2	16.3
Cancer, all sites	77.2	89.2	109.7	138.0	93.9
Lung, bronchia, and trachea cancer only	8.1	4.9	23.5	28.2	7.1
Circulatory diseases	109.1	98.4	167.4	219.9	342.1
IHD only	16.2	24.6	81.0	119.1	169.4
Cerebrovascular only	45.0	30.0	29.5	65.9	126.7
All respiratory diseases	25.9	16.1	31.3	61.6	52.9
Chronic bronchitis, emphysema, and asthma only	3.9	4.0	4.6	6.6	14.3
All digestive diseases	12.4	18.9	15.5	16.9	17.2
Cirrhosis only	4.9	8.5	5.3	4.7	—
All injuries and poisonings	21.3	34.4	28.2	28.1	46.7

IHD = ischemic heart disease; — = data not available
[a]Data from 1989.
[b]Life expectancy at birth 76.2 years for men and 82.5 years for women.
[c]Life expectancy at birth 72.9 years for men and 81.3 years for women.
[d]Life expectancy at birth 71.6 years for men and 78.6 years for women.
[e]Life expectancy at birth 70.6 years for men and 76.2 years for women.
[f]Life expectancy at birth 64.7 years for men and 73.4 years for women.
Source: World Health Organization, World health statistics annual 1990. Geneva: WHO, 1991.

sample of 2000 people, with an overall response of approximately 65 percent. The data presented are from Haute Garone (France), Stanford (the United States), Glasgow (Scotland), and Kaunas (the former Soviet Union). The only non-MONICA data come from Tanushimaru (Japan) [26]. Risk factor data for Japan were not available from the MONICA project, so we have taken values from the Seven Countries Study, which utilized similar criteria. To show

the relationship between CHD mortality rates and levels of important CHD risk factors, we have tabulated relevant data in Table 6-3 for men and Table 6-4 for women.

Table 6-3 shows the gradient of CHD risk factors for men from these countries, highlighting three important aspects: first, the contrast of very high rates of smoking and hypertension with the lowest CHD mortality rate in Japan, which supports the hypothesis that high blood

Table 6-3.   CHD mortality rates and risk factors in men aged 35 to 64 from selected industrialized countries

	Japan	France	United States	Scotland	Soviet Union
CHD rate, per 100,000	29.9[a]	63.0[a]	158.8[a]	250.6[a]	297.5[a]
Regular smoker,[b] percent	71.0[c]	36.5	40.0	52.4	38.1
Median cigarettes/day	18.0[c]	20.0	25.0	20.0	15.0
Hypertension,[d] percent	36.0[e]	25.7	23.5	32.0	30.4
Total cholesterol, mg/dl	169.5[c]	228.3	205.1	240.0	228.3
BMI, kg/m², fiftieth percentile	22.7[c,f]	25.5	25.6	25.4	27.5

IHD = ischemic heart disease; BMI = body mass index.
[a]Data from the WHO World Health Statistics Annual 1990.
[b]Defined as person who smokes every day.
[c]Data from the Seven Countries Study of men aged 40–59.
[d]Defined as systolic and/or diastolic blood pressure ≥ 159/94 mm Hg.
[e]For men at age 60. Data from the Collaborating Center for Research on Primary Prevention of Cardiovascular Diseases, Izumo, Japan.
[f]Approximate calculation from a relative body weight of 91.3 percent.
Source: WHO MONICA Project, Risk factors. Int J Epidemiol 18(Suppl 1):S46–S55, 1989.

Table 6-4.   CHD mortality rates and risk factors in women aged 35 to 64 from selected industrialized countries

	Japan	France	United States	Scotland	Soviet Union
IHD rate, per 100,000[a]	16.2	24.6	81.0	119.1	169.4
Regular smoker,[b] percent	—	17.4	36.8	50.2	3.8
Median cigarettes/day	—	10.0	20.0	20.0	7.0
Hypertension,[c] percent	—	17.6	16.7	25.4	30.7
Total cholesterol, mg/dl	—	220.6	201.2	247.7	232.2
BMI, kg/m², fiftieth percentile	—	23.6	23.5	25.5	29.3

IHD = ischemic heart disease; — = data not available; BMI = body mass index.
[a]Data from the Who World Health Statistics Annual 1990.
[b]Defined as person who smokes every day.
[c]Defined as systolic and/or diastolic blood pressure ≥159/94 mm Hg.
Source: WHO MONICA project, Risk factors. Int J Epidemiol 18(Suppl 1):S46–S55, 1989.

cholesterol levels may be the necessary precondition for hypertension and smoking to become multiplicative factors in the coronary atherosclerotic process; second, the very low CHD mortality rate in France, despite high blood cholesterol levels, which might possibly reflect a beneficial effect of moderate alcohol intake (mainly wine) [27, 28]; and third, the multiplicative effect of the known risk factors on CHD mortality rates. Table 6-4 shows a similar pattern in women, although there are no available data from Japan.

Cardiovascular disease is rapidly increasing in many nonindustrialized countries [13, 29]. The latest available data for CHD mortality rates

among selected Latin American countries are shown in Table 6-5. Cuba, Venezuela, and Costa Rica have the highest rates, whereas Ecuador, Peru, and Guatemala have the lowest. However, even among countries such as Ecuador (Figure 6-4), there has been a large increase in the incidence of CHD mortality rates over the last two decades. Similar trends have also been observed in other countries of the region [29].

In a country such as Costa Rica, where infectious disease largely has been controlled, recent data indicate that diseases of the heart are now the leading cause of death [29]. An increase of 24 percent in CHD mortality rates from 1973

Table 6-5. Deaths from ischemic heart disease[a] in selected Latin American countries

Country	Year	Death rate, per 100[b]
Cuba[c]	1982	69.8
Venezuela[c]	1983	56.9
Costa Rica[c]	1983	53.8
Puerto Rico[c]	1983	48.9
Argentina[c]	1981	43.4
Chile	1983	42.0
Panama	1984	39.0
Ecuador	1986	24.9
Mexico	1982	24.0
Peru	1982	15.0
Guatemala	1981	8.5

[a]ICD 9th Revision, pages 410–414.
[b]Age adjusted and for both sexes.
[c]Diseases of the heart (ICD 9th Revision, pages 390–429) are the leading cause of death.
Source: Pan American Health Organization. Health Conditions in the Americas. Scientific Publication no. 500. Vol. 2 Annex III:203–30, 294–368, 1986.

to 1984 has been reported. This is probably due to progressively increasing habits of affluence [30]. Despite the importance of the diseases of underdevelopment, nonindustrialized countries need to be aware that a significant proportion of their population is increasingly at risk for the harmful effects of coronary and cerebrovascular disease.

Specific Risk Factors

Diet, Cholesterol, and Overweight

In 1932 a review was published that described on an international level the relationship of dietary dairy product intake to the presence of atherosclerosis, emphasizing the importance of and the need for further international investigations [31]. Two years later, S. R. Rosenthal carried out an extensive literature analysis in which he observed the close relationship of a high cholesterol diet to the development of atherosclerosis in various countries [32].

More recently (although still several decades ago) several populations, some of them black African, were described that had a very low dietary salt intake and little or no rise in blood pressure with age [33]. These typically remote populations often have a diet resembling that of

preindustrial societies, low in fat and consisting primarily of foods of vegetable origin [34]. More modern nonindustrialized countries, however, tend to have diets increasingly higher in fat and more dependent on single grains such as rice [35].

The natural experiment suffered by European countries during World War II demonstrated that there was a decrease in cardiovascular disease mortality rates associated with changes in dietary and smoking habits caused by severe economic hardship. Concomitant changes in body weight, physical activity, and blood pressure were also observed. Within two years after the war, mortality rates from CVD had returned to prewar levels [36, 37]. These changes in mortality, occurring within relatively brief periods of time, are similar to changes in CHD morbidity observed in the Lipid Research Clinics Coronary Primary Prevention Trial (LRC-CPPT) [38, 39], the Helsinki Trial [40], and the Oslo Diet-Heart Study [41]. This evidence suggests that major alterations in dietary intake can lead to important changes in the rate of progression of the atherosclerotic process.

Studies from living population samples have been very valuable. The Seven Countries Study [12, 42] showed that the percent of calories derived from saturated fatty acids was significantly correlated with ten-year CHD death rates, as well as with incidence rates of nonfatal MI and coronary death.

The strongest evidence for diet-disease relationships almost always comes from cross-national or interpopulation comparisons. This is because the range of relevant dietary predictors is too small within a given population. For example, in the United States, 90 percent of all adults eat between 30 and 42 percent of calories as fat, whereas in the 153 countries of the world for which we have food disappearance data, 90 percent of all country mean values lie in a much broader range, between 11 and 43 percent (Figure 6-5) [15].

The dietary changes in animal fat consumption seen during the most recent 15-year period in 27 countries corroborate the view that marked decreases or increases in CHD mortality are correlated with reductions or increases, re-

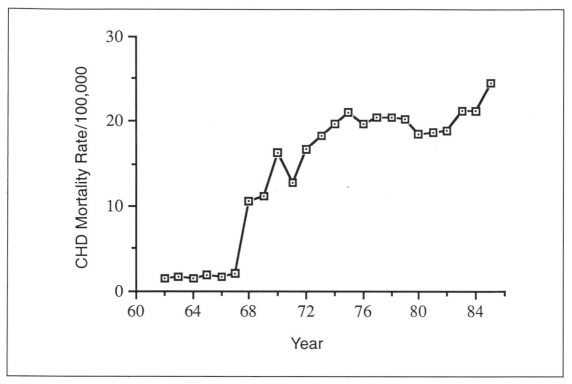

Figure 6-4.   Mortality trend from IHD in Ecuador 1968–1986. (Source: Suárez J, López R, Laspina I, et al. Situación de Salud en el Ecuador 1962–1985. Quito: Ministry of Public Health, 1987; 112.)

spectively, in the intake of animal fats. CHD mortality declines of lesser degree are less obviously related to dietary changes and may be due as much to other primary or secondary prevention efforts [43].

There is a widely accepted appreciation that total blood cholesterol levels are positively associated with the risk of CHD. The evidence from the large number of studies in which this association has been observed has been reviewed extensively [43, 44, 45] (see Chapters 1, 3, and 4). No population having mean total cholesterol (TC) levels under 200 mg/dl is reported to have a high CHD mortality rate [46, 47].

There are at least four types of interpopulation comparisons that associate diet, blood cholesterol levels, and the risk of CHD:

• autopsy series (comparison of at-risk population risk factor profiles)
• classical ecological studies

• comparison of levels of cardiovascular risk and dietary assessment
• migrant studies

The first type of comparison is exemplified by the International Atherosclerosis Project [17]. In this study carried out in the 1960s, autopsy records of 23,000 people from 12 countries were reviewed, and the severity of atherosclerosis was compared with population serum cholesterol levels and dietary survey data. The percent of calories consumed as fat ranged from 10 to 15 percent in Costa Rica and Guatemala to nearly 50 percent among certain population subgroups in the United States. The percentage of calories from fat was related both to the severity of atherosclerosis ($r = .67$) and to population levels of blood cholesterol ($r = .74$).

The second type of comparison utilizes the nutrient and food products data from the FAO food balance sheets, which have been compared with WHO CHD mortality data for certain sets

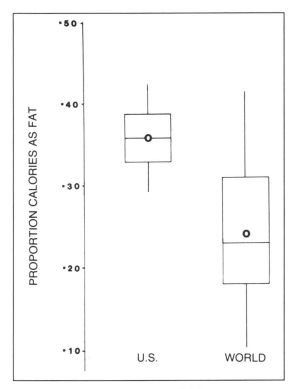

Figure 6-5. The proportion of calories consumed as fat in the United States and worldwide. Notes: The circles in the boxes indicate mean values, the end of the upper tail indicates the ninety-fifth percentile value, the upper limit of the box the seventy-fifth percentile value, the line through the box the fiftieth percentile value, the lower limit of the box the twenty-fifth percentile value, and the end of the lower tail the fifth percentile value. Values for the United States are based on data for individuals from the National Health and Nutrition Examination Survey II, which have been adjusted to exclude sources of variation within individuals according to the findings of Beaton et al. Values for the world are derived from mean levels of nutrients in the various countries, based on food disappearance. (Source: With permission from the New England Journal of Medicine 1987; 317:165–6.)

of countries. Stamler [48] compared the consumption levels of several dietary variables among adult males with cardiovascular mortality data from 20 countries. Saturated fat intake was associated with increased mortality, whereas polyunsaturated fat consumption appeared to be protective. Significant associations were found between CHD mortality and intake

of total fat, saturated fat, and animal products (poultry, eggs, meat, and dairy products).

Another type of interpopulation comparison is the direct measurement of cardiovascular risk factors and dietary intake. In the Seven Countries Study [26], 12,000 people from 18 populations in seven countries were studied. Seven-day food records were supplemented by direct analyses of the diet consumed by participants. Results showed that saturated fat intake was highest in Finland, the United States, and the Netherlands: 12 to 22 percent of total calories as saturated fat compared to 5 to 9 percent in the other countries. Saturated fat intake and five-year CHD incidence rates for these populations were very highly correlated (r = .84), as were saturated fat and serum cholesterol levels (r = .89) and blood cholesterol levels and CHD incidence rates (r = .81).

Migrant studies are the fourth type of cross-population study. Comparison of a stable population with a population that emigrates to another country or location provides a special opportunity to evaluate changes in risk factors among persons sharing similar genetic and cultural backgrounds. If this move involves a higher consumption of dietary fat and saturated fat, the population distribution of serum cholesterol shifts upward and CHD rates also rise. There are several examples of this type of international comparison. The Ni-Hon-San Study (*Nippon-Honolulu-San* Francisco) showed intakes of saturated fat of 7 percent, 12 percent, and 14 percent of calories in Japanese men living in Japan, Honolulu, and San Francisco respectively. There was also a concomitant difference in mean body weight of 55, 63, and 66 kg, respectively [49]. The serum cholesterol was 12 percent and 21 percent higher in Honolulu and San Francisco, respectively, than in Japan. CHD mortality was 1.7 times higher in Hawaii and 2.8 times higher in San Francisco compared to Japan [50].

The Ireland-Boston Heart Study, which focused on male siblings and offspring of Irish descent in Boston and Ireland, found that the incidence of CHD death was significantly higher in the Boston cohort and that individuals who died of CHD had a higher intake of saturated fatty acids and cholesterol and a lower intake of polyunsaturated fatty acids. Mean total fat intake also was higher (39.4 percent vs. 38.5 percent) and fiber intake lower (.75 percent vs. .81 percent) in the group who died of CHD compared with the group where no CHD deaths were observed [51].

We have compared the CHD risk factor distribution among Indians living in a rural area of the Andes Mountains in Ecuador (n = 118) with that of their first-degree relatives who migrated (n = 186) and currently work and live in Quito, the large, urbanized capital [52]. Unfavorable changes in coronary risk factors occurred over a short interval of time (44±24 months) in the migrant group compared to their relatives who stayed in the rural area, with significant increases in both sexes in blood pressure, body mass index, the percent of calories taken in as fat, and smoking rates among women. Results of this study are shown in Table 6-6.

Obesity results when habitual energy intake exceeds habitual energy output for an extended period. An increased prevalence of obesity and redistribution of fat from the extremities to the trunk occurs with age and with changes from rural to urban lifestyles [53, 54, 55]. General and abdominal (central, or upper body) obesity has been associated with an increased risk of CHD and of death from all causes in both sexes and in several populations [56, 57, 58, 59]. Indicators of body fat distribution have also been related to an atherogenic lipid profile in both men and women [60, 61]. Some studies have reported interpopulation differences in the association between fat distribution and blood lipids [62, 63]. The levels of high-density lipoprotein (HDL) cholesterol and triglyceride among Mexican Americans are different from their Anglo counterparts, and it has been suggested that this ethnic difference may be explained, in part, by their different distribution of body fat [64].

In a sense, exercise is the other half of the energy balance equation that governs body weight and obesity. However, like diet, it is an aspect of lifestyle that can be very difficult to change. Among the more affluent portions of the industrialized nations there has been a trend toward more physical exercise, while at the same time these same groups of people have progressively adopted a more healthful diet. Exercise exerts a beneficial effect independent of

Table 6-6. Blood pressure, blood cholesterol, and selected anthropometric and dietary results in men and women from the Quito Migrants Study, 1989

	Men		Women	
	Rural[b]	Migrant[a]	Rural[b]	Migrant[a]
Age	52.3±15.7[c]	40.1±16.0	46.4±15.1[c]	39.5±14.3
Daily caloric intake Kcal	1171±269	1728±251[c]	981±260	1539±207[c]
Calories as fat%	19.9±3.4	26.2±5.7[c]	22.4±6.4	26.6±4.9[c]
BMI Kg/m2	24.3±2.2	25.4±4.4	24.0±3.1	27.8±4.7[c]
Triceps skin fold mm	7±2.4	9±1.7[c]	8.8±2.6	16.3±3.5[c]
Subscapular skin fold mm	11.1±2.3	16.8±3.2[c]	12.7±3.1	24.6±4.8[c]
Blood cholesterol mg/dl	177.2±20.8	179.9±16.2	183.1±15.9	195.0±31.4[b]
Systolic blood pressure mm Hg	122.9±12.3	133.7±12.5[c]	120.4±13.2	128.6±11.8[c]
Diastolic blood pressure mm Hg	67.2±6.9	78.7±9.5[c]	66.8±11.0	69.3±12.0
Smoking prevalence %	39.5	37.6	0.0	27.1[b]

[a] mean ± standard deviation
[b] p <.005
[c] p <.0001

Source: Zevallos JC, Ockene I S, Callay S, Baca, MC. The impact of urbanization on cardiovascular risk factors in an indigenous population of the highlands of Ecuador. Circulation 1991; 84(suppl II):II-118

its role in regulating body weight, that is, it increases the relative concentration of HDL cholesterol [65].

Hypertension

Hypertension is a known risk factor for CHD. In some industrialized countries, such as the United States, the prevalence of hypertension (diastolic blood pressure above 90 mm Hg) is as high as 25 percent among adults. Similar rates have been described in some nonindustrialized countries [66].

The INTERSALT Study, which used uniform procedures in 52 population samples from 32 countries of Africa, Asia, Europe, North America, and South America [67, 68], found a significant relationship between median 24-hour sodium excretion and the slope of systolic blood pressure increase with age. From this study it is easy to quantify the expected rise in median systolic blood pressure as a population ages if one knows the level of sodium intake per day over a 30-year period from age 25 to age 55.

Environmental factors that increase the incidence of hypertension include high sodium intake, obesity, and psychogenic stress. However, a genetic predisposition also exists and interacts with the environmental risk factors. There is about a twofold higher incidence of hypertension among those individuals who have a close relative who is hypertensive. Racial factors have also been implicated in hypertension — hypertension appears in black Americans almost twice as often as it does in whites [69].

The increase of blood pressure with age is similar in most of the populations surveyed. The mean systolic blood pressure increases from approximately 110 to 120 mm Hg at age 20 to 150 to 160 mm Hg at age 70. Interestingly, studies of a number of populations living a relatively isolated lifestyle have shown that such an increase does not necessarily have to take place. These populations include groups living at high altitudes in the Andean region, Indian tribes of Brazil [70, 71] and Costa Rica [72], and certain African populations described earlier in this chapter, among others.

Data compiled from a variety of clinical, epidemiologic, and pathologic sources suggest that hypertension is now the most prevalent cardiovascular disorder on the African continent [73]. Table 6-7 shows the prevalence rates of high blood pressure among middle-aged males and females in several countries of the region. Half a century ago, however, several studies found that high blood pressure was rare among Africans [74].

Low-blood pressure communities, which are common in rural Africa, are characterized by the absence of hypertensive subjects and a lack of increase in blood pressure values with age. Such communities share a number of similarities: high-carbohydrate diets, low salt consumption, lean body makeup, and high levels of physical activity [75].

A recent controlled longitudinal observational study by Poulter and colleagues demonstrates the magnitude, timing, and possible causes of changes in blood pressure among Kenyan Luo migrants from a low blood pressure community who move to Nairobi, the largest urban center of Kenya. The authors found a statistically significant increase in systolic blood pressure and a mean systolic and diastolic blood pressure distribution increase over time among those individuals living in the urbanized area compared to those individuals who remained in the rural zone, with these changes becoming evident as soon as one month after migration. Sodium-to-potassium ratio, body weight, and stress might be important predictors of the shift in the blood pressure distribution during the urbanization process, and these factors may play a role in the development of hypertension [76].

Cigarette Smoking

Ecologic analyses have shown a relationship between cigarette and tobacco consumption and CHD mortality, with correlation coefficients between mean per capita tobacco consumption for the late 1950s and the early 1960s and CHD mortality rates in 1971 and 1973 for men and women in 19 countries being in the range of .44 to .50 [45]. In the United States, the decline in CHD mortality rates correlates with the decreasing prevalence of cigarette smoking in

Table 6-7. Prevalence of hypertension in men and women aged 40 to 55 from selected countries in Africa

Country	Population basis	Year of survey	Hypertension measurement	Men (%)	Women (%)
Ethiopia	Rural	1983	A	11	3
Zambia	Rural	1979	A	11	9
Zaire	Urban	1983–1984	B	33	15
South Africa	Urban	1976	B	20	41

A = diastolic blood pressure ≥90 mm Hg; B = systolic and/or diastolic blood pressure ≥160/95 mm Hg.
Source: World Health Organization. Hypertension in Developing Countries. In: World Health Statistics Quarterly Report 1988; 41:141.

men, although in women the relationship is more difficult to demonstrate [5].

Exposure to tobacco is also related to other unhealthy lifestyle practices, including diets high in fat and low in protective nutrients [77, 78]. In the more affluent countries of the West, smoking rates in recent years have fallen rapidly, especially among males and in those persons with high levels of educational attainment [79].

Changes in aggregate smoking exposures, however, are not very highly correlated with changes in CHD mortality rates on an international level [46]. This lack of association may be due in part to the skewed nature of the available tobacco data, which is based on import and export data rather than on actual cigarette smoking patterns of the population [9]. Because ecologic studies rely on estimates of mean population values as a meaningful summary statistic for population rates of exposure, they are more likely to produce erroneous results when distributions are skewed. In a prior publication we have described how this might explain why dietary fat is a stronger predictor of lung cancer mortality than is tobacco in analyses based on ecologic data [9].

A synthesis of the available data suggests that the relationship of smoking to CHD is such to suggest that smoking is an accelerator of CHD and an initiator of clinical events, not a primary causal agent of atherosclerosis. As discussed in Chapter 4, the evidence favors dyslipidemia as the causal necessity in CHD, with other risk factors important as risk-modifying agents. Thus, in countries like the United States, where blood cholesterol levels are generally high, cig-

arette smoking is the single most important modifiable aspect of lifestyle for CHD risk modification [80]. In other countries where cigarette smoking rates are high but blood cholesterol levels generally are low, such as Japan, the association of smoking and CHD is weak [26]. Even in these countries, however, tobacco use is associated with increased mortality from noncardiac causes.

OTHER ASPECTS OF TOBACCO CONSUMPTION

Tobacco damages soil and displaces food crops urgently needed for proper nutrition by poor farmers and their families as well as to avoid food emergencies in many parts of the world. It is also known that there is an effect of nicotine on basal metabolic requirements and levels of essential nutrients that may be related to disease risks [81, 82]. For these reasons, this section deals with some of the other problems related to tobacco consumption in nonindustrialized countries and in the poor populations in more affluent countries.

Despite their poverty people of lower socioeconomic status constitute a very large tobacco market. The Third World offers exceptional future marketing opportunities for the international tobacco industry. By the year 2000 the projected population of low-income (e.g., China, India, Bangladesh), lower-middle (e.g., Egypt, the Philippines, Nigeria), and upper-middle income countries (e.g., Malaysia and Brazil) will account for 80 percent of the world's population. In 1988 Chinese smokers smoked 29.3 percent of all the cigarettes consumed in the world, or 1.5 trillion cigarettes [83]. It has been predicted that in China alone 50 million individuals now under 20 years of age will ultimately die of tobacco-related diseases [84]. Despite the large body of accumulated evidence about the devastating consequences of tobacco consumption for both active and passive smokers, in the non-industrialized countries there is a remarkable lack of fundamental knowledge organized in a form to help antismoking campaigns. Tobacco not only causes great morbidity and mortality, but in many countries it is an important deficit item in balance of trade sheets, as shown in Table 6-8.

From the perspective of the international tobacco industry, there are only "victims" and "dominating" nations. The recent episode in which the United States attempted to coerce several Asian countries into accepting tobacco importation quotas in order to receive favored-nation trading status is an example in support of this point of view [85]. The tobacco industry has developed a sophisticated global organization to misinform the general public about the dangers of smoking. The industry often uses any available resource to control government policies on antismoking campaigns. Such pol-

icies are strongly influenced by publicity statements regarding the economic benefits of tobacco growing, manufacture, trade, and use. Many governments of non-industrialized countries see tobacco as an immediate cash crop with economic benefits; for them promoting legislation against tobacco is an economically unrealistic position.

Although the prevalence of current adult smokers in the United States has declined since 1965, the United States is still the number-one exporter of tobacco in the world [86]. In the United States the percentage of men who smoke has decreased from an estimated 53 percent in 1964 to less than 33 percent in 1985. The percentage of female adult smokers was 28 percent in 1985, having declined from 34 percent in 1965. In 1985 the United States spent approximately 65 billion dollars on direct health care and indirect lost productivity costs related to smoking [87]. A survey of cigarette smoking habits conducted in 1971 in eight cities of Latin America demonstrated a smoking prevalence that ranged from 45 percent to 58 percent, compared to 42 percent at that time in the United States [88].

Other Risk Factors

Differing mortality and morbidity profiles among social classes have been noted for some time [89]. As CHD mortality rates begin to increase in industrialized countries, the change first affects the more affluent classes and is then disseminated to the rest of the population. Marmot also showed that the more recent decline in CHD mortality rates in England and Wales first began in the most affluent part of the population [90] (Figure 6-6). A differential response to preventive education [91] may play a role in this class difference in the CHD decline rate, e.g., more educated people have given up smoking more rapidly and in greater numbers and are more likely to have diets closely approximating those recommended for CHD prevention [92].

A number of reports from industrialized countries have shown that CHD mortality rates are now higher among the lower socioeconomic classes; other studies have shown that the de-

Table 6-8.   Selected countries with negative tobacco trade balances, 1984–1985

Country	Thousands of U.S. dollars		
	Imports	Exports	Balance
Africa			
Egypt	178,850	920	−177,930
Libya	47,660	—	−47,760
Morocco	35,402	—	−35,402
Asia/Pacific			
Taiwan	66,239	4,852	−61,387
China	44,705	443	−44,262
Malaysia	44,030	740	−43,290
Latin America			
Trinidad and Tobago	6,723	318	−6,405
Haiti	4,100	—	−4,100
Ecuador	1,900	993	−907

Source: Food and Agriculture Organization of the United Nations Trade and Production Year Book. Rome FAO, 39; 1986

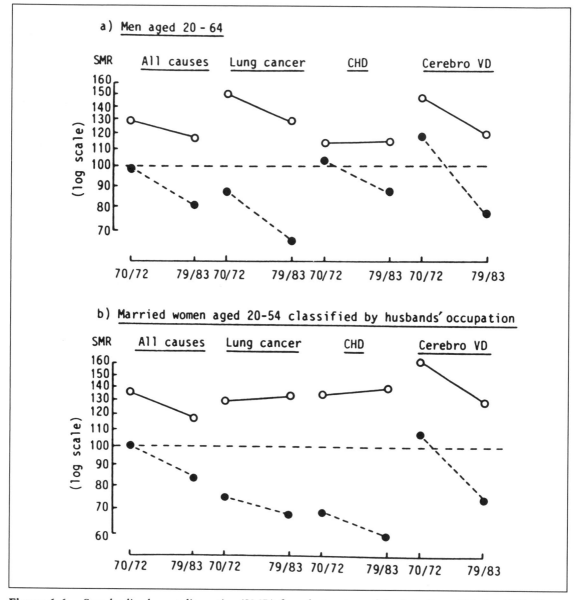

Figure 6-6. Standardized mortality ratios (SMR) for select causes of death in Great Britain, 1970–72 and 1979–83, for manual and nonmanual groups. Note: For each cause the SMR in 1979–1983 is 100 for each sex. ○———○ = manual; ●- - -● = nonmanual. (Source: Marmot, M. Socioeconomic determinants of CHD mortality. Int J Epidemiol 1989, 18:Suppl 1:S196–202, with permission.)

cline in CHD has been greatest in the higher socioeconomic groups defined in either occupational or educational terms [93, 94, 95, 96]. Feldman and colleagues [96] from the National Center for Health Statistics in the United States used educational levels instead of occupational

levels (i.e., manual or nonmanual labor) and demonstrated trends similar to those found in the United Kingdom [90].

Thus we are faced with the apparent paradox that although CHD is more common in affluent than in less affluent countries, in affluent countries it is more common in the less affluent subgroups, whereas in nonindustrialized countries it is more common in the higher socioeconomic strata. This reflects differing attitudes toward coronary risk factors: in nonindustrialized countries cigarettes, high-saturated-fat foods, and a sedentary lifestyle are all seen as signs of wealth and status, whereas in countries such as the United States the opposite is now true.

Stress, as defined by type A personality or type A behavior pattern (TABP), has been associated with CHD morbidity and mortality. Such studies on an international level are greatly limited, however, since standardized procedures or methods to evaluate and classify behavior patterns from an international perspective are largely lacking. Despite this limitation several studies have been performed in Europe [97], the United States [98], and Japan [99] that suggest a link between TABP and CHD.

Another issue of interest from the international perspective is the possible inverse relationship between alcohol intake and the risk of CHD. Data exist to suggest that the ingestion of two to three drinks of an alcoholic beverage per day reduces the rate of nonfatal MI and mortality from CHD [65]. A report from the Yugoslavia Cardiovascular Disease Study found a statistically significant inverse relationship of alcohol consumption to CHD incidence that persisted even after controlling for blood pressure, serum cholesterol levels, and cigarette smoking [100]. A prospective study performed in 87,500 women over a four-year period suggested that among middle-aged women moderate alcohol consumption decreases the risk of CHD and ischemic stroke [101]. Similar results were obtained for both sexes in a study in New Zealand [102]. The mechanism by which moderate alcohol intake protects an individual from CHD remains unclear. It has been suggested that this effect is mediated by increasing HDL levels. On the other hand, it should be stressed that once hepatic damage occurs in alcoholics, plasma HDL levels may actually be lower than normal [28]. However, high population rates of alcohol consumption, specifically of wine, may help to explain the unusually low rates of CHD in France. High rates of cirrhosis are also seen in this country [24].

Dietary and alcohol consumption data from 18 countries were examined by Hegsted and Ausman [103]. Saturated-fat intake had a simple correlation with CHD of .71; polyunsaturated fat, − .34; and total alcohol consumption, − .58. Despite these suggestive results, the apparent beneficial effect of moderate alcohol intake on CHD needs further verification.

Japan — A Special Example

Japan has one of the lowest rates of CHD mortality among the industrialized countries [24] and so has been extensively studied to determine if the coronary risk factor patterns seen here differ from those of other countries and thus can provide clues into the aetiology of CHD and the manner in which risk factors interact. With progressive industrialization, many changes in lifestyles (acculturation) have occurred (and continue to occur) in Japan. Thus, we have a unique and important opportunity to witness a natural experiment in a population with very low rates of CHD mortality.

In Japan, traditionally, the diet has been rich in salt and carbohydrates, relatively low in protein, and very low in fat. As much as 80 percent of the male population used to smoke in the 1970s, and for 1985 to 1986 the percentage of cigarette smoking in men was 60 to 65 percent [104]. Obesity has been rare, and the Japanese lipid profile has been characterized by very low levels of total and LDL-cholesterol compared to many countries of the world.

Rural and national surveys in Japan [105] strongly suggest that in recent years there has been a rapid acculturation to Western eating patterns and lifestyles, departing from centuries-old traditions and resulting in an elevated consumption of total fat, saturated fatty acids, cholesterol, animal fats, and protein and a decreased consumption of carbohydrates (rice) and salt. These changes, together with a vigorous hypertension control program, have been related to a major decline in both mean blood pressure and stroke — primarily cerebral hemorrhage — between the 1960s and the 1980s [106].

It has been suggested that the rise in serum cholesterol levels that has occurred in Japan and the decline in hemorrhagic stroke are related, with individuals having the combination of hypertension and blood cholesterol levels of under 160 mg/dl being especially susceptible to cerebral hemorrhage. This relationship of very low cholesterol levels in hypertensive individuals to cerebral hemorrhage has also been reported in other studies [107, 108]. It has been hypothesized that hypertension in the presence of very low serum cholesterol levels causes angionecrosis and the weakening of the small cerebral arteries [109].

Overall mortality from CHD remains at a relatively constant level in Japan, despite the progressive increase in dietary saturated fat and cholesterol intake and mean serum cholesterol levels. Shimamoto [110], however, suggests that population exposure to atherogenic lipoproteins may not yet have been of sufficient magnitude and duration to result in mass atherosclerosis and CHD. After a 20-year follow-up of a cohort of rice-farming people in rural Japan, there was no change in the CHD incidence rate, a 60 percent decrease in stroke in men and women aged 40 to 69, and an average serum cholesterol increase of 27 mg/dl from a mean of 155 mg/dl to 180 mg/dl. The population had a community-based hypertension control program that was established at the time of the onset of the study, and salt intake decreased from 20±7 grams to 14.2±5 grams during the study period.

Other reports suggest differences between rural and urban Japanese CHD mortality, with an increase in the urban rate [111]. A recent report from an urban population in Japan suggests that cholesterol levels are progressively increasing and may be the cause for the increased CHD incidence [112]. Similarly Ueshima [113] states that increased CHD mortality in urban areas may be partly attributed to elevated levels of serum cholesterol due to an increased fat intake.

A study using data from long-term epidemiologic and pathologic studies conducted between 1963 and 1984 in urban and rural populations [114] demonstrated that MI incidence rates increased in urban men but did not change in rural men. Serum cholesterol levels were positively correlated with MI incidence. The age-adjusted incidence rate of MI for men with serum cholesterols of 220 mg/dl and over was 4.9 times higher than that for men with serum cholesterol levels of 180 mg/dl or less. Also, the age-adjusted incidence rate of MI for men who smoked 20 cigarettes or more per day was 7.4 times higher than that of nonsmokers, and alcohol intake was inversely associated with CHD incidence. Similar findings have been reported by Kiyohara from a study in a rural community [115]. These results are entirely compatible with findings in the United States and in European countries.

Some interesting pathologic findings in men with infarcts were also obtained from this study: massive necrosis of the heart, as a gross pathologic type, was found in 73 percent of the urban men but in only 9 percent of the rural men, with the opposite proportion for the scattered necrosis type. Conversely, a high proportion of rural men showed atherosclerosis in their cerebral arteries, whereas in urban men the proportion was smaller.

In the urban men significant risk factors for MI were hypertension, hypercholesterolemia, smoking, and hyperglycemia. In the rural men only hypertension was identified as a risk factor for MI. In this study, however, the decrease in blood pressure was marked and the increase in blood cholesterol was relatively modest in both groups.

This apparent rural-to-urban gradient of CHD mortality in Japan has been associated with the Western acculturation process. Further information toward the acculturation thesis has been derived from the Ni-Hon-San migration study [50] discussed earlier. Marmot [116] also hypothesized that social and cultural differences may contribute to the CHD gradient observed in that study. In a study of 3800 Japanese Americans, he found that individuals with the most traditional lifestyles had a CHD prevalence similar to that observed in Japan, whereas those individuals most acculturated to a Western lifestyle had a three- to fivefold increase in CHD incidence, a finding that could not be accounted for by the observed differences in the classical risk factors.

Thus, in Japan today we have a situation of rapidly changing risk factors for CHD. The content of saturated fat and cholesterol in the diet is rapidly increasing, and the percentage of smokers remains very high. On the other hand, another important CHD risk factor, hypertension, has been dramatically altered in a favorable direction by decreased dietary salt content and a vigorous treatment program. To date this balance has resulted in only modest changes in CHD incidence rates. How this changing risk factor pattern will affect CHD in Japan in the future is the subject of intense interest and scrutiny, since we should be able to learn much from this fascinating natural experiment.

Recommendations

If the underlying causes of disease are to be changed and a population strategy is to be applied, appropriate actions need to be taken by the public, by government and policymakers, and by the producers of goods and services. The role of public health workers, teachers, and parents is also crucial to achieving success. (See Chapter 4 for a discussion of the advantages and disadvantages of a population-based strategy.)

In 1981 the WHO Expert Committee on the Prevention of Coronary Heart Disease recommended that each country should prepare a plan of action [117] identifying specific targets and establishing a deadline for their achievement. Plans of action should be reviewed regularly and the incidence of CHD monitored over time. Moreover, the Expert Committee emphasized the importance of beginning intervention early in life. Preventive efforts should start among children and adolescents. There are two major reasons for focusing preventive efforts on these age groups. First, because this is the time when the atherosclerotic process begins, intervention may stop further development of the disease. Second, this is the period when lifestyle habits that lead to the development of risk factors for CHD (e.g., smoking, inactivity, and high-fat, high-calorie, high-salt diets) begin and tend to progress into adulthood. Thus, preventive ef-

forts should be targeted at children and adolescents to discourage them from adopting harmful and hard-to-change lifestyle habits.

In industrialized countries, excess intake of fat, salt, and simple sugar leads to obesity and increased levels of blood lipids and sugar, which, in turn, are risk factors for many conditions, including CHD, adult-onset diabetes, and hypertension [118, 119]. Many nonindustrialized countries are simultaneously facing problems related to underdevelopment — malnutrition, infections, parasitic diseases — and increasing rates of CHD related to development — tobacco smoking, excess dietary fat and salt, and stress.

Central, state, and district governments, non-government organizations, voluntary agencies, and international organizations can play important roles in motivating healthful change in the different categories of risk factors. Price subsidies, taxes, and other economic incentives and disincentives can be used to modify the production and usage of tobacco and various foodstuffs. In the nonindustrialized countries, with their massive debts and heavy reliance on foreign exchange, the International Monetary Fund (IMF) and the World Bank (WB) have a potentially important role to play in linking economic development and the rescheduling of debt with health policy.

Faced with mounting health care costs and limits on productivity due to avoidable morbidity, governments and international organizations have begun to realize that health policy planning that includes a strong preventive component must be an integral part of overall economic and development planning. Often subunits of the overall decision-making body correctly identify health-related priorities, but their recommendations may run counter to the current goals of the greater governing body. In the United States the branch of federal government concerned with health policy, the Department of Health and Human Services (formerly the Department of Health, Education, and Welfare), recognizes the untoward effects of tobacco on health but is forced to work at cross-purposes with a Department of Agriculture policy that subsidizes the growing of tobacco. In the United Nations, UNICEF and WHO have promulgated positions that have run counter to the predominating views of the United Nations Development Program and, more important, because they control the flow of funds, the IMF and the WB. In both instances it took decades for the role of prevention in overall public policy planning to be appreciated and then translated into meaningful policies. The role of advocate for preventive medicine is the necessary social step in creating national and international climates that are sensitive to the need for mass action to promote healthy lifestyles.

Any public health message designed to alter behavior to modify known risk factors must be based on an understanding of the determinants of prevailing habits in the target populations. "Bad" eating habits may be reinforced by tradition in a certain population or by status in another, which may also be true for smoking. The simple statement that "animal fat is not good for your heart" may not be enough to lead to behavior modification.

CHD is one of the greatest health problems in the world. International studies have indicated important CHD risk factors on which to focus to develop better methodologies to prevent this disease in differing populations, and provide us with a broader perspective of the nature of this disease.

References

1. World Health Organization Regional Office for Europe. Myocardial infarction community registers. Public Health in Europe no. 5. Copenhagen, 1976.
2. Elveback LR, Connolly DC, Kurland LT. Coronary heart disease in residents of Rochester, Minnesota. II. Mortality, incidence and survivorship 1950–1975. Mayo Clin Proc 1981; 56:661–4.
3. Puska P, Tuomilehto J, Nissinen A, et al. The North Karelia Project: 15 years of prevention of coronary heart disease. Annals of Medicine 1989; 21:169–73.
4. U.S. National Center for Health Statistics. 1986 summary: National Hospital Discharge Survey advance data. No. 145. Sept. 30, 1987.
5. Higgins M, Thom T. Trends in CHD in the United States. International Journal of Epidemiology 1989, 18:Suppl 1:S58–S66.
6. Dawson DA, Adams PF. Current estimates from the National Health Interview Survey, United States, 1986. Vital and Health Statistics, National Center for Health Statistics, series 10, no. 164. DHHS publ. no. (PHS) 87-1592, 1987.
7. U.S. National Center for Health Statistics. Monthly vital statistics report (37) 1, April 25, 1988.
8. Armstrong B, Doll R. Environmental factors and cancer incidence and mortality in different countries with special reference to dietary practices. Int J Cancer 1975; 15:617–31.
9. Wynder EL, Hebert JR, Kabat GC. Association of dietary fat and lung cancer. JNCI 1987; 79:631–7.
10. Food and Agriculture Organization of the United Nations. Trade yearbook, vol. 13. Rome: FAO, 1959.
11. The World Bank. World Development Report. Washington DC: The World Bank, 1984.
12. Keys A, ed. Coronary heart disease in seven countries. Circulation 1970; 41:Suppl 1:1–211.
13. Williams OD. Methodological issues in international comparisons. Int J Epidemiol 1989; 18:Suppl 1:S166–8.
14. Greenland S, Morgenstern H. Ecological bias, confounding, and effect modification. Int J Epidemiol 1989; 18:269–74.
15. Hebert JR, Wynder EL. Dietary fat and the risk of breast cancer. N Engl J Med 1987; 317:165–6.
16. World Health Organization. World health statistics annual 1983. Geneva:WHO, 1983.
17. International Atherosclerosis Project. General Findings of the International Atherosclerosis Project. Laboratory Investigation 1968; 18:5:38–42.
18. Pooling Project Research Group. Relationship of blood pressure, serum cholesterol, smoking habits, relative weight and ECG abnormalities to incidence of major coronary events: final report of the Pooling Project. J Chron Dis 1978; 31:201–306.
19. Dawber TR. The Framingham Study. The epidemiology of atherosclerotic disease. Cambridge: Harvard University Press, 1980.
20. Kimura N. Analysis of 10,000 postmortem examinations in Japan. In: Keys A, White PD, eds. World trends in cardiology. I. Cardiovascular epidemiology. New York: Hoeber-Harper, 1956; 22–33.
21. Uemura K, Piša Z. Trends in cardiovascular disease mortality in industrialized countries since 1950. Wld Hlth Stat Qtly 1988; 41: 155–78.

22. Harlan W. CHD trends in the United States: overview. Int J Epidemiol 1989; 18:Suppl 1:S56-7.

23. World Health Organization. Proposal for the multinational monitoring of trends and determinants in cardiovascular disease and protocol (MONICA Project). Geneva: WHO/MNC/82.1, 1983.

24. World Health Organization. World health statistics annual 1990. Geneva: WHO, 1991.

25. WHO MONICA Project. WHO MONICA Project: risk factors. Int J Epidemiol 1989; 18:Suppl 1:S46-55.

26. Keys A. Seven countries: a multivariate analysis of death and coronary heart disease. Cambridge: Harvard University Press, 1980.

27. Ghalim N, Hugot-Puchois A, Puchois A, et al. Influence of alcohol on plasma lipids and atherogenesis. Epidemiological and biochemical aspects. Presse Medicale-Paris 1991; 20(11):507-12.

28. Steinberg D, Pearson TA, Kuller LH. Alcohol and atherosclerosis. Ann Intern Med 1991; 114:967-76.

29. Pan American Health Organization. Health conditions in the Americas. Scientific publ. no. 500, 1986; vol. I; 65-8.

30. Jiménez JG, Rojas MT. Análisis del cambio de las enfermedades cardiovasculares en Costa Rica. Rev Cost Cienc Med 1987; 8(3).

31. Raab W. Alimentare factoren in der enstenhung von arteriosklerrose und hypertonie. Med Klin 1932; 28:487, 521.

32. Rosenthal SR. Studies in atherosclerosis. Chemical, experimental and morphologic. Arch Path 1934; 18:473-506, 660-98.

33. Shaper AG. Communities without hypertension. In: Shaper AG, Hutt MSR, Fejfar Z. Cardiovascular disease in the tropics. London: British Medical Association, 1974; 77-83.

34. Eaton SB, Konner MJ. Paleolithic nutrition: a consideration of its nature and current implications. N Engl J Med 1985; 312:283-9.

35. Eaton SB, Nelson DA. Calcium in evolutionary perspective. Am J Clin Nutr 1991; 54:Suppl 1:281S-7S.

36. Malmros H. The relation of nutrition to health. A statistical study of the effect of the wartime on arteriosclerosis, cardiosclerosis, tuberculosis and diabetes. Acta Med. Scand 1950; Suppl:246:137-50.

37. Strom A, Jensen RA. Mortality from circulatory disease in Norway 1940-1945. Lancet 1951; 1:126.

38. Lipid Research Clinics Program. The Lipid Research Clinics Coronary Primary Prevention Trial results. I. Reduction in incidence of coronary heart disease. JAMA 1984; 251: 351-64.

39. Lipid Research Clinics Program. The Lipid Research Clinics Coronary Primary Prevention Trial results. II. The relationship of reduction in incidence of coronary heart disease to cholesterol lowering. JAMA 1984; 251:365-74.

40. Frick MH, Elo O, Haapa D, et al. Helsinki Heart Study: primary prevention trial with gemfibrozil in middle-aged men with hyperlipidemia. N Engl J Med 1984; 317:1237-45.

41. Leren P. The Oslo Diet-Heart Study: eleven-year report. Circulation 1970; 42:935-42.

42. Keys A, Aravanis C, Blackburn HW, et al. Epidemiological studies related to coronary heart disease: characteristics of men aged 40-59 in seven countries. Acta Med Scand 1966; Suppl:460:1-392.

43. Epstein FH. The relationship of lifestyle to international trends in CHD. Int J Epidemiol 1989; 18:S203-9.

44. Levy RI. Cholesterol and cardiovascular disease: no longer whether, but rather when, in whom, and how? Circulation 1985; 72:686-91.

45. Stamler J. Opportunities and pitfalls in international comparisons relate to patterns, trends and determinants of coronary heart disease mortality. Int J Epidemiol 1989, 18:Suppl 1:S3-18.

46. Keys A. Seven countries: death and coronary heart disease in ten years. Cambridge: Harvard University Press, 1980.

47. Blackburn H, chairman. Conference on the Health Effects of Blood Lipids: optimal distribution for populations. Workshop Report, Epidemiological Section. American Health Foundation, April 1979. Prev Med 1979; 8:612-78.

48. Stamler J. Population studies. In: Levy RI, Rifkind BM, Dennis BH, Ernst N, eds. Nutrition, lipids, and coronary heart disease. New York: Raven, 1979; 25-88.

49. Kato H, Tillotson J, Nichaman MZ, et al. Epidemiologic studies of coronary heart disease and stroke in Japanese men living in Japan, Hawaii, and California. Serum lipids and diet. Am J Epidemiol 1973; 97:372-85.

50. Marmot MG, Syme SL, Kagan A, et al. Epidemiologic studies of CHD and stroke in Japanese men living in Japan, Hawaii and California. Prevalence of coronary and hypertensive heart disease and associated risk factors. Am J Epidemiol 1975; 102:514.

51. Kushi LH, Lew RA, Stare FJ, et al. Diet and 20-year mortality from coronary heart disease: the Ireland-Boston Diet-Heart Study. N Engl J Med 1985; 312:811-8.

52. Zevallos JC, Ockene IS, Callay S, Baca ML.

The impact of urbanization on cardiovascular risk factors in an indigenous population of the highlands of Ecuador. Circulation 1991; 84(Suppl 2):II-118.

53. Okeke EC, Nanyelugo DO, Ngwu E. The prevalence of obesity in adults by age, sex, and occupation in Anambra State, Nigeria. Growth 1983; 47:263–71.

54. Mueller WH. The changes with age of anatomical redistribution of fat. Soc Sci Med 1982; 16(2):191–6.

55. Ramírez ME, Mueller WH. The development of obesity and anatomical fat patterning in Tokelau children. Human Biol 1980; 52:675.

56. Donahue RP, Abbott RD, Bloom E, et al. Central obesity and coronary heart disease in men. Lancet 1987; 1:821–4.

57. Larsson B, Svördsudd K, Welin L, et al. Abdominal adipose tissue distribution, obesity, and risk of cardiovascular disease and death: 13 year follow-up of participants in the study of men born in 1913. Br Med J 1984; 288:1401–4.

58. Higgins M, Kannel W, Garrison R, et al. Hazards of obesity — the Framingham experience. Acta Med Scand 1988; Suppl:723:23–26.

59. Lapidus L, Bengstoon C, Larsson B, et al. Distribution of adipose tissue and risk of cardiovascular disease and death: a 12 year follow up of participants in the population study of women in Gothenberg, Sweden. Br Med J 1984; 289:1257–61.

60. Garn SM, Sullivan TV, Hawthorne VM. Fatness dependence of skinfold ratios and its implications to fat patterning. Ecology Food Nutr 1987; 21:151–8.

61. Després JP, Allard C, Tremblay A, et al. Evidence for regional components of body fatness in the association with serum lipids in men and women. Clin & Exp Metab 1985; 34:967–73.

62. Durnin JVGA, Womersley J. Body fat assessed from total body density and its estimation from skinfold thickness: measurements on 481 men and women aged from 16 to 72 years. Br J Nutr 1974; 32:77–92.

63. Seidell JC, Giocolini M, Charzewska J, et al. Indicators of fat distribution, serum lipids, and blood pressure in European women born in 1948. The European Fat Distribution Study. Am J Epidemiol 1989; 130:53–65.

64. Haffner SM, Stern MP, Hazuda HP, et al. Role of obesity and fat distribution in non-insulin dependent diabetes mellitus in Mexican American and non-Hispanic whites. Diabetes Care 1986; 9:153–61.

65. Gartside PS, Khoury P, Glueck CJ. Determinants of high-density lipoprotein cholesterol in blacks and whites: the Second National Health Nutrition Examination Survey. Am Heart J 1984; 108:641.

66. Marmot MG. Geography of blood pressure and hypertension. Br Med Bull 1984; 40:380–6.

67. INTERSALT Cooperative Research Group. INTERSALT Study: an international cooperative study on the relation of blood pressure to electrolyte excretion in populations. I. Design and methods. J Hypertension 1986; 4:781–7.

68. INTERSALT Cooperative Research Group. INTERSALT: an international study of electrolyte excretion and blood pressure: results for 24 hour urinary sodium and potassium excretion. Br Med J 1988; 297:319–28.

69. Joint National Committee. The 1988 report of the joint national committee on detection, evaluation and treatment of high blood pressure. Arch Int Med 1988; 148:1023–38.

70. de Costa E, et al. Salt and blood pressure in Rio Grande do Sul, Brazil. Bull Pan Am Health Organ 1990; 24:159–76.

71. The INTERSALT Cooperative Research Group. Appendix tables. Centre-specific results by age and sex. Hypertension 1989; 3:331–407.

72. Ruiz L, Dunbar JB, Horan MJ. Hypertension in Latin America. Special report. Interamerican Society Proceedings. Hypertension 1988; Suppl I:II:2.

73. World Health Organization Hypertension in developing countries. Wld Hlth Stat Qtly 1988; 41:141.

74. Donnison CP. Blood pressure in the African natives: its bearing upon the aetiology of hyperpiesia and arterio-sclerosis. Lancet 1929; 1:6, 7.

75. Watkins LO. Coronary heart disease and coronary disease risk factors in black populations in underdeveloped countries: the case for primordial prevention. Am Heart J 1984; 108:850–62.

76. Poulter NR, Khaw KT, Hopwood BE, et al. The Kenyan Luo migration study: observations on the initiation of a rise in blood pressure. Br Med J 1990; 300:967–72.

77. Schoenborn CA, Benson V. Relationships between smoking and other unhealthy habits: United States, 1985. NCHS Advanced Data 1988; 154:1–8.

78. Hebert JR, Kabat GC. Differences in dietary intake associated with smoking status. Eur J Clin Nutr 1990; 44:185–93.

79. Kabat GC, Wynder EL. Determinants of quitting smoking. Am J Public Health 1987; 77:1301–5.

80. U.S. Department of Health and Human Services. Reducing the health consequences of smoking: 25 years of progress. A report of the Surgeon General. Public Health Service, Cen-

ters for Disease Control, Center for Chronic Disease Prevention and Health Promotion, Office on Smoking and Health. USDHHS publ. no. (CDC) 89-8411, 1989.

81. Stryker WS, Kaplan LA, Stein EA, et al. The relation of diet, cigarette smoking, and alcohol consumption to plasma beta-carotene and alpha tocopherol levels. Am J Epidemiol 1988; 127:283–96.

82. Perkins KA, Epstein LH, Stiller RL, et al. Acute effects of nicotine on resting metabolic rate in smokers. Am J Clin Nutr 1989; 50:545–50.

83. Tobacco. Cigarette sales are on the up. Tobacco Sept. 1989.

84. Peto R. Future mortality from tobacco in China. Paper presented to the Shanghai Symposium on Smoking and Health, Shanghai, China, Nov. 1987; 14–7.

85. Chen TTL, Winder AE. The opium wars revisited as U.S. forces tobacco exports on Asia. Am J Public Health 1990; 80:659–62.

86. Chapman S, Leng WW. Tobacco control in the Third World: a resource atlas. Malaysia: International Organization of Consumers Unions, 1990; 35–44.

87. U.S. Congress. Office of Technology Assessment. Smoking-related deaths and financial costs. Staff memo. Sept. 1985: 48,55.

88. Pan American Health Organization. Encuesta sobre las características del hábito de fumar en América Latina. Washington: PAHO. Publicación científica no. 337, 1977.

89. Marmot MG, McDowall ME. Mortality decline and widening social inequalities. Lancet 1986; 1:274–6.

90. Marmot M. Socioeconomic determinants of CHD mortality. Int J Epidemiol, 1989, 18:Suppl 1:S196–202.

91. Liu K, Cedres LB, Stamler J, et al. Relationship of education to major risk factors and death from CHD, cardiovascular diseases and all causes. Circulation 1982; 66:1308–14.

92. Kushi LH, Folsom AR, Jacobs DR Jr, et al. Educational attainment and nutrient consumption patterns: the Minnesota Heart Study. Am Diet Assoc J 1988; 88:1230–4.

93. Marmot MG, McDowall ME. Mortality decline and widening social inequalities. Lancet 1986; 2:274–6.

94. Gibberd RW, Dobson AJ, du Ve Florey C, et al. Differences and comparative declines in ischemic heart-disease mortality among subpopulations in Australia 1969–1978. Int J Epidemiol 1984; 13:25–31.

95. Rosengren A, Wedel H, Wilhelmsen L. Coronary heart disease and mortality in middle aged men from different occupational classes in Sweden. Br Med J 1988; 297:1497–1500.

96. Feldman JJ, Makuc DM, Kleinman JC, et al. National trends in educational differential in mortality. Am J Epidemiol 1989; 129:913–33.

97. Wrsesniewski K, Forgays DG, Bonaiuto P. Measurement of the Type A behavior pattern in the adolescents and young adults: cross-cultural development of AATAB. J Behavioral Med, April 1990; 13(2):111–35.

98. Eaker ED, Castelli WP. Type A behavior and mortality from coronary disease in the Framingham Study. N Engl J Med 1988; 319: 1480–1.

99. Maeda S, Ito T. Type-A behavior pattern as a risk factor for coronary heart disease. Jap Circ J 1990; 54:457–63.

100. Kozarevic D, Demirovic J, Gordon T, et al. Drinking habits and coronary heart disease: the Yugoslavia cardiovascular disease study. Am J Epidemiol 1982; 116:748–58.

101. Stampfer MJ, Colditz GA, Willett WC, et al. A prospective study of moderate alcohol consumption and the risk of coronary disease and stroke in women. N Engl J Med 1988; 319:267–73.

102. Scragg R, Stewart A, Jackson R, et al. Alcohol and exercise in myocardial infarction and sudden coronary death in men and women. Am J Epidemiol 1987; 126:77–85.

103. Hegsted M, Ausman LM. Diet, alcohol and coronary heart disease in men. J Nutr 1989; 118:1184–9.

104. Kawane H. Tobacco smoking in Japan. Med J Australia 1987; 146:503–4.

105. Ueshima H, Tatara K, Asakura A. Declining mortality from ischemic heart disease and changes in coronary risk factors in Japan, 1956–1980. Am J Epidemiol 1987; 125:62–72.

106. Ueshima H, Tatara K, Asakura S, et al. Declining trends in blood pressure level and the prevalence of hypertension, and changes in related factors in Japan, 1956–1980. J Chron Dis 1987; 40:137–47.

107. Yano K, Reed DM, Maclean CJ. Serum cholesterol and hemorrhagic stroke in the Honolulu Heart Program. Stroke 1989; 20:1460–5.

108. Iso H, Jacobs DR, Wentworth D, et al. Serum cholesterol levels and six-year mortality from stroke in 350,977 men screened for the Multiple Risk Factor Intervention Trial. N Engl J Med 1989; 320:904–10.

109. Blackburn H, Jacobs DR Jr. The ongoing natural experiment of cardiovascular diseases in Japan. Circulation 1989; 79:718–20.

110. Shimamoto T, Komachi Y, Inada H, et al. Trends for coronary heart disease and stroke and their risk factors in Japan. Circulation 1989; 79:503–15.

111. Komachi Y, Iida M, Shimamoto T, et al. Geo-

graphical and occupational comparisons of risk factors in coronary heart disease in Japan. Jap Circ J 1971; 35:189–207.

112. Sakurai T, Matsuda T. Increased incidence of sudden death in an urban area in Japan (abstract). Circulation 1988; 78:suppl II: II-89.

113. Ueshima H, Iida M, Shimamoto T. Dietary intake and serum total cholesterol level: their relationship to different lifestyles in several Japanese populations. Circulation 1982; 66:519–26.

114. Konishi M, Iso H, Iida M, et al. Trends for coronary heart disease and its risk factors in Japan — epidemiologic and pathologic studies. Jap Circ J 1990; 54:428–35.

115. Kiyohara Y, Ueda K, Fujishima M. Smoking and cardiovascular disease in the general population in Japan. Hypertension 1990; 8:S9–15.

116. Marmot MG, Syme L. Acculturation and coronary heart disease in Japanese-Americans. Am J Epidemiol 1976; 104:225–47.

117. WHO Expert Committee. Prevention of coronary heart disease: a report. WHO Technical Report Series no. 678, 1982.

118. Black D, chairman. Royal College of Physicians. Obesity. Journal of the Royal College of Physicians of London 1983; 17:5–65.

119. Gurney M, Gorstein J. The global prevalence of obesity — an initial overview of available data. Wld Hlth Stat Qtly 1988; 41:251–4.

II

CLINICAL INTERVENTION

7

Helping Patients to Reduce Their Risk for Coronary Heart Disease: An Overview

JUDITH K. OCKENE
IRA S. OCKENE

EDITORS' INTRODUCTION

With this chapter we come to the essence of this book. It is our purpose to provide not only knowledge — the "why" of intervention — but also skills — the "how" of intervention. Physicians and other health care providers want to help their patients make lifestyle changes for the modification of CHD risk, but most lack the counseling skills needed for such intervention. This chapter provides an overview of the counseling process, emphasizing that a patient-centered counseling approach, in which the resources of the patient are elicited, need take no more time than less effective methods of physician-patient interaction. The chapter also discusses the theoretical background needed for an understanding of physician-patient interactions. Physicians must take an active role in the counseling process; it is important that they understand the need for and be able to participate in an integrated approach that takes advantage of the different skills available on the health care team.

The later chapters in Part II discuss the approach to specific risk factors on an individual basis. Chapter 7 provides a synthesis of current understanding of effective approaches to counseling for risk factor modification and is the foundation for the succeeding chapters.

Changing such lifestyle behaviors as smoking, high-fat eating patterns, sedentary habits, and ineffective methods for dealing with stress can significantly decrease the risk of coronary heart disease (CHD) (see Chapter 4). Likewise, improved adherence to therapeutic regimens for the treatment of hypertension, diabetes, and hyperlipidemia can prevent the development and/or progression of CHD [1] (see Table 7-1). By some estimates over 50 percent of the recent decline in CHD mortality is attributable to behavioral change [2]. However, changing a behavior that is detrimental to health requires knowledge, skills, and active involvement by the at-risk individual in the planning and learning process [3, 4].

The Importance of Physician Intervention

Physicians who focus on lifestyle changes with their patients have demonstrated that they can significantly affect a patient's efforts to alter behaviors like smoking [5], diet [6], and adherence to medical regimens [7, 8, 9]. Physicians and other members of the health care team are uniquely and powerfully situated in their routine office practice to educate patients about the relationship of certain behaviors to CHD and to help them develop the skills required to make behavioral changes. Thus, they play a pivotal role in the prevention of CHD. Doctors have always been expected to teach their patients

Table 7-1.   Suggested target behaviors for risk factor modification

---

Smoking
Dietary behaviors related to CHD
   High sodium intake (high blood pressure)
   High saturated-fat intake (atherosclerosis, obesity, diabetes)
   Low fiber intake (diabetes mellitus, cardiovascular disease)
Physical inactivity
Poor medication adherence (e.g., for high blood pressure, diabetes)
High stress levels and type A personality
Poor-quality relationships/supports

---

about their illnesses (the word *doctor* derives from the Latin *docere,* meaning "to teach") [10, 11]. It is only a logical extension of this role that doctors should educate patients about behaviors that might cause illness in the future.

There are several reasons why physicians and other members of the health care team can and should play a major role in helping patients make behavioral changes. First, physicians are perceived by the general public as the most reliable and credible source of health information and advice [12, 13, 14]. Patients generally prefer to receive as much information as possible from physicians, who often do not appreciate this desire and underestimate how much information patients actually want [15, 16, 17, 18]. Second, physicians and the health care system have contact with at least 75 percent of the adults in the United States each year [19] and are thus an immediately available and potent source of information regarding the prevention of CHD for over 120 million individuals. Data from the National Health Interview Survey (NHIS) also indicate that Americans visit a physician an average of 5.3 times per year [19]. Third, people think more seriously about their health and the impact of their lifestyle on it when they are in a physician's office or a hospital than at any other time. Fourth, primary care physicians, such as internists, family physicians, gynecologists, and general pediatricians, provide a continuity of care, which allows them to reinforce messages to their patients. Thus, these physicians are particularly well suited to educate, intervene, and follow up with patients who need to alter lifestyle behaviors [20].

Finally, patients generally do not want to go to a special program for help in altering unhealthy behaviors. More than 90 percent of smokers who have quit smoking have done so on their own, without formal smoking-intervention programs [21]; most current smokers would prefer to stop without such a program. Physicians and other providers in the health care setting are not perceived as special programs. They are part of the natural environment of individuals who may require help for reduction of risk for CHD [22].

Given the high credibility level of physicians

and other providers in the health care system as a source of needed health information, their high contact rate with the population at a time when people are particularly aware of their health and lifestyle behaviors, and the continuity of care that they provide, physicians and other providers can have a significant impact on the prevention of CHD.

Overcoming Barriers to Physician Interventions

Although physicians are generally aware of the benefits of implementing preventive interventions with their patients, national surveys of both patients and physicians indicate that a large percentage of physicians often do not intervene with lifestyle behaviors [20]. Physicians report several barriers to providing such intervention, including a belief that they are not effective in their health behavior interventions, poor intervention skills, a belief that patients do not want intervention when they are being seen for other problems, and little time to fit such intervention into their practices. Other factors more broadly associated with the practice of medicine also inhibit preventive interventions, such as nonreimbursement for these services. Also, physicians' practices generally are not set up to cue them to intervene and to facilitate integration of prevention activities with other more traditional medical needs. Finally, even though behavioral intervention for risk factor modification is of exceptional importance, there will never be the same immediate gratification as with other interventions such as giving penicillin for a streptococcal throat infection or resuscitating a patient who has arrested.

These barriers to implementing physician-delivered interventions can be overcome. Physicians can achieve the skill level necessary for effective interventions with very little training. These interventions can be relatively brief (three to four minutes) if they are focused and utilize the back-up services of office staff, consultants, special programs, and supportive aids such as self-help materials. They can also be easily integrated into the outpatient encounter if effective office systems are set up to facilitate integration with other services (see Chapter 17).

Surveys have demonstrated that patients welcome their physicians' input for health behavior change; in fact, even those patients who do not alter their behaviors are more satisfied with [23] and more likely to refer other patients to those physicians who do intervene than to those who do not [24].

Many patients and physicians are understandably concerned about the lack of reimbursement for prevention-oriented visits. However, there are legitimate billable diagnoses that physicians can use to receive reimbursement. In most cases, for example, physicians can receive reimbursement from third-party payers for patients with smoking-related problems (e.g., bronchitis). Reimbursement policies vary from state to state and among different insurers and types of policies. It is likely that the recently proposed resource-based relative-value reimbursement scales [25] will place a higher value on the time-intensive counseling required for preventive cardiology interventions.

Finally, physicians must have realistic expectations about the possibilities of health behavior change and adopt a new (or at least modified) mind set when dealing with behavioral change for risk-factor reduction. Change often comes slowly, and sometimes it seems as though little is accomplished. For example, smokers often quit three or four times over a period of about five years before they are successful in the long term [26]. From a population perspective, there have been remarkable changes in both smoking [26] and diet [27, 28] in the United States over the last 20 years, and the health professions have played an important role. Throughout this chapter we present information to address barriers to intervention and help physicians to acquire the knowledge and skills needed to intervene effectively.

Physicians as Part of an Integrated Approach to Intervention

Although physicians and other providers in the health care system have a major role in the prevention of CHD, their intervention efforts do not exist in a vacuum. Rather, they occur in combination with health promotion education efforts implemented through the media, worksites, schools, and voluntary organizations and via legislation covering areas such as smoking in public places and food labeling. Physicians, other health care providers, and the health care system as a whole are an integral and important part of these combined efforts [29].

The first section of this chapter is an overview of the determinants of human behavior and behavior change and the principles and procedures of behavior modification that physicians can use to educate patients and facilitate behavior change. Although physicians are not expected to become experts in psychological and behavioral theories, a general understanding of the development of behavior and the factors that affect its alteration can enhance a physician's ability to help patients alter harmful behaviors. The second section addresses the practical aspects of physician-delivered interventions and the skills needed in the practice of clinical preventive cardiology. It presents strategies ranging from those that are relatively simple and can be used by providers who have minimal availability of time and staff to do preventive interventions to those that are more involved and require more of the provider's time as well as that of other staff to coordinate activities and referrals. The last section addresses the special issues the provider needs to be aware of when implementing preventive interventions with special populations.

Determinants of Behavior and Behavior Change

A large body of literature regarding the determinants of health behavior development and change has evolved, driven by the need to provide empirical and theoretical guidelines for developing effective interventions. In this section we present four important theories. The first, Consumer Information Processing theory, explains the effects of knowledge on health behavior and on the factors that influence its processing. The other three theoretical models — Social Learning Theory, the Health Belief Model, and the Stages of Change Model — present the cognitive, attitudinal, and behavioral determinants of health behavior. The four theories taken together help us to understand how to promote changes in health behavior.

In this book we are interested in strategies for increasing CHD-preventive behaviors and decreasing CHD-promoting behaviors. CHD-preventive behaviors, or health-promoting behaviors, are defined here in a manner similar to Russell's [30] definition of health behaviors. They are actions or activities that contribute to the maintenance of current good cardiac health and a reduction in the likelihood of developing CHD, or to the favorable alteration of the rate of progression of already-present CHD. These activities include the elimination or reduction of undesirable CHD-promoting behaviors, such as cigarette smoking. Examples of CHD-preventive behaviors are the cessation of cigarette smoking, the alteration of eating patterns that contribute to increased weight or hyperlipidemia, and the reduction of certain types of stress responses. CHD-preventive behaviors also would include the initiation or increase in the frequency of healthy activities as part of the patient's daily routine. These activities might include an exercise or meditation routine or adherence to a medication-taking regimen. The definition of a CHD-preventive behavior emphasizes that it is the patient who has responsibility for performing the action, which often requires special skills.

Consumer Information Processing (CIP) theory [31] states that information is necessary for rational decision making and has an important influence on human behavior. It does not, however, explain the full range of lifestyle behaviors; although information is necessary, it is not sufficient to guide health actions and promote health-enhancing behaviors [32]. Thus, 87 percent of current smokers report that they understand that smoking is harmful to their health [33], but they continue to smoke. Most smokers also express a great desire to stop smoking but find it difficult to do so. Similarly, surveys indicate that three-quarters of U.S. adults believe that cholesterol reduction would have an effect on CHD [34], yet many continue to eat high-fat diets. Several minimum conditions are necessary for individuals to make use of information: information must be available; it must be wanted or believed to be useful by the consumer; it must be able to be processed within the time, energy, and comprehension levels of the consumer; and it must not be too confusing to process [32].

Thus, the clinician must make information available and present it in such a way that it is at the level of the patient's comprehension, and the patient must be ready to hear the information and act on it. Once individuals have the necessary information, they often lack the motivation, skills, environmental support, or resources needed to use it and to establish a new behavior as a habit or to eliminate undesirable behaviors. These mediating factors are explained more fully by the social learning theory and the health belief model, described next.

Social Learning Theory (SLT) (also referred to as social cognitive theory) is one of the best theoretical models for understanding lifestyle behaviors and methods to promote behavioral change. SLT assumes that most behaviors are learned and can therefore be unlearned or altered; that a person is able to self-manage behavior; that active participation is needed in the learning and the application of behavior-changing skills; and that health is dynamic and is constantly interacting with and being influenced by multiple determinants (*reciprocal determinism*) [35, 36, 37], with no single factor being sufficient to totally influence the behavior (see Table 7-2). Some theorists go a step beyond positing an interactive relationship and assume a person-in-environment perspective, which posits that each determinant of behavior mutually defines the others and none would be the same without the others [38].

The multiple and reciprocal interacting determinants of behavior include four groups of factors: personal characteristics of the individual (cognitive factors, personality, and demographic factors); environmental influences (the social, cultural, and economic environment, including advertising and policy); other associated behaviors (e.g., drinking a cup of coffee triggers the behavior of eating a piece of cake or smoking a cigarette); and physiologic and/or pharmacologic factors that affect addictive and/or ha-

Table 7-2. Multiple and interacting determinants that affect health behavior

Personal Characteristics/Cognitions
Demographics
Personality
Education/information
   Availability
   Believed to be useful
   Wanted by consumer
   Can be processed by consumer
Cognitions (thoughts, beliefs, fears)
   Belief in personal vulnerability and perceived risks of the behavior
   Belief in capability of changing the behavior
   Belief that behavior change will decrease risk
   Belief that benefits from change outweigh costs
Skills
   Self-management skills
   Stress reduction skills
Stage of change (readiness)
Environment
Social
Cultural
Economic
Political
Other Behaviors (e.g., use of alcohol in a person trying to stop smoking)
Physiologic Factors (e.g., nicotine addiction)

bitual behaviors, such as smoking, dietary patterns, alcohol intake, and other drug addictions. Cognitive factors include knowledge, thoughts, attitudes or beliefs, and skills. SLT also assumes that cognitive conditioning, or attaching thoughts or feelings to a specific behavior, occurs as behaviors become habits. An individual may eat whenever he has a thought that makes him anxious, because in the past he found that eating reduced his anxiety. This urge to eat may appear so rapidly that the person is no longer aware of the triggering association. Thus, thoughts and feelings are often associated with and conditioned to behaviors targeted for change.

SLT incorporates easily applied behavior modification strategies that address the cognitive, interpersonal, and environmental influences on behavior [37]. (The specific strategies are discussed in the next section.) The clinician using these strategies can help the patient identify the triggers and reinforcements of behaviors, understand how and when they operate, and learn how to control these triggers and find reinforcements for CHD-preventive behaviors.

Three concepts in SLT are of particular importance for physicians and other health care providers seeking easily used interventions to help patients develop the skills and attitudes necessary to facilitate development of health-promoting behaviors. These concepts are self-efficacy, behavioral self-management, and shaping. *Self-efficacy,* the degree to which a person is confident of his ability to successfully change a specific behavior (e.g., to stop smoking), has an effect on his performing that behavior independent of actual skill or knowledge. Self-efficacy is affected by past experiences of success and is important not only because it affects behavior [39, 40] but also because it has been demonstrated to be alterable through behavior modification strategies [41, 42] such as reaching small goals, monitoring, and self-reward.

Behavioral self-management (BSM) requires that an individual be aware that behavior is not an arbitrary occurrence but occurs as a result of identifiable factors (antecedents) that trigger, or cue, it and the consequences that reinforce it. The triggers can become linked, or conditioned, to the behavior, depending on the consequences that follow it. The consequences, in operant conditioning terms, are either positive (pleasurable) and reinforce the occurrence of the behavior or negative (aversive) and decrease the likelihood of its occurrence. If a stressful situation triggers smoking and the smoker then feels more relaxed, the result reinforces the continued use of cigarettes. Alternatively, a stressful situation may trigger the consumption of a cup of coffee and palpitations immediately follow. In this case, the individual may decrease coffee use as a result of the aversive consequence.

Behavioral self-monitoring — the use of a special log to record occurrences of a behavior, its triggers, and consequences — can help an individual become aware of his behaviors. He can then decide whether to avoid the trigger, alter it, or substitute a CHD-preventive behav-

ior when the trigger occurs. Alternatively, he can alter the consequences or reinforcements of the undesirable behavior to the extent that an alternative behavior is elicited and supported instead.

Shaping involves initially setting realistic, often small, attainable goals for change, so that reinforcement can be achieved quickly, in preparation for moving toward the final desired behavior [36, 37]. This gradual shaping helps facilitate the development of self-efficacy and subsequent motivation for the patient to continue to work on change. As specific steps toward the desired behavior are performed, the criterion for success and reinforcement is increased. For example, an individual who has the ultimate goal of smoking cessation may begin by cutting her number of cigarettes by 25 percent each week for one or two weeks before quitting completely.

The *Health Belief Model (HBM)* focuses on cognitive and attitudinal variables [43, 44, 45] as a way of understanding a patient's motivation and the likelihood of his adhering to a particular medical regimen or implementing a health behavior change. The HBM proposes that several factors affect the likelihood that a patient will implement preventive action. The model proposes that individuals are more likely to take action if they believe they are personally vulnerable or susceptible to a given condition, such as CHD; if there will be potentially serious consequences if they do not take action; if they are capable of taking action that will decrease their risk; and if the potential costs (barriers) of their taking action will be outweighed by the benefits [45]. The concepts of susceptibility and perceived risks help to explain why individuals who have already had a myocardial infarction are more likely to stop smoking or change their eating behavior than are individuals who do not yet have evidence of illness [26]. Providing information to the patient about the atherosclerotic process and its personal relevance to him, prior to the manifestation of signs and symptoms of cardiac disease, is important in helping the patient develop a realistic perception of personal risks and vulnerabilities.

The *Stages of Change Model* facilitates the development of more realistic expectations of what can be achieved in one encounter with a patient. This model emphasizes that behavior change is not a one-time event but a process that occurs in stages, often over an extended period of time [46, 47]. Smoking cessation, for example, often takes five to ten years and three to four attempts before long-term success is achieved [46, 47]. The stages of behavior change include precontemplation (not yet considering change), contemplation (thinking about and making plans to change a behavior), action (alteration of the behavior), and maintenance of the altered behavior (usually defined as having maintained the altered behavior for at least six months) or relapse (see Table 7-3). The stages are cyclical rather than linear, so if an individual relapses to the old behavior, he will generally cycle back to either precontemplation or contemplation.

The stages of change model has two important implications for interventions by health care providers. First, because change is a process of several stages before eventful action takes place, physicians and other providers in the health care system, by their persistent efforts over repeated contacts, can be important resources to individuals who are at different points in the change process. Their assistance can help move the precontemplator to contemplation and the contemplator to action. Second, providers need to be aware of this process so they do not become discouraged or alienate the often defensive precontemplator or embarrassed relapser. A single counseling interaction is not likely to move a precontemplator to action, but it may move him to the next stage, contemplation. The patient who quit smoking for three months and then resumed the behavior is not a failure; he is someone learning about what he needs to succeed and finding the path a bit difficult. While every patient may not completely succeed at altering a CHD-related behavior, every patient can be reached at some level through persistent efforts. Individuals not ready or willing to change can still benefit from a brief intervention during their medical encounters to move them closer to the final goal.

Interventions need to be different depending on the stage of the patient. Treatment must be realistic for the patient, given the behavior targeted for change, his level of education and skills, and the social, financial, and cultural context.

The four theoretical models discussed here indicate that provision of usable information is necessary but not sufficient for behavioral change to occur (see Table 7-2). Whether an individual modifies a particular health behavior depends on several sets of factors: environmen-

Table 7-3. Stages of behavior change and strategies to help the patient move to the next stage

Stage	Strategies
Precontemplation: Patient not yet considering change	Provide more information. Help patient develop belief in ability to change (self-efficacy). Personalize assessment/feedback.
Contemplation: Patient thinking about and making plans to change behavior	Help patient develop skills for behavior change. Provide support. Help patient develop plan for behavior change. Provide self-help materials.
Action: Patient changing behavior	Provide support. Help patient prepare for possible problems.
Maintenance: Patient maintaining behavioral change	Help patient prepare for possible problems.
Relapse: Patient returning to old behavior	Help patient understand reasons for relapse. Provide information about process of change. Help patient make plans for next attempt. Facilitate patient's belief in ability to change again. Provide unconditional support.

tal, personal/cognitive, behavioral, and, in some cases, physiologic. These factors interact and determine whether an individual is ready to consider using the information available to make a change. No one factor is sufficient by itself to affect behavior. Such cognitive factors as belief in personal susceptibility, capability to make the needed change, and comprehension of the risk of disease strongly affect behavior.

Our understanding of the multiple and interacting factors that affect behavior determine the strategies clinicians can use to help patients develop CHD-preventive behaviors. These strategies, which are discussed in the next section, include methods designed to promote a patient's self-efficacy, or confidence in his ability to regulate his own behavior, self-management skills, and an understanding of personal risk.

The Practice of Clinical Preventive Cardiology

The physician's role in patient's lifestyle modification for the prevention of CHD involves a sequence of activities: diagnosis/assessment, treatment/intervention, plan for change, and monitoring/followup (Table 7-4). This sequence is similiar to the physician's actions when faced with a patient with more conventionally defined medical problems such as hypertension or chest pain. Not all risk factors can receive the same attention, given time availability, known effective interventions, patients'

openness to action, and the physician's personal interests. *Physicians and other providers need to decide what they are willing and capable of doing and set themselves up to succeed at that level.* They also need to develop an office system that will be conducive to implementing preventive interventions.

Diagnosis/assessment involves the evaluation of CHD risk factors, medical and family history, and relevant psychosocial, physiologic, behavioral, and demographic variables. *Treatment/intervention* involves, at a minimum, the physician advising the patient of the need to increase CHD-preventing behaviors and to alter CHD-promoting behaviors. When appropriate and desired by the physician, treatment/intervention also involves an interactive counseling process where both the patient and the physician ask questions, provide information, and discuss the use of possible behavioral and pharmacologic interventions. The eventual outcome of counseling is the collaborative development of a *plan for change.* Whether or not the physician decides to provide brief counseling, someone else in the office should be able to provide more comprehensive assistance, or the patient could be referred outside the office for assistance with behavioral change. In any case, the physician's role is crucial and one that requires coordination and a level of energy that indicates to the patient that risk reduction is of primary importance for his health. *Monitoring/follow-up* involves further assessment to determine whether goals have

Table 7-4. Steps to clinical preventive cardiology

Step	*Physician's role*
Step 1: Diagnosis/assessment	Assess health and risks using: Medical interview Questionnaires Laboratory tests
Step 2: Treatment/intervention	Advise need for behavioral change Provide information/personalize risk Help patient to establish motivation, understand strengths, and deal with barriers.
Step 3: Plan for change	Negotiate goals with patient and plan strategies to achieve them.
Step 4: Follow-up/maintenance	Schedule follow-up visits. Provide support.

been met and whether the treatment plan developed has been implemented by the patient and is adequate to reach the goals set. Further development of goals and refinement of the treatment plan can then occur, again with the provision of continued follow-up.

Diagnosis/assessment, treatment/intervention, and monitoring/follow-up are often cyclical and ongoing. Even when risk factor control has occurred, periodic monitoring is necessary.

The physician can carry out each phase in the practice of clinical preventive cardiology. It is unlikely, however, that she will want or have the time and/or skills to be intensively involved in the treatment of each patient. To limit the physician's involvement, office staff can intervene at each step, or professionals outside the office can be used for referrals. Because the cycle can become rather complex, it is important for the physician to set up an adequate office reminder and follow-up system and communication links to ensure efficiency of patient management.

There are four basic models for physician involvement, which can be used in various combinations: (1) brief physician advice; (2) brief physician counseling; (3) brief counseling with referral for comprehensive individual counseling; and (4) brief counseling with referral for group education (either one session or multiple sessions) [48]. The following comprehensive overview of what the physician can do in the behavior modification process can be adapted to each physician's own needs, time, interests, and circumstances.

Step 1: Diagnosis/Assessment

The first step in the physician's role in the prevention of CHD is an assessment of the patient's health and risk status, his perception of the problem(s), and his knowledge regarding the relationship of lifestyle to CHD. This first step of diagnosis/assessment in clinical preventive cardiology parallels the first step in diagnostic and therapeutic medicine [49] (see Table 7-4). Such an assessment uses the medical interview, questionnaires, the physical examination, and laboratory tests. Self-administered questionnaires have the advantage of increasing effi-

ciency and standardization, are widely available, and have a high level of patient acceptability. Questionnaires can also facilitate communication. Although most of the needed information for determining a risk profile can be obtained without laboratory tests, data regarding factors such as total blood cholesterol and lipid profiles require blood tests.

A substantial number of patients are likely to have multiple risk factors, which will be identified during the risk assessment. For patients with multiple risk factors, the patient and the physician need to decide which factor to address first. (The possible options are discussed in the final section of this chapter.) The assessment process is one of mutual education for the patient and the physician. It provides the physician with information regarding the patient's CHD risk and an understanding of who the patient is — his needs, knowledge, motivations, resources, barriers to change, and concerns. The same process provides the patient with information about himself and the prevention of CHD and the physician's perceptions, concern, and support for risk factor change. Education of the patient begins during this initial assessment, as the physician and the patient engage in an interactive process.

During this interactive exchange between physician and patient, in which the patient provides much of the information, the physician provides feedback, at times paraphrasing what the patient has said, and provides additional information as required. These interviewing behaviors, which are appropriate and valuable for all physician-patient encounters, inform the patient that the physician is listening, understands his needs and concerns, and cares about him. They also allow the physician to help the patient use all the available information to eventually develop goals and a plan for altering the CHD-promoting behaviors and for maintaining these changes. A patient who is invited to express his concerns, beliefs, and perceptions can be freed up to hear what the physician is saying. This "guided-questioning" process leads to increased satisfaction for both the physician and the patient. It requires little extra time in the long-term care of the patient: if the physician carefully facilitates the discussion, greater understanding results and less time is needed later to clear up misconceptions and conflicts.

Step 2: Treatment/Intervention

Treatment/intervention by the physician is of crucial importance, and it is the physician's responsibility to ensure that it is carried out effectively. With a highly motivated patient who has personal resources and a positive history of change, such treatment by the physician usually requires very little time. However, additional time for education is needed for even the most motivated patient if he has few resources, little support, substantial problems in daily living, low confidence in his ability to alter behavior, and multiple risk factors. For the patient with poor motivation for change, treatment may be time-consuming. The physician needs to decide how much time preventive intervention will take, how much time he is willing to devote, and whether a referral to a specialist is appropriate. At the very least, the physician must emphasize the patient's risk and the importance of the need for change. Even when making a referral, the physician needs to take at least a few minutes to make sure the patient understands the reason for the referral and that the physician plans to continue to follow the progress made and will be available if problems occur.

Whether the physician himself works with the patient or refers the patient to an outside resource, he needs to convey several consistent brief messages that have a strong scientific basis:

- Behavior change is a *process,* not a one-time event. It often proceeds through several gradual changes from first becoming aware of the need to change to finally making the complete change.
- Behavior change often takes several attempts before long-term maintenance of the change occurs.
- A return to an old behavior is not a failure. It can be used as a learning experience to help you prepare for the next time you make the change.
- Many methods can help you change a behav-

ior. The best method to use is the one you choose for yourself, based on your own experiences.

The major intervention strategy used in treatment to help patients make lifestyle changes is education, which is more than just the delivery of information or the transfer of facts [10]. The National Task Force on Training Family Physicians in Patient Education [50] defined patient education as a process of influencing patient behavior to produce the changes in knowledge, attitudes, and skills needed to maintain or improve health. This process includes providing information and interpreting and integrating it in such a way as to bring about attitudinal or behavioral changes to benefit patient health.

Attention to factors such as the social, political, and cultural environment, cognitions (thoughts), and skills, each of which mediate the relationship between knowledge and action, is needed if maximal change is to occur. This attention requires the use of a wide variety of strategies in patient education, including providing information, patient-centered counseling, discussion, and behavior modification. Although this may sound somewhat forbidding, the strategies are easily learned and can fit into the framework of the typical office encounter. While not likely to use all approaches in her encounters with patients, it is important that the physician be aware of which approaches have been demonstrated to be efficacious in behavioral interventions. Physicians must also accept that for some patients problems in their social environment and difficulties in their daily lives may preclude their ability and desire to make CHD-preventing changes. The physician may need to divert her energies to help the patient obtain the assistance he needs to deal with his environment and his difficult life situation. Of course, final responsibility for change lies with the patient, who may have priorities at the time of the encounter other than changing lifestyle behaviors.

PROVIDING INFORMATION

If the physician does nothing else, a necessary step in treatment/intervention is to use the information gathered during assessment and advise the high-risk patient of the value of reducing his CHD risk by modifying certain behaviors. An understanding of the patient can be used to personalize the approach and make it particularly relevant to the patient and his situation. By knowing the patient's concerns, beliefs, and perceptions, the physician is better able to provide information in a manner to which the patient is likely to respond positively. Thus, the most important information needed for advising a patient to change lifestyle behaviors comes from the patient.

The physician can provide information verbally or through written self-help materials. Alternatively the patient can be referred to other health professionals for additional information or more intensive intervention. Depending on the preference and the needs of the patient, the physician, and the health care setting, the physician can use a combination of these approaches to provide information. A wide variety of informational and self-help materials regarding changes in various health behaviors is available for distribution to patients free of charge or for a nominal cost. These materials are published by several agencies, including the American Heart Association (AHA), the American Cancer Society (ACS), the National Heart Lung and Blood Institute (NHLBI), the American Lung Association (ALA), and the National Cancer Institute (NCI). (See the chapters on specific behaviors for lists of organizations from which to obtain these materials.) The materials used should correspond to the social, cultural, and educational level of the patient. The AHA, ACS and ALA have state and regional offices, which can provide assistance and information.

PATIENT-CENTERED COUNSELING

The physician who desires to go beyond a two-minute personal advice session and the provision of information can engage in brief patient-centered behavioral counseling. If the physician does engage in such counseling, advice giving and the provision of information can be integrated into the counseling approach and do not need to precede it. Patient-centered counseling can take anywhere from two to three additional minutes, if it is focused on a particular concern and ancillary materials or resources are used, to 10 to 15 minutes for the physician who wishes to or is able to spend more time with the patient. The most important aspect of patient-centered counseling, no matter how much time is spent, is that it emphasizes the importance of the patient's input in developing an effective plan for change and strategies for altering behaviors.

It is difficult to separate the assessment from the counseling intervention process, which largely entails further exploration of the patient's resources, motivations, strengths, problem areas, and behavioral patterns in relation to the targeted behavior. However, the goal shifts from simple assessment to a facilitative role for the physician. Through discussion and exploration of the way in which the patient can make the needed changes, the physician can help the patient gain greater self-awareness and can act as a catalyst for change. Table 7-5 summarizes the topics that should be covered in patient-centered counseling.

The counseling process provides a systematic approach for working with a patient in which the physician asks a series of questions that focus on the development of positive self-efficacy in the patient (i.e., a belief in one's ability to implement the behavioral change) and on the development of a plan for change. Every individual has strengths, resources, and past experiences that can be used to help make the needed health-related changes. If necessary, further information can be provided regarding effective behavioral strategies to be used to promote the target behavior. The effect of these strategies can be monitored in follow-up, and the treatment plan can be adjusted as needed.

The physician-patient interaction is different in the counseling-for-behavior-change encounter than that which typically occurs in traditional medical treatment. In the latter situation the patient's role is often one of cooperation and dependence; in the counseling relationship the patient is actively involved in diagnosis and treatment, and the relationship is collaborative. Despite the active involvement of the patient, the physician must still assume clinical responsibility. He sets the tone for the encounter — a

Table 7-5.   Physician-delivered counseling steps and sample questions

Step	Sample questions
1. Advise change. Personalize risks of CHD and benefits of altering behaviors.	
2. Assess motivation.	How do you feel about your diet? About the stresses in your life? How do you feel about changing this? What reasons or motivations would you have for changing this? Are you thinking about altering your diet in the next six months?
3. Assess past experiences with behavioral change.	Did you ever (stop smoking) before? *If yes:* When and why did you stop? How did you stop? What problems did you have? What helped? When and why did you start again? *If no:* Have you made any other positive changes in your lifestyle (diet, exercise)? How? Any problems? What helped you?
4. Discuss problems/barriers.	In what situations do you most want to eat sweets? What possible problems are you concerned about if you stop?
5. Discuss resources.	What might you do to help deal with possible problems? What might you do instead of overeating in situations when you usually overeat or eat unnecessarily?
6. Develop plan for change. *If patient decides to change behavior:* Negotiate behavioral goals. Set timeline. Review strategies for change. Provide self-help materials (discuss these at next regularly scheduled visit). Refer patient to outside resource if indicated. *If patient decides not to change or is unsure:* Discuss other related goals (e.g., relaxation approaches, exercise program) instead of end-point goal (e.g., diet change). Provide self-help materials (discuss these at next regularly scheduled visit).	Now that we have discussed your exercise, what plans would you like to make now to increase it?
7. Schedule follow-up contact. Monitor progress to determine if goals have been met. Determine future goals and revise plan.	What part of your plan was helpful? What part did you have problems with?

mutual exchange of information where both the physician's and the patient's participation is optimal [51]. The physician also needs to remain ultimately in control of the process to facilitate progression along a sequence of interchangeable steps designed to help the patient make the needed changes. The success of counseling depends on the collaboration between patient and physician and on the physician's ability to facilitate the process and help keep the patient on target.

The collaborative patient-centered approach

is equally useful in the traditional medical encounter. Physicians often prescribe therapeutic or medication-taking regimens without engaging the patient in such a dialogue. The regimens are often not followed, because of complexity, lack of understanding by the patient, or a difficult social setting that impedes adherence and, ultimately, maintenance of the desired change [52, 53].

TOPICS IN PATIENT-CENTERED COUNSELING

The topics to be addressed in patient-centered counseling are suggested in a particular sequence. However, the sequence and the emphasis can be changed to fit the style of the physician and those needs and factors unique to the patient. For example, intervention in smoking often emphasizes exploring past changes, while counseling for alteration in eating patterns might be more effective if present patterns are emphasized. As the physician becomes more comfortable with the counseling approach, he should adapt it to his own needs, time constraints, and style.

The first topic that might be addressed is the patient's desire and motivation to change her behavior. It is important to determine the patient's reasons for wanting to change, which may be different from the physician's reasons for wanting the patient to make a change. For example, the patient may be more concerned about the impact of her eating behavior on her weight than on the risk of disease. Without a clear motivation for making the needed changes, it is unlikely that change will take place. For some patients, however, lack of motivation may be related to a lack of confidence in their ability to make the needed change. Therefore, even for the patient who does not express strong motivation for change, it may be useful to go to the second topic, exploration of past experiences with change, to help the patient focus on past successes, no matter how small.

Most individuals who have made lifestyle changes in the past have returned to their old behaviors. For example, 80 percent of all smokers have stopped in the past [26]. The past behavior modification should be positively reinforced, no matter how brief the period of change. The physician can help the patient focus on the resources she used and the positive feelings that came from being a nonsmoker. This can help the patient become aware of her ability to stop smoking and help motivate her to try again. Thus, it is common for women to discount previous periods of smoking cessation associated with a pregnancy rather than realize that they were able to make it through stressful times without smoking by using other coping strategies; therefore, they could be successful again. After addressing past experiences with the patient who was not initially motivated to make a change, the physician can return to assessing motivation and determine whether the patient is now motivated to make a smaller change. Small successes help to shape positive self-efficacy.

Exploration of past experiences with change can also reveal problems that need to be prepared for and dealt with and the resources available to handle problems. What led to the stopping of an exercise program? What was most difficult about starting one? How did the patient try to overcome lack of motivation when she was exercising regularly? What worked? What didn't?

The third and fourth topics, problems experienced and resources utilized, should be used to provide information about resources for the current effort. Ask the patient what most concerns her about making the change at the present time. Once again, it is important for the physician to focus initially on the patient's perspective and then add his own perspective, as needed. A reticent patient can be asked open-ended questions about behaviors that she might substitute for an unwanted behavior: "What do you do to relax besides eating sweets?" If the patient cannot think of anything, a more focused question such as "Have you ever used exercise to help you relax?" or "Have you ever used deep breathing as a relaxation approach?" is useful.

The counseling approach should lead to a plan for change. No encounter should end without a plan, no matter how small the goal. The plan may focus on immediate goals: not shopping when hungry, walking ten minutes each morning, or simply learning a relaxation technique. Optimally this plan should be written and signed (see Figure 7-1), indicating commitment from both the physician and the patient. Finally, end with an arrangement for follow-up.

BEHAVIOR MODIFICATION STRATEGIES

During the treatment/intervention phase the patient may need assistance in developing new skills. Several behavior modification strategies can be used to help the patient develop the skills and new behaviors needed for alteration of CHD-promoting behaviors. Changes that depend only on the provision of information or personal support alone often do not result in long-lasting behaviors [54]. When the information is no longer remembered or when the personal contact in the professional relationship is ended, the individual often returns to the previous comfortable behavior, and little long-

My reasons for (losing weight, exercising, stopping smoking) are:

1. _____

2. _____

3. _____

4. _____

Steps I will take to help me (lose weight, exercise, stop smoking) are:

1. _____

2. _____

3. _____

4. _____

I am responsible for this decision and understand that my own commitment to

_____ is of primary importance.

I will return in _____ weeks or I will be telephoned in _____ weeks to see/to speak

to Dr. _____ on _____ at _____.
                                         (DATE)   (TIME)

_____   _____
(MY SIGNATURE)   (TODAY'S DATE)

_____
(PHYSICIAN'S SIGNATURE)

Figure 7–1. Sample plan for change. Source: PDSIP Training Manual. © 1990

term change remains. As noted previously, behavior modification strategies are based on social learning theory (SLT) concepts [35, 36, 37] of self-efficacy, shaping, and behavioral self-management. Health care providers can use the following five key strategies as treatment options with the patient who needs to make lifestyle changes. Not all strategies are appropriate for each patient or problem. Deciding on the appropriate strategy for a given patient comes from knowledge of the patient and an understanding of the problem.

Behavioral Self-Monitoring. The individual uses a special log (behavioral record) to record each occurrence of the behavior that has been targeted for change (e.g., smoking), the triggers (antecedents) that cue the urge to perform the behavior, and the rewards or incentives (consequences) that follow it (Figure 7-2). Self-monitoring by the patient provides both the patient and the physician with additional information and insight about the behavior targeted for change and allows the individual to engage in behavioral self-management. The individual can then choose to avoid or alter the trigger in some way, that is, control the stimuli that often trigger the behavior or substitute a CHD-preventive behavior when the trigger occurs (e.g., do slow, deep breathing instead of eating) and/or develop rewards or incentives for substituting CHD-preventive behaviors.

Stimulus Control. The information from the self-monitoring records can be used to identify situations or thoughts that have been conditioned to the unwanted behavior and now serve to trigger it. The patient can then decide how to avoid that trigger, as a way to change the behavior. For example, an individual who eats sweets when they are available in the home may decide not to buy any for a week and request that other household members help by not bringing any into the home. A person who snacks a lot when watching television may decide to substitute walking or reading for watching television.

Incentives. Rewards, or incentives, are developed for meeting predefined behavioral goals.

Investigators have demonstrated that self-reward strategies, when used as consequences of the performance of a specific behavior, reinforce its occurrence and maintenance better than do self-punishment strategies [55]. Rewards should be provided close to the time that the goal is met. If a patient's goal is to walk ten minutes each day for the next three days, a reward might be to purchase a magazine which he likes but usually does not allow himself to buy after he has completed the three days. Incentives must be developed by the patient, be pleasurable, and be used often and repeatedly to reinforce and shape the desired behavior.

One of the difficulties of discontinuing a CHD-promoting behavior or initiating a CHD-preventive behavior is that most of the positive consequences of the healthy behavior are often experienced only in the future (e.g., good health or feeling better), whereas the immediate consequences are often negative (e.g., feeling anxious). Conversely the positive consequences of an unhealthy behavior (e.g., drinking alcohol) are often immediate (e.g., being able to forget stressful events), and the negative consequences are experienced only in the long term (e.g., dying prematurely). This pattern often makes it difficult for patients to reach their desired behavioral goals because they lack the necessary reinforcements for behavior change [30]. It is important for the physician to briefly explore with the patient immediate positive and meaningful consequences of the CHD-preventive behavior. For example, a parent of a young child may see being a good role model as a positive short-term consequence of smoking cessation.

Substituting CHD-Preventive Behaviors. The vast majority of individuals offer the need to increase relaxation or reduce stress or boredom as a primary reason for smoking or overeating. Even individuals who can readily identify other ways of relaxing, such as exercise, reading, or socializing, may not think they are capable of doing without cigarettes or food to handle the moment-to-moment stressors from which smoking or eating provide quick relief. Deep breathing, simple meditation exercises, and physical exercise are relaxation techniques that

Name: _____ Date: _____

Record each time you snack between meals (exercise) (smoke)

	Time	Place	Activity	With Whom	Need* Rating

1. _____

2. _____

3. _____

4. _____

5. _____

6. _____

7. _____

8. _____

9. _____

10. _____

11. _____

12. _____

13. _____

14. _____

15. _____

16. _____

17. _____

18. _____

19. _____

20. _____

* Estimate how much you need the snack (cigarette) on a scale of 1–5.
1 = very important (cannot do without), 5 = least important (can do without).

Figure 7–2. Behavioral record.

can be used as substitutes and serve as effective functional equivalents for smoking or food in that they provide brief breaks from ongoing concerns, can be used under many circumstances, and seem to be physiologically effective. Training in stress-reduction techniques can be done relatively quickly, particularly if aided by the use of an audiotape. (See Chapter 10 and Chapter 11 for a presentation of how the physician can assist the patient in developing exercise regimens and stress reduction skills, respectively.)

Contracts. After a review of goals and the means by which to reach these, putting the details into a written behavioral plan for change may help the individual to keep them in mind, particularly if no further treatment contact is possible. Such a plan or contract underlines the seriousness of the endeavor and provides the patient with something to refer to after the encounter. The plan should indicate the steps for change, the timetable proposed, the reasons for changing the behaviors, and a plan for follow-up (see Figure 7-1.).

Step 3: Negotiate a Plan for Change

The patient-centered counseling sequence ends in a collaborative plan for change. Since most of the changes involved in risk reduction and prevention require the patient's voluntary cooperation and assumption of responsibility, successful outcomes require the patient to take a more active role in decision making and planning for change than usually occurs in a physician-patient interaction, with the physician acting as educator and counselor [56, 57]. The need for active involvement by the patient was first stated in Lewin's involvement principle [4], which indicates that individuals are more likely to initiate and maintain changes in their behavior if they have participated actively in developing the goals and plans for change [3, 58].

Some patients may be ready to change, and the patient and the physician may decide that the time is right for the patient to put effort into changing a particular behavior. In other cases they may decide that the time is not appropriate. A patient may have pressing social or financial problems that make it difficult for him to attend to health behavior alteration. He may want to wait until he is able to bring these problems under control. Alternatively he may decide that attending to the health behavior problems will provide him with a better sense of self, since he may be able to do something positive for his health while he may not be able to do anything about his other problems. For the patient who decides that the time is not right for change, the physician may want to set up a subsequent appointment two to three months later to discuss the problem again. It is important not to let the issue drop or be deferred for too long. The patient with pressing life problems may also benefit from a referral to a specialized social service agency.

REFERRING PATIENTS FOR ASSISTANCE

The physician's assessment of the patient during the diagnosis/assessment and the treatment/intervention phases may lead him to conclude that specialized attention or more advanced, time-consuming efforts are needed to help the patient make the necessary behavioral changes or deal with other life problems. Such patients may be very dependent on food or cigarettes for relief of negative feelings; they may in general be having such problems of daily living as unemployment, marital difficulties, drug abuse, or chronic depression or anxiety; or they may be slower in learning and require the services of a specialist. For example, a very obese individual may require a highly structured long-term program to lose weight and maintain the loss, which would be beyond the resources of most physicians' offices. The physician can still fill a very important role, however, by providing continued support and continuity of follow-up. Some problems requiring referral can be identified easily during the initial session, while others may take more than one visit to recognize.

When making a referral, the physician needs to indicate to the patient the reason for the referral, and should emphasize his continued involvement in the patient's care. Patients are often hesitant to obtain specialized help because they are concerned that this need indicates that they are "sick" or too incompetent to handle their own problems. Discussion of these concerns is necessary if a successful referral is to be made. Specialists in prevention, such as health psychologists involved in intervention with medical patients, are often affiliated with medical clinics. Many patients would prefer to see a specialist such as a psychologist in a medical setting rather than a mental health setting. The physician needs to write out a referral to the specialist or agency indicating the specific problems, the information that has been gathered, and the reason for the referral. He also needs to develop a mechanism in his office practice system to ensure that he is kept aware of what occurs as a result of the referral.

It is important for physicians to have psychologists, nutritionists, nurses, and other health care providers and special intervention programs identified for appropriate referral. In general such programs and specialists are available in medical centers and medical schools, often in specialized departments of behavioral medicine or nutrition. Psychologists specializing in behavioral medicine can also be found in universities or colleges with psychology departments that have a concentration in health psychology. Names of individuals who specialize in interventions for risk factor–related changes can be obtained through local voluntary organizations. Most communities also have special group programs that help patients make health-related changes and local offices of the AHA, ACS, and ALA often have group programs available for risk-factor modification. In addition, many local hospitals, health departments, and community health centers sponsor programs for smoking cessation, dietary change, exercise, and stress reduction.

A member of the physician's staff can develop a listing of programs or specialists in particular programs in the geographic area to provide to patients. While the effort is initially time-consuming, the long-term payoff is substantial. Only those programs consistent with the physician's message should be included on this list. If the patient is referred to a program, it is necessary for the physician to know if the patient kept the appointment, what recommendations were made, and the outcomes.

Step 4: Follow-up/Monitoring

Follow-up by the physician or a staff person should occur within a few weeks of the initial visit, ideally in person, but follow-up by telephone is acceptable. The time frame for follow-up is determined by the behavioral goals. If achievements are to be reinforced and problems identified, follow-up must be done while motivation to change is still high. Successful behavior change is not easy, and if follow-up does not occur for several months, it is likely that the process will need to be started over. Sending a letter that reiterates the goals and the plan immediately after the visit can be a useful procedure. (Figure 7-3 shows a sample letter.) This letter serves as a reminder to the patient and reinforces how important the physician thinks the behavior change is. Follow-up permits the physician and the patient to determine whether the plan for change is helpful and whether there are problems in meeting the negotiated goals. As part of this encounter, problem solving can occur and negotiation can again take place for new or revised goals and plans. The patient with multiple risk factors will need considerable follow-up to work through all the problem areas.

A major problem in behavioral change is that relapse or a return to old behaviors often occurs. For example, 70 percent of all smokers who stop smoking return to smoking within six months [47]. Implementation of new behaviors is generally easier than their long-term maintenance. For most patients it is not realistic to expect that brief one-session interventions will produce successful long-term outcomes. Hypertension control is a more traditional medical example of the need for continued intervention of some type. It would be unusual for a physician to treat a patient's hypertension and then not follow up to evaluate the treatment plan and its effects. Continued follow-up and reinforcement of some kind are likewise important for behavioral risk factors. The behavioral and counseling strategies used in the intervention phase can also be used in maintenance or relapse prevention. A relapse prevention strategy as a specific treatment component was developed by Marlatt, Gordon, and McClellan [59] to deal with preventing relapse in alcohol abuse and has been extended to other behaviors.

Relapse prevention is an approach that is consistent with social learning theory concepts and encourages patients to strengthen coping, self-management, and problem-solving skills. Five key elements, which are summarized below, can provide preparation for maintaining new behaviors. The physician can review these elements with the patient; they are also often addressed in self-help materials.

Sample Follow-up Letter for Preventive Interventions

Note: This letter is addressed to patients with high cholesterol. Followup letters can be used for any behaviors.

Dear

At your recent visit we discussed the importance of finding a method to decrease your intake of foods high in cholesterol and saturated fat. Any method you choose can be helpful to you as long as you make a firm decision to alter your eating pattern. At the visit you indicated that you would:

1. (note steps agreed upon) _____

2. _____

3. _____

   When you lower your cholesterol, important health benefits can be achieved. Your risk of developing heart disease will be decreased. If you would like further assistance, please call _____ at our office. As your physician, I encourage all efforts that you may want to make to lower your cholesterol. I wish you success.

Sincerely,

_____
(Physician's Name)

Figure 7–3.   Sample follow-up letter for preventive interventions.

IDENTIFYING TRIGGERS OF HIGH-RISK SITUATIONS

Situations formerly associated with the behavior can trigger urges to return to the behavior, even though initial change has occurred. Thus, identification of high-risk situations can help patients predict problems and prepare for them. The following types of situations are ones in which individuals are most likely to slip:

- situations involving negative emotional states such as anger, frustration, or stress
- situations involving positive emotional states — being relaxed and in a good mood and often involving the consumption of alcohol
- situations in which the individual sees others engaging in the old behavior, such as smoking cigarettes

Patients should be reassured that cravings or urges to reengage in the old behavior are normal and are to be expected rather than an indication of poor motivation or lack of will power. Patients who deny any significant difficulties may find themselves much more vulnerable to urges to return to their earlier behaviors.

COPING REHEARSAL

The outcome of exposure to high-risk situations is determined by whether the individual produces a healthy coping response that does not involve the old behavior. Use of imagery or hypnotherapy techniques may be valuable if the patient cannot easily visualize handling the high-risk situations. Once the individual has identified high-risk situations, he can develop and mentally rehearse specific strategies that can prevent a slip that might lead to a full-blown relapse.

IDENTIFYING AND COMBATING RESUMPTIVE THINKING

Patients may have habitual rationalizations to justify behavioral lapses or resumption of old behaviors. Identification of these rationalizations ahead of time can help guard against relapse by increasing awareness and by returning a sense of control to the patient. The following rationalizations are examples of resumptive thinking:

- Nostalgia: "I remember how nice it was when I didn't feel like I had to take a walk and could just sit and relax before dinner."
- Testing oneself: "I bet I could eat just one cookie with my coffee."
- Crisis: "I know I'll deal with this better if I take a drink."

Combating resumptive thinking may require rehearsal of counterthoughts:

- Challenging: "Taking just one cookie may be an excuse for returning to overeating. I do not need to test myself."
- Visualization of benefits: "I want to be able to play tennis without collapsing."
- Distractions: "I think I'll go call a friend instead."

AVOIDING THE ABSTINENCE VIOLATION EFFECT

The abstinence violation effect (AVE) is a common emotional response to a slip or a lapse in the face of personal commitment to change. Accompanying thoughts such as "I blew it" appear to predict a decision to give up the commitment entirely and to resume the avoided behavior. Discussion with a patient of this predictable response appears to decrease the problem. Consequently patients should be acquainted with the following points:

- Anticipating the AVE will help to reduce its impact.

- A slip is not the same as a relapse.
- A slip can be a learning experience.

ENCOURAGING SUPPORT

Other relapse prevention strategies include encouraging the patient to enlist the support of family, friends and coworkers. The stronger the patient's support system, the more likely it is that he will maintain the new behavior. The patient's spouse may benefit from encouragement to provide positive rather than nagging support.

It is important that neither the physician nor the patient become discouraged or angry if relapse occurs. A characteristic of successful long-term maintenance is that there is a history of having made changes in the past [47]. Each attempt can be viewed as a small gain on the way to final success.

Summary of the Practice of Clinical Preventive Cardiology

As noted in the introduction to this section, the physician may be able to and desirous of implementing each of the phases of the practice of clinical preventive cardiology. Alternatively, part of each phase can be carried out by referrals to consultants, programs or agencies, or other office personnel can assist. Considering the various possible combinations of professionals who may assist in assessment and intervention, it is necessary that an adequate communication and office monitoring system be set up to assure that there are no gaps in the process and that all required communications occur (See Chapter 17).

For the patients who have only one risk factor to change, good skills, strong motivation to make changes, and strong support systems, much of the preventive sequence can be accomplished in 3 to 10 minutes, depending on the level of physician involvement and use of ancillary materials, during two or three visits. The first visit would include diagnosis/assessment and possible treatment/intervention. If laboratory tests are used then treatment/intervention and development of a plan for change will need to take place during visit two. However, there are likely to be enough data available during visit one for an initial plan to be negotiated and strategies for change identified. Visits two and three and possibly a fourth visit are needed to address follow-up and assessment and possible revision of the negotiated plan for change. Patients with multiple risk factors or more difficult patients will require more time and/or greater reliance on other intervention specialists.

Physicians with little practice can quickly learn the skills needed for the practice of preventive cardiology. (Chapter 22 discusses programs and materials available for the learning of such skills.) Studies have demonstrated that the development of such skills can occur within one to two hours and can lead to more effective patient intervention [60].

Clinical Preventive Cardiology for Special Populations

Difficult-to-Reach Patients

Patients of lower socioeconomic status (SES) who may also be unemployed or homeless are generally difficult to reach for CHD-preventive interventions and often face multiple obstacles to making needed changes. Patients with psychiatric disorders and drug and alcohol abusers are also difficult to intervene with and require special attention. Individuals in each of these groups have difficulty seeing beyond the needs of the day and have little energy to make changes that would lead to health benefits in the more distant future. Minimal resources and poor skills may also make it difficult for these individuals to obtain the help they need. Poor comprehension may make it difficult for them to apply health-related information to themselves, and disrupted social and family environments make it hard for them to adhere to programs and plans that require focused attention. These substantial obstacles require attention and an approach that is sensitive to the patient's needs.

Preventive efforts aimed at homeless individuals are especially important since they have a high prevalence of CHD-promoting behaviors, such as smoking, recently found by Geldberg and associates to have a prevalence of 74 percent in this population [61]. Results of a recent study by Dr. Lori Fantry, an internist who provided medical services in the shelters in Worcester, Massachusetts, demonstrated that there is a subgroup of homeless individuals with a high desire to stop smoking and a high confidence level in their ability to do so [62]. Similar results were found with a largely lower SES, unemployed population in Springfield, Massachusetts [63]. Health-related intervention efforts for the homeless population should be specifically targeted toward their needs and can be successful if provided at sites such as shelters, city hospital clinics, and soup kitchens, which are easily accessible to them [62].

The physician in encounters with hard-to-reach patients can become aware of their special problems and belief systems and help to direct them to appropriate agencies for assistance if indicated. It is important for the physician not to be pulled into a sense of hopelessness and helplessness. He can help the patient see that options are available, including obtaining the help needed for dealing with problems in daily living. The physician must also not make the assumption that a patient with difficult problems would not be interested in making health-related changes. To do so is to reinforce the message of hopelessness and to discount the patient's decision-making ability. Some patients in difficult life situations actually view health behavior change as something positive that they can do for themselves, no matter how small. For those patients with chronic life problems who make small changes, there is an increase in their self-efficacy and belief in their ability to effect change. Such an increase in self-efficacy can help patients make other changes in their lives as well. Some of these individuals may want referrals to health promotion specialists to help them develop the skills needed for health behavior changes.

Patients with chronic psychiatric problems and drug or alcohol abusers present special problems. Research examining treatment options for health behaviors in these populations has not been done in spite of the substantial evidence of an unusually high incidence of poor health behaviors. Treatment of health behaviors in these complicated patients usually requires much individualized attention and longer follow-up. Regarding alcohol abuse, there is no clear indication that smoking cessation prompts relapse back to drinking among individuals who are alcohol dependent [64]. In fact, it may be associated with better outcomes [65, 66].

Minority Patients

Patients from minority groups are often at greater risk for obesity, non–insulin-dependent diabetes, and hypertension than those from white populations. However, patients from minority groups are often also more difficult to reach because of the physician's lack of awareness of their health beliefs and cultural values and because these individuals often have fewer financial and educational resources. Patients from black and Hispanic cultures in the United States are likely to consume a diet relatively rich in high-fat meats and other high-fat foods. The physician must be aware of and sensitive to the needs, environment, and beliefs of these individuals. Providers should familiarize themselves with the health-belief systems of the minority populations they serve so they can provide these patients with adequate information.

Elderly Patients

Risk factor modification in the elderly patient has been demonstrated to be beneficial [67, 68, 69, 70]. However, elderly patients often present with special needs that may interfere with CHD-preventive interventions. Some elderly individuals have poor social support systems, difficulty exercising, the need to adhere to regimens for other medical problems, depression, and other chronic problems. These possible obstacles require attention and a sensitive approach. The physician can direct the patient to the appropriate services for assistance. It is important not to assume that the elderly patient, especially the vigorous healthy individual, is not interested in risk factor modification. The elderly patient experiencing other chronic problems is also a possible candidate for risk factor modification, and this possibility needs to be assessed.

Patients with Multiple Risk Factors

Patients with multiple risk factors require special consideration for intervention decisions. The presence of multiple risk factors may pose obstacles to change or, alternatively, may increase the individual's motivation and subsequent improvement in each of the behaviors. Several studies have found that individuals who quit smoking are also more likely to lower their cholesterol and blood pressure and practice other health-promoting behaviors than those individuals who continue to smoke [71, 72, 73]. Of course the former may be more health-conscious at the outset. However, changes in some behaviors, for example, increased exercise or use of meditation, can help individuals implement changes in other behaviors such as smoking cessation and reduced food intake.

For the patient with multiple problems the patient and the physician need to decide which behavior to address first, following one of three approaches:

- Start with alteration of one risk factor; once that is under control, focus on another risk factor.
- Work equally on all risk factors at the same time.
- Focus attention on one risk factor and at the same time make small changes in another risk factor.

With the first approach an optimal way to proceed is to work first with the behavior the patient believes he is most capable of changing and most interested in changing. However, if the physician thinks a particular behavior has a significantly greater effect on the patient's health, for example, smoking 40 cigarettes a day compared to being ten pounds overweight, then the physician needs to indicate this to the patient and negotiate regarding the first risk factor to be addressed. It has been our experience that many patients who smoke and are also overweight most commonly choose weight control as their initial target, because they perceive it to be easier; in reality long-term success rates are much greater for smoking cessation [47]. The second approach requires a highly motivated patient with good resources and a supportive environment. The third approach is useful for the patient who may need to stop smoking and at the same time alter his eating patterns because of a concern for possible weight gain. The patient may decide that along with stopping smoking he will monitor his sweets intake and start an exercise program but not focus on weight loss.

Whatever approach is chosen, the physician and the patient must weigh the costs against the benefits. The physician's role is to express what he sees as optimal and help direct the patient to set realistic goals. He must also be sensitive to the fact that for some patients the cost of change may outweigh any benefits.

Costs of Lifestyle Change

For some patients behavioral change can lead to deleterious consequences as well as benefits. Altering lifelong habits can, for a small number of patients, cause anxiety, irritability, and, in the case of smoking cessation, weight gain (which is generally moderate [47]), especially for the patient with poor resources and other problems in daily living. Important social networks can be disrupted by the cessation of smoking or alcohol abuse or by the implied criticism of others seen in such actions as the initiation of a vigorous diet-alteration and exercise program. For some individuals these detrimental effects may outweigh the benefits of change, at least in the short term, and make such change difficult. The physician can take the following steps to minimize such difficulty:

- Identify clearly the target goals that are likely to decrease risk.
- Analyze both the benefits and the expected costs of a particular lifestyle change.
- Identify a range of alternative approaches that might reduce the cost of achieving particular goals.
- Negotiate with the parties involved to reach consensus on the importance of a change and the best approach(es) to achieve maximum benefit based on the energy and the resources available.
- Identify the conditions under which interven-

tion to achieve a particular goal is not warranted because of an anticipated high cost/benefit ratio or because it produces irreconcilable social dilemmas.
- Monitor progress periodically to reassess the balance of costs and benefits in light of changing circumstances and the response to the intervention.

Larger-scale approaches can make individual change less costly. A worksite with a smoking cessation program makes individual change more acceptable; the presence of healthful choices in a cafeteria or a fast-food restaurant allows an individual to eat well without being labeled as an oddball. These macro-level interventions will be covered in later chapters of this book.

As we encourage patients to make lifestyle changes beneficial to their health, it is equally important to avoid creating a nation of people who are hypochondriacal and overly health-conscious. Barsky points out that although life expectancy has increased remarkably (a 6.5-year increase from 1950 to the mid-1980s), the proportion of people living in the United States who are satisfied with their health has fallen from 61 percent in the 1970s to 55 percent in the mid-80s [75]. People now report more frequent and longer-lasting episodes of serious disability than they did 60 years ago, and there has been a continuous decline in the proportion of people who report no symptoms. Dr. Barsky concludes, "There appears to have been a progressive decline in our threshold and tolerance for mild disorders and symptoms."

This is not a simple problem. An almost inevitable consequence of continuously reminding people to think about their health, to eat better, to avoid various noxious behaviors, and to run to the emergency room for thrombolytic therapy at the first hint of chest pain is a nation of people preoccupied with the state of their bodies. As we encourage people to make beneficial changes, we must also avoid using scare tactics, and we should emphasize a patient's current state of health rather than the dire potential for disease. It is at times a difficult balance to achieve, but an important one.

Summary

We began this chapter by noting that while physicians are aware of the benefits of preventive interventions they often do not provide such interventions. The reasons for such failures include:

- low perceived efficacy
- lack of skills
- concern that patients do not welcome such interactions
- lack of time
- lack of reimbursement
- lack of practice organization to facilitate such interventions
- little self-gratification from such efforts

Throughout this chapter we have presented information that indicates that physicians can be effective by using brief interventions that are direct and supportive of the patients' efforts. This approach accepts that patients do welcome physician interventions, that they usually want to make the needed changes, and that they often have the resources to do so. The physician's role as counselor and educator is to help the patient become aware of the need for change and of his own personal resources and to help him find ways to make the needed changes. The physician must also learn to enlist the services of other office staff, consultants, and outside programs. She must be aware of the available services and able to make an effective referral. To close the intervention loop and ensure that prevention is addressed, an office system must be set up that facilitates support, integration with other services, and follow-up. While reimbursement for these services is not likely to change in the near future, there are legitimate billing practices that allow for reimbursement of risk factor intervention. Physicians need to become aware of how to maximize such reimbursement.

Regarding gratification for the physician's prevention efforts, the physician must have realistic expectations of what can be accomplished. Behavioral change is often a slow process as people move through stages of change. It is important to be aware that significant risk factor changes have occurred in this country and that the physician is an important part of the national effort.

The ability to think in terms of large numbers of patients as well as the individual patient, a public health perspective often foreign to usual physician practice, is very helpful. A 5 percent decrease in the blood cholesterol level is small and often ungratifying when seen from the perspective of the individual physician-patient relationship. However, a 5 percent decrease in cholesterol yields a 10 percent decrease in risk [28], and a 10 percent decrease in risk in a disease that causes 500,000 deaths a year is an annual savings of 50,000 lives. Gratifying indeed when seen from such a population perspective. Similarly if increased physician efforts double or triple smoking cessation rates (i.e., from 5 percent to 15 percent), a magnitude of impact found in several physician-delivered intervention studies, such an effect is of tremendous clinical and public health importance. The physician, however, may be more aware of the 85 percent of his smoking patients who continue to smoke.

It is also necessary to accept that once a patient becomes ill, all medicine usually has to offer is palliation. We cure very few adult diseases, and the knowledgeable physician understands that the cost of such therapy is extraordinary. The patient who remains healthy because the physician successfully helped him to stop smoking may never appreciate that because of the counseling, he is well and active instead of having prematurely suffered a myocardial infarction. However, for the prevention-oriented physician who understands the positive consequences of risk factor modification, the rewards can be great.

Suggested Further Readings

Bandura A. Social foundation of thought and action. A social cognitive theory. Englewood Cliffs, NJ: Prentice-Hall, 1986.

Branton SA. Physicians as patient teachers. Western J Med 1984;141:855-60.

Prochaska JO, DiClemente CC. Stages and processes of self-change: Toward an integrative model for change. J of Counseling and Clinical Psychology 1983;51:390-5.

Roemer MI. The value of medical care for health

promotion (Commentary). Amer J of Public Health 1984;74:243-8.

Russell ML. Behavioral counseling in medicine. Oxford, NY: Oxford University Press, 1984.

References

1. Stamler J. Coronary heart disease: doing the "right things" (editorial). N. Engl J Med 1985; 12:1053-5.
2. Goldman L, Cook EF. The decline in ischemic heart disease mortality rates. Ann Intern Med 1984; 101:825-36.
3. Haggerty RJ. Changing lifestyles to improve health. Prev Med 1977; 6:276-89.
4. Lewin K. Group decision and social change. In: Maccoby EE, Newcomb THE, Hartlet H, eds. Readings in social psychology. New York: Holt, Rinehart & Winston, 1958.
5. Ockene JK, Quirk ME, Goldberg RJ, et al. A residents' training program for the development of smoking intervention skills. Arch Intern Med 1988; 1039-45.
6. Mojonnier ML, Hall Y, Berkson DM, et al. Experience in changing food habits of hyperlipidemic men and women. J Am Diet Assoc 1988; 77:140-8.
7. Dunbar J. Assessment of medication compliance: a review. In: Haynes RB, Mattson ME, Engebretson TO, eds. Patient compliance to prescribed antihypertensive medication regimen. USDHHS publ. no. (NIH) 81-2101, 1988.
8. Greenfield S, Kaplan SH, Ware JE, et al. Patients' participation in medical care: effects on blood sugar control and quality of life in diabetes. J Gen Int Med 1988; 3:448-57.
9. Schulman BA. Active patient orientation and outcomes in hypertensive treatment: application of a socio-organizational perspective. Med Care 1979; 17(3):267-80.
10. Canfield RE. Role preparation: the physician as a teacher of patients. J Med Ed 1973; 48(12):79-87.
11. Brunton SA. Physicians as patient teachers. West J Med 1984; 141:855-60.
12. U.S. Department of Health, Education and Welfare. Healthy people. The Surgeon General's report on health promotion and disease prevention. USDHHS publ. no. (ADM) 79-800.
13. Glynn TJ, Manley MW, Cullen JW, Mayer WJ. Cancer prevention through physician intervention. Seminars in Onc 1990; 17:391-401.
14. Ford AS, Ford WS. Health education and the primary care physician: the practitioner's perspective. Soc Sci Med 1983; 17:1505-12.
15. Waitzkin H. Information giving in medical care. J Hlth & Soc Beh 1985; 26:81-101.
16. Davis F. Passage through crisis. Indianapolis: Bobbs-Merrill, 1963.
17. Faden RR, Becker C, Lewis C, et al. Disclosure of information to patients in medical care. Med Care 1981; 19:718-33.
18. Joos SK, Hickam DH. How health professionals influence health behavior: patient-provider interaction and health care outcomes. In: Glanz K, Lewis FM, Rimer BK, eds. Health behavior and health education: theory, research and practice. San Francisco: Jossey-Bass Publishers, 1990;216-41.
19. National Center for Health Statistics. Health, United States 1987. U.S. Department of Health and Human Services, Public Health Service. USDHHS publ. no. (PHS) 88-1232, 1988.
20. Ockene JK. Physician-delivered interventions for smoking cessation: strategies for increasing effectiveness. Prev Med 1987a; 16:723-37.
21. Fiore M, Novotny T, Lynn W, et al. Methods used to quit smoking in the United States. Do cessation programs help? JAMA 1990; 263:2760-5.
22. Ockene JK. Toward a smoke-free society. Am J Pub Hlth 1984; 74:1198-1200.
23. Bertakis KD. The communicating of information from physician to patient: a method for increasing patient retention and satisfaction. J Fam Prac 1977; 5:217-22.
24. Ockene JK, Kristeller JK, Goldberg R, et al. Increasing the efficacy of physician-delivered smoking interventions: a randomized trial. J Gen Int Med 1991; 6:1-8.
25. Hsiao WC, Braun P, Douwe Y, et al. Estimating physicians' work for a resource-based relative-value scale. N Engl J Med 1988; 319:835-41.
26. U.S. Department of Health and Human Services. Reducing the health consequences of smoking: 25 years of progress. A report of the surgeon general. Centers for Disease Control, Office of Smoking and Health. USDHHS publ. no. (CDC) 89-8411, 1989.
27. National Center for Health Statistics, National Heart, Lung and Blood Collaborative Lipid Group. Trends in serum cholesterol levels among US adults aged 20 to 74 years: data from the national Health and Nutrition Examination Surveys, 1960 to 1980. JAMA 1987; 257:937-42.
28. Lipid Research Clinic Program. The Lipid Research Clinics Coronary Primary Prevention Trial results. I. Reduction in incidence of coronary heart disease. JAMA 1984; 251:351-464.
29. Ockene JK. Smoking intervention: the expanding role of the physician. Am J Pub Hlth 1987b; 77:782-3.
30. Russell ML. Behavioral counseling in medicine. New York: Oxford University Press, 1984.
31. Bettman JR. An information processing theory

of consumer choice. Reading, Mass.: Addison-Wesley, 1979.

32. Rudd J, Glanz K. How individuals use information for health action: consumer information processing. In: Glanz K, Lewis FM, Rimer BK, eds. Health behavior and health education: theory, research and practice. San Francisco: Jossey-Bass Publishers, 1990.

33. American Lung Association. Survey of attitudes toward smoking. Princeton, NJ: Gallup Organization, July 1985.

34. Schucker B, Bailey K, Heimbach JT, et al. Change in public perspective on cholesterol and heart disease: results from two national surveys. JAMA 1987; 258:3521-6.

35. Mischel W. Toward a cognitive social learning reconceptualization of personality. Psych Rev 1973; 80:252-83.

36. Bandura A. Social learning theory. Englewood Cliffs, NJ: Prentice-Hall, 1977.

37. Bandura A. Social Foundation of thought and action. A social cognitive theory. Englewood Cliffs, NJ: Prentice-Hall, 1986.

38. Quick M, Wapner S. Notes on an organismic-developmental systems perspective for health education. Hlth Educ, Res 1991; 6:203-10.

39. Condiotte MM, Lichtenstein E. Self-efficacy and relapse in smoking cessation programs. J Consult & Clin Psych 1981; 49:648-58.

40. DiClemente CC. Self-efficacy and smoking cessation maintenance: a preliminary report. Cogn Ther Res 1981; 5:175-87.

41. Bandura A. Self-efficacy: toward a unifying theory of behavioral change. Psych Rev 1977: 84:191-215.

42. Bandura A. Schunk DH: Cultivating competence, self-efficacy and interests through proximal self-motivation. Journal of Personality and Social Psychology 1981; 41:586-98.

43. Rosenstock IM. What research in motivation suggests for public health. Amer J Pub Hlth 1960; 50:295-301.

44. Becker MH, ed. The health belief model and personal health behavior. Hlth Ed Mono 1974; 2:324-473.

45. Rosenstock IM. The health belief model: explaining health behavior through expectancies. In: Glanz K, Lewis FM, and Rimer BK, eds. Health behavior and health education: theory, research and practice. San Francisco: Jossey-Bass Publishers, 1990.

46. Prochaska J, DiClemente C. Stages and processes of self-change of smoking: toward an integrative model of change. J Counseling and Clinical Psych 1983; 51:390-5.

47. U.S. Department of Health and Human Services. The health benefits of smoking cessation. A report of the surgeon general. Centers for Disease Control, Office of Smoking and Health. USDHHS publ. no. (CDC) 90-8416, 1990.

48. Glanz K. Nutrition education for risk factor reduction and patient education: a review. Prev Med 1985; 14:721-52.

49. Stokes J, Noren J, Shindell S. Definition of terms and concepts applicable to clinical preventive medicine. J Comm Hlth 1982; 8:33-40.

50. Fass MF, Vahldieck LM, Meyer DL. Teaching patient education skills: a curriculum for residents. Kansas City, Mo.: Society of Teachers of Family Medicine, 1983.

51. Lazare A, Eisentral S, Frank A. A negotiated approach to the clinical encounter. II. Conflict and negotiation. In: Lazare A, ed. Outpatient psychiatry: diagnosis and treatment. Baltimore: Williams and Wilkins, 1979.

52. Horwitz RI, Viscoli CM, Berkman L, et al. Treatment adherence and risk of death after a myocardial infarction. Lancet 1990; 336:542-5.

53. Editorial. Are you taking the medicine? Lancet 1990; 335:262-3.

54. Stunkard AJ. Behavioral medicine and beyond: the example of obesity. In: Pomerleau OF, Brady JP, eds. Behavioral medicine: theory and practice. Baltimore: Williams & Wilkins, 1979.

55. Mahoney MJ, Moura NCM, Wade TC. Related efficacy of self-reward, self-punishment, and self-monitoring techniques for weight loss. J Consult and Clin Psych 1973; 40:404-7.

56. Demak MM, Becker MH. Current perspectives on the changing patient-provider relationship: charting the future of health care. Patient Ed Couns 1987; 9:5-24.

57. Carter WB, Belcher DW, Inui TS. Implementing preventive care in clinical practice: problems for managers, clinicians, and patients. Med Care Rev 1981; 38:195.

58. Green LW. Modifying and developing health behavior. Ann Rev Pub Hlth 1984; 5:215-36.

59. Marlatt A, Gordon J, McClellan W. Current perspectives: patient education in medical practice. Patient Ed Couns 1986; 8:151-63.

60. Ockene JK, Quirk MA, Goldberg RJ, et al. A residents' training program for the development of smoking intervention skills. Arch Intern Med 1988; 148:1039-45.

61. Geldberg L, Linn LS, Usatine RP, Smith MH. Health, homelessness and poverty: a study of clinic users. Arch Intern Med 1990; 150:2325-30.

62. Fantry LS. Unpublished report. 1990.

63. Miller DR, Ockene JK, Hebert J, et al. Racial differences in smoking-related factors among participants in a physician-based smoking intervention trial. Submitted for publication.

64. Kozlowski LT, Ferrence RG, Corbit T. Tobacco use: a perspective for alcohol and drug researchers. Brit J Addiction 1990; 85:245.

65. Hughes JR, Hatsukami D. Signs and symptoms of tobacco withdrawal. Arch Gen Psych March 1986; 43 (3):289-99.

66. Miller WR, Hedrik KE, Taylor CA. Addictive behaviors and life problems before and after behavioral treatments of problem drinkers. Addictive Beh 1988; 8:403-12.

67. Castelli WP, Wilson PWF, Levy D, et al. Cardiovascular risk factors in the elderly. Am J Cardiol 1989; 63:12H-9H.

68. Gordon DJ, Rifkind BM. Treating high blood cholesterol in the older patient. AM J Cardiol 1989; 63:48H-52H.

69. Hermanson B, Omenn GS, Kronmal RA, et al. Beneficial six year outcome of smoking cessation in older men and women with coronary artery disease: results from the CASS registry. N Engl J Med 1988; 319:1365-9.

70. Kafonek SD, Kwiterovich PO. Treatment of hypercholesterolemia in the elderly. Ann Int Med 1990; 112:723-5.

71. Orleans CT, Shipley RA, Wilbur C, et al. Wide-ranging improvements in employee health lifestyle and well-being accompanying smoking cessation in the Live for Life program. Paper presented at annual meeting of Society of Behavioral Medicine, Baltimore, Md., 1983.

72. Schoenenberger J. Smoking change in relation to changes in blood pressure, weight and cholesterol. Prev Med 1982; 11:441-53.

73. Tuomilehto J, Nissinen A, Puska P, et al. Long-term effects of smoking cessation on bodyweight, blood pressure and serum cholesterol in the middle-aged population with high blood pressure. Addictive Beh 1986; 11:1-9.

74. Ockene JK, Sorensen G, Kabat-Zinn J, et al. Benefits and costs of lifestyle change to reduce risk of chronic disease. Prev Med 1988; 17:224-34.

75. Barsky AJ. The paradox of health. N Engl J Med 1988; 318:414-8.

8

Smoking Intervention: A Behavioral, Educational, and Pharmacologic Perspective

JUDITH K. OCKENE

EDITORS' INTRODUCTION

Tobacco use is a major risk factor for CHD and also for many other serious illnesses, including cancer, chronic bronchitis, and emphysema. One of every six deaths in the United States is attributable to this noxious agent. Most smokers wish to quit, and the methodologies described in Chapter 7 can be successfully applied to this problem. There is certainly reason for optimism: smoking prevalence in the United States has dropped sharply in the last 25 years. Health care providers are often discouraged by what they perceive to be a lack of success in helping patients to stop smoking, yet in the population at large dramatic changes have occurred, and there is good evidence that even minimal intervention by a respected health care professional can have an important impact. This chapter provides the tools the physician needs to approach the smoking patient with confidence and suggests a practical, time-efficient approach to the problem.

Cigarette smoking has been strongly established as a major cause of coronary heart disease (CHD) [1, 2, 3], the leading cause of death in the United States; its elimination can produce a substantial reduction in premature morbidity and mortality. Estimates indicate that up to 30 percent, or 170,000, of all CHD deaths in the United States each year are attributable to cigarette smoking, with the risk being strongly dose-related [1, 2, 3]. Smoking acts synergistically with other risk factors, substantially increasing the risk of CHD.

Clinical and epidemiologic studies have also consistently demonstrated that cigarette smokers are at increased risk for cerebrovascular and peripheral vascular disease, as well as cancers of most sites, chronic lung disease, and many other chronic diseases [2, 3, 4, 5]. Cigarette smoking is the single most alterable risk factor contributing to premature morbidity and mortality in the United States, accounting for approximately 390,000 or 18 percent, of all deaths annually [2].

The Benefits of Smoking Cessation

Prospective investigations have demonstrated a substantial decrease in CHD mortality for former smokers compared with continuing smokers. This diminution in risk occurs relatively promptly following cessation of smoking, and increasing intervals since the time one last smoked are associated with progressively lower mortality rates from CHD [1, 6, 7, 8, 9, 10]. However, unlike the relatively prompt decrease in risk for CHD among former smokers, mortality from lung cancer begins to move toward that of nonsmokers only after five years of abstinence and does not approach that of never-smokers until 15 to 20 years after cessation [11].

Investigations also have demonstrated benefits from cessation for smokers who have already developed smoking-related diseases or symptoms. Individuals with diagnosed CHD experience reduced risks of reinfarction, sudden cardiac death, and total mortality if they quit after the initial infarction [3, 12, 13, 14]. In some

studies this reduction in risk approaches or is as much as 50 percent [14, 15].

Benefits from quitting are seen in former smokers even after many years of heavy smoking [3]. A primary conclusion of the 1990 Surgeon General's Report on Smoking and Health: The Health Benefits of Smoking Cessation was that smoking cessation has major and immediate health benefits for men and women of all ages with and without smoking-related diseases [3]. In addition to medical health benefits, some studies have demonstrated that after several months of abstinence former smokers have better psychosocial functioning and are more likely to practice more health-promoting and disease-preventing behaviors than continuing smokers [16, 17] and most nicotine withdrawal symptoms disappear. For some former smokers, however, increased appetite and the continued urge to smoke remain problematic. These problems are addressed later in this chapter.

The Prevalence of Cigarette Smoking Among Adults

The proportion of current male cigarette smokers, defined as persons who have smoked at least 100 cigarettes in their lifetime and are smoking at the time of the interview, declined from 50 percent in 1965 to 43 percent in 1970, to 35 percent in 1983, and to 32 percent in 1987 for all U.S. males over age 18 [1, 2, 3, 18, 19]. For females the overall decline in current smokers is less pronounced, from 34 percent in 1965 to 30 percent in 1970, with a subsequent increase in the late 1970s and then a decrease to 27 percent in 1987. By 1987 nearly half of all living adults who had ever smoked had quit [2]. Over 80 percent of current smokers indicate that they would like to quit. The greatest changes in smoking occurred in the second half of the 1970s, coinciding temporally with an observed decline in CHD mortality. Much of the decline in smoking can be attributed to the strong educational campaign that has taken place in the United States over the last two decades, to the anticigarette advertising campaigns of the mid-1960s, and to increased taxation of cigarettes [2].

Quit rates adjusted for differential mortality and smoking initiation increase progressively with each age cohort [20]. For example, in the late 1960s men in the seventh decade of life quit at a rate of about 7 percent per year, while men in their 50s quit at a rate of about 3 percent per year. The quit rate was between 4.0 percent and 4.5 percent per year for all males during this period. In each decade quit rates were substantially lower for women. Thus, while the overall declines are encouraging, the change has been greater for males than for females, for older rather than younger individuals, and for those with higher levels of educational achievement [21].

Data limitations do not permit one to draw definitive conclusions about the effects of smoking cessation on the declining CHD mortality rate. However, associations in the data do suggest certain conclusions. The documented changes in risk factors prior to and during the period of CHD decline, which occurred between 1968 and 1976 and since, indicate that the decrease in the prevalence of cigarette smoking, which affected the greatest number of people, may have contributed more to the CHD decline than did changes in most other risk factors. The effect of smoking cessation on the declining CHD mortality rate during this period has been estimated in several ways by Goldman and Cook, who obtained a mean estimate of a 5-percent reduction in coronary mortality, which would represent about 24 percent of the overall 21 percent decline, or about 150,000 lives saved, between 1968 and 1976 [22].

Pathophysiologic Framework of Smoking and the Development of CHD

The complex pathogenesis of CHD is mediated by multiple mechanisms [23], which have been discussed in Chapters 1, 3, and 5. Atherosclerosis, thrombosis, reduced blood oxygen-carrying capacity, coronary artery spasm, and cardiac arrhythmias may all contribute to the clinical manifestations of angina, myocardial infarction (MI), and sudden death, and there is substantial evidence that smoking influences many if not all of these steps [3].

Physiologic Effects of Cigarette Smoke

Cigarette smoke has hundreds of potentially toxic components, and the quantitative contributions of many of these remain to be elucidated [1, 3, 24]. Nicotine and carbon monoxide, however, have been implicated in several processes.

Toxic materials in cigarette smoke exist in both the gas and the particulate phases. Carbon monoxide (CO), a gas component, has a strong affinity for hemoglobin, displacing oxygen and causing the smoker to lose as much as 15 percent of his blood oxygen-carrying capacity, depending on such factors as the amount smoked and the depth of inhalation. It is clear that such a loss can exacerbate angina and may also provoke MI, arrhythmias, and sudden death. The decrease in tar and nicotine content in many cigarettes over recent years has not been accompanied by any reduction in the amount of CO produced by cigarettes and inhaled [2]. In fact, as smokers inhale more deeply from lower-tar and -nicotine cigarettes in an attempt to derive the same flavor dose, their CO exposure may increase.

Also present in cigarette smoke are such toxic gases as acrolein, hydrogen cyanide, hydrogen oxide, nitrogen oxide, and ammonia; inhalation of these gases produces coughing and bronchial narrowing. Ciliary action is paralyzed, thickening of the bronchial epithelium occurs, and with time a progressive inflammatory response results, leading to a destructive bronchiolitis. As this process continues, the lungs lose their normal elasticity, airways become hyperreactive, and there is a progressive destruction of alveoli. Finally the patient presents with the fully developed clinical syndrome of chronic obstructive pulmonary disease [3, 4].

Toxic particulates consist of tars and nicotine. In cigarettes manufactured in the United States over the last three decades tar yield has decreased from an average of 37 mg per cigarette to 12 mg; nicotine has decreased from 2.5 mg to 1.1 mg. Among the many toxic organic compounds found in the tar phase are nonvolatile

N-nitrosamines and aromatic amines, both known human carcinogens. Sidestream smoke — the smoke coming off of the burning end of the cigarette — contains higher amounts of the carcinogenic aromatic amines than the smoke inhaled by smokers and has thus been implicated in causing disease in individuals who do not smoke themselves but who are exposed to environmental tobacco smoke produced by smokers [2, 3].

Nicotine produces a number of potent cardiovascular effects. It causes the release of epinephrine and norepinephrine, resulting in increases in blood pressure, heart rate, cardiac output, coronary blood flow, and myocardial oxygen consumption. In individuals with coronary artery narrowings, this can result in myocardial ischemia and cardiac arrythmias [1, 3].

Carbon monoxide and nicotine thus produce a variety of adverse cardiovascular effects, augmented by the contribution of numerous other recognized and unrecognized toxins in cigarette smoke. In addition to the major clinical manifestations of CHD, they also lead to all the other known harmful sequelae of smoking: cough, sputum production, shortness of breath, skin wrinkling, poor dentition and gum disease, and tooth staining.

The harmful constituents of cigarette smoke affect essentially every organ of the body and cause excess morbidity and mortality from all major diseases. The more that the physician or other health care provider is able to relate a patient's symptoms and illnesses to smoking and is confident that the patient understands and is able to use this information, the greater the likelihood that the smoker will be motivated to attempt cessation and successfully accomplish it.

The Importance of Physician-Delivered Smoking Intervention

More than 90 percent of the 30 million smokers who gave up cigarettes between 1964 and 1982 did not use an organized program to help them stop smoking, and most smokers who continue to smoke state that they would prefer to stop without the aid of a formal smoking-cessation program [3, 25]. It is with this large group of smokers that the physician can have a major impact. Seventy-five percent of the adult population has at least one contact per year with a physician, with the average yearly number of contacts being five per adult. Thus, the physician as educator, facilitator, or counselor has the potential to be a powerful agent for smoking cessation [26, 27]. Individuals probably think more seriously about their health and smoking's effect on it when they are in a physician's office or in a hospital than at any other time. This opportunity for health promotion with smokers, ex-smokers, and would-be smokers should not be overlooked.

Evidence from both observational studies [28, 29] and randomized trials [30, 31, 32, 33, 34, 35, 36, 37, 38] indicates that physicians who intervene with their smoking patients have a significant impact on the patients' cigarette smoking behavior. Smokers also report that physicians' interventions can have a powerful effect on their smoking [39]. Recent reviews [26, 40, 41, 42] summarizing the smoking intervention literature suggest that simple advice by one's physician to stop smoking is more effective than no advice at all and that as the physician-delivered smoking intervention becomes more extensive, the effects are greater. These studies have also demonstrated that special training of physicians to deliver brief interventions [30, 37] and general office practice procedures to help cue the physician to intervene with smokers and provide follow-up [30, 31, 43] increase the likelihood that physicians will intervene with smokers and that they will have a favorable impact on patients' smoking behavior. To keep the interventions brief and to meet the special needs of patients, physicians can also refer patients to special programs or have someone in their office provide intervention and follow-up.

Almost any intervention strategy can be effective, given a commitment by both the smoker and the physician and realistic expectations of what can be accomplished. As a supportive authority figure and role model, the physician can promote change in a majority of cigarette smokers at one of the levels listed in Table 8-1. The physician's potential impact can

Table 8-1. The physician's potential impact on smokers

Motivation of the patient to think about possible efforts to stop smoking

Reduction of smoking

Immediate cessation

Support and reinforcement of a cessation program in which the smoker is already involved or to which she is being referred

Support maintenance of cessation

be brought about by direct interventions or by reinforcement and encouragement for the smoker to go to a special program for help.

A physician's effect on a patient's smoking varies greatly with the context for change [44]. The patient who is symptomatic or already ill, e.g., post-MI or with newly diagnosed respiratory disease, is more likely to respond to the physician's advice. The patient may show immediate interest in change when some acute symptoms caused by smoking occur; the smoking pattern of the patient will be least affected when he feels well and has few if any symptoms or abnormal findings [45, 46]. Studies have shown high quit rates (50 to 63 percent) for patients who are advised to quit smoking after suffering an MI [45, 47] or who have been diagnosed as having CHD [39, 46]. These rates are directly related to the severity of disease [39, 45, 46]. Cessation rates fall to 30 to 40 percent when intervention is directed at those smokers at high risk for infarction [48]. This relationship between cessation and disease status is consistent with the principles of the health belief model (discussed in the following section), which hold that the patient who perceives that he is vulnerable to the actual effects of smoking and that the benefits of cessation outweigh the costs will be more motivated to quit.

Barriers to Physician-Delivered Smoking Intervention

Most physicians are generally aware of the health benefits of smoking cessation; however, national surveys of patients and physicians indicate that a large percentage of physicians often do not intervene with their smoking patients

[27]. Physicians report several barriers to their doing smoking intervention, including a belief that they are not effective, poor intervention skills, a belief that patients do not want their physicians to intervene, and little time to fit intervention into their practices, especially when reimbursement for these services is often a problem.

These barriers can all be dealt with adequately. Physicians can quickly acquire the skills needed to work effectively with patients to help them quit smoking. These skills can be used to deliver brief (three to four minutes) interventions that require a minimal input of time and that utilize office staff, the back-up services of consultants and special programs, and supportive aids such as self-help materials. Surveys have demonstrated that even patients who do not make behavioral changes welcome their physicians' input for health behavior change; in fact, they are more satisfied with their physicians [49] who intervene than with those who do not. Regarding reimbursement, there are legitimate billable diagnoses for smokers that can often be used for the physician services provided. Reimbursement policies vary among states and carriers.

The first section of this chapter is an overview of the determinants of smoking behavior and those factors that influence its change. The second section addresses the steps and the skills providers need for intervening with smokers. The last section gives information on how to intervene with special populations of smokers.

Determinants of Smoking Behavior and Change

Cigarette smoking is a complex behavior pattern that, like most behavior patterns, is affected by multiple and interacting factors: physiologic factors, personal characteristics (cognitive factors, information, personality, and demographic factors), environmental influences (social, cultural, and economic environment), and other behaviors (e.g., drinking a beer triggers taking a cigarette). The behavior goes through a sequence of phases from initiation to regular smoking to possible cessation and maintenance of cessation or relapse. During the initiation phase, individuals start experimenting with cigarettes, generally before they are 20. They then move into the transition phase, in which environmental, psychologic, and physiologic factors influence their becoming smokers or nonsmokers. The sequence then proceeds through the phases of regular smoking, possible cessation, and maintenance of cessation. Relapse occurs at very high rates among those individuals who have stopped smoking (often as many as 70 to 80 percent return to smoking within one year) [2]; thus, maintenance of cessation is often a difficult phase.

In each phase different motives, needs, and environmental factors operate to determine whether an individual will move into the next phase [2]. Initiation of smoking is strongly associated with social influences extrinsic to the individual, e.g., peer pressure, as well as with psychologic variables such as self-esteem, status needs, and other personal needs. The sociologic variables that are so important during the formation of the behavior seem to play a minor role in its maintenance once smoking has become part of the lifestyle of the individual. As the behavior continues, it becomes more and more tied to psychologic and physiologic needs and becomes a habit that is an intrinsic part of the person's life, having many functions.

Theories of Behavioral Change

The consumer information processing theory [50], which explains the effects of the availability of information on behavior and the factors that influence its processing, and theories of health behavior, which include social learning theory [51, 52], the health belief model [53, 54], and the stages of change model [55], provide a strong basis for understanding smoking and for facilitating the development of effective treatments. These theories are briefly touched on here and are discussed more fully in Chapter 7.

The *consumer information processing (CIP)* theory [50] states that several minimum conditions are necessary for individuals to make use of information: information must be made available; it must be wanted or believed to be useful by the consumer; it must be able to be processed within the time, energy, and comprehension levels of the consumer; and it must not be too confusing to process [56]. Thus, for information about smoking and health to influence action, the clinician must make it available and present it at the level of the patient's comprehension, and the patient must be ready to hear the information and act on it.

Social learning theory (SLT) (also referred to as social cognitive theory) is an excellent theoretical model for understanding smoking and other lifestyle behaviors and methods to promote behavioral change. SLT holds that most behaviors are learned and can therefore be unlearned or altered; that an individual needs to participate actively in the learning of behavior-change skills [51, 52, 57]; and that behavior is dynamic and is constantly interacting with and being influenced by multiple determinants, no one of which is sufficient to totally influence the behavior by itself [52]. The multiple and reciprocal interacting determinants of smoking include the four aforementioned groups of factors: physiologic factors, personal characteristics, environmental influences, and other behaviors (Table 8-2).

The SLT concepts of self-efficacy and behavioral self-management are of particular importance for physicians and other health care providers who are seeking easily used interventions to help patients develop the skills and attitudes necessary to facilitate smoking cessation. *Self-efficacy,* the degree to which a person is confident of his ability to successfully change a specific behavior (e.g., to stop smoking), has been demonstrated in many studies to have an effect on smoking cessation separate from actual skill or knowledge. Past experiences of success in smoking cessation increase self-efficacy. Self-efficacy is important not only because it affects behavior [58, 59] but also because it is modifiable through behavior modification strategies [60, 61], such as meeting small goals and self-reward. *Behavioral self-management (BSM)* requires that an individual become aware of the triggers that cue a behavior and the consequences that reinforce it. The individual can

Table 8-2. Multiple and interacting determinants that affect smoking

Physiologic factors (nicotine addition)
  Conditioning of smoking to activities, thoughts or
    feelings
Personal characteristics/cognitions
  Demogaphics
  Personality
  Education/information
   Availability
   Believed to be useful
   Wanted by consumer
   Can be processed by consumer
  Cognitions (thoughts, beliefs, fears)
   Belief in personal vulnerability and perceived risks
     of smoking
   Belief in capability of stopping smoking
   Belief that stopping smoking will decrease risk
   Belief that benefits from cessation outweigh costs
  Skills
   Self-management skills
   Stress-reduction skills
  Stage of change (readiness)
Environment
  Social
  Cultural
  Economic
  Political
Other behaviors (examples)
  Drinking alcohol
  Drinking coffee
  Eating

then decide whether to avoid the trigger, alter it, or substitute a CHD-preventive behavior when the trigger occurs.

The health belief model (HBM), another model for understanding health-related behaviors, focuses on cognitive factors [53, 54, 62] that affect a smoker's motivation and the likelihood of his implementing a preventive action such as smoking cessation. In general, the HBM has demonstrated that, to some extent, individuals will take action if they believe they are personally vulnerable or susceptible to a given condition such as CHD; there will be potentially serious consequences if they do not take action; they are capable of taking action; the action they are capable of will decrease their risk; and the potential costs (barriers) of their taking action will be outweighed by the benefits [62]. An indi-

vidual's perceptions of his vulnerability, risk, ability to change, and costs associated with change are in turn affected by his environment, personal resources, habits, and educational level. This multiplicity of determinants again indicates that many factors affect change.

The HBM has implications for interventions that can be used by physicians and other health care providers with patients who need to stop smoking. For example, an individual's personal vulnerability to CHD and the benefits of alltering CHD-promoting behaviors must be communicated in a way acceptable to the patient. Providing personalized information to the patient about the atherosclerotic process and the effects of his smoking on it, prior to the manifestation of signs and symptoms, is a necessary step in facilitating the development of a realistic perception of personal risk. Health care providers need to personalize the damage of smoking, feed back the symptoms reported by the patient who may think she is in a disease-free state, and discuss the costs and benefits of cessation specific to the individual.

The *stages of change model* describes smoking cessation as a process of change over time which takes place in stages, and thus it is not realistic for physicians to expect cessation to occur as the result of one encounter [55]. Smoking cessation often takes five to ten years and three to four attempts before long-term success is achieved [3, 55]. The stages of change model helps to guide intervention and defines four stages of change: precontemplation, when the smoker is neither considering stopping nor actively processing smoking and health information; contemplation, when the smoker is thinking about stopping and is processing information about the effects of smoking and ways to stop; action, when the smoker is no longer smoking and has been without cigarettes for up to six months; and maintenance, which involves the establishment of long-term abstinence, or leads to relapse, the eventual resumption of smoking. When relapse occurs, the smoker recycles to any one of the three previous stages.

Smokers at each stage benefit from different approaches. The precontemplator's tendency to ignore quitting strategies and information may need to be met with an assessment of his perceptions regarding disease risk, vulnerability, and capability for change, continued personalized information on smoking and health, and correction of misperceptions. The contemplator may need support to attempt cessation and help to develop effective cessation strategies. The abstainer may need help that emphasizes the development of relapse-prevention skills.

In summary, whether an individual modifies his smoking depends on several major factors. Provision of usable information is necessary but not sufficient in itself for behavioral change. Belief in personal susceptibility to disease, the benefits of change, smoking as a risk for disease, and personal capability to make the needed change (self-efficacy) strongly affect whether an individual will attempt to stop smoking. The four major groups of factors that affect smoking — physiologic factors, personal factors, environmental influences, and other behaviors — interact to determine whether an individual is ready to consider making a change and able to use the information available to him.

Determinants of Smoking and Cessation

PHYSIOLOGIC FACTORS OF SMOKING: ADDICTION AND CONDITIONING

The three major conclusions of the 1988 surgeon general's Report on Smoking and Health: Nicotine Addiction were: (1) cigarettes and other forms of tobacco are addicting; (2) nicotine is the drug in tobacco that causes addiction; and (3) the pharmacologic and behavioral processes that determine tobacco addiction are similar to those that determine addiction to heroin and other drugs of addiction [63]. Thus, while physiologic dependence is an important aspect of nicotine addiction, it is the interplay between social, behavioral, and physiologic factors that define nicotine addiction, as is the case with dependence on other drugs [63].

After a short period of time, patterns of tobacco use become regular and compulsive, and a withdrawal syndrome often accompanies tobacco abstinence. The nicotine withdrawal syndrome is a psychiatric diagnosis described in the Diagnostic and Statistical Manual of Mental Disorders (DSM III R) of the American Psychiatric Association [64]. (Table 8-3 lists the diagnostic criteria.) After a few months of abstinence all of the withdrawal symptoms, except in some cases craving for nicotine and increased appetite, disappear.

Conditioning mediates the role of the physiologic effects of nicotine in cessation. Numerous environmental stimuli, activities, thoughts, feelings, and behaviors are likely to be conditioned to or attached to the use of nicotine and evoke urges or cues to smoke. This conditioning ties smoking to the rituals of daily life and contributes to the difficulty of breaking this addiction [63]. Recent work by Abrams and colleagues demonstrates that former smokers manifest psychophysiologic reactivity to smoking cues long after they have quit [65, 66]. Conditioned responses to environmental cues, then, may have more influence in the later stage of maintenance of cessation, after withdrawal symptoms have subsided.

Many individuals who are dependent on nicotine, as with alcohol or other drugs, are able to give it up without special treatment programs, while others may require outside help. For the individual who is physiologically ad-

Table 8-3. Diagnostic criteria for nicotine withdrawal syndrome

Daily use of nicotine for at least several weeks

Abrupt cessation of nicotine use or reduction in the amount of nicotine used followed by at least four of the following signs:

- Craving for nicotine
- Irritability, frustration, or anger
- Anxiety
- Difficulty concentrating
- Restlessness
- Decreased heart rate
- Increased appetite or weight gain

Source: Condensed from American Psychiatric Association DSM III R (1987) [64].

dicted to nicotine, treatments may require behavioral interventions with adjunctive pharmacologic treatment such as nicotine replacement therapy or other medication.

Even when involved in intervention programs, the heavier, more dependent smokers are less likely to quit than are lighter, less dependent smokers [67, 68, 69] and are more likely to experience withdrawal symptoms and to relapse once they do quit. As noted in the 1988 Surgeon General's Report on Nicotine Addiction, "Withdrawal symptoms, whether elicited by acute deprivation or by conditioned stimuli, are hypothesized to be the link between dependence and relapse" [63]. Further evidence of the influence of addiction comes from intervention studies that evaluated nicotine-containing gum (NCG). Several studies have found that NCG is effective primarily because it reduces withdrawal symptoms frequently noticed in the first days and weeks of abstinence [70, 71].

PERSONAL CHARACTERISTICS
Prospective studies indicate that educational level, income, self-efficacy (belief in one's own ability to change), social support, stress, and skills in self-management or personal coping of stress are significantly related to smoking and to success in self-initiated efforts to stop smoking [2, 4, 72, 73, 74], as well as to success in specialized intervention programs [74]. These findings have strong implications regarding the intervention strategies that physicians can use to assist patients with smoking cessation. Assistance needs to include helping the patient to focus on constructive ways to handle stress without the use of cigarettes, alcohol, or increased food intake. (These strategies are discussed in Chapter 11.)

Stress appears to be a factor that especially influences smoking cessation in women [75, 76], as well as their initiation of smoking [77]. High levels of anxiety [78] and self-reported tendencies to smoke to relieve depression, anger, or anxiety [79] also have been associated with reduced success in stopping. The link of smoking to stress and the role of social support in buffering stress [80] suggest that women may benefit from interpersonal support in their cessation efforts more than men [81].

Women's concerns about weight gain associated with smoking cessation have received much recent attention [3]. Women often indicate that weight concerns or actual gains in weight are related to their return to smoking. In actuality the average weight gain after smoking cessation is about 5 pounds (2.3 kg) [3]. While this weight gain poses a minimal health risk, it is important not to discount its importance to the smoker. The physician must acknowledge the concern over weight gain and help the smoker use strategies to prevent or decrease the likelihood of its occurrence. Strategies for preventing or decreasing weight gain will be discussed later in this chapter.

ENVIRONMENTAL INFLUENCES
Social, political, cultural, and economic influences are related to whether an individual becomes a smoker and whether or not he is likely to stop smoking. Individuals who experience more social support for cessation and have fewer smokers in their environment are more successful at cessation attempts [68]. Similarly individuals who work in an environment with smokers are more likely themselves to be smokers [82]. Different cultural groups also provide different degrees of support for smoking. For example, in the recent past smoking rates among Hispanic and black females have been relatively low, much lower than among white females [2, 83]. This rate has recently begun to increase, however, while smoking rates in general have gone down in most other groups. Physicians and other providers need to become familiar with the cultural norms of the people they most often treat.

Since the social environment has a significant effect on smoking, the changing of norms by using policies and programs in large social networks such as the workplace is attracting considerable attention. Worksites differ widely with regard to the prevalence of smoking and rates of cessation as well as norms for supporting cessation attempts [82]. Programs aimed at changing worksite norms and providing general support for nonsmoking have reported substantial quit rates, even among smokers who did not participate in cessation clinics offered at the worksite. (The use of the worksite as an effective channel for health behavior change is discussed in Chapter 19.)

The Practice of Clinical Preventive Cardiology: Physician-Delivered Smoking Intervention

Intervention for smoking involves the sequence of activities — diagnosis/assessment, treatment/intervention, plan for change, and monitoring/follow-up — described in Chapter 7. (See Table 7-4.) This sequence of activities is the same no matter which disease-related behavior is intervened with — smoking, diet, stress, or lack of exercise [85].

Not all smokers will respond and not all physicians will be interested in intervening to the same extent. Physicians and other providers must decide on their level of willingness to intervene and then set themselves up to succeed. Physicians must also set up a work environment that facilitates intervention. (Chapter 17 discusses how to set up an office for the practice of clinical preventive cardiology.)

Diagnosis/assessment involves evaluation of the patient's smoking, medical, and family history and relevant psychosocial, behavioral, and demographic variables. *Treatment/intervention* involves, at a minimum, the provision of brief personalized advice by the physician of the need for the patient to stop smoking. When appropriate and within the time constraints of the physician, treatment/intervention also involves an interactive counseling process in which the eventual outcome is the collaborative development of a *plan for change*. The physician can also have someone in the office or an outside program or consultant provide more comprehensive assistance. If the patient is referred, the physician's role is still critical and requires coordination, with the help of an effective office system, and a level of energy and commitment that tells the patient that smoking cessation is important for his health. *Monitoring/follow-up* involves continued assessment to determine whether negotiated goals have been met, whether the patient used the strategies agreed on, and whether the strategies were adequate to reach the goals. Further discussion and development of the treatment plan may also take place, with the likely need for continued follow-up. Follow-up can be by telephone and can be accomplished by someone other than the physician. An adequate office system and communication links will ensure efficiency and coordination of patient management.

The physician or someone else in the intervention loop can carry out each phase in the smoking-intervention process. It is unlikely that the physician will want or be able to be intensively involved in the treatment of each patient.

There are four basic models for physician involvement, which can be used in various combinations: (1) brief physician advice, (2) brief physician counseling, (3) brief counseling with referral for comprehensive individual counseling, and (4) brief counseling with referral for group education (either one session or multiple sessions) [84]. The following overview of what the physician can do in the smoking-cessation process must be adapted to the individual physician's own needs and situation.

Step 1: Diagnosis/Assessment

The first step is assessment of the patient's smoking and health, his perception of the problem(s), and his knowledge regarding the relationship of smoking to CHD (see Table 7-4). Information for this assessment comes from the medical interview, questionnaires (Appendix A is an example of a brief questionnaire), the physical examination, and possible diagnostic tests. The latter can include the use of a CO meter to demonstrate to the smoker the presence of elevated CO levels. A CO meter is relatively inexpensive to purchase (about $800), and the valuable feedback and information about the effects of CO on CHD can help to increase motivation for change if used in a nonconfrontational, information-sharing manner.

It is likely that some smokers have other lifestyle behaviors that put them at additional risk for CHD. These behaviors will be uncovered as part of an overall risk factor assessment. The patient and the physician need to decide together on priorities for change and on the best strategies. It is during the initial assessment that education of the patient begins as the physician and the patient engage in an interactive process.

Step 2: Treatment/Intervention

It is important that the physician take an active role in the treatment/intervention of smoking. The role can be minimal (two to three minutes) or comprehensive, depending on the patient's and the physician's resources and needs. The physician will need to decide how much time she is willing to devote and whether a referral to a behavioral or smoking specialist is appropriate. At the very least, emphasis on the patient's risk and the importance of smoking cessation is required. A referral requires that the physician take at least a few minutes to ensure that the patient understands the reason for the referral and what he needs to do in following up with the specialist.

No matter who eventually works with the patient, the physician needs to deliver several consistent brief messages that have a strong scientific basis:

- Quitting smoking is a *process,* not a one-time event. It moves from becoming aware of the need to stop smoking, to taking action, to maintaining cessation.
- Quitting smoking often takes several attempts before long-term cessation occurs.
- A return to smoking is not a failure. It can be used as a learning experience to help you prepare for the next time.
- Many methods can help you to stop smoking. The best method is the one you choose for yourself, based on your own experiences.

The major intervention strategy used in treatment to help patients stop smoking is education, which is more than just the delivery of information or the transfer of facts. (See Chapter 7 for a definition and discussion of patient education.) The multiple and interacting determinants of behavior discussed in the previous section and the patient's skills mediate the re-

lationship between what the patient knows and the action he takes. A wide variety of strategies in patient education can help the patient make the connection between knowledge and action. These strategies include provision of the needed information, patient-centered counseling, discussion, and behavior modification strategies. When working with a smoker, the physician also needs to know how to use pharmacologic interventions, such as the prescription of nicotine-containing gum or nicotine patches for the physiologically addicted smoker.

As discussed in Chapter 7, patient-intervention strategies are easily learned and can be integrated into the framework of the typical office encounter.

PROVIDING INFORMATION

Using the information gathered during assessment, the physician must advise the patient of the need to stop smoking. It is most effective to make the advice relevant to the patient, his situation, his concerns, beliefs, and perceptions, so that the patient can hear and make use of that advice.

The physician can provide information either verbally or through written self-help materials, or she can refer the patient to other health professionals for additional information. A variety of smoking-cessation informational and self-help materials are available free of charge or for a nominal cost for distribution to patients. Table 8-4 lists some self-help smoking materials and their sponsoring organizations.

PATIENT-CENTERED COUNSELING

Brief patient-centered behavioral counseling can be used by the physician who wants to and is able to go beyond the two to three minutes of personalized advice given to the patient. As noted earlier, patient-centered counseling helps patients to develop plans for change and strategies to alter behaviors and has been demonstrated to be significantly more efficacious in helping patients to alter smoking than advice alone [30]. It emphasizes the importance of the patient's input in developing an effective plan for change and can be accomplished using an additional three to five minutes of the physi-

Table 8-4. Self-help guides for smoking cessation
(Materials are free unless otherwise indicated. Prices shown may be subject to change.)

Area/title	Contact	Area/title	Contact
General Information			
Fifty Most Often Asked Questions about Smoking and Health	ACS	Nicotine Addiction to Cigarettes	ALA
The Decision Is Yours	ACS	Smokeless Tobacco	ALA
ALA Fact Series: Cigarette Smoking Second Hand Smoke	ALA	Is There a Safe Tobacco?	ALA
Specialized Information			
Why Start Life under a Cloud?	ACS	ALA Facts Series: Emphysema Chronic Bronchitis	AHA
Cigarette Smoking and Cardiovascular Disease ($4.25/50)	AHA		
Facts on Lung Cancer	ACS	Children and Smoking, A Message to Parents ($2.19/50)	AHA
Self-Help Materials			
Clear the Air (English and Spanish)	NCI	Freedom From Smoking Self-Help Kit ($7.00/kit) 1) Freedom from Smoking in 20 Days	ALA
Quit for Good Kit	NCI	2) A Lifetime of Freedom from Smoking	
Why Do You Smoke?	NCI	Quitting with the Help of Nicorette	Marion Merrell Dow, Inc.
Smart Move	ACS		
Calling It Quits ($16.20/25)	AHA	Weight Control Guidance In Smoking Cessation ($4.08/100)	AHA

Selected Summaries

Quit for Good Kit/Clearing the Air. The kit contains enough materials for 50 patients. Included are smoker identification chart stickers, posters, desk display cards, and 50 copies of Clearing the Air. Contains many suggestions for behavioral self-management during both the quitting process and maintenance.

Why Do You Smoke? A three-stage self-scoring pamphlet that helps patients identify patterns of smoking and then provides specific suggestions for coping strategies tailored to each person's need. Short enough to complete in the waiting room.

Freedom from Smoking. A more extensive self-help kit, in two clearly written and illustrated booklets, that provides a structured plan for stopping and maintaining abstinence. The maintenance manual (A Lifetime of Freedom from Smoking) provides particularly good information on remaining abstinent.

Quitting with the Help of Nicorette. Provided by Marion Merrell Dow, Inc., to accompany prescription of Nicorette gum, with guidelines for effective use. It emphasizes the importance of behavioral self-management.

ACS = American Cancer Society; ALA = American Lung Association; AHA = American Heart Association; NCI = National Cancer Institute. Contact the state or regional office for your area.
Source: PDSIP (Physician-Delivered Smoking Intervention Program) Training Manual [30].

cian's time. Of course more time can be spent if desired and available. (For a full discussion of patient-centered counseling, see Chapter 7.) (Table 8-5 is a summary of topics that should be covered in patient-centered counseling.)

While the process of patient-centered counseling is collaborative, the physician (provider) must still set the tone for the encounter — a mutual exchange of information where both the physician's and the patient's participation are optimal [86]. The physician remains ultimately in control of the process by utilizing a sequence of steps designed to help the patient make the needed changes.

TOPICS IN PATIENT-CENTERED COUNSELING

The sequence of topics presented here is interchangeable and should be adapted to the physician's needs and style and the needs of the patient. The patient's desire and motivation to stop smoking are often the first topic to be addressed. The patient's reasons for wanting to stop may be different from the physician's reasons for wanting her to do so. A patient may be more concerned about the impact of her smoking on her children than on her risk for disease. For some patients lack of motivation may be related to a lack of confidence in their ability to stop smoking. The second step, exploration of past experiences with cessation, helps patients focus on possible past successes, no matter how small, and encourages them to believe that they are capable of cessation.

Eighty percent of all smokers have stopped sometime in the past [2]. The physician can help patients focus on the resources they used and the positive feelings they had about themselves when they were nonsmokers.

Past experiences with cessation also reveal problems to be prepared for and resources that were used in the past and can be used in the present to handle problems. The third and fourth topics, problems experienced and resources utilized, help to identify possible problems and resources for the current cessation effort. A patient who has difficulty articulating can be asked open-ended questions about substitute behaviors: "What do you do to help you avoid smoking?" If the individual cannot think of anything, a more focused question such as, "Have you ever used exercise to help you avoid smoking?" or "Have you ever used deep breathing as a relaxation approach?" is useful.

During this step of assessing possible problems it is also important to determine whether the smoker is physiologically addicted to nicotine. The physician assessing the patient's past experiences with cessation needs to determine whether the patient had experienced symptoms of nicotine withdrawal (see Table 8-3). The more intense the withdrawal symptoms were in previous quit attempts, the more likely they will be a problem again. Assessment of withdrawal and the use of a specially developed scale for measuring addiction, the Fagerstrom Addiction Scale [87] (Appendix B) can help the physician to decide whether to suggest the use of pharmacologic therapy, in addition to educational and behavioral interventions, which include tapering of cigarette usage. Another sensitive indicator of possible difficulty in quitting is the length of previous attempts. On the average, withdrawal symptoms peak at three to four days, so a pattern of multiple attempts to quit with return to smoking after only a few days suggests that nicotine dependency is highly related to relapse for that individual.

The physician should also alert the smoker to the various symptoms associated with withdrawal, and should point out that these symptoms decrease quickly, and that a variety of approaches, such as tapering nicotine intake before stopping "cold turkey" or use of a nicotine replacement such as nicotine-containing gum or nicotine patches can be used to handle them. With nicotine replacement the smoker is able to attend to the psychologic and behavioral factors of cessation while the drug is gradually discontinued [88]. Table 8-6 lists nicotine withdrawal symptoms and suggestions for dealing with them.

The counseling sequence leads to a plan for change. The plan may focus on immediate goals: not staying at the table after completing dinner; changing cigarette brands; or learning a relaxation technique. It can also focus on goals closer to the end point: using nicotine-contain-

Table 8-5. Physician-delivered smoking intervention counseling and sample questions

Step	*Sample questions*

1. Advise change.
   Personalize risks of CHD and benefits of
   stopping smoking.	

2. Assess motivation.	How do you feel about your smoking?
	How do you feel about changing this?
	What reasons or motivations would you have for
	   stopping smoking?
	Are you thinking about stopping smoking in the
	   next six months?

3. Assess past experiences with smoking behavior
   change.
	Did you ever stop smoking before?
	   If yes: When and why did you stop? How did
	   you stop? What problems did you have? What
	   helped?
	   If no: Have you made any other positive changes
	   in your lifestyle (diet, exercise)? How? Any
	   problems? What helped you?

4. Discuss problems/barriers.	In what situations do you most want to smoke? What possible problems are you concerned about if you stop?

Assess nicotine dependency.
    (If high dependency, discuss tapering or
    possible use of nicotine-replacement therapy.)
	Use Fagerstrom Addiction Scale.
	Determine length of past periods of abstinence.

5. Discuss resources.	What might you do to help deal with possible
	   problems?
	What might you do instead of smoking in
	   situations when you usually smoke?

6. Develop plan for change.	Now that we have discussed your smoking what
	   plans would you like to make now to stop
	   smoking?

If patient decides to stop smoking:
    Negotiate behavioral goals.
    Set timeline.
    Review strategies for stopping.
    Provide self-help materials (discuss these at
      next regularly scheduled visit).
    Refer patient to outside resource if indicated.
    If patient decides not to stop or is unsure:
    Discuss other related goals (e.g., relaxation
      approaches, exercise program) instead of
      end-point goal of smoking cessation.
    Provide self-help materials (discuss these at
      next regularly scheduled visit).	

7. Schedule follow-up contact.
   Monitor progress to determine if goals have
      been met.
   Determine future goals and revise plan.
	What part of your plan was helpful?
	What part did you have problems with?

Table 8-6. Symptoms of nicotine withdrawal and methods for dealing with them

Stopping smoking produces a variety of symptoms associated with physical and psychological withdrawal. Most symptoms decrease sharply during the first few days of cessation followed by a continued, but slower rate of decline in the second and third weeks of abstinence. Most symptoms disappear within two to four weeks after stopping.

Symptom	Cause	Average duration	Relief
Irritability	Craving for nicotine	2–4 weeks	Walks, hot baths, relaxation techniques, nicotine replacement.
Fatigue	Nicotine is a stimulant.	2–4 weeks	Naps, do not push yourself; nicotine replacement.
Insomnia	Nicotine affects brain wave function, influences sleep patterns. Coughing and dreams about smoking are common.	1 week	Avoiding caffeine after 6 p.m., relaxation techniques.
Cough, dry throat, nasal drip	Respiratory tract beginning to function normally again.	A few days	Drinking plenty of fluids, cough drops.
Dizziness	Normal oxygenation of brain restored.	1–2 days	Changing positions slowly.
Lack of concentration	Brain needs time to adjust to not having constant stimulation from nicotine.	A few weeks	Planning workload accordingly; avoiding additional stress during first few weeks.
Tightness in the chest	Probably due to tension created by withdrawal of nicotine; may be caused by sore muscles from coughing.	A few days	Relaxation techniques, especially deep breathing. Nicotine replacement may help.
Constipation, gas, stomach pain	Intestinal movement decreases for a brief period.	1–2 weeks	Drinking plenty of fluids, adding fiber to diet, (e.g., fruits, vegetables, whole grain cereals).
Hunger	Craving for a cigarette can be confused with hunger pangs. Oral craving/desire for something in the mouth is common.	Up to several weeks.	Drinking water or low-calorie liquids, having low-calorie snacks available.
Craving for a cigarette	Withdrawal from nicotine, a strongly addictive drug.	Most frequent first 2 or 3 days; can happen occasionally for months or years	Waiting out the urge, which lasts only a few minutes. Distractions: exercise, walk around the block

Source: Adapted from materials from NCI and KM Cummings et al, Addictive Behaviors. 10:373–81, 1985.

ing gum or patches in place of cigarettes or not smoking and using relaxation exercises and physical exercise in its place. A written plan often indicates commitment from both the physician and patient. Finally, end with an arrangement for follow-up.

BEHAVIOR MODIFICATION STRATEGIES

As part of treatment for smoking the patient may need assistance in developing new skills. Several behavioral modification strategies can be used to help the patient develop these skills. (See Chapter 7 for an in-depth discussion of these strategies.)

These strategies, based on SLT concepts, help the patient develop the skills and new behaviors needed for behavioral change [50, 51]. Five key strategies used by smoking intervention specialists can also be used by the physician as treatment options with the patient who needs to stop smoking.

Behavioral Self-Monitoring. The smoker uses a special log (behavioral record) to record the times he takes a cigarette, the cues (antecedents) that trigger the urge to smoke, and the rewards (consequences) that follow smoking (Figure 7-2). The smoker can choose to control the stimuli that often trigger smoking, substitute a CHD-preventive behavior when the trigger occurs (e.g., do slow, deep breathing instead of smoking), and/or develop incentives for substituting CHD-preventive behaviors.

Stimulus Control. Based on the information from the logs, situations or thoughts that trigger smoking can be identified, and the smoker can decide how to avoid those triggers, in order to change the behavior. An individual who smokes whenever he sits at the kitchen table after a meal may decide to get up immediately after the meal and take a walk. A smoker who smokes whenever she drinks coffee at the kitchen table may decide to not drink coffee for a while or to drink it in a different place in order to break its conditioned attachment to smoking.

Incentives. Rewards or incentives can be developed for meeting predefined behavioral

goals. Self-reward strategies, when used to reinforce the performance of a specific behavior, can facilitate maintenance of change better than self-punishment strategies [89]. Rewards must be decided on by the patient and used often and repeatedly to reinforce and shape the desired behavior.

Substituting CHD-Preventive Behaviors. Most individuals say that their primary reason for smoking is to reduce stress and boredom and increase relaxation. Relapse is often caused by boredom or difficulty in handling stress. For women, fear of weight gain also prompts relapse. Simple meditation exercises and physical exercise are relaxation techniques that can be substituted for smoking. Like cigarettes they provide brief breaks, can be used in many circumstances, and seem to be physiologically effective. Exercise, especially walking, is often easy to integrate into a regular day. Many individuals have had experiences using stress reduction techniques in the past but have not identified them as an aid for smoking cessation. Chapters 10 and 11 describe how the physician can assist the patient in developing exercise regimens and stress reduction skills.

Contracts. Putting the goals and strategies into a written behavioral plan for smoking cessation or reduction can help the smoker to keep them in mind and emphasizes the seriousness of smoking cessation. Included in the plan should be the strategies to be used, the timetable proposed, the reason for stopping smoking, and a plan for follow-up. Figure 7-1 is a sample form of a plan for behavioral change which can be used for smoking.

Interventions for Reducing Nicotine Withdrawal Symptoms. The more physiologically addicted smoker, in addition to using the above strategies to develop new skills, may need help to deal with difficult withdrawal symptoms. Several strategies are available for reducing nicotine withdrawal symptoms.

Over-the-counter (OTC) drugs purported to aid in smoking cessation have been available for some time, but they generally have been found to be no more effective than placebos. The major pharmacologic treatment approach involves nicotine-replacement therapy. The general principle of this approach for nicotine or any other drug dependence is to provide the user with a safer and more manageable form of the drug that can decrease withdrawal symptoms such as anxiety, difficulty concentrating, and irritability while the drug of addiction is gradually discontinued [90]. A variety of nontobacco-based delivery systems provide potentially effective means for nicotine replacement and can be used for direct treatment application.

Nicotine-containing gum (NCG) (nicotine polacrilex) is the most researched nontobacco delivery system to date. The only form of nicotine gum presently available is Nicorette, manufactured by Marion Merrell Dow, Inc. In 1984 the Food and Drug Administration (FDA) approved the use of a 2 mg dosage of nicotine gum as a prescription for tobacco dependency to be used in combination with behavioral treatment. Nicorette, when used in combination with behavioral intervention, has been shown to be effective in aiding cessation [91]. It seems to be most effective in increasing short-term abstinence, less so for long-term abstinence [67, 92, 93]. Several trials have demonstrated the effectiveness of Nicorette when it is used with behaviorally oriented brief counseling delivered by a physician trained in counseling intervention [30, 37]. Most patients using this gum are able to withdraw from it easily within six months, partly because the delivery of nicotine is slow and gradual, rather than the sharp spike of nicotine obtained from cigarettes, which may account for much of their psychoactive appeal. After 20 to 30 minutes of proper chewing, the release of 90 percent of the nicotine occurs [94], although the gum does not generally lend itself to full replacement of the nicotine provided by smoking. The urge to smoke, as opposed to other withdrawal side effects, is not reliably decreased by the use of nicotine gum [95].

Some patients reject the NCG because of its purposefully unappealing flavor, their dislike for chewing, the lack of a nicotine high, or their concern for replacing one drug of addiction with another. The often inadequate instructions given by providers in the use of NCG also limit the efficacy of this approach. It is important to inform patients of the need to stop smoking cigarettes completely before using the gum, to plan strategies to deal with the social and psychological aspects of smoking, and to provide the necessary instructions for its correct use. (Proper instructions can be found in the package insert; they are also listed in Table 8-7.) Physicians should keep in mind that patients are more likely to use too little gum for too short a time than to overuse it. There are certain contraindications for using Nicorette: recent MI, increasing angina, severe arrhythmia, pregnancy, lactation, and temporomandibular joint disease. Except for the last, these are also contraindications for the use of nicotine. Although the gum may be safer in the noted cases than continued use of cigarettes, such individuals should explore other means to stop smoking.

A *transdermal nicotine patch,* which provides continuous systemic delivery of nicotine over 24 hours and can be worn unobtrusively under clothing on the upper trunk or arms, is also available. It has been demonstrated to be an efficacious nicotine delivery system when used in the context of behavioral intervention [88, 96, 96a and 96b]. This form of nicotine replacement, compared with the use of NCG, could improve compliance with the use of the drug, provide a more steady-state concentration of

Table 8-7. Instructions to patients on the use of nicotine-containing gum

Use only after complete cessation of cigarettes.

Follow instructions included in package.

Do not chew gum continuously. Chew *slowly* and periodically place between gum and teeth. This is how nicotine is absorbed. After 30 minutes all of the nicotine will be absorbed.

Do not drink most beverages (coffee, tea, juices, sodas) while using the gum. The acid does not allow absorption of the nicotine through the mouth.

Use as many pieces as needed each day, up to 30 pieces. Most people underuse the gum.

Side effects of the gum are often caused by using it incorrectly or chewing too fast.

Report any problems to your physician.

nicotine, provide early-morning nicotine levels, which may suppress the desire to smoke upon awakening, and alleviate any chewing problems. It may also be seen as more socially acceptable. A patch, however, does not allow for as-needed use in response to urges to smoke, does not have the same behavioral benefits as the gum, and in a small percentage of patients has been reported to have been associated with moderate to intense erythema at the site of application [96]. One study demonstrated that the patch produces significant cessation effects up through six months of follow-up [96b], although no long-term data are available at this time. Two pharmaceutical companies have patches that became available in January 1992. Two other companies may also have patches available later in 1992.

Nicotine patches are available in three sizes (21mg, 14mg, 7mg) which deliver different dose levels of nicotine over a 24 hour period. The 21 mg/day patch has been demonstrated to be most effective for decreasing withdrawal symptoms. Most smokers can start with the 21 mg/day patch. However, physicians may want to start with the lower doses for smaller patients, lighter smokers (< 10 cigs/day) or smokers with cardiovascular disease. After four to eight weeks on the 21 mg/day dose the smoker can be down-titrated to a lower dose and remain on each of the lower doses for two to four weeks. Down-titration is important, making it easier to eventually stop the use of the patch. The dosing schedule can best be determined after an initial one or two weeks of treatment. As with any intervention it is important for follow-up and monitoring to take place. Follow-up which occurs within the first two weeks after a smoker initiates use of the patch is optimal. This schedule allows the physician and smoker to discuss any possible problems that may occur. The contraindications for use of the patch are similar to those for using nicotine-containing gum except for jaw problems. In addition, patients with sensitivity to the components of the patch system should not use it.

To date there have been no studies to determine which patients would benefit more from the use of NCG or the patch. Individual choice is the most important factor, along with knowledge of whether a smoker has a temporomandibular joint problem or sensitive skin. It is possible that individuals who desire to have more control over their smoking habit and have a greater need for oral gratification may prefer the gum, while smokers who do not want to give much thought to their smoking may prefer the patch. In the use of both nicotine replacement therapies it is important for the physician to help the smoker develop strategies to handle social and psychological aspects of smoking and to provide adequate follow-up.

A *nasal nicotine solution (NNS)*, which is applied as a nasal spray [97], is another delivery system for nicotine replacement. This replacement therapy has only undergone preliminary evaluation in an exploratory trial. Results indicated that NNS decreased some withdrawal symptoms and could potentially be helpful in achieving cessation of smoking. However, irritation of the nose and eyes was commonly reported, and the form of administration is obtrusive in social settings. Other products undergoing investigation include nicotine vapor inhalers that mimic the nicotine high of a cigarette, and nicotine lozenges. Further studies are clearly needed before NNS, nicotine vapor inhalers or lozenges can be considered for nicotine-replacement therapy.

In addition to nicotine replacement therapies, several pharmacologic approaches developed for other forms of drug dependence have been applied to nicotine dependence. Clonidine hydrochloride, an antihypertensive medication, has alpha-2-adrenergic effects and appears to alter nicotine withdrawal symptoms through its effects on the locus coeruleus [98]. Glassman and colleagues [98] compared clonidine to placebo and found cessation rates significantly greater in the clonidine condition at four weeks and six months. However, this finding was seen only in women; no effect was observed for men. A recent study found no benefit for clonidine when compared to a placebo and used in a general medical setting [99]. Before any definitive judgment can be made regarding clonidine, more investigations are necessary. It is also important to consider such possible side effects of this antihypertensive medication as sedation and possible severe rebound hypertension with abrupt cessation of the drug [63].

Tapering the number of cigarettes smoked is another method that can be used by patients who do not want to use or who are not good candidates for pharmacologic interventions, to reduce their nicotine levels and nicotine-withdrawal symptoms before they stop smoking entirely. Tapering, when used as part of a plan to stop smoking, should follow certain guidelines (Table 8-8).

Step 3: Plan for Change

The patient-centered counseling sequence ends in a plan for change, a collaborative decision or negotiation between patient and physician. If smoking cessation is to be attained, the patient's voluntary cooperation and assumption of responsibility are necessary, and the patient must take a more active role in decision making and planning for change than usually occurs in a physician-patient interaction, with the physician acting as educator and counselor [100, 101].

REFERRING PATIENTS FOR ASSISTANCE

Specialized attention or more advanced, time-consuming efforts may be needed to help a patient stop smoking or to deal with other life problems such as unemployment, marital difficulties, drug abuse, or chronic depression and anxiety. Patients who have difficulty learning new information or skills may also require the services of a specialist. Some problems may be identified during the initial session, while others may take more than one visit to be recognized.

When making a referral the physician needs to clearly indicate his continued interest to the patient, the reason for the referral, where the patient is being referred to, and his plan for ongoing involvement in the patient's care.

Local offices of the AHA, the ACS, and the ALA often sponsor group programs for smoking cessation/modification. Local hospitals, medical clinics, health departments, and community health centers may also have programs for smoking cessation. A referral list of smoking programs or specialists in the area should be provided to the patient upon request (Table 8-9). This listing can be developed by someone in the physician's office and should include only those programs consistent with the physician's message.

Step 4: Follow-up/Monitoring

Follow-up optimally should occur in person within a few weeks of the initial visit. If this is not possible, follow-up by telephone by the physician or someone in the office is acceptable. It is critical that follow-up occur at least within a few months of the initial visit; otherwise, the whole intervention process is likely to need to begin anew. Immediately following the initial visit it is useful to send a letter reiterating the goals for smoking-behavior change and the plan developed to achieve them. This serves as a reminder to the patient of the importance the physician attaches to smoking cessation. During follow-up the physician and the patient can determine whether the patient was able to meet the negotiated goals, and new or revised goals and plans can be negotiated. Considerable follow-up likely will be needed for the patient with multiple risk factors.

Many patients and physicians are understandably concerned about the possible costs to the patient of follow-up visits for smoking cessation. In many cases smokers have billable diagnoses of smoking-related diseases (e.g.,

Table 8-8. Suggestions for designing a nicotine-tapering program

Tapering schedule should not be drawn out too long. A period of 3–5 weeks is optimal — long enough not to produce withdrawal symptoms and short enough to maintain motivation.

Tapering should not go below 6–10 cigarettes per day. Too few cigarettes makes them more pleasurable and reinforcing.

Begin by cutting out low-need cigarettes. Need can be assessed on the behavioral record (see Figure 7-2).

Tapering or brand switching is only an intermediate goal; cessation is the eventual goal.

Source: Physician-Delivered Smoking Intervention Program Training Manual [30].

Table 8-9. Local resources for smoking cessation programs

Most communities have programs to help smokers stop smoking. Contact the local affiliates of the American Cancer Society (ACS), the American Lung Association (ALA), and the American Heart Association (AHA) to develop a list of current area programs. Local hospitals, health departments, and community health centers may also sponsor programs for smoking cessation.

A list of programs or contact numbers in the area can be given to patients who request outside referrals. Update this list annually.

Organization	Address	Phone number
ALA	————————	————————
ACS	————————	————————
AHA	————————	————————
Local heart association	————————	————————
Local health department	————————	————————
Hospitals	————————	————————
————————	————————	————————
————————	————————	————————
Private programs or practitioners	————————	————————
————————	————————	————————
————————	————————	————————
Community health centers	————————	————————
————————	————————	————————
————————	————————	————————

Source: Physician-Delivered Smoking Intervention Program Training Manual [30].

bronchitis, small airways disease, CHD) that allow reimbursement by third-party payers. If the visit is not covered, it may be useful to point out to the smoker that the visit is cheaper than most smoking treatment programs or than continued smoking.

Relapse often occurs in smoking, as with other addictive agents, with 70 percent of all smokers who stop returning to smoking within six months [3]. Brief one-session preventive interventions will not produce long-term outcomes for most patients. Continued follow-up and reinforcement of some kind is as important for smoking cessation as it is for more traditionally treated medical problems such as hypertension. The behavioral and counseling strategies used in the intervention phase can also be used to assist patients to maintain cessation and to prevent relapse. In addition, Marlatt and Gordon [102] have developed a relapse prevention strategy as a specific treatment component, and have identified the five key elements sum-

marized below. (For full discussion of these approaches, see Chapter 7.)

IDENTIFYING TRIGGERS AND HIGH-RISK SITUATIONS
Patients can be helped to predict specific situations that might cause difficulty.

COPING REHEARSAL
An important goal, once the individual has identified high-risk situations, is to develop and mentally rehearse specific strategies that can prevent a slip that might lead to a full-blown relapse.

IDENTIFYING AND COMBATING RESUMPTIVE THINKING
Identification ahead of time of habitual rationalizations to justify the resumption of smoking can increase awareness and help guard against relapse by returning a sense of control to the patient.

AVOIDING THE ABSTINENCE VIOLATION EFFECT

The abstinence violation effect (AVE) is a common emotional response to the occurrence of a slip or a lapse to old behavior in the face of personal commitment to change. Helping patients to anticipate this predictable response and to accept that a slip is not the same as a relapse should decrease the problem.

ENCOURAGING SUPPORT

Other relapse prevention strategies include encouraging the patient to enlist the support of family, friends, and coworkers.

The physician and the patient must not become discouraged or angry if relapse occurs. The majority of successful long-term maintainers of smoking cessation have a history of having stopped several times in the past [3]. Each attempt can be reinforced and viewed as a small gain on the way to final success.

With a minimal amount of practice, physicians can quickly learn the skills needed for smoking intervention. (Chapter 22 discusses programs available for the learning of such skills and how to implement such programs.) We and other investigators have demonstrated that the development of such skills requires only two hours of time, and can lead to effective smoking interventions with patients [103].

Smoking Intervention with Special Populations

Patients Concerned with Weight Gain

Many smokers often note that the reason they do not want to stop smoking is their fear of weight gain [3, 63, 104, 105]. Weight gain is also a reason for returning to smoking. While weight gain is an important concern, the average gain associated with cessation is about 5 pounds, with only a very small percentage of individuals gaining 20 pounds or more [3]. Both physiological and behavioral factors contribute to this weight gain. Nicotine appears to affect metabolism and appetite. Smoking deadens taste buds. Withdrawal of nicotine may slow metabolism, increase appetite, and increase craving for sweets. Food may taste better. Due to the change in metabolism, some individuals may gain small amounts of weight even if they do not eat more.

While weight gain is likely to be small, the physician must acknowledge this concern, often particularly important to young women, and assist the patient in developing strategies to prevent weight gain or keep it at a minimum. These strategies can encourage weight-conscious smokers to attempt cessation and help successful abstainers remain abstinent. Weight gain often varies directly with the number of cigarettes smoked [3]. Behavioral patterns play an important role in weight gain. Typical patterns include substitution of eating for smoking, increased intake of high-sweet, high-fat snacks, and use of food instead of cigarettes as a way to manage negative feelings, such as anxiety, boredom, anger, or depression. If these changes occur and persist, then excess weight gain is much more likely.

Several investigators have demonstrated that smokers can stop smoking without significant weight gain. These studies are of particular interest since they included subjects who were at high risk for CHD and who were participating in multicomponent CHD risk reduction trials [17, 106]. The interventions focused on smoking cessation and improvement in eating patterns. Thus, strategies that combine dietary and smoking intervention can be effective. Table 8-10 gives recommendations for preventing weight gain.

Smokers should also be alerted to the idea that nicotine does alter metabolism and that weight gain after smoking cessation may be a result of a decreased metabolic rate. Therefore, smokers concerned with weight gain can also be instructed to use exercise instead of sweets in place of cigarettes and to make regular exercise a strategy for cessation. There is substantial support for the fact that nicotine is the factor in tobacco that causes changes in body weight [63]. Therefore nicotine replacement, as with the use of NCG or a transdermal nicotine patch, has been demonstrated in some studies to reduce postcessation weight gain [88, 107, 108, 109, 110]. In one study the weight gain seemed to

Table 8-10. Recommendation to prevent weight gain during smoking cessation

Assess which factors seem to be contributing to weight gain. An increased craving for sweets? Eating more snacks in general? Larger portions at meals? Eating compulsively to deal with negative feelings? Assist the patient in making a plan designed to help with those problem situations.

A craving for sweets is often satisfied with very small amounts of sweets, such as hard candies or chewing gum. Even sugarless candy or gum may help. Nonsweet foods such as carrot sticks may help substitute for a need to have something in one's mouth, but they do not necessarily satisfy a sweet craving.

If part of the problem is a need to keep your hands busy or something in your mouth, there are other choices besides food: fiddling with an object, doodling, keeping a toothpick handy, chewing gum or cinnamon sticks.

If compulsive eating becomes a substitute for smoking in order to deal with negative emotions, it is even more important to learn other methods. Attend a weight management class, seek counseling, or use a relaxation technique.

Exercise regularly if possible. Exercise can counter the purely metabolic effects of stopping smoking, and it can be very rewarding to become more active as breathing capacity improves. Many people also find exercise helpful in managing how they are feeling emotionally.

Source: Physician-Delivered Smoking Intervention Program Training Manual [30].

be postponed rather than prevented [109]. While research in nicotine replacement to prevent weight gain is preliminary, we recommend that the physician explore its possible use with the patient who is addicted to nicotine.

Patients Who Are Nicotine Addicted

Patients who are physiologically addicted to nicotine also present a special problem for the physician. Use of combined behavioral and pharmacologic therapy is recommended.

Patients Who Relapse

Patients who relapse often become discouraged and have a difficult time reconsidering cessation if they view themselves as failures. It is necessary to help the patient identify what triggered the relapse and problem solve for future cessation attempts. Remind the patient that relapse is a normal part of the cessation process and that most smokers have stopped several times before they are eventually successful.

Research on relapse indicates that the physiologic, personal, and environmental factors that affect smoking and cessation also affect relapse. Primary triggers of relapse include stress, interpersonal conflict, dysphoria, presence of other smokers, and alcohol consumption [111,

112]. Although the data are primarily retrospective reports from relapsed or tempted subjects, there is convincing consistency on the importance of stress and negative affect in determining maintenance or relapse [63, 68, 111, 112, 113, 114]. The mechanism whereby a lapse becomes a full return to smoking is usually a high-risk occasion that triggers a smoking lapse (that is, a brief return to smoking) and a subsequent interpretation of the lapse that may lead to abandoning the cessation effort and returning to regular smoking. Patients must be alerted to the fact that a lapse does not need to lead to a full return to smoking. Much recent attention has been paid to the importance of coping responses in dealing with both high-risk situations and lapses [115, 116]. The available data suggest that smokers who have not developed strategies for coping with these are more likely to relapse [115], supporting the important role of physicians in instructing smokers of the need to learn how to deal with stressful situations without cigarettes.

Minority Patients

Patients from minority groups are often more difficult to reach because of the physician's lack of awareness of their health beliefs and cultural values. Providers should familiarize themselves with the cultural norms and beliefs of the differing populations they serve so they can provide information that their patients can and will use.

Difficult-to-Reach Patients

Patients of lower socioeconomic status who may also be unemployed or homeless, patients with psychiatric disorders, and drug and alcohol abusers are generally difficult to reach for implementing smoking interventions and often face multiple obstacles to stopping smoking [117, 118, 119]. This topic is discussed fully in Chapter 7.

Although there is substantial evidence of an unusually high incidence of tobacco dependence among patients who have chronic psychiatric problems or who abuse drugs or alcohol, there has been little investigation of the treatment of smoking in these complicated patients. Such treatment will likely require much individualized attention and longer follow-up. Regarding alcohol abuse, there are no strong indications that smoking cessation prompts relapse back to drinking among individuals who are alcohol dependent [120]. In fact, some studies indicate that among smokers trying to stop smoking permanently, alcohol use decreases substantially [70], and smoking cessation does not impair the course of treatment for alcohol problems and may be associated with better outcomes [121]. However, the clinical rule of thumb for alcoholics has been to wait at least six months after stopping drinking before treating smoking, if appropriate when considering their health status. Nonetheless, some smokers may benefit from immediate cessation (e.g., those preparing for bypass surgery), and this option will need to be considered.

Elderly Patients

There are data to support the benefit of smoking cessation in the elderly patient [3, 122, 123, 124, 125]. A healthy man aged 60 to 64 who smoked one pack or more of cigarettes per day reduces his risk of dying during the next 15 years by 10 percent if he stops smoking. However, elderly patients often present with special needs that may interfere with smoking intervention, and they often are not aware of the benefits of cessation.

Patients with Multiple Risk Factors

The presence of multiple risk factors may pose ostacles to change or they may increase the individual's motivation and improvement in each of the behaviors [16, 106, 126].

The physician's role is to express what he sees as optimal and to help direct the patient to set realistic goals. He must also be sensitive to the fact that for some patients the cost of change may outweigh the benefits. (See Chapter 7 for a discussion of cost and benefits of risk factor changes.)

Summary

The physician's intervention role with smokers is to, at the very least, educate them about their risk for heart disease and advise them of the need to stop smoking. As a next step, the physician who is interested and able may want to help patients to become aware of their own personal strengths and resources and help them plan an approach to stopping smoking. Intervention can be brief, and the physician can provide patients with effective self-help materials and refer more difficult or needy patients to personnel in his office or to outside consultants. To ensure that smoking is addressed, that adequate follow-up and monitoring of patients are provided, and that the intervention loop is closed, an adequate office system must be set up. Physicians must also become aware of legitimate billing practices for smoking-related problems to maximize reimbursement for their efforts.

The physician must also be aware that smoking cessation is a continuous process and often takes several attempts before the smoker stops long-term. From a public health perspective physicians can help a large number of people with their smoking cessation efforts by just taking a few minutes of their time.

Appendix A.   Smoking History Questionnaire

Name: _____ Date _____

1. What is your smoking status? (Check one)
   ___ Ex-smoker ___ Current smoker ___ Never-smoker

2. If ex-smoker:
   a. When did you stop smoking? _____
   b. How did you stop? _____

3. If current smoker:
   a. How many cigarettes a day do you smoke? _____
   b. What brand of cigarette do you usually smoke? _____
   c. How soon after you wake up do you smoke your first cigarette?
      _____ within 15–30 minutes _____ 30 minutes to 1 hour _____ over 1 hour
   d. Do you find it difficult to refrain from smoking in places where it is forbidden, such as the library, theater, doctor's office?
      _____ Yes   _____ No
   e. Do you smoke when you are so ill that you are in bed most of the day?
      _____ Yes   _____ No
   f. How many times have you stopped smoking cigarettes for more than 1 day?
      _____ Never _____ Once _____ 2–3 times _____ 4 or more times
   g. When did you last stop? _____
   h. Why did you decide to stop smoking on your last attempt? _____
   i. If you have stopped smoking cigarettes in the past, which methods have helped you?
      (Check as many as apply.)
      ___ Individual or group counseling   ___ Hypnosis
      ___ Self-help materials   ___ Acupuncture
      ___ Gradual reduction   ___ Physician advice
      ___ Special filters   ___ Cold turkey
      ___ Exercise   ___ Nicotine-containing gum
      ___ Other (please specify): _____
   j. The last time you stopped smoking cigarettes, how difficult was it?
      _____ Very difficult _____ Difficult _____ Easy _____ Very easy
   k. Why did you start smoking again? _____
   l. How interested are you in stopping again?
      _____ Not at all _____ A little _____ Some _____ A lot _____ Very much
   m. If you decided to stop smoking during the next two weeks, how confident are you that you would succeed?
      _____ Not at all _____ A little _____ Some _____ A lot _____ Very much

Appendix B. Fagerstrom Nicotine Dependency Assessment

	0 points	*1 point*	*2 points*	*Your score*
1. How soon after you wake do you smoke your first cigarette?	After 30 min.	Within 30 min.	—	
2. Do you find it difficult to refrain from smoking in places where it is forbidden, such as the library, theater, doctor's office?	No	Yes	—	
3. Which cigarette would you hate most to give up?	Any, other than the first one in the morning	The first one in the morning	—	
4. How many cigarettes do you smoke a day?	1–15	16–25	26 or more	
5. Do you smoke more during the morning than the rest of the day?	No	Yes	—	
6. Do you smoke if you are so ill that you are in bed most of the day?	No	Yes	—	
7. How often do you inhale the smoke from your cigarette?	Never	Often	Always	

TOTAL SCORE:

HOW TO INTERPRET NICOTINE DEPENDENCY SCORES:

Score of 6 or higher: Indicates high nicotine dependency and represents individuals who would be particularly likely to benefit from instruction in tapering and/or nicotine replacement therapy to decrease nicotine withdrawal symptoms* as an adjunct to standard counseling.

Score of 5 of less: Suggests a low to moderate dependency.

*Craving tobacco, restlessness, irritability, difficulty concentrating, increased appetite.

Suggested Readings

Fielding JE. Smoking: Health effects and control (Part I). N Engl J Med 1985;313:491-8.

Ockene JK, Kristeller J, Goldberg R, et al. Increasing the efficacy of physician-delivered smoking intervention: A randomized clinical trial. J Gen Int Med 1991;6:1-8.

Schwartz SL. Review and evaluation of smoking cessation methods: The United States and Canada, 1978-1985. U.S. Department of Health and Human Services, PHS, NIH publ. no. 87-2940, 1987.

US Department of Health and Human Services. The Health Benefits of Smoking Cessation. A Report of the Surgeon General. USDHHS, Centers for Disease Control. Office of Smoking and Health. USDHHS publ. no. (CDC) 90-846, 1990.

Wilson D, Taylor W, Gilbert, et al. A randomized trial of a family physician intervention for smoking cessation. JAMA 1989;160:1570-4.

References

1. U.S. Department of Health and Human Services. The health consequences of smoking. A report of the Surgeon General. Public Health Service, Centers for Disease Control, Center for Chronic Disease Prevention and Health Promotion, Office on Smoking and Health. USDHHS publ. no. (PHS) 84-50204, 1983.

2. U.S. Department of Health and Human Services. Reducing the health consequences of smoking: 25 years of progress. A report of the Surgeon General. Public Health Service, Centers for Disease Control, Center for Chronic Disease Prevention and Health Promotion, Office on Smoking and Health. USDHHS publ. no. (CDC) 89-8411, 1989.

3. U.S. Department of Health and Human Services. The health benefits of smoking cessation. A report of the Surgeon General. Centers for Disease Control, Office on Smoking and Health. USDHHS publ. no. (CDC) 90-8416, 1990.

4. U.S. Department of Health, Education and Welfare. Healthy people. The Surgeon General's report on health promotion and disease prevention. USDHHS publ. no. (ADM) 79-800, 1979.

5. Holbrook JH, Grundy SM, Hennekens CH, et al. Cigarette smoking and cardiovascular diseases. A statement for health professionals by a task force appointed by the steering committee of the American Heart Association. Circulation 1984; 70:1114A-1117A.

6. Hammond EC, Horn D. Smoking and death rates. Report on forty-four months of follow-up of 187,783 men. II. Death rates by cause. JAMA 1958; 166:1294-1308.

7. Doll R, Peto R. Mortality in relation to smoking: twenty years' observations on male British doctors. Br Med J 1976; 2:1525-36.

8. Friedman GD, Petitti DB, Bawal RD, et al. Mortality in cigarette smokers and quitters: effect of base-line differences. N Engl J Med 1981; 304:1407-10.

9. Gordon T, Kannel WB, McGee D, et al. Death and coronary attacks in men giving up cigarette smoking: a report from the Framingham Study. Lancet 1983; 2:1345-8.

10. Ockene JK, Kuller LH, Svendsen KH, Meilahn E. The relationship of smoking cessation to coronary heart disease and lung cancer in the Multiple Risk Factor Intervention Trial (MRFIT). Am J Pub Hlth 1990; 80(8):954-8.

11. Kahn HA. The Dorn study of smoking and mortality among U.S. veterans: report on eight and one-half years of observation. In: Haenszel W, ed. Epidemiological approaches to the study of cancer and other chronic diseases. U.S. Department of Health, Education, and Welfare, Public Health Service, National Cancer Institute. NCI monograph no. 19, January 1966; 1-125.

12. Sparrow D, Dawber TR, Colton T. The influence of cigarette smoking on prognosis after a first myocardial infarction. A report from the Framingham Study. J Chronic Dis 1978; 31:425-32.

13. Wihelmsson C, Vedin JA, Elmfieldt D, et al. Smoking and myocardial infarction. Lancet 1975; 1:415-20.

14. Salonen JT. Stopping smoking and long-term mortality after acute myocardial infarction. Br Heart J 1980; 43:463-9.

15. Mulcahy R, Hickey N, Graham IM, MacAirt J. Factors affecting the 5 year survival rate of men following acute coronary heart disease. Am Heart J 1977; 93(5):556-9.

16. Orleans CT, Shipley RA, Wilbur C, et al. Wide-ranging improvements in employee health lifestyle and well-being accompanying smoking cessation in the Live for Life program. Paper presented at Annual Meeting of Society of Behavioral Medicine, Baltimore, MD, 1983.

17. Gerace T, Hollis J, Ockene JK, Svendsen K. Relationship of smoking cessation to diastolic blood pressure, body weight, and plasma lipids. Prev Med 1991; 20:602-28.

18. Shopland DT, Brown C. Changes in cigarette smoking prevalence in the United States: 1955 to 1983. Ann Behav Med 1985; 7:5-8.

19. Thornberg OT, Wilson RW, Golden PM. Health promotion data from the 1990 objectives: estimates from the National Health In-

terview Survey Health Promotion and Disease Prevention, United States, 1985. Public Health Service, U.S. National Center for Health Statistics. Advance data from vital and health statistics, no. 126. USDHHS publ. no. (PHS) 86-1250, Sept. 19, 1986.

20. Stoto MA. Changes in adult smoking behavior in the United States: 1955-1983. Discussion paper series, Institute for the Study of Smoking Behavior and Policy. Cambridge: Harvard University Press, 1986.

21. Ockene JK. The influence of medical care on smoking cessation: treatment of smoking to prevent coronary heart disease. In: Higgins MW, Luepker RV, eds. Trends in coronary heart disease mortality: the influence of medical care. New York: Oxford University Press, 1988.

22. Goldman L, Cook EF. The decline in ischemic heart disease: comparative effects of medical interventions and changes in lifestyle. Ann Intern Med 1984; 101:825-36.

23. Munro JM, Cotran RS. The pathogenesis of atherosclerosis: atherogenesis and inflammation. Laboratory Investigation 1988; 58(3):249-61.

24. U.S. Department of Health and Human Services. The health consequences of smoking. The changing cigarette. A report of the Surgeon General. Public Health Service, Office on Smoking and Health. USDHHS pub. no. (PHS) 81-50156, 1981.

25. Fiore M, Novotny T, Lynn W, et al. Methods used to quit smoking in the United States. Do cessation programs help? JAMA 1990; 263:2760-5.

26. Ockene JK. Physician-delivered interventions for smoking cessation: strategies for increasing effectiveness. Prev Med 1987; 16:723-37.

27. Ockene JK. Smoking intervention: the expanding role of the physician. Am J Pub Hlth 1987; 77:782-3.

28. Handel S. Change in smoking habits in a general practice. Grad Med J 1973; 49:679-81.

29. Porter AMW, McCullough DM. Counseling against cigarette smoking. Practitioner 1972; 209:686-9.

30. Ockene JK, Kristeller J, Goldberg R, et al. Increasing the efficacy of physician-delivered smoking intervention: a randomized clinical trial. J Gen Int Med 1991; 6:1-8.

31. Cohen SJ, Stookey GK, Katz BP, et al. Encouraging primary care physicians to help smokers quit. Ann Int Med 1989; 110(8):648-52.

32. Ewart CK, Li VC, Coates TC. Increasing physician antismoking influence by applying an inexpensive feedback technique. J Med Educ 1983; 58:468-73.

33. Fagerstrom KO. Effects of number of follow-up sessions and nicotine gum in physician based smoking cessation. Presented at the Fifth World Conference on Smoking and Health, Winnipeg, Canada, July 14, 1983.

34. Jamrozik K, Fowler G, Vessey M. Placebo controlled trial of nicotine chewing gum in general practice. Br Med J 1984; 289:794-7.

35. Russell MAH, Merriam R, Stapleton J, Taylor W. Effects of nicotine chewing gum as an adjunct to general practitioner's advice against smoking. Br Med J 1983; 287:1782-5.

36. Russell MA, Wilson C, Taylor C, Baker CD. Effect of general practitioners' advice against smoking. Br Med J 1979; 231-5.

37. Wilson D, Taylor W, Gilbert R, et al. A randomized trial of a family physician intervention for smoking cessation. JAMA 1988; 260:1570-4.

38. Wilson D, Wood G, Johnston N, Sicuvella J. Randomized clinical trial of supportive followup for cigarette smokers in a family practice. Can Med Assoc J 1982; 126:127-9.

39. Ockene JK, Lindsay E, Berger L, Hymowitz N. Health care providers as key change agents in the Community Intervention Trial for Smoking Cessation (COMMIT). Int Quart Commun Health Ed 1991; 11:223-38.

40. Kottke TE, Battista RN, DeFriece GH, Brekke ML. Attribution of succccessful smoking cessation interventions in medical practice: a meta-analysis of 39 controlled trials. JAMA 1988; 259:2883-9.

41. Schwartz JL. Review and evaluation of smoking cessation methods: the United States and Canada, 1978-1985. U.S. Department of Health and Human Services, Public Health Service, National Institutes of Health, USDHHS publ. no. (NIH) 87-2940, 1987.

42. Stokes J, Rigotti NA. The health consequences of cigarette smoking and the internist's role in smoking cessation. Advances in Med 1987; 33:431-60.

43. Kottke TE, Brekke ML, Solberg LI, Hughes JR. A randomized trial to increase smoking intervention by physicians: doctors helping smokers, round 1. JAMA 1989; 261(14):2101-6.

44. Ockene JK. Cigarette smoking. In: Greene HL, Glassock RJ, Kelley MA, eds. Introduction to clinical medicine. Philadelphia: BC Decker, Inc., 1990

45. Shipley RH, Orleans CS. Treatment of cigarette smoking. In: Boudewyns PA, Keefe FJ, eds. Behavioral medicine in general medical practice. Menlo Park, CA: Addison-Wesley 1982; 237-68.

46. Ockene JK, Kristeller JL, Goldberg RL, et al. Smoking cessation and severity of disease: the

Coronary Artery Smoking Intervention Study. Hlth Psych 1992 (In Press).

47. Croog SH, Richards NP. Health beliefs and smoking patterns in heart patients and their wives: a longitudinal study. Am J Pub Hlth 1977; 67:921-30.

48. Rose G, Hamilton PJS. A randomized controlled trial of the effect on middle-aged men of advice to stop smoking. J Epidemiol Community Health 1982; 36:102-8.

49. Bertakis KD. The communicating of information from physician to patient: a method for increasing patient retention and satisfaction. J Fam Prac 1977; 5:217-22.

50. Bettman JR. An information processing theory of consumer choice. Reading, MA: Addison-Wesley, 1979.

51. Bandura A. Social learning theory. Englewood Cliffs, NJ: Prentice-Hall, 1977.

52. Bandura A. Social foundation of thought and action. A social cognitive theory. Englewood Cliffs, NJ: Prentice-Hall, 1986.

53. Rosenstock IM. What research in motivation suggests for public health. Amer J Pub Hlth 1960; 50:295-301.

54. Becker MH, ed. The health belief model and personal health behavior. Hlth Ed Mono 1974; 2:324-473.

55. Prochaska JO, DiClemente CC. Stages and processes of self-change of smoking: toward an interactive model of change. J Consult Clin Psych 1983; 51(3):390-5.

56. Rudd J, Glanz K. How individuals use information for health action: consumer information processing. In: Glanz K, Lewis FM, Rimer BK, eds. Health behavior and health education: theory, research and practice. San Francisco: Jossey-Bass Publishers, 1990.

57. Mischel W. Toward a cognitive social learning reconceptualization of personality. Psych Rev 1973; 80:252-83.

58. Condiotte MM, Lichtenstein E. Self-efficacy and relapse in smoking cessation programs. J Consult Clin Psych 1981; 49:648-58.

59. DiClemente CC. Self-efficacy and smoking cessation maintenance: a preliminary report. Cogn Ther Res 1981; 5:175-87.

60. Bandura A. Self-efficacy: toward a unifying theory of behavioral change. Psych Rev 1977b; 84:191-215.

61. Bandura A, Schunk DH. Cultivating competence, self-efficacy and interests through proximal self-motivation. J Personality and Social Psych 1981; 41:586-98.

62. Rosenstock IM. The health belief model: explaining health behavior through expectancies. In: Glanz K, Lewis FM, and Reimer BK, eds. Health behavior and health education: theory, research and practice. San Francisco: Jossey-Bass Publishers, 1990.

63. U.S. Department of Health and Human Services. The health consequences of smoking: nicotine addiction. A report of the Surgeon General. Public Health Service, Centers for Disease Control, Center for Health Promotion and Education, Office on Smoking and Health, USDHHS publ. no. (CDC) 88-8406:523, 1988.

64. American Psychiatric Association. Diagnostic and statistical manual of mental disorders (revised), 3d ed. (DSM III R). Washington, DC: American Psychiatric Association, 1987.

65. Abrams DB, Monti PM, Carey KB, et al. Reactivity to smoking cues and relapse: two studies of discriminant validity. Beh Research and Therapy 1988; 26:225-33.

66. Abrams DB. Roles of psychosocial stress, smoking cues, and coping in smoking-relapse prevention. Hlth Psych 1986; 5:Suppl:91-2.

67. Hall SM, Tunstall C, Gensberg D, et al. Nicotine gum and behavioral treatment: a placebo controlled trial. J Consult Clin Psych 1987; 55:603-5.

68. Ockene JK, Benfari RC, Hurwitz I, et al. Relationship of psychosocial factors to smoking behavior change in an intervention program. Prev Med 1982; 11:13-28.

69. Hughes GH, Hymowitz N, Ockene JK, et al. The Multiple Risk Factor Intervention Trial (MRFIT). Prev Med 1981; 10(4):476-500.

70. Hughes JR, Hatsukami D. Signs and symptoms of tobacco withdrawal. Arch Gen Psych 1986; 43(3):289-99.

71. West RJ, Jarvis MJ, Russell MAH, et al. Effect of nicotine replacement on the cigarette withdrawal syndrome. Br J of Addiction 1984; 79:215-9.

72. Blair A, Blair SN, Howe HG, et al. Physical, psychological, and sociodemographic differencs among smokers, exsmokers, and nonsmokers in a working population. Prev Med 1980;9(6):747-59.

73. Gritz ER, Carr CR, Marcus AC. Unaided smoking cessation: Great American Smokeout and New Year's Day quitters. J of Psychosocial Oncology 1988; 6(3/4):217-34.

74. Perri MG, Richards CS, Schultheis KR. Behavioral self-control and smoking reduction: a study of self-initiated attempts to reduce smoking. Beh Therapy 1977; 8:360-5.

75. Abrams DB, Monti PM, Pinto RP, et al. Psychosocial stress and coping in smokers who relapse or quit. Health Psychology 1987; 6(4):289-303.

76. Sorensen G, Pechacek TF. Attitudes toward smoking cessation among men and women. J of Beh Med 1987; 10(2):129-37.

77. Mitic WR, McGuire DP, Neumann B. Perceived stress and adolescents' cigarette use. Psych Rep 1985; 57:3, Part 2:1043-8.

78. Schwartz JL, Dubitzky M. Psycho-social factors involved in cigarette smoking cessation. Final report of the smoking control research project. Berkeley, CA: Institute for Health Research, Permanente Medical Group, Kaiser Foundation Health Plan, September 1968.

79. Pomerleau O, Adkins D, Pertschuk M. Predictors of outcome and recidivism in smoking cessation treatment. Add Beh 1978; 3:65-70.

80. Cohen SJ, Syme SL. Social support and health. Orlando: Academic Press, 1985.

81. Fisher EB, Lowe MR, Levenkron JC, Newman A. Reinforcement and structural support of maintained risk reduction. In: Stuart RB, ed. Adherence, compliance, and generalization in behavioral medicine. New York: Brunner/Mazel, 1982; 145-68.

82. Sorensen G, Pechacek TF, Pallonen U. Occupational and worksite norms and attitudes about smoking cessation. Am J Pub Hlth 1986; 76(5):544-9.

83. Novotny TE, Warner KE, Kendrick JS, Reminton PL. Smoking by blacks and whites: socioeconomic and demographic differences. Am J Pub Hlth 1988; 78(9):1187-9.

84. Glanz K. Nutrition education for risk factor reduction and patient education: a review. Prev Med 1985; 14:721-52.

85. Stokes J, Noren J, Shindell S. Definition of terms and concepts applicable to clinical preventive medicine. J Comm Hlth 1982; 8:33-40.

86. Lazare A, Eisentral S, Frank A. A negotiated approach to the clinical encounter. II. Conflict and negotiation. In: Lazare A., ed. Outpatient psychiatry: diagnosis and treatment, Baltimore: Williams & Wilkins, 1979.

87. Fagerstrom KO. Measuring degree of physical dependence on tobacco smoking with reference to individualization of treatment. Addictive Beh 1978; 3(3):235-41.

88. Jarvik ME, Henningfield JE. Pharmacological treatment of tobacco dependence. Pharmacology, Biochemistry and Behavior 1988; 30:279-94.

89. Mahoney MJ, Moura NCM, Wade TC. Related efficacy of self-reward, self-punishment, and self-monitoring techniques for weight loss. J Consult Clin Psych 1973; 40:404-7.

90. Jaffe JH. Drug addiction and drug abuse. In: AG Gilman, LS Goodman, TW Rall, F Murad, eds. The pharmacologic basis of therapeutics, 7th ed. New York: MacMillan, 1985; 532-81.

91. Schneider NG, Jarvik ME, Forsythe AB, et al. Nicotine gum in smoking cessation: a placebo-controlled, double-blind trial. Addictive Beh 1983; 8(3):253-61.

92. Fagerstom KO. Efficacy of nicotine chewing gum: a review. In: Pomerleau OF, Pomerleau CS, eds. Nicotine replacement: a critical evaluation. New York: Alan R Liss, Inc., 1988; 109-28.

93. Hughes JR, Gust SW, Keenan RM, et al. Nicotine vs. placebo gum in general medical practice. JAMA 1989; 26:1300-5.

94. Ferno O, Lichtnechert S, Lundgren C. A substitute for tobacco smoking. Psycho Pharmacologia 1973; 31:201-4.

95. Henningfield JE, Jasinski DR. Pharmacologic basis for nicotine replacement. In: Pomerleau OF, Pomerleau CS, eds. Nicotine replacement: a critical evaluation. New York: Alan R Liss, Inc., 1988.

96. Abelin T, Ehrsam R, Bühler-Reichert A, et al. Effectivness of a transdermal nicotine system in smoking cessation studies. Meth and Find Exp Clin Pharmacol 1989; 11(3):205-14.

96a. Tonnesen P, Norregaard J, Simonsen K, Säwe U. A double-blind trial of a 16-hour transdermal nicotine patch in smoking cessation. N Engl J Med 1991: 5(325):311-5.

96b. Transdermal Nicotine Study Group. Transdermal nicotine for smoking cessation: Six-month results from two multicenter trials. JAMA 1991:22(266):3133-8.

97. Russell MAH. Nicotine replacement: the role of blood nicotine levels, their rate of change, and nicotine tolerance. In: Pomerlau OF, Pomerlau CS, eds. Nicotine replacement: a critical evaluation. New York: Alan R. Liss, Inc., 1988; 63-94.

98. Glassman AH, Stetner F, Walsh BT, et al. Heavy smokers, smoking cessation, and clonidine. JAMA 1988; 259:2866-71.

99. Frank P, Harp J, Bell B. Randomized controlled trial of clonidine and smoking cessation in a primary care setting. JAMA 1989; 262: 3011-33.

100. Demak MM, Becker MH. Current perspectives on the changing patient-provider relationship: charting the future of health care. Pat Ed Couns 1987; 9:5-24.

101. Carter WB, Belcher DW, Inui TS. Implementing preventive care in clinical practice: problems for managers, clinicians, and patients. Med Care Rev 1981; 38:195.

102. Marlatt GA. Relapse prevention: theoretical rationale and overview of the model. In: Marlatt GA, Gordon JR, eds. Relapse prevention: maintenance strategies in the treatment of addictive behaviors. New York: Guilford Press, 1985.

103. Ockene JK, Quirk ME, Goldberg RJ, et al. A residents' training program for the development

ment of smoking intervention skills. Arch Intern Med 1988; 148:1039-45.

104. Grunberg NE. Behavioral and biological factors in the relationship between tobacco use and body weight. In: Katkin ES, Manuck SB, eds. Advances in behavioral medicine. Vol. 2. Greenwich, CT: JAI Press, 1986; 97-129.

105. Klesges RC, Meyers AW, Klesges LM, LaVasque ME. Smoking, body weight, and their effects on smoking behavior: a comprehensive review of the literature. Psych Bull 1989; 106(2):204-30.

106. Schoenenberger JC. Smoking change in relation to changes in blood pressure, weight, and cholesterol. Prev Med 1982; 11:441-53.

107. Emont SL, Cummings KM. Weight gain following smoking cessation: a possible role for nicotine replacement in weight management. Addictive Beh 1987; 12(2):151-5.

108. Fagerstrom KO. Reducing the weight gain after stopping smoking. Addictive Beh 1987; 12(1):91-3.

109. Gross J, Stitzer ML, Maldonado J. Nicotine replacement: effects of post-cessation weight gain. J Consult Clin Psych 1989; 57(1):87-92.

110. Hajek P, Jackson P, Belcher M. Long-term use of nicotine chewing gum. Occurrence determinants, and effect on weight gain. J Consult Clin Psych 1989; 260(11):1593-6.

111. Marlatt GA, Gordon JR. Determinants of relapse: implications for the maintenance of behavior change. In: Davidson PO, Davidson SM, eds. Behavioral medicine: changing health lifestyles. New York: Brunner/Mazel, 1980; 410-52.

112. Shiffman S. Relapse following smoking cessation: a situational analysis. J Consult Clin Psych 1982; 50(1):71-86.

113. Baer JS, Lichtenstein E. Classification and prediction of smoking relapse episodes: an exploration of individual differences. J Consult Clin Psych 1988; 56(1):104-10.

114. Niaura RS, Rohsenow DJ, Binkoff JA, et al. Relevance of cue reactivity to understanding alcohol and smoking relapse. J of Abnormal Psych 1988; 97(2):133-52.

115. Shiffman S. Coping with temptations to smoke. J Consult Clin Psych 1984; 52:261-7.

116. Brandon TH, Tiffany ST, Baker TB. The process of smoking relapse. In: Tims FM, Leukefeld CG, eds. Relapse and recovery in drug abuse. NIDA Research Monograph 72. U.S. Department of Health and Human Services, Public Health Service, Alcohol, Drug Abuse, and Mental Health Administration, National Institute on Drug Abuse. USDHHS publ. no. (ADM) 86-1473, 1986;104-17.

117. Geldberg L, Linn LS, Usatine RP, Smith MH. Health, homelessness and poverty: a study of clinic users. Arch Intern Med 1990; 150:2325-30.

118. Fantry LS. Unpublished report. 1990

119. Miller DR, Ockene JK, Hebert J, et al. Racial differences in smoking-related factors among participants in a physician-based smoking intervention trial. (Submitted for publication.)

120. Kozlowski LT, Ferrence RG, Corbit T. Tobacco use: a perspective for alcohol and drug researchers. Brit J Addiction 1990; 85:245.

121. Miller WR, Hedrik KE, Taylor CA. Addictive behaviors and life problems before and after behavioral treatments of problem drinkers. Addictive Beh 1988; 8(4):403-12.

122. Castelli WP, Wilson PWF, Levy D, et al. Cardiovascular risk factors in the elderly. Am J Cardiol 1989; 63:12H-19H.

123. Gordon DJ, Rifkind BM. Treating high blood cholesterol in the older patient. Am J Cardiol 1989; 63:48H-52H.

124. Hermanson B, Omenn GS, Kronmal RA, et al. Beneficial six year outcome of smoking cessation in older men and women with coronary artery disease: results from the CASS registry. N Engl J Med 1988; 319:1365-9.

125. Kafonek SD, Kwiterovich PO. Treatment of hypercholesterolemia in the elderly. Ann Int Med 1990; 112:723-5.

126. Tuomilehto J, Nissinen A, Puska P, et al. Long-term effects of cessation of smoking on bodyweight, blood pressure and serum cholesterol in the middle-aged population with high blood pressure. Addictive Beh 1986; 11:1-9.

9

Nutritional Intervention: A Behavioral and Educational Perspective

KAREN GLANZ

EDITORS' INTRODUCTION

If it is true that abnormal serum lipids are the *sine qua non* of the atherosclerotic process, then the modification of diet to lower serum cholesterol and LDL levels is a crucial part of any program to lower CHD risk. Yet dietary modification can be difficult. The smoker who wants to quit need deal with only one goal, stopping smoking, and must make decisions relating to only one substance, the cigarette. But one cannot stop eating, and the variety of foods is enormous. Decisions must be made many times a day regarding food choices, amounts, and preparation. Not only is the patient often at a loss how to successfully alter diet, the physician, too, often feels inadequate to the task. In this chapter Dr. Glanz reviews the theoretical framework underlying dietary behavior change and presents assessment and treatment options designed to fit into a busy practice. She also discusses the important topic of physician–dietitian collaboration, as well as dietary intervention in special populations.

Nutrition plays an important role in reducing the risk of coronary heart disease (CHD) and other chronic illnesses. Serum cholesterol and low-density lipoprotein (LDL) cholesterol are causally related to the development and progression of CHD, and control of cholesterol and lipoprotein levels can reduce both the risk of coronary artery disease and the severity of its consequences [1, 2]. Excess dietary intake of fat, especially saturated fat and cholesterol, and excess caloric intake, contribute to the increased risk and progression of CHD through their effect on lipid abnormalities [1, 3, 4, 5]. Obesity and excessive sodium intake contribute to the development and maintenance of hypertension in some individuals; weight reduction and sodium restriction may help to control elevated blood pressure [3, 5] (See Chapters 1, 3, and 13 for detailed discussions of these topics.)

In addition to CHD, eating patterns contribute substantially to four other of the ten leading causes of death in the United States — cancer, stroke, diabetes mellitus, and atherosclerosis. [3, 3a]. Nutritional risk factors for chronic illness include obesity, elevated serum cholesterol, and overconsumption of fats, sugar, sodium, and highly refined foods [3, 6]. Reduction of such consumption can help in the prevention of chronic diseases.

The Benefits of Changing Dietary Behavior

Dietary change is a treatment goal for a broad spectrum of chronic diseases. Effective nutritional management can reduce the need for long-term medication in hypertension, dyslipidemia, and diabetes [7, 8]. One study has shown regression of coronary artery lesions using only dietary and other nonpharmacologic lifestyle changes [9], and another well-controlled recent study has suggested that a low-fat vegetarian diet is of value in rheumatoid arthritis [9a].

Changes in eating patterns may yield psychosocial and economic benefits as well. Dietary changes leading to achievement of desirable body weight can enhance feelings of self-confidence, physical comfort, and attractiveness.

Health-enhancing nutritional habits may improve physical performance, both in athletic and work-related activities. Dietary modification that obviates the need for medication, surgery, and/or hospitalization can result in significant financial savings. With consistent and effective nutritional management, patients and their families may be spared the distress of disability and/or rehabilitation, and employers can reap economic benefits through decreased morbidity- and mortality-related benefit expenses and employee turnover.

The Role of Health Care Providers in Dietary Intervention

The primary treatment approach for high blood cholesterol levels is dietary change, making nutritional intervention a central component of cholesterol management [10]. The American public perceives physicians and dietitians as the most useful sources of information on nutrition, although they cite physicians as sources of information four times as often as dietitians [11, 12]. Current public health recommendations in the United States give high priority to including nutrition education in all routine health care contacts [5, 13].

Physicians and other health care professionals have a potentially large role in the screening and management of patients with abnormal lipid levels. Approximately 70 percent of adults have contact with the health care system each year [14]. Public interest in and concern about high cholesterol levels have increased in recent years [15]. While physician surveys in 1983 and 1986 indicate greater willingness to initiate diet therapy for adults with elevated blood cholesterol levels [16], studies using patient chart audits and surveys between 1985 and 1989 revealed large incongruities between physician practices and recommended guidelines [17, 18, 19].

Physicians give a number of reasons for their limited adoption of nutritional intervention in reducing CHD risk. Only half of the physicians in national surveys stated that they felt prepared to provide diet counseling to lower blood cholesterol levels [16]. They further cited lack of time, lack of knowledge, lack of confidence in their counseling skills [16, 20, 21], and perceived lack of patient interest as reasons for not counseling or referring patients whose treatment involves nutritional modification [22]. The lack of financial incentives is an additional barrier [23].

For office-based nutrition intervention to be feasible for physicians in busy practices, providers need a continuum of models for patient management. The most easily adopted strategies should cause little disruption in office routines, require minimal additional office staff expertise, and not require a centrally located multidisciplinary team [24]. This chapter presents simple strategies that can be implemented by practitioners with time and staff limitations, as well as more elaborate models involving detailed counseling, referral, and coordination of multiple sources of nutritional care.

Physicians' roles in nutritional intervention are pivotal because of their centrality in health care and credibility as patient educators. At a minimum they can serve as agenda setters, emphasizing the patient's risk and the importance of further management by other health professionals, and provide positive reinforcement for change [25].

Dietary behavior changes are truly effective in preventing cardiovascular disease and/or its complications only when they are sustained over the long term and outside the clinical setting. To be effective in nutritional intervention, health care providers need to understand both the principles of nutrition management and a variety of behavioral issues. This chapter first discusses the National Cholesterol Education Program's recommended evaluation and treatment guidelines for cholesterol and then examines the determinants of dietary behavior and the processes of change. Next, it presents assessment and treatment options and special situations for intervention.

Treatment Guidelines and General Dietary Principles

The current guidelines for the treatment of elevated cholesterol levels in adults were estab-

lished by an expert panel convened by the National Cholesterol Education Program (NCEP) and released in 1988 [26]. The NCEP was established in 1985 by the National Heart, Lung, and Blood Institute (NHLBI) as a coordinated effort to improve professional and public knowledge, awareness, and behaviors related to cholesterol [27, 28]. The NCEP adult treatment guidelines were designed to be authoritative, scientifically based, and practical for clinical implementation. They advise that total cholesterol levels should be measured in all adults age 20 and over and that initial classification should be based on total blood cholesterol levels as follows: levels below 200 mg/dl are considered desirable, levels 200 to 239 mg/dl are considered borderline high, and levels of 240 mg/dl or above are considered high [29].

For individuals with borderline-high cholesterol levels who do not have definite CHD or two other CHD risk factors, the Adult Treatment Panel (ATP) report recommends provision of dietary information and annual reassessment of total cholesterol.* Adults with borderline-high cholesterol and other CHD risk factors and those with high cholesterol levels need additional evaluation, including repeat testing, complete lipoprotein analysis including assessment of LDL cholesterol (the major atherogenic component of cholesterol), and evaluation of other risk factors for CHD. Following a complete evaluation, decisions about treatment should be made [26, 29].

The LDL-cholesterol level is the basis for decisions about initiating nutritional or pharmacologic therapy. LDL-cholesterol levels less than 130 mg/dl are considered desirable, levels of 130 to 159 mg/dl are borderline high, and levels of 160 mg/dl or higher are considered high-risk. Patients with borderline-high levels who do not have definite CHD or two other CHD risk factors should receive dietary information and annual reassessment. Those with borderline-high levels and other CHD risk fac-

---

*CHD risk factors as defined in the ATP report include cigarette smoking, hypertension, diabetes mellitus, severe obesity, family history of premature CHD, low HDL-cholesterol concentration, history of cerebrovascular or occlusive peripheral vascular disease, and male sex [26].

tors and those with high-risk LDL–cholesterol levels should have complete clinical evaluations and be given cholesterol-lowering treatment [26, 29].

Although a low HDL–cholesterol is considered to be a risk factor in the NCEP guidelines, the program has been criticized for the relatively modest weight given to this lipid abnormality [29a, 29b, 29c]. An anticipated revision of the guidelines is likely to place greater emphasis on the importance of this risk marker.

The primary treatment approach for high blood cholesterol is dietary change. Dietary modification is advised in two steps, with referral to a registered dietitian for instruction and monitoring as necessary and as feasible. For most patients who follow the recommended dietary changes, therapeutic goals can be reached within three to six months, with many patients showing significant reductions within four to six weeks. Initiation of drug therapy is indicated only when LDL–cholesterol remains above goal levels after maximal efforts at dietary treatment (Figure 9-1). Even when cholesterol-lowering drugs are used, nutritional intervention should be continued [26, 29].

The NCEP Step 1 and Step 2 Diets

The NCEP recommends that dietary modification be taken in two steps. The step 1 and step 2 diets share four central characteristics: reduction of total fat intake to less than 30 percent of total calories, restricted consumption of saturated fatty acids, restricted intake of dietary cholesterol, and reduced caloric intake, if necessary, to achieve desirable weight level. The step 2 diet, which is recommended when adherence to the step 1 diet does not result in achievement of cholesterol-reduction goals, is more restrictive with respect to the intake of saturated fatty acids (less than 7 percent of total calories versus less than 10 percent of total calories for step on2) and dietary cholesterol (less than 200 mg/day versus less than 300 mg/day) [26, 29]. Table 9-1 details both diets.

In comparison to the average American adult's diet, the most striking difference of the NCEP diets is the reduction of the proportion of calories derived from fat, from about 37 per-

cent to 30 percent. Figure 9-2 is a comparison of the step 1 diet and the average American diet with regard to macronutrients and dietary cholesterol [30]. The step 2 diet is different in terms of the dietary proportion of saturated fatty acids and also more restricted in dietary cholesterol intake. It is important to note that the step 1 diet is essentially identical to the prudent diet recommended to the entire population for health maintenance and disease prevention in the reports of authoritative scientific bodies such as the National Academy of Sciences [4] and the National Cancer Institute [31]. It is thus considered a realistic goal that should not require radical alteration of most individuals' diets. It can be tasty and filling, so that patients, families, and friends can enjoy the same foods. At continuing medical education and other physician meetings and programs, meals based on the step 1 diet are often served [32].

Restriction of Dietary Fats

Restriction of dietary fat intake is central to cholesterol-lowering diets. The major dietary influence on blood cholesterol is saturated fat intake, which has been shown to raise both total plasma cholesterol levels and LDL–cholesterol levels [33]. The saturated fats that are hypercholesterolemic are found primarily in animal products and in some vegetable fats, usually referred to as tropical oils (palm oil, palm kernel oil, and coconut oil) [33, 34, 35]. Because saturated fatty acids raise blood cholesterol more than any other dietary constituent, reduction of saturated fat is the most important dietary change for controlling blood cholesterol. The foods that contribute the most saturated fat to the average American diet are meat and dairy products: butter, cheese, whole milk, ice cream, and the white fatty streaks surrounding the muscle of meat (marbling). Poultry, fish, and shellfish contain saturated fat but less than red meats per same-size servings. Tropical oils are often used in commercially processed foods (although their use is rapidly decreasing) and can usually be identified by a careful reading of package labels. The importance of tropical oils as a contributor of saturated fat to the diet has in any case probably been overemphasized —

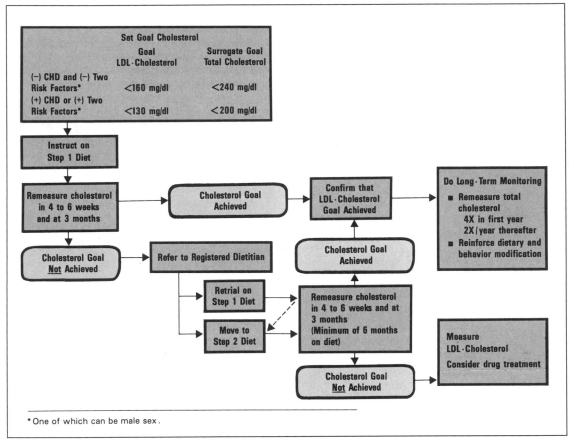

Figure 9-1.   Dietary treatment guidelines (National Cholesterol Education Program).

Table 9-1.   Dietary therapy of high blood cholesterol

Nutrient	Recommended intake	
	Step 1 diet	*Step 2 diet*
Total fat	Less than 30% of total calories	Less than 30% of total calories
Saturated fatty acids	Less than 10% of total calories	Less than 7% of total calories
Polyunsaturated fatty acids	Up to 10% of total calories	Up to 10% of total calories
Monounsaturated fatty acids	10 to 15% of total calories	10 to 15% of total calories
Carbohydrates	50 to 60% of total calories	50 to 60% of total calories
Protein	10 to 20% of total calories	10 to 20% of total calories
Cholesterol	Less than 300 mg/day	Less than 200 mg/day
Total calories	To achieve and maintain desirable weight	To achieve and maintain desirable weight

Source: NCEP Adult Treatment Panel guidelines [29].

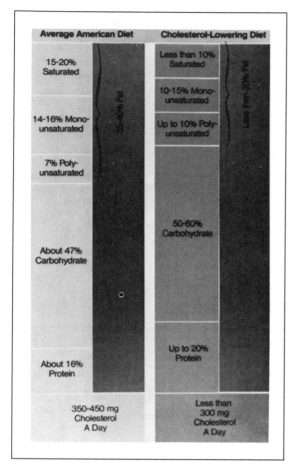

Figure 9-2. Cholesterol-lowering diet compared to the average American diet.

it has been estimated that they provide less than 2% of total energy [35a, 35b].

Some vegetable oils are treated by a process known as hydrogenation, which makes the fats largely saturated and therefore solid at room temperature. Hydrogenated vegetable oils are used for hard margarines and shortenings. Similar products in soft or tub forms are less hydrogenated and contain less saturated fat.

Monounsaturated fatty acids are a type of unsaturated fatty acid that is neutral in its effect on plasma cholesterol levels; that is, it neither raises nor lowers the plasma cholesterol level [33, 34]. The major monounsaturated fatty acid is oleic acid, which is found in olive oil, rapeseed (canola oil), and some forms of safflower oil

and sunflower seed oil. While monounsaturated fats are neutral in their effect on total plasma cholesterol levels, recent evidence indicates that oleic acid may help to decrease LDL-cholesterol levels when substituted for saturated fatty acids [28, 36]. Monounsaturated fatty acids should constitute 10 to 15 percent of total calories in both the step 1 and the step 2 diets.

Polyunsaturated fatty acids are of two types: omega-6 and omega-3 fatty acids [33]. The major omega-6 fatty acid is linoleic acid, found primarily in common cooking oils, such as safflower, corn, sesame, soybean, cottonseed, and sunflower oils. This fatty acid is known to have a cholesterol-lowering action for both total plasma cholesterol and LDL-cholesterol [34, 35, 36]. It is particularly useful in managing dyslipidemia when substituted for part of the saturated fat intake [36]. Omega-3 fatty acids are found in high concentrations in fish oils. They do not appear useful for reducing LDL-cholesterol levels, although they have been found useful in lowering triglycerides [33]. More generally, fish is a good choice for low-fat diet plans because it is low in saturated fat and has been shown to be associated with a reduction in CHD risk [26, 28].

Nutritional management of elevated blood lipid levels should include restriction of total dietary fat intake, with an emphasis on substituting unsaturated fatty acids for saturated fatty acids within a limit of 30 percent of total calories from fat. For patients who need to lose weight, it is also important to remember that all fats, irrespective of fatty acid composition, are equally high in calories: 9 kcal/gm, or 100 kcal/tablespoon.

The implementation of these principles is complicated by emerging research and the fact that many foods contain combinations of various types of fatty acids. Not all saturated fats raise cholesterol; stearic acid is a saturated fatty acid that either lowers or negligibly affects the levels of total plasma cholesterol and LDL cholesterol [37]. Significant sources of stearic acid include cocoa butter, chocolate, and red meat. However, these food products contain other significant sources of saturated fatty acids that are hypercholesterolemic. Thus, the new data on stearic acid would not warrant recommendations to increase consumption of chocolate and red meat. Another recent development involves a process for preparing ground beef (heating it in vegetable oil and rinsing it in boiling water) that greatly reduces the saturated fat content [38]. This process has not yet been introduced on a wide scale, however, and may turn out to be more costly and troublesome than simply eating foods that naturally contain less saturated fat [39].

Dietary Cholesterol

The step 1 diet recommends a dietary cholesterol intake of less than 300 mg/day; the step 2 diet calls for less than 200 mg/day of dietary cholesterol [26]. Clinical, animal, and epidemiologic studies indicate that dietary cholesterol raises serum total cholesterol and LDL-cholesterol levels and increases the risk of CHD [4]. However, dietary cholesterol appears to produce variable responses in total plasma cholesterol and LDL-cholesterol levels both within and between individuals [4, 26]. Dietary modifications to lower saturated-fat intake usually lower cholesterol intake at the same time. Dietary cholesterol is found only in animal products — particularly rich sources of cholesterol include egg yolks and organ meats (liver, kidney, sweetbread, brain). Other important sources include high-fat dairy products, meat, poultry, and some kinds of shellfish. While current scientific data warrant limiting dietary cholesterol in lipid-lowering diets, it is important that patients not be left with the misconception that reducing major sources of dietary cholesterol is the crux of recommended eating-pattern modifications [28].

CHOLESTEROL-SATURATED FAT INDEX (CSI) OF FOODS

The greatest cholesterol-lowering benefits come from a dietary reduction in both cholesterol and saturated fatty acids. To make it easier to identify foods that are low in both, Connor and associates have devised the cholesterol-saturated fat index (CSI) [40, 41]. The CSI reflects findings that emphasize the contribution of both saturated fat and dietary cholesterol to dietary control of total cholesterol and LDL-cholesterol [40, 41].

The CSI helps translate nutritional recommendations about sources of dietary fat into appropriate advice about foods. Shellfish (e.g., shrimp, crab, lobster), although they contain cholesterol, have a saturated-fat content near zero, and thus have a CSI of 6, similar to that of poultry and other fish. On the other hand, beef, pork, and lamb have CSI scores of 9 to 18, depending on the percentage of fat [41]. Table 9-2 lists the CSI of various common sources of dietary fat.

Complex Carbohydrates and Fiber

An increase in the consumption of carbohydrates to 50 to 60 percent of caloric intake is recommended in both the step 1 and the step 2 diets [26]. Specifically the recommendations suggest eating more complex carbohydrates (starches and fiber), emphasizing sources such as whole-grain foods, cereal products, vegetables, and fruits. These guidelines are consistent with current healthy-eating recommendations from several authoritative scientific and government bodies [3, 4, 6, 31]. Diets high in plant foods are usually low in fat, high in vitamins, and high in complex carbohydrates [24, 42]. This type of diet is associated with lower occurrence rates of CHD as well as lower occurrence rates of some cancers [4], although the specific mechanisms are not entirely understood.

Dietary fiber, which is the indigestible portion of plant foods, has been a focus of interest for its possible protective effect against CHD. There are several types of dietary fiber, and studies have examined their effects on lipid levels. It is difficult to interpret and compare many of the studies; it appears, however, that soluble fiber sources can significantly lower serum total cholesterol and LDL-cholesterol, while insoluble fibers produce variable results [24]. Soluble fibers that have been found to reduce cholesterol include pectin, guar gum, locust bean gum, oat gum, and psyllium. They are found in food

Table 9-2. Cholesterol-saturated fat index (CSI) and caloric content of selected foods

Food	CSI	Calories
Fish, poultry, red meat (3.5 ounces, or 100 grams, cooked)		
White fish (snapper, sole, cod, etc.), water-packed tuna, some shellfish (clams,		
oysters, scallops)	4	91
Shellfish (shrimp, crab, lobster)	6	104
Poultry, no skin	6	171
Beef, pork, and lamb:		
10% fat (ground sirloin, flank steak)	9	214
20% fat (ground chuck, pot roasts)	13	286
30% fat (ground beef, ribs, pork and lamb chops, roasts)	18	381
Cheese (3.5 ounces, or 100 grams)		
Cottage cheese (not low-fat)	6	139
Cheddar, Roquefort, Swiss, American cheeses	26	386
Whole eggs (2)	29	163
Peanut butter (¼ cup)	5	353
Fats (4 tablespoons, or ¼ cup)		
Soft vegetable margarines	10	423
Hard-stick margarines	15	432
Butter	37	430
Coconut oil, palm oil, cocoa butter (chocolate)	47	530
Milk (1 cup)		
Skim milk (0.1% fat)	<1	88
2% milk	4	144
Whole milk (3.5% fat)	7	159

Adapted from: Connor SL and Connor WE. The new American diet. New York: Simon and Schuster, 1986.

sources such as oatmeal, oat bran, barley, and legumes [24, 28]. Both oat bran [43, 44] and rice bran [44] have been found to be useful dietary sources of soluble fiber.

Weight Control: Caloric Intake and Energy Expenditure

Obesity is associated with elevated LDL-cholesterol levels and is also a risk factor for CHD and hypertension, as well as a number of other chronic illnesses, including diabetes mellitus, gallbladder disease, and osteoarthritis [4, 6, 45]. Overweight patients should reduce their total caloric intake and increase their energy expenditure through exercise to achieve a desirable weight. Weight control is an important part of nutritional intervention for high cholesterol in patients who are overweight [26, 42]. Also, weight loss promotes cholesterol lowering for many overweight patients [46]. Adherence to low-fat eating patterns with special attention to

moderate caloric restriction is congruent with safe weight-loss regimens.

Alcohol

Alcohol is not harmful when consumed in moderation; a high intake, however, is known to have adverse effects on health and safety. Alcohol is also high in calories and may contribute to excess weight in many individuals [47].

A number of studies indicate that moderate alcohol consumption can increase HDL-cholesterol concentrations [48, 49, 50]. However, the findings of a possible protective effect of alcohol aginst CHD remain uncertain and do not warrant the advice that consuming alcoholic beverages is desirable. The high caloric content of alcoholic beverages and the numerous social and health problems associated with excess drinking make it imprudent to encourage drinking in any given quantity. The use of alcohol in diets for prevention of CHD is not recommended [26]. On the other hand, the patient who normally drinks in moderation can be told that this is certainly within the bounds of an acceptable CHD-preventing diet.

Caffeine

Several studies have suggested that coffee drinking increases cholesterol and is associated with an increased incidence of myocardial infarction (MI), whereas other studies have shown just the opposite. No such association has been found with drinking tea, which also contains caffeine (though usually in somewhat lower concentrations). Most of the studies that have found an association indicate that drinking more than four to five cups of coffee per day increases risk of CHD mortality [51, 52]. Recent papers have more specifically identified a cholesterol-raising factor in boiled coffee that does not pass through a paper filter, and have described decaffeinated coffee as having a cholesterol-raising effect [52a, 52b].

It has been suggested that all or most of the excess incidence of MI in coffee drinkers is due to the smoking and/or other dietary habits of heavy coffee drinkers [53, 54]. Overall, there appears to be little evidence that coffee drinking in moderation is harmful. Moderation seems warranted because of the stimulant effects of high doses of caffeine.

Sodium Restriction

Restriction of sodium intake, in addition to weight reduction when warranted, has been recommended for the treatment of hypertension. The recommendation to limit the intake of salt is based on the epidemiologic association between high-salt diets with elevated blood pressure and the possibility of a dietary alternative to long-term drug treatment [4, 8, 55, 56]. It appears that those who are susceptible to salt-induced hypertension (i.e., they are salt sensitive) benefit most from this recommendation [4]; however, no test is currently available to identify such individuals. A recent review concluded that salt restriction should be prescribed only in "selected cases . . . when efficacy is demonstrated" [57]. Despite inconclusive evidence for the benefits of salt restriction in blood pressure control of individuals, recommendations for generally healthy individuals to consume fewer salty and highly processed foods remain in the current guidelines for healthy nutrition [3, 4, 6]. (See Chapter 13 for further discussion of this topic.)

The Role of Very Strict Diets

Diets even more restrictive than the step 2 diet have gained attention for their potential to reverse heart disease. The best known of these diet programs are part of lifestyle modifications based on the Pritikin program [58] and Dr. Dean Ornish's Lifestyle Heart Trial [9, 59]. The lifestyle programs include a diet very low in fat and high in complex carbohydrates, aerobic exercise, group support, stress management training, and smoking cessation [9]. The Lifestyle-Intervention Program at the Pritikin Longevity Center is a three-week residential program [58].

The diet in both these programs contains less than 10 percent of calories from fat, about 15 percent from protein, and the remainder from carbohydrates, with dietary cholesterol intake below 5 mg/day (the Ornish program) and 25 mg/day (the Pritikin program) [9, 58]. Both programs have resulted in substantially lower serum lipid levels, and in the Lifestyle Heart Trial, coronary angiography revealed partial regression of severe coronary atherosclerosis [9].

Such strict diets, as part of significant lifestyle modification programs, may be useful for patients who are highly motivated and have been unsuccessful at making gradual changes in their usual environments. If they can participate in and afford a residential center when beginning such a program, these programs are more likely to succeed. The physician should help the patient to evaluate available services, maintain communication with medical personnel, and resume careful supervision of the patient after the intensive phase. Careful supervision is also important to ensure nutritional adequacy in such diets. Extremely strict diets are not suitable for all patients, but when they are warranted the physician should work closely with the patient and other involved health care professionals.

The Nutritional Adequacy of Cholesterol-Lowering Diets

The low-fat, low-saturated-fat, low-cholesterol, low-calorie diet for hyperlipidemia is consistent with prudent diets for the population at large and carries little known risk in adults [60]. Traditionally, adequate diets have been defined as providing the types of foods that would contain sufficient amounts of essential nutrients to prevent deficiency diseases [3]. Clinical criteria of adequacy include nutrient intakes that avoid clinically detectable signs of deficiency and maintain normative tissue levels of nutrients in metabolic pools [61].

It is possible that some patients will alter their eating patterns to the extent that they will consume insufficient amounts of calcium and iron, or ingest complex carbohydrates in quantities that interfere with nutrient absorption. Patients should be encouraged to eat a variety of foods, which will help to ensure dietary adequacy. Adolescent girls and women should receive supervision and/or counseling regarding adequate calcium and iron intake, and pregnant and lactating women (in whom cholesterol levels are physiologically elevated) should receive specific nutritional guidelines for fetal and maternal health [5]. The benefits and risks of lipid-lowering diets require special attention in individuals with very low caloric intakes and in pregnant and lactating women. If the clinician or office staff have inadequate time or skills to provide intensive counseling, these patients should be referred to a qualified registered dietitian for additional consultation [5].

Controversies About Nutritional Intervention

The rapid pace of cholesterol reduction initiatives in the 1980s has given rise to considerable controversy in the medical community and the lay press. The critiques concern the scientific rationale for attempting large-scale efforts to detect elevated blood cholesterol levels, the use of nutritional intervention, the translation of the scientific data into the NCEP adult treatment guidelines, charges of profit-driven cholesterol-reduction campaigns, and concerns over public health policy in terms of resource allocation and the cost-benefit ratio of clinical prevention efforts [62].

The importance of high serum cholesterol levels as a risk factor for CHD and the benefits of cholesterol reduction for lowering risk are being increasingly accepted. However, the precise impact of lipid management through diet is not yet known in certain populations nor is the proportion of people who can respond adequately to dietary change [42]. Continuing research is needed along with clinical and public health efforts in cholesterol control.

Clinicians need to be familiar with the debates that reach the public and patients, support continued research to elucidate remaining questions, and understand the methodological limitations of cardiovascular nutrition research. They also need to be able to balance public health advice with clinical experience, understand the factors that affect individual eating patterns, and know practical strategies for incorporating the principles of cardiovascular risk-reducing diets into patient care.

To effect successful nutritional intervention with patients, clinicians need to be continually aware of the patient and the context of his world, remembering, in particular, that patients choose *foods* in their daily lives, not nutrients. Dietary behavior is complex and results from a series of actions, including food purchase, preparation, and ingestion. These actions are determined by multiple factors in the individual and the environment. The next section focuses on factors that affect dietary behavior and changes in such behavior.

Dietary Behavior: Determinants and Change Processes

Attempts to reduce risk by promoting dietary change pose several unique challenges to practitioners. Most diet-related health problems develop gradually and do not present immediate or dramatic symptoms. Eating patterns are habitual lifestyle behaviors, requiring long-term behavior change for the successful reduction of CHD risk. Recommendations for dietary change are usually restrictive, are often only one aspect of a complex medical regimen, and may be incompatible with individual or family eating habits. In addition, there may be barriers such as food costs, access, and the skill, time, and effort necessary for food preparation, which constrain compliance with therapeutic diets [63]. For many patients consistent and long-term adherence to a low-fat diet requires dramatic changes in shopping, meal planning, and cooking and eating habits [64].

The Multiple Determinants of Dietary Behavior

Many social, cultural, and economic factors contribute to the development, maintenance, and change of dietary patterns. No single factor or set of factors has been found to adequately account for why people eat as they do [65]. Physiologic and psychologic factors, acquired food preferences, and knowledge about foods are important individual determinants of food intake. Social factors are also important: families and other primary relationships influence food purchase, preparation, and consumption in many situations [66]. Socioeconomic status, economic change, and social support have been extensively studied in relation to eating patterns and the prevalence of chronic disease [67].

The influence of culture, geography, and food availability on eating habits can be quite dramatic, as shown in studies of Japanese-Americans who migrated to Hawaii and California and developed diet-related diseases as they adopted Western eating styles [68]. Cultural factors influence people's typical food choices in both qualitative and quantitative ways. People living in the United States may consider three ounces of shrimp to be adequate, but would be quite upset with a three-ounce steak. However, the same individuals willingly accept smaller amounts of red meat as it is prepared in a Chinese restaurant, mixed with vegetables, rice, and so on. Family customs and ethnic and religious celebrations also involve traditions that are deeply rooted in many people's ideas about what to eat and when and how to enjoy food.

Factors in the social and physical environment also affect food choices. These include the availability of healthful foods, point-of-choice in-formation about nutritional quality, policies and incentives for dietary behavior change, and access to sound nutritional advice in the medical care system and in the community [69].

Factors That Influence Changes in Dietary Behavior
KNOWLEDGE AND CONCERN ABOUT DIET AND CHRONIC DISEASE

Several national consumer surveys have recently found that Americans are more aware now of the relationship between food and health and are more concerned about what they are eating than at any other time in recent history [70, 71, 72, 73]. A 1982 survey of 4000 adults found that cardiovascular disease was identified as the most important diet-related problem in the nation [74]; an even greater proportion in a 1988 survey correctly identified excess cholesterol and saturated-fat intake as contributors to heart disease [71]. Results of the 1986 Cholesterol Awareness Survey showed that 72 percent of adults believe that reducing elevated cholesterol levels would have a large effect on preventing CHD [15].

Although Americans are more nutrition-conscious than in the past, this awareness may not be translated into changes toward healthy eating patterns. The FDA's Diet and Health Survey revealed several common misconceptions about food sources of dietary fat and cholesterol [71]. One review of several national surveys of nutrition attitudes and knowledge suggests that although basic nutrition knowledge has increased, most people lack an understanding of how to apply *specific* nutrition advice to the foods and ingredients they eat every day [75]. This suggests that, while awareness of and concern about nutrition have grown, many people either don't know how or are not yet motivated to apply nutritional guidance to their food choices. Thus, effective nutritional intervention with patients requires their understanding of how to apply specific knowledge to their dietary behavior [64, 76]. The following theories have been developed to help explain factors that affect behavior change. (For a more detailed discussion of these theories, see Chapter 7.)

PERSONAL HEALTH CONCERNS

Knowledge alone is not sufficient to change dietary behavior. Strategies for changing dietary behavior must also address individual, social, and environmental factors. For patients on lipid-lowering diets, it is usually safe to assume that a health concern, rather than cosmetic or social factors, is providing the impetus for dietary change [77]. The concept of personal vulnerability or susceptibility, as formulated in the health belief model (HBM), has been found predictive of a variety of positive health-related behaviors [78], including desirable changes in eating patterns [79]. Thus, it is important to emphasize an individual's specific risks, in terms of both lipid levels and coexisting CHD risk factors.

SOCIAL LEARNING FACTORS AND SELF-EFFICACY

In addition to models concerned with information use and health beliefs, efforts to assist in modifying eating behavior have drawn on social science theories [63, 77]. Strategies for dietary behavior change have often employed principles of behavior modification, including goal setting, behavioral contracting, monitoring, and reinforcement [63, 80]. Recently the most prominent models have used the social learning theory (SLT), or social cognitive theory, as a framework for understanding dietary change and organizing eating strategies for behavior change [81]. SLT incorporates behavior modification methods and also addresses cognitive (knowledge and attitude), interpersonal, and environmental influences on eating [82].

The basic components of behavioral approaches are (1) self-monitoring and analysis of behavior; (2) self-management, which includes stimulus control, that is, control of external cuse, or triggers, that set the occasion for eating high-fat foods; (3) the replacement of eating high-fat foods with such healthful behaviors as stress reduction techniques and exercise; and (4) reinforcement of desirable behaviors [63]. These strategies have been widely used in weight management programs and are a central component of comprehensive counseling for low-fat eating [77, 83].

SLT provides a model for change in which interpersonal and environmental factors receive attention. For example, there may be real support of or barriers to dietary change in family and work situations. These opportunities and constraints can be addressed and modified, thus improving the chances for healthier eating patterns.

The SLT concept of self-efficacy is also useful as a basis for fostering behavior change [84, 85]. Self-efficacy is defined as an individual's perception of his or her chances of success at mastering a given type of behavior; it is synonymous with self-confidence about performing a specific type of behavior. Behavioral and cognitive strategies such as setting small goals, monitoring, and self-reward can be used to increase self-efficacy and improve the motivation to attempt or maintain recommended dietary changes.

THE PROCESS OF DIETARY BEHAVIOR CHANGE: STAGES OF CHANGE

Dietary change involves multiple actions and adaptations over time. Some patients may not be ready to attempt changes, while others may be well along in implementing diet modifications. Psychologists in the areas of substance abuse and smoking cessation have developed a model of *stages of change,* which it may be fruitful to apply to nutritional change as well [86]. The model suggests that people are at various points along a continuum of change: precontemplation (unaware, not interested in change), contemplation (thinking about and making plans to change a behavior), action (actively modifying behvior and/or environment), and maintenance (maintaining the new, healthier behaviors) or relapse (returning to the old behavior) [87, 88]. People often recycle and repeat certain stages, such as individuals who relapse and go back to any of the preceding stages depending on their level of motivation and self-efficacy.

The stages of change model has a unique implication for the way success is defined in health counseling: it suggests that the traditional end points of behavior change and/or maintenance are not the only successes but that *movement through the stages* is also a mark of success. Thus, a wider range of intermediary steps can be viewed as successful, or at least positive, outcomes, which eventually lead to the desired behavior change.

The maintenance of a nutritional change can be strengthened with a strategy for behavior change known as *relapse prevention,* which encourages patients to develop problem-solving skills to help strengthen their commitment and ability to continue new behaviors. Its primary focus is the maintenance of the behavioral change through self-management or self-control procedures [89]. Examples of relapse prevention skills and attitudes for improving dietary self-management include skills to deal with stressful or challenging situations, positive cognitions (attitudes, attributions) concerning one's ability to control behaviors, and health-promoting behaviors such as exercise and stress reduction techniques as part of a daily lifestyle [89].

Most of the precedents for applying these behavior change models to healthy behavior come from smoking cessation and weight management studies. They require some adaptation for nutritional intervention and counseling for CHD prevention, but they offer promising strategies for clinically based intervention. For example, studies suggest that self-management materials based on the stages of change model, self-help nutrition programs using minimal contact, and brief physician counseling [90] can improve the feasibilty of delivering effective nutritional intervention in health care.

An important caveat in applying these models is in order. Dietary change for cardiovascular risk reduction involves *qualitative* dietary change, and lipid abnormalities do not share the recognized cosmetic or addictive properties of changes in body weight or smoking. There may be less reason to pay attention to *intra*psychic factors in low-fat dietary intervention (e.g., emotional eating, self-esteem, stress as a trigger) than for behaviors related to weight control and smoking cessation. In this situation, the knowledge/information component is more prominent. Clinicians need to be aware of the wide variety of individual factors involved in patients' efforts to make dietary changes.

The Practice of Nutritional Intervention in Preventive Cardiology

Comprehensive nutritional intervention involves a cyclical sequence of diagnosis/assessment; treatment; and evaluation, monitoring, and follow-up [63, 77, 91, 92]. Thorough *assessment* for diagnosis and treatment includes evaluation of lipids and other CHD risk factors, dietary evaluation, and assessment of relevant psychosocial, behavioral, and educational factors. *Treatment* includes dietary advice and nutrition counseling; if dietary management alone is ineffective, it may be supplemented by pharmacologic agents (see Chapter 12). During counseling intervention the patient and the physician negotiate a plan for change with specific goals and strategies to achieve them. *Evaluation, monitoring, and follow-up* involve assessment of compliance and treatment effectiveness, negotiation of new goals, adjustment of regimens as indicated, and periodic monitoring once risk factor control is achieved.

Each phase of the cycle of nutrition intervention can be carried out by a variety of health professionals. The physician, however, should be involved to some extent in all phases, establishing office systems and communication mechanisms that maximize coordination and providing for medical supervision when necessary.

A traditional model of nutrition intervention includes physician evaluation, referral to a dietitian, a one-to-one counseling relationship between patient and dietitian, repeated counseling sessions over a period of time, and periodic medical follow-up. However, this model is not feasible for many physicians and their patients. Application of the guidelines for management of dyslipidemia are likely to be based on the judgment of the physician, the preferences of the patient, and the context of the health care situation [93]. Thus, it is essential to consider alternative models for nutritional intervention to reduce CHD risk.

Basic models of intervention, along a continuum of intensity, range from simple and brief physician advice to intensive and long-term counseling by a nutritionist. This chapter emphasizes the availability of various options and encourages clinicians to consider developing and/or adapting systematic and structured methods that they can implement in their practices.

Step 1: Diagnosis/Assessment

Thorough assessment is the foundation of effective nutrition intervention. Patient assessment should include evaluation of the following:

- lipids and other CHD risk factors
- dietary intake
- relevant behavioral, psychosocial, and educational factors

The results of these assessments should then be used to tailor therapy and establish treatment goals and expectations. Assessment of dietary intake and behavioral, psychosocial, and educational factors is discussed next.

ASSESSMENT OF DIETARY INTAKE

Measurement of dietary intake for clinical evaluation and planning nutritional intervention is a mainstay of nutritional management, and helps to focus initial dietary advice and to evaluate adherence to a regimen [80]. In choosing a method for assessing dietary intake, it is important to consider *why* the assessment is being done, what factors are of interest, and how detailed the assessment must be [94]. In clinical settings dietary assessment may differ from measurement for research purposes — the focus is primarily to identify the needed areas of emphasis of dietary advice for individual patients, identify specific deviations from the regimen, and evaluate progress [80]. Although no dietary assessment method is perfect, clinicians should use approaches that are feasible and that elicit reproducible, valid data representative of the usual diet over time [95, 96].

Much concern has been expressed about the validity of self-reports of eating behavior, due to problems of clients' willingness and ability to record or recall exactly what they eat and the difficulty of accurately interpreting the nutrient implications of reported intakes [97]. Most patients, however, are willing to report what they eat and to disclose problems with their regimens if they are asked questions in a nonthreatening, nonjudgmental way [98]. Also, the use of scoring/analysis methods that involve patients in interaction with the provider where the patient provides much of the necessary information promotes awareness of the eating pattern and fosters a patient-centered approach to nutritional management [80]. (See Chapter 7 for discussion of a patient-centered approach.)

The most common types of dietary assessment methodologies are 24-hour-diet recalls, food frequency questionnaires (FFQs), detailed diet histories, and food diaries or records, usually for three, four, or seven days [94]. Computerized analysis systems may also be useful for detailed nutrient analyses. These programs and detailed diet histories are very time-consuming, however, and are more likely to be used by consulting dietitians than by physicians. In assessing diets of individual patients, the two most important considerations are usual intakes and correct interpretation as a basis for intervention [94]. Thus, FFQs are likely to be most practical in clinical intervention.

One dietary assessment method, used in the Multiple Risk Factor Intervention Trial (MRFIT), was the Food Record Rating (FRR) tool. This instrument has established validity based on blood lipid effect and combines patient self-evaluation with counselor evaluation [99, 100]. The FRR was administered by trained nutritionists. It is too time-consuming for some clinical settings, and shorter measures have been reported or are currently being studied. One brief measure is an eight-item questionnaire developed by Heller and colleagues in Great Britain [101] which was found to have criterion validity relative to cholesterol response.

The Eating Pattern Assessment Tool (EPAT) is an FFQ that can be self-administered or counselor-administered. The EPAT was developed and has been tested in the Physician-Based Nutrition Program (PBNP) in Minnesota. Studies of the reliability and validity of the EPAT indicate that it can be used repeatedly over several months without significant loss of reliability [102] and that it provides a reasonably valid indicator of an individual's usual fat and cholesterol intake [103].

Another brief FFQ, the Dietary Risk Assessment (DRA), was developed as a culturally specific assessment tool for low-income southern populations. It can be easily administered and scored by a nonnutritionist in 10 to 15 minutes. The DRA identifies both positive and problematic dietary behaviors, is easy to interpret, and assesses potential barriers to dietary change. Validation of the DRA using a Keys score revealed a significant positive correlation (r = .60, p < .001) [104]. An abbreviated version of the DRA was used in a trial of resident education for cholesterol management (the Cholesterol and Diet Resident Education Project (CADRE)) [105]. This "Food and Your Heart" tool, shown as Figure 9-3, is easy to use and can be self-administered by the patient or completed with a physician, nutritionist, or other office staff.* It can be self-scored and linked directly to dietary change goals (see Figure 9-5, p. 254). A version of this instrument adapted for a middle-class population has also been developed [105a].

Additional work is in progress to develop valid, reliable, and practical tools for assessing eating patterns related to CHD prevention. Dissemination of current work should occur in the near future. In addition, scientists working in diet and cancer control have developed brief screening tools to assess high intakes of dietary fat, which may have applications in clinical prevention settings [106, 107, 107a].

A final consideration in the choice of dietary assessment methods is the personnel needed to administer and score the assessments. Most FFQ methods can be self-administered, although some patients require assistance in completing the forms. Some tools are best administered by a qualified nutritionist or a specially trained nurse, but others can be managed effectively by

*Source: Alice Ammerman, DrPH, RD, Department of Nutrition, University of North Carolina at Chapel Hill, CB 7400, Chapel Hill, NC 27599

other office staff (e.g., medical assistant, receptionist). Scoring systems should be efficient, and the physician should, at a minimum, provide key nutritional advice based on the assessment.

ASSESSMENT OF BEHAVIORAL, PSYCHOSOCIAL, AND EDUCATIONAL FACTORS

While some form of assessment of dietary intake has long been routine in nutritional intervention, a thorough problem diagnosis, which includes investigation of behavioral, psychosocial, and educational factors, is conducted much less often [63, 108]. This type of assessment explores the factors that contribute to dietary patterns and those that are most relevant in promoting behavior change. Tools to examine antecedents to eating behaviors have become accepted practice in behavior modification strategies for weight reduction [77, 109], but few such tools have been reported for low-fat dietary management.

In-depth behavioral diagnosis should assess as much of the following information as possible: previous dietary-change experience, views about coexisting risk factors, involvement in food purchase and preparation, other significant individuals (family, friends, roommates) who influence the patient's eating patterns, belief in the need for and the importance of modifying eating patterns, interest in and readiness to attempt dietary changes, potential barriers to change, self-efficacy or self-confidence for making dietary changes, educational sophistication, and preference for various types of intervention modalities. Many of these factors are interrelated. Prior dietary-change experience, and views about coexisting risk factors can have a major impact on the patient's efforts to make dietary changes and are worth taking the time to consider at the outset [81].

Dietary-Change Experience. Many adults, particularly those with a history of being overweight, have made multiple attempts to modify their eating patterns. Others have been involved in dietary-change or therapeutic diets through

Food And Your Heart
(Circle the number or word to the right)

Meat

How many times a week do you eat...

Meat for breakfast?	0	1 2 3	4+
Hot dogs or lunch meat? (like bologna)?	0	1 2 3	4+
Chicken or fish?	4+	3 2	1 0
• Is the fish usually fried?	No	Sometimes	Yes
• Is the chicken usually fried?	No	Sometimes	Yes
• Do you usually eat the chicken skin?	No	Sometimes	Yes
Supper without meat?	3+	2 1	0

Eggs

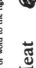

How many eggs a week do you eat? 0 1 2 3 4 5+

Dairy

How many times a week do you eat or drink...

Whole milk	0 1	2	3+
Cheese—including on sandwiches or in mixed dishes	0 1 2	3 4	5+
Ice cream	0 1	2	3+

Invisible Fats

How many times a week do you eat...

Sweets: pies, cakes, cookies, donuts, sweet rolls, or chocolate candy	0 1 2	3 4	5+
Biscuits	0 1	2 3	4+
French fries, fried potatoes, or hash browns	0 1 2	3 4	5+

Cooking

When you eat fried food at home, what is it usually fried in?	Veg. oil	Margarine Veg. short. (solid, in can)	Meat grease Butter
How are your vegetables usually seasoned, especially greens?	Nothing Salt/pepper Herbs/spices Veg. oil Vinegar	Margarine Ham	Butter Fat back Side meat Bacon
Do you usually eat margarine or butter?	Margarine	Both	Butter
If you use margarine, what type is it?	Soft/diet	Stick	
What kind of shortening is usually used for baking in your home?	Veg. oil Margarine	Veg. short. (solid, in can)	Butter Lard

Snacks, Starches

How many times a week do you eat...

Snack chips like potato chips, corn chips, pork skins, or cheese snacks	0 1 2	3 4	5+
Snack crackers, like "Nabs"	0 1 2	3 4	5+
Rice, potatoes, or noodles	5+	4 3	2 1

How many times a day do you eat...

Fruits or vegetables	4+	3 2	1 0

> Now, please go back and look at the things you circled in the middle and the right hand column. Mark 2 of these foods or habits that you would be willing to work on with your doctor.

What do you think?
(Circle the answer you agree with most)

Does food that is good for your heart taste good and satisfy you?	Yes	Not sure	No
Would it be easy or hard for you to give up foods that aren't good for you?	Easy	Not sure	Hard
Is it better for your heart to stay away from starchy foods (like bread, potatoes, or rice)?	No	Not sure	Yes
Do you think all foods that say "cholesterol free" on the label are OK for your heart?	No	Not sure	Yes

Figure 9-3. "Food and your heart" dietary assessment.

a family member or close friend. Their personal efforts, involvement with others' dietary changes, and experiences of success and failure set the stage for their motivation and confidence in the present situation.

After assessing dietary behavior and determining possible problem areas that contribute to high dietary-fat intake, the patient should be asked about past experiences, the nature of the change effort(s), and the level of success or experience with that (those) efforts. An example of a more in-depth line of questioning follows:

• Have you ever thought about reducing your intake of red meat?
• Have you ever tried to do so?
• How did you do it? Did you seek outside help? What kind?
• How successful were you in making this change?
• What problems did you encounter?
• What did you do to deal with those problems?
• What do you think you can do now to be successful at reducing your intake of red meat?

These questions, adapted from a brief clinical approach for smoking cessation counseling [90], allow both patient and clinician to learn from and build on prior experiences. The focus in the encounter is on overcoming the stumbling blocks, or barriers, to change in a personally relevant manner. The patient provides much of the information, which can be used collaboratively by the patient and the physician to help the patient develop goals and plans for change.

Coexisting Risk Factors. The existence of other risk factors may affect patient motivation and ability to change eating patterns in paradoxical ways. On the one hand, they may make the need for change compelling for the patient (for example, after bypass surgery or an MI). On the other hand, they may overwhelm the patient with the many needed aspects of lifestyle modification. In the MRFIT, men with concurrent cardiovascular disease risk factors (smoking and/or hypertension) were less successful at adhering to low-fat diets and reducing their lipids

[110]. Of course, the patient's interest in attempting dietary change should be considered along with the practitioner's clinical judgment, with both based on an understanding of the total risk factor profile. One option is to postpone dietary intervention until other changes have been accomplished (for example, stopping smoking). Another option is to emphasize only those dietary changes the patient believes will be easier to make (for example, eating more fish and poultry instead of red meat). A third approach is to focus on diet modification and deemphasize reduction of other risks in the interim.

USE OF ASSESSMENT FOR TAILORING TREATMENT GOALS

Nutritional intervention is more likely to be effective if it includes not only biochemical and clinical evaluation but targeted dietary assessment and behavioral-psychosocial-educational assessment as well. Comprehensive assessment of the patient's situation sets the stage for realistic treatment goals, and a patient-centered approach is most likely to garner the patient's motivation for risk reduction.

Step 2: Treatment/Intervention
DIETARY ADVICE

The NCEP adult treatment guidelines are intended for use by health professionals. Patients need concrete, practical information about the foods they eat to adhere to a prescribed regimen. Adoption of a cholesterol-lowering diet requires that patients master a large body of knowledge related to their daily food choices [111]. In addition patients need to learn behavioral and cognitive skills to support their efforts to adapt to a modified eating pattern.

In time-limited informational sessions most health professionals tend to focus on core concepts, i.e., the nutrients that are the foundation of the therapeutic diet. While it is true that patients who learn these concepts and their applications will be best equipped for long-term compliance, this may not be the best place to start. Patients need to believe that they can master the information they receive; thus, examples of foods to be limited, avoided, and emphasized should be the focus of brief dietary advice. Everyone can relate to, and most people can remember, concrete suggestions. Supplementary teaching, print educational materials, and in-depth counseling and classes should be provided for those who are willing and able to seek and/or attend them.

This section focuses on practical elements of delivering nutritional intervention for CHD prevention. First, the role of print educational materials and considerations in selecting them is addressed. Dietary counseling, especially brief counseling that a physician can implement, is discussed next, followed by a section addressing referral for counseling and classes and collaboration with consulting dietitians.

Written Educational Materials. Even the best oral communication with a patient can result in misunderstanding and memory failure over time [112]. Thus, an important adjunct to education and counseling for changing dietary behavior is written cholesterol education materials. Since these aids to self-management are taken by patients when they leave the office, the provider should pay attention to developing and/or selecting them.

It is essential that educational materials be accessible and understandable to the individuals for whom they are intended. All too often in nutrition education concern about technical accuracy of content has taken priority over readability and understandability [113]. Educational materials may be written at too sophisticated a level in terms of wording and concepts. A recent analysis of readability levels of 38 printed, publicly available sets of cholesterol education materials revealed that the average reading grade level was close to grade 11, which is too difficult for many adults [114].

Numerous off-the-shelf cholesterol education pamphlets and brochures are available from voluntary health agencies, professional associations, government organizations, and corporations in quantity and at low or no cost to health professionals [114]. Dietary goal sheets that are coordinated with the previously described dietary assessment forms are available as part of the "Food and Your Heart" tool de-

scribed on pages 246 and 254 (Figures 9-3 and 9-5). The NCEP's "Physician's Kit on High Blood Cholesterol" contains background information, posters for office use, and samples of patient brochures. Table 9-3 lists other sources of nutrition education information. Educational materials are more useful when they are suitable for and appealing to the type of patients seen in a given practice.

Physicians, their office staff, and other collaborating health professionals should be familiar with their patients' average reading levels and cultural backgrounds and evaluate print educational materials with these in mind. Any new materials developed in-house should be pretested on people similar to the patients who will receive them. (If current staff are unfamiliar with pretesting methods, health educators or communications consultants can help.) Also, in the course of counseling, the physician or other counselor can go through, mark, and "translate" some difficult words, so the patient will not be confused later. For patients who want more information about the cholesterol-lowering diet, including details about disease processes, brand-name product lists, and recipes, many books are available in bookstores. Several useful and scientifically credible books are listed at the end of this chapter.

BEHAVIORAL AND EDUCATIONAL TECHNIQUES: PHYSICIAN-DELIVERED DIETARY INTERVENTION

In a busy office practice a variety of models for patient nutrition counseling are possible [91]. The four basic models, along a continuum from simple and brief to intensive and long-term, are (1) brief physician advice, (2) brief individual physician counseling, (3) brief counseling with referral for comprehensive individual counseling, and (4) brief counseling with referral for group education, either one session or long term. Combinations of these models and of individual and group counseling are also possible.

Brief Physician Advice. In the model of brief physician advice, the physician informs patients with elevated cholesterol who require dietary treatment about their CHD risk and the initial

Table 9-3.   Sources of information for nutrition intervention

Source	What they provide
National Sources	
National Cholesterol Education Program (NCEP)	Physician's kit on high blood cholesterol
	Guidelines for screening, treatment
Sponsored by: National Heart, Lung, and Blood Institute (NHLBI)	Written educational materials
	Reports and examples of programs
NHLBI Information Center 4733 Bethesda Ave., Suite 530 Bethesda, MD 20814–4820 (301) 951-3260	
American Dietetic Association 216 W. Jackson Blvd., Suite 800 Chicago, IL 60606–6995 (312) 899-0040	Referral to local dietitians
	Information about dietitians specializing in sports and cardiovascular nutrition (SCAN practice group)
	Written educational materials
	Professional journal with current policies and research
American Medical Association 535 North Dearborn Street Chicago, IL 60610 (312) 645-5000	Catalog of nutrition publications
	Continuing education programs
Society for Nutrition Education 2001 Killebrew Drive, Suite 340 Minneapolis, MN 55425–1882 (612) 854-0035 or (800) 235-6690	Referral to local nutrition educators
	Written educational materials
	Professional journal with current educational research
Local Sources	
American Heart Association	
American Dietetic Association (state and local offices)	
Society for Nutrition Education (large metropolitan areas)	

treatment approach with diet. Without in-depth discussion, the provider emphasizes the risk of high blood cholesterol and the potential effectiveness of dietary management. This can be followed by providing print materials about the diet, answering any questions, establishing the need for periodic follow-up, and designating a member of the office staff who is available to answer additional questions. The physician's role is that of educator, motivator, and adviser. The estimated time for brief nutritional advice and provision of written materials is two to five minutes.

Brief Dietary Counseling. Brief counseling requires more time than does simply giving advice. Counseling can be implemented by a physician or other trained health professional such as a nutritionist, nurse, or patient health educator. It can stand alone when a patient is unlikely to return for further counseling, or it can be a first step toward comprehensive counseling. (See Chapter 7 for an in-depth discussion of counseling.) The three major components are assessment of readiness for change, motivation or action planning, and follow-up [81]. Thus further assessment and follow-up are part of the counseling process. A unique feature of this approach is that it does not assume that all patients are equally motivated, ready, or interested in attempting dietary changes. Through continued assessment, the physician or a counselor decides how to help move the patient toward change.

Figure 9-4 illustrates a model that can be used

Figure 9-4.   Brief dietary counseling for low-fat eating. (Source: Adapted from Glanz, K, In: Kris-Etherton PM, ed. Cardiovascular Disease: Nutrition for Prevention and Treatment. Chicago: The American Dietetic Association, 1990.)

A.   Assess Risks

CONCURRENT RISKS: **FAMILY HISTORY:**

[ ]   Obesity   [ ] Coronary Heart Disease
[ ]   Hypertension   [ ] Hypertension
[ ]   Diabetes   [ ] High Cholesterol
[ ]   Little Physical Activity   [ ] Diabetes
[ ]   Smoking

RISK INDICATORS: **DIETARY BEHAVIORS:**

Total Cholesterol _____ mg/dl   [ ] Vegetarian
LDL Cholesterol _____ mg/dl   [ ] Eats fish/poultry ≥3/wk
HDL Cholesterol _____ mg/dl   High Intake of:
Triglycerides _____ mg/dl   ___ red meat   ___ dairy products
                                                ___ eggs   ___ baked goods

---

B.   Counsel
        ASK: Are you interested in working on decreasing your dietary fat intake?

              [ ] Yes or Maybe   [ ] No

1.   ASSESS HISTORY OF CHANGE   MOTIVATE:
       EFFORTS:
"Have you decreased your dietary fat   PERSONALIZE the benefits of
intake in the past?"   adopting low-fat eating behaviors

[ ] Yes; tried...   [ ] No
       [ ] on my own   1. Reduce current health risks
       [ ] with family/friend   2. Avoid hereditary health problems
       [ ] through a health   3. Feel better
             ed/counseling program
       [ ] to lose weight only; no other
             low-fat change tried

"What changes did you make?"   INCREASE AWARENESS:
   Decreased or reduced fat in: INFORMATION, BEHAVIOR
   ___ red meat   ___ dairy products
   ___ eggs   ___ baked goods   1. Reinforce "+" habits
                                                2. Note available sources of information
What problems did you have in   3. Suggest ways to identify opportunities
changing?   in everyday life for choosing low-fat
                                                   foods
REINFORCE: Encourage to continue
                with changes

2. ASSESS OBSTACLES TO ADOPTING A LOW-FAT EATING PATTERN:

FOLLOW-UP

[ ]   I like the foods I eat now, would have to give up favorites.

[ ]   Don't know how to fit low-fat foods into the way I eat.

[ ]   Don't know which foods I can eat on a low-fat diet. There are too many things to remember.

[ ]   Too rushed, too much work to buy or fix low-fat foods.

[ ]   Eating out a lot

[ ]   Someone else buys and prepares [most of] my food.

If not motivated to change, check on motivation at next visit or call.

3. HELP PATIENT ADDRESS CONCERNS AND CONSIDER SUITABLE INTERVENTION MODALITY/IES (see Table 9–4)

4. SUGGEST A SPECIFIC APPROACH TO CHANGE

Advise person to attempt changes gradually; each change will help.
Suggest signing up for a class, reading, or meeting with a nutritionist for individualized counseling.

Suggest keeping track of eating patterns most closely related to low-fat eating pattern: meat, dairy, eggs, poultry, fish, alcohol, etc.

Reinforce positive habits.
Encourage the person to discuss changes s/he is trying to make with family and friends.
Remind the person that s/he can learn easy ways to adopt low fat eating patterns.

GIVE OUT WRITTEN EDUCATIONAL MATERIAL

FOLLOW-UP
Check on change at next visit or call.
Reinforce/encourage and counsel if problems arise.

for nutritional counseling. Alternative sequences and questions can be used and should be tailored to the constraints and needs of the physician and the patient. The step before treatment, *assessment of risks,* includes review of the patient's risk indicators, including comorbidity, CHD risk factors, lipid profile, past and present dietary behavior, and positive dietary habits (to the extent that this information is available). A brief discussion of the patient's risks, along with verification that he understands the health problems and anticipates the multiple behavioral changes that may need to be faced (e.g., the need to stop smoking as well as reduce dietary fat) establishes the point for initiating treatment.

Assessment of readiness for change is an important step in brief dietary counseling. After explaining that a diet low in dietary fat will reduce the patient's cardiac risk, the practitioner needs to determine if the patient is interested in working on making changes at this time. This can be asked by a question such as "Are you willing to work on reducing yor dietary fat intake at this time?" If the patient replies "Yes" or "Maybe," the provider proceeds to assessment of past dietary change experience, helping the patient to identify possible problems that may occur, and possible steps to take to counter them. If the patient replies "No," the provider can help the patient develop the necessary motivation and then follow up at a later visit. Most patients are willing and able to make some changes.

If the patient is interested in improving his eating pattern, discussion and planning for possible problems when making changes are important next steps. Planning builds on a review of past experiences. When asking about previous efforts to make dietary changes, the practitioner should determine what the changes were, whether outside help was sought, and the successes and problems encountered. This information is a foundation for the next step, helping patients to address concerns.

Addressing concerns involves engaging the patient in a discussion about the obstacles or problems that might interfere with adopting a low-fat eating pattern. Problem-solving assistance can help the patient develop his own solutions. The practitioner can also be prepared with sugestions of ways to overcome the most common concerns, such as those listed in Table 9-4.

For the person not yet considering change, the precontemplator, it is necessary to increase motivation by personalizing the benefits of change and increasing awareness and opportunities for thinking about change efforts. A key approach is to emphasize the benefits of dietary change rather than the risks of not changing. To increase awareness, available sources of information can be suggested (e.g., labels on packaged foods), and everyday opportunities for trying small changes can be pointed out (e.g., trying frozen yogurt the next time the urge for ice cream strikes). The patient should be encouraged to think about what — not whether — he is willing to change. Follow-up can be a phone call or can occur at the next visit.

As part of planning for change, a few suggestions for initiating dietary modifications can be given. The provider should recommend suitable intervention modalities for the patient, such as printed educational materials, comprehensive individual counseling with a dietitian, group education, or a combination of these. The effectiveness of behavioral approaches is usually enhanced by negotiating a plan for change (see Chapter 7) and agreeing on at least one specific patient goal. The goal might involve reduction of dietary fat intake in one food area such as red meats or follow-through on a referral for further education and counseling. The goal and/or referral should be written, not only in the medical chart but also on a page or card that the patient can take home. An example of a tool that can be used for goal setting appears in Figure 9-5. This two-sided information sheet is linked directly to the dietary assessment (see Figure 9-3) and is perforated for the patient to take home. To help both the provider and the patient to remember the eating patterns that need attention, it uses the acronym MEDICS: Meat, Eggs, Dairy, Invisible fats, Cooking, and Snacks/Starches [105].

Follow-up to brief dietary counseling can be done by a phone call from the physician or office staff or by flagging the patient's chart for atten-

Table 9-4. Possible responses to patients' concerns

Patient concern	Physician response
"I like the foods I eat now and would have to give up my favorite foods."	"Even though adopting a low-fat eating pattern means making changes in how you eat, you don't have to give up the foods you like. You might have to cut down on them or plan for those choices, though."
"I don't know how to fit low-fat foods into the way I eat."	"Small, gradual changes are the key." "Often you can eat the same type of foods; you have to change only the way the food is prepared or the portion size."
"I don't know which foods I can eat on a low-fat diet — there are too many things to remember."	"It seems complicated at first, but once you learn some basic ideas and begin to pay attention to what you eat, choosing foods will get easier." "Some of the guides, books, manuals, or classes you can attend will include convenient wallet-size reminder cards; the tipsheet from our office should be helpful also." "Learning to read labels can go a long way in helping you choose low-fat foods."
"I'm too rushed; it's too much work to buy or fix low-fat foods." "I eat out a lot."	"It's easy to learn ways to cook low-fat foods without too much work; once you pick out some low-fat foods that are your favorites, you will find it even easier." "Often you can fix foods partially in advance and save time in the long run." "Some of the foods need *less* preparation; for example, fresh fruit and not making heavy sauces or fried foods." "Once you learn some basic ideas and tips, you will find it easy to choose low-fat foods when eating out."
"Someone else buys and prepares (most of) my food."	"In that case, you will want to have that person work with you as you try to develop a low-fat way of eating."

Source: Glanz, K. In Kris-Etherton PM, ed. Cardiovascular Disease: Nutrition for Prevention and Treatment. Chicago: The American Dietetic Association, 1990.

tion to nutrition at the next scheduled visit. A designated follow-up appointment should be scheduled if indicated.

Brief Physician Counseling with Referral for Comprehensive Individual Counseling. Most physicians are unable to devote long patient counseling sessions to nutritional intervention. Brief counseling can help to identify patients who are ready for action and motivated to work toward dietary change. Those patients often benefit from in-depth nutritional counseling or group education sessions. Referral does not signal the end of the physician's nutritional man-

agement of the patient; rather, it supplements and extends her efforts. The physician, along with support from office staff, should make specific suggestions about referral sources, establish communication with the consulting provider, and obtain follow-up reports. Referral to counseling can involve referral to a qualified counselor in the office practice or to a consulting dietitian. Individual counseling gives the patient personal attention and follow-up over an extended period of time. The counselor can also work closely with the patient to deal with challenging situations and answer technical food-related questions. There is more time to

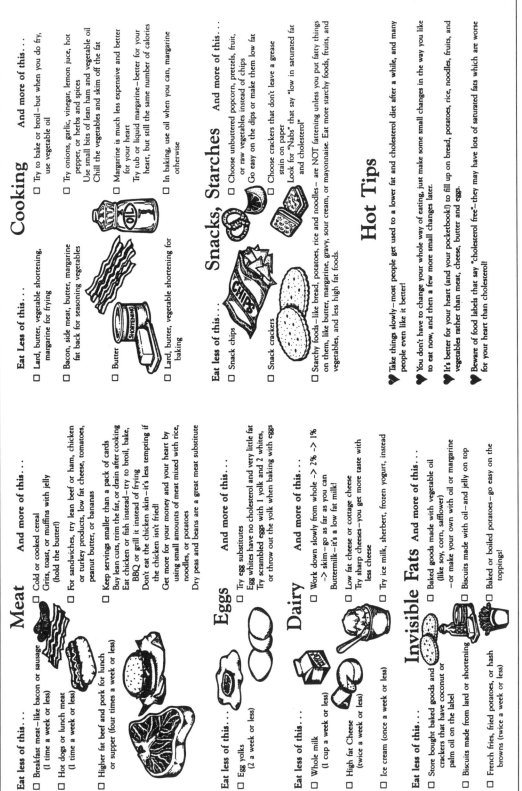

Meat

Eat less of this...

- ☐ Breakfast meat—like bacon or sausage (1 time a week or less)
- ☐ Hot dogs or lunch meat (1 time a week or less)
- ☐ Higher fat beef and pork for lunch or supper (four times a week or less)

And more of this...

- ☐ Cold or cooked cereal
  Grits, toast, or muffins with jelly (hold the butter!)
- ☐ For sandwiches, try lean beef or ham, chicken or turkey products, low fat cheese, tomatoes, peanut butter, or bananas
- ☐ Keep servings smaller than a pack of cards
  Buy lean cuts, trim the fat, or drain after cooking
  Eat chicken or fish instead—try to broil, bake, BBQ or grill it instead of frying
  Don't eat the chicken skin—it's less tempting if the chicken isn't fried!
  Get more for your money and your heart by using small amounts of meat mixed with rice, noodles, or potatoes
  Dry peas and beans are a great meat substitute

Eggs

Eat less of this...

- ☐ Egg yolks (2 a week or less)

And more of this...

- ☐ Try egg substitutes
  Egg whites have no cholesterol and very little fat
  Try scrambled eggs with 1 yolk and 2 whites, or throw out the yolk when baking with eggs

Dairy

Eat less of this...

- ☐ Whole milk (1 cup a week or less)
- ☐ High fat Cheese (twice a week or less)
- ☐ Ice cream (once a week or less)

And more of this...

- ☐ Work down slowly from whole –> 2% –> 1% –> skim—go as far as you can
  Buttermilk—it's a low fat milk!
- ☐ Low fat cheese or cottage cheese
  Try sharp cheeses—you get more taste with less cheese
- ☐ Try ice milk, sherbert, frozen yogurt, instead

Invisible Fats

Eat less of this...

- ☐ Store bought baked goods and crackers that have coconut or palm oil on the label
- ☐ Biscuits made from lard or shortening
- ☐ French fries, fried potatoes, or hash browns (twice a week or less)

And more of this...

- ☐ Baked goods made with vegetable oil (like soy, corn, safflower) —or make your own with oil or margarine
- ☐ Biscuits made with oil—and jelly on top
- ☐ Baked or boiled potatoes—go easy on the toppings!

Cooking

Eat Less of this...

- ☐ Lard, butter, vegetable shortening, margarine for frying
- ☐ Bacon, side meat, butter, margarine fat back for seasoning vegetables
- ☐ Butter
- ☐ Lard, butter, vegetable shortening for baking

And more of this...

- ☐ Try to bake or broil–but when you do fry, use vegetable oil
- ☐ Try onions, garlic, vinegar, lemon juce, hot pepper, or herbs and spices
  Use small bits of lean ham and vegetable oil
  Chill the vegetables and skim off the fat
- ☐ Margarine is much less expensive and better for your heart
  Try rub or liquid margarine–better for your heart, but still the same number of calories
- ☐ In baking, use oil when you can, margarine otherwise

Snacks, Starches

Eat less of this...

- ☐ Snack chips
- ☐ Snack crackers

And more of this...

- ☐ Choose unbuttered popcorn, pretzels, fruit, or raw vegetables instead of chips
  Go easy on the dips or make them low fat
- ☐ Choose crackers that don't leave a grease stain on paper
  Look for "Nabs" that say "low in saturated fat and cholesterol"
- ☐ Starchy foods–like bread, potatoes, rice and noodles– are NOT fattening unless you put fatty things on them, like butter, margarine, gravy, sour cream, or mayonnaise. Eat more starchy foods, fruits, and vegetables, and less high fat foods.

Hot Tips

- ➤ Take things slowly—most people get used to a lower fat and cholesterol diet after a while, and many people even like it better!
- ➤ You don't have to change your whole way of eating, just make some small changes in the way you like to eat now, and then a few more small changes later.
- ➤ It's better for your heart (and your pocketbook) to fill up on bread, potatoes, rice, noodles, fruits, and vegetables rather than meat, cheese, butter and eggs.
- ➤ Beware of food labels that say "cholesterol free"–they may have lots of saturated fats which are worse for your heart than cholesterol

Figure 9–5. "Food and your heart" dietary advice and goal sheet.

address interpersonal relationships (family, work, and community) as part of the totality of the individual's food environment that aids, reinforces, and rewards behavior change.

Referral for Counseling and Classes. Comprehensive nutritional counseling by a counselor or dietitian includes assessment, treatment, evaluation [63, 77], and a therapeutic alliance between the patient/client and the counselor. It reflects a continuum of approaches from a single, full-length encounter of 30 to 45 minutes to regular and repeated individual sessions over a period of six months or more. The aim of comprehensive nutrition counseling is to work with the patient to set goals, solve problems, and take action to make dietary changes that reduce cardiovascular risk. The process is, ideally, one in which responsibility is shared, the patient is an active participant, and eventually the patient adopts and maintains new behavior patterns so that counseling is no longer needed [115, 116]. Negotiating a plan for change is a central feature, as discussed above and in Chapter 7.

Referral for Group Education. Group programs for nutrition education that emphasize CHD risk reduction are available in many communities and health care organizations. They range from informational and behavioral skill development groups to low-fat cooking classes. Group programs may be single-session lectures and/or demonstrations, or they may be a series of classes. They may also vary in whether they are open to the general public or only to individuals diagnosed as having dyslipidemia and their families. The health professional's recommendation for participation in group education should be based on a preliminary investigation of the types of programs available and their costs and suitability for the patient's needs. It is helpful to know about the possibility of third-party payment for participation in group programs, as well.

Group and Family Counseling. One-to-one counseling methods may be combined with group education; for example, group education sometimes includes one or more individual sessions for setting and monitoring personal goals. Family members can be invited to participate in counseling and group programs. This may enhance social support, both practical and emotional, for putting dietary changes into action. Family involvement can mobilize group support by encouraging changes in group dietary norms [117].

COLLABORATING WITH DIETITIANS

Professionally trained dietitians and nutritionists are important resources in nutritional management to prevent CHD. They extend physicians' efforts and can answer technical questions about high blood cholesterol and cholesterol-lowering diets. Nutrition services are integral to the delivery of comprehensive health services [118]; one study found that the majority of family practice residency training programs have registered dietitians available to them [119]. However, referral to a nutritionist is infrequent in the medical follow-up of individuals with high blood cholesterol levels [120].

The term *dietitian* connotes a professionally trained nutrition specialist who has fulfilled the requirements for becoming a registered dietitian (R.D.). The label *nutritionist* refers to a broader category of professionals with training in human nutrition [63]. People with a wide variety of backgrounds refer to themselves as "nutritionists"; not all have completed a uniform course of training or become formally affiliated with the nutrition profession. They include skilled nutrition educators and bona fide research nutritionists who work mainly with animals, as well as self-styled nutritionists without formal training. (A check on credentials and experience should be conducted.) In addition, some states now have licensure laws; dietitians who qualify for licensure are known as L.D.s, or licensed dietitians.

Dietitians often specialize, and not all are equally skilled or experienced at nutrition counseling. Appropriate referrals may be identified through the clinical dietetics department at a hospital or through state and local affiliates of the American Dietetic Association. The Division of Practice of the American Dietetic Association (telephone number 312/899-0040) can also help in locating registered dietitians in your area.

When a health care provider makes a referral to a dietitian or a nutritionist, communication is essential, much the same as in a referral to a physician subspecialist. The consulting dietitian should receive all pertinent information before the first patient visit, and expectations about the timetable and the amount of feedback should be established clearly at the outset.

Referrals for counseling, whether within a medical office practice or to an outside source, carry the practical concern of reimbursement and third-party payment coverage. Third-party payment systems vary in their coverage of nutritional counseling [121]. If insurance, HMO, or government health care coverage does not reimburse for dietitians' services, patients may not follow through on referrals. In most states dietitians cannot certify the need for medical treatment or obtain provider numbers, and CPT-4 billing codes are proprietary for physician use [121]. The American Dietetic Association has developed information resources related to coverage and reimbursement [122, 123]. Physicians and their office administrators should explore the prevailing local policies that apply to their third-party payers when they anticipate making referrals to dietitians.

Nonnutritionist counselors. In some health care settings, particularly in rural areas, the number of trained nutritionists is limited. Also, their mandate may be to provide maternal and child nutrition services, leaving them unavailable for chronic disease control activities. For these situations, alternative approaches should be considered. The Food for Heart Program (FFHP) in North Carolina was designed for use by physicians in busy clinical settings where nutrition services were not readily available. The program can be delivered by other professionals, such as nurses and health educators, with back-up technical support and supervision from a nutritionist [104, 124]. Models such as this should be further developed and disseminated. It may be possible to arrange for office staff training through a local Heart Association chapter, a

university medical center, or an experienced consulting dietitian and/or psychologist.

Step 3: Follow-up and Evaluation

Assessment of adherence and lipid reduction are the basis for ongoing treatment decisions. For most people who are diet sensitive, both total cholesterol and LDL-cholesterol levels begin to drop two to three weeks after the start of a cholesterol-lowering diet [94]. For patients who make gradual changes but do not follow the step 1 diet faithfully, reductions occur more slowly. Blood cholesterol reduction levels are especially closely tied to saturated-fat consumption [33, 94]. The step 2 diet is more restrictive and thus more difficult to follow; in general the decision to prescribe this regimen should be made only if excellent adherence to the originally recommended diet is not effective for achieving progress toward cholesterol level goals. However, the well-motivated patient with markedly elevated lipid levels may benefit from being placed directly on a step 2 diet.

For patients who successfully reduce their risk through nutritional changes, initial behavior change is only the first step in achieving health improvement. Maintaining behavior change is crucial to CHD prevention over the long term. Such change deserves medical attention in the same manner as if drugs had been prescribed, though lifestyle change may not prompt follow-up consultation as routinely as medication use.

A major challenge in promoting long-term adherence to low-fat, low-cholesterol eating patterns is the prevention of relapse to former eating habits [64]. We cannot realistically expect long-term behavior changes with short-term programs. It has been found repeatedly that when an intervention is not sustained, improved eating habits and reduced lipid levels do not persist [63]. Use of self-management techniques such as those included in relapse prevention training [89] and periodic reinforcement from health professionals (by telephone and/or in person) are the most promising methods for enhancing maintenance. The use of support groups and related strategies like the buddy system are additional ways to extend the supportive aspect of counseling beyond the initial treatment period.

Training in self-management techniques to prevent relapse can be built in to the end of counseling programs or used in post-counseling booster sessions. These techniques can include behavioral rehearsal (i.e., practicing skills for coping with difficult or challenging eating situations, such as stressful times, traveling, and holidays) and methods to avoid letting small slips turn into full relapses or returns to old behaviors [89]. (See Chapter 7 for an in-depth discussion of relapse prevention.)

Just as there are organizational, administrative, financial, and situational barriers to physicians and other health care providers implementing comprehensive counseling, there are often such obstacles to implementing maintenance strategies. It is worth the effort to devise methods to overcome these barriers, because nutritional intervention yields long-term health benefits only when dietary changes are sustained. Individual practitioners may need to enlist the aid of other health professionals to propose and establish creative strategies for facilitating maintenance procedures that are feasible in their practice settings.

Setting Up the Office Practice to Facilitate Dietary Intervention

In the practice setting the responsibility for nutritional intervention for CHD is divided among physicians, nurses, dietitians, other health professionals, and ancillary personnel. These team members must work together to coordinate patient evaluation, treatment, and follow-up. A health team approach makes efficient use of the physician's time [125] and the skills and roles of other staff members.

Practice management for nutritional intervention includes staffing within the office and identification of sources for nutritional consultation and intensive intervention; organizing protocols to specify the process of patient management and follow-up procedures; developing information systems; and acquiring, providing, and/or using community resources [69, 126].

An office practice system is needed that creates a work environment conducive to implementing nutritional interventions. (See Chapter 17 for an in-depth discussion of the elements of designing and managing a prevention-oriented practice.)

The medical chart is an important part of integrated office systems for nutrition-related CHD risk assessment and dietary management [69]. A modified chart form or an additional form for dietary counseling may be helpful because it cues practitioners to record relevant points that may not be written up for many encounters. Several other kinds of office practice tools are helpful to facilitate dietary intervention. Chart stickers or flags can help cue physicians, nurses, and other office staff as to when lipid measures are needed and to the fact that a patient is receiving dietary treatment. Patient-tracking systems, including reminder postcards and telephone follow-up scripts, make the follow-up process more routine. Patient education materials, including posters, brochures, and even books for browsing, can be left in the reception area.

Office systems for nutritional management may be slow to develop, may require some experimentation before they work smoothly, and may be perceived as difficult to implement [127, 128]. However, the practice can benefit beyond the focus of CHD prevention, because counseling about healthy nutrition is recommended as a routine part of patient contact in overall health care [5].

A Public Health View of Clinical Nutritional Intervention

In the past decade, at least ten authoritative health and government organizations in the United States have issued dietary guidelines to promote good health consistent with cholesterol-lowering treatment recommendations. Similar suggestions have been adopted in at least nine nations in Europe and Asia [129]. Indeed, adoption of low-fat eating patterns and weight control are population-wide goals, not limited to adults who are found to have elevated blood cholesterol levels [130]. The adult treatment guidelines [29] and most of this chapter focus on a patient-based approach but acknowledge the complementarity of population-based and clinical approaches.

Both patient-based strategies, designed to help those with the highest cholesterol levels, and population-based strategies, which seek to reach all citizens, are needed [131]. As Remington points out, "Prevention cannot be embedded within a purely clinical framework . . . we will never reach public health or community level prevention one case at a time" [132, p. 110]. Physicians and other health professionals have important roles in building support for population-based dietary changes [132b]. They can work with community organizations, educational programs, government agencies, the food industry, and in research and surveillance to help reduce diet-related risk in the population at large [130].

Treatment of Special Populations

Obese Patients

Adjustment of caloric intake and expenditure is an integral part of cholesterol-lowering diets [94, 42]. For many obese patients weight loss promotes a lowering of cholesterol. Weight loss also effectively helps to control blood pressure in overweight hypertensives [4]. The presence of a measurable heart disease risk factor can be a motivator for individuals who have previously regarded weight loss only as a cosmetic matter.

Severely obese patients ($\geq$ 30% above desirable weight) often present with multiple risk factors. For these patients dietary treatment combined with other therapies (e.g., inpatient treatment, very low calorie diets) should be considered. These options should be explored with bariatric specialists, and careful medical supervision and follow-up are necessary.

Many obese patients have extensive experience at attempting dietary changes. They may have more knowledge about nutrition than those who have not attempted modifications in the past. At the same time they may be discouraged due to previous failures to lose weight or maintain weight loss. These factors should

be considered carefully in designing a regimen with good chances for success. Because weight-loss and weight-gain cycles can be physically dangerous as well as psychologically distressing [133], the combination of referral and monitoring deserves special attention in obese patients with CHD risk factors.

Low Socioeconomic Status Patients

Low socioeconomic status (SES) patients often face multiple obstacles in CHD prevention generally and specifically with respect to nutrition management. Poverty may be linked to the inability to obtain food in optimal quantity and/or quality. Inadequate health care coverage may inhibit patients from following through on referrals and obtaining periodic monitoring. Disrupted family environments make it difficult to adhere to a dietary regimen that requires frequent vigilance. Illiteracy may inhibit understanding of educational materials and application of nutritional concepts to daily food choices. In general the person who has difficulty seeing beyond the needs of the day has little energy to devote to making changes that lead to benefits only in the future.

These very real practical obstacles require attention if nutritional intervention is to be successful with low-SES patients. It is important to be sensitive to these concerns and to assist patients in coping with them. In addition to the physician's intervention, someone in the medical office should review the patient's situation and provide information and assistance or referral to social services and public health programs as appropriate.

The Elderly

The strength of the association between elevated serum cholesterol and increased CHD mortality appears to diminish with advancing age, although studies of adults over age 80 are not available (but see discussion of relative versus attributable risk in Chapter 4) [134]. This issue continues to be a matter of debate, but current treatment guidelines call for managing older adults in essentially the same way as younger adults [42]. Altered eating patterns and therapeutic diets are widespread among the elderly, which should be considered in tailoring a treatment plan. Many elderly are already following what amounts to a cholesterol-lowering diet for other conditions such as obesity, hypertension, or diabetes.

Common nutrition-related problems of the elderly include overweight, fluid imbalance (especially dehydration), osteoporosis, hypertension, food-drug interactions, and oral health problems [135]. The elderly are often prone to digestive disturbances, vitamin and mineral supplement abuse, altered appetite, declining sensory abilities (taste and smell), and interrupted nutrient absorption [136]. Hospitalized patients and those living alone or in nursing homes are at increased risk for malnutrition [137]. A thorough nutritional assessment of older adult patients beginning therapeutic diets for CHD prevention should evaluate the presence and extent of these factors.

Social factors that influence adherence to prescribed diets and that are common among the elderly include difficulty in purchasing and preparing food and reliance on food assistance programs such as Meals on Wheels and congregate meals at senior citizen centers. Nutritional counseling with attention to these matters is important to promote adherence. Referral to social services and community programs for the aging is warranted if these problems are apparent.

Children

The process of atherosclerosis occurs over many years, and atherosclerotic lesions related to serum lipoprotein levels are identifiable in adolescents and young adults [138]. However, the use of cholesterol measurements in children as a basis for treatment decisions remains controversial [139, 140]. The risks and benefits of nutritional intervention in children should be carefully weighed.

For children nutritional intervention to reduce CHD risk may be indicated for one or more of several conditions: high serum cholesterol or triglyceride levels, obesity, or borderline hypertension. The step 1 and step 2 diets for children over the age of two have the same nutrient composition as cholesterol-lowering diets for adults. (See Chapter 16 for a more

detailed discussion of the safety of therapeutic diets for children.)

Several special considerations should be noted regarding dietary management of nutrition-related CHD risk in children [1]. Adequate nutrition is important in childhood to facilitate normal growth and development; therefore, counseling and medical supervision to avoid overrestriction are essential. Overrestrictive diets can have deleterious effects on normal growth and development and can also set the stage for eating disorders.

Another concern relates to childhood obesity, which is associated with increased lipid levels and hypertension in children. Much of childhood obesity has been attributed to inactivity as well as to excess food intake. Exercise should be encouraged as an integral part of the dietary management of obese children.

Finally, the involvement and influence of the family are integral to effective dietary modification in children. Family-based treatments have been found to be the most effective available approaches [128]. A family history of CHD signals a greater need for early intervention. The family's eating and food preparation environment affects the child's diet, although older children make more food choices that are beyond their parents' control (e.g., school lunches, snacks). These eating occasions require attention to help improve nutritional status.

Summary

Nutrition plays an important role in reduction of the risk for CHD and other leading chronic diseases. The primary treatment approach for high blood cholesterol levels is dietary change; thus, nutritional intervention is a central part of cholesterol management and CHD prevention. Efficacious and efficient nutritional intervention requires that health professionals understand the principles and concepts of nutritional management and have the skills needed to address behavioral and educational issues.

Dietary behavior is influenced by a variety of psychological, social, cultural, environmental, and economic factors. Patients need specific, relevant information, as well as a sense of personal health concern and the confidence that they can successfully follow a therapeutic diet. The process of dietary-behavior change may be gradual, and not all patients are equally ready to attempt important changes.

For most patients who require nutritional management for CHD prevention, the NCEP treatment guidelines are the basis for intervention. After initial risk assessment patients requiring therapy should be treated with a step 1 diet, which is a low-fat diet emphasizing restriction of saturated fatty acids, total fat, and dietary cholesterol. If progress toward cholesterol-lowering goals is not achieved after adherence to the step 1 diet, a step 2 diet should be attempted before considering pharmacologic therapy. The step 2 diet is more restrictive in the proportion of saturated fatty acid intake and limits dietary cholesterol to 200 mg/day.

Nutritional intervention should include thorough patient assessment, treatment, and monitoring and follow-up. Assessment includes lipid and risk factor evaluation; assessment of dietary intake; and assessment of relevant behavioral, psychosocial, and educational factors. The results of assessment should be used to tailor treatment goals and expectations.

In a busy office practice setting patient nutrition counseling can follow one of several models: brief physician advice, brief individual physician counseling, brief counseling with referral for comprehensive counseling, referral for group education, or a combination of these models. Negotiating a treatment plan in collaboration with the patient is an important component of each counseling model. Collaboration with professional dietitians and other medical professionals and office staff and the use of available community resources help to extend physician time and effort for dietary management.

Follow-up and evaluation are the basis for ongoing treatment decisions. Attention to maintenance of eating behavior changes is necessary for effective disease prevention. Office systems to facilitate dietary management should be developed to improve efficiency and serve patient needs. Physicians also have important roles as advocates and advisers in supporting population-based dietary changes.

Suggested Readings for Patients

American Heart Association. American Heart Association Cookbook. New York: David McKay Company, 1984.

Connor, W, and Connor, S. The New American Diet. New York: Simon and Schuster, 1986.

Goor, R, and Goor, N. Eater's Choice: A Food Lover's Guide to Lower Cholesterol (rev. ed.) New York: Houghton Mifflin Company, 1989.

Ornish, D. Dr. Dean Ornish's Program for Reversing Heart Disease. New York: Random House, 1990.

References

1. Consensus Department Conference. Lowering blood cholesterol to prevent heart disease. JAMA 1987; 258:3527–31.
2. Roussow JE, Lewis B, Rifkind BM. The value of lowering cholesterol after myocardial infarction. N Engl J Med 1990; 323:1112–9.
3. U.S. Department of Health and Human Services. Nutrition and Health. A report of the Surgeon General. USDHHS publ. no. (PHS), 88-50210 1988.
3a. Bal DG, Foerster SB. Changing the American diet — impact on cancer prevention policy recommendations and program implications for the American Cancer Society. Cancer 1991;67:2671–80.
4. National Research Council, National Academy of Sciences. Diet and health: implications for reducing chronic disease risk. Washington, DC: National Academy Press, 1989.
5. U.S. Preventive Services Task Force. Guide to clinical preventive services. Baltimore: Williams & Wilkins, 1989.
6. U.S. Department of Health and Human Services and U.S. Department of Agriculture. *Nutrition and your health*; dietary guidelines for Americans (2nd ed.). USDA and USDHHS, (Home and Garden Bulletin; #232) 1985.
7. Cohen M, Zimmet P. Self-monitoring of blood glucose levels in non-insulin-dependent diabetes mellitus. Med J Austral 1983; 2:377–81.
8. Trevisan M, Cooper R, Stamler R, et al. Dietary salt and blood pressure. Prev Med 1983; 12:133–7.
9. Ornish DM, Brown SE, Scherwitz LW, et al. Can lifestyle changes reverse coronary heart disease? Lancet 1990; 336:129–33.
9a. Kjeldsen-Kregh J, Haugen M, Borchgrevink CF, et al. Controlled trial of fasting and one-year vegetarian diet in rheumatoid arthritis. Lancet 1991; 338:899–902.

10. Glanz K. Patient and public education for cholesterol reduction; a review of strategies and issues. Pat Educ Couns 1988; 12:235–57.

11. How are Americans making food choices? Chicago: The American Dietetic Association and the International Food Information Council, 1990.

12. Yankelovich, Skelly, and White, Inc. The General Mills American Family Report 1978–1979: family health in an era of stress. Minneapolis: General Mills, 1979; 44.

13. Sullivan LW. Healthy people 2000. N Engl J Med 1990; 323:1065–7.

14. U.S. Department of Health and Human Services. Vital and health statistics. Physician visits: volume and interval since last visit, United States. DHHS publ. no. (PHS) 185–1572, 1983.

15. Schucker B, Bailey K, Heimbach JT, et al. Change in public perspective on cholesterol and heart disease: results from two national surveys. JAMA 1987; 258:3527–31.

16. Schucker B, Wittes JT, Cutler JA, et al. Change in physician perspective on cholesterol and heart disease: results from two national surveys. JAMA 1987; 258:3521–6.

17. Otradovek K, Blake RL, Parker BM. An assessment of the practice of preventive cardiology in an academic health center. J Fam Pract 1985; 21:125–9.

18. Madion-Kay DJ. Family physician recognition and treatment of severe hypercholesterolemia. J Fam Pract 1987; 24:54–6.

19. Shea S, Gemson DH, Mossel P. Management of high blood cholesterol by primary care physicians. J Gen Int Med 1990; 5:327–34.

20. Wechsler II, Levine S, Idelson RK, et al. The physician's role in health promotion — a survey of primary care practitioners. N Engl J Med 1983; 308:97–100.

21. Mann KV, RW Putnam. Physicians' perceptions of their role in cardiovascular risk reduction. Prev Med 1989; 18:45–58.

22. Kottke TE, Foels JK, Hill C, et al. Nutrition counseling in private practice: attitudes and activities of family physicians. Prev Med 1984; 13:219–25.

23. Demak MM, and Becker MH. The doctor-patient relationship and counseling for preventive care. Pat Educ Couns 1987; 9:5–24.

24. Kupper NS, Blondell RD, Aspy CB. Hypercholesterolemia: a plea for a practical solution. J Nutr Educ 1989; 21:104–5.

25. Owen AL. What patients need to know about nutrition. J Nutr Educ 1988; 20,1:S25–S29.

26. National Cholesterol Education Program Expert Panel. Report on detection, evaluation and treatment of high blood cholesterol in adults. Arch Int Med 1988; 148:36–69.

27. Rifkind BM, Lenfant C. Cholesterol lowering and the reduction of coronary heart disease risk. JAMA 1986; 256:2872–3.

28. Ernst N, Cleeman J. Reducing high blood cholesterol levels: recommendations from the National Cholesterol Education Program. J Nutr Educ 1988; 20:23–9.

29. National Cholesterol Education Program. Highlights of the report of the National Cholesterol Education Program Expert Panel on Detection, Evaluation and Treatment of High Blood Cholesterol in Adults. National Heart, Lung and Blood Institute. NIH publ. no. (NIH) 88–2926, 1987.

29a. Glueck CJ, Sanghvi VR, Laemmle P, et al. Lack of concordance in classification of coronary heart disease risk: high-risk HDL cholesterol less than 35 mg/dl in subjects with desirable total serum cholesterol, less than 200 mg/dl. J Lab Clin Med 1990; 116:377–85.

29b. Genest JJ, McNamara JR, Salem DN, et al. Prevalence of risk factors in men with premature coronary artery disease. Am J Cardiol 1991; 67:1185–9.

29c. Ginsburg GS, Safran C, Pasternak RC. Frequency of low serum high–density lipoprotein cholesterol levels in hospitalized patients with desirable total cholesterol levels. Am J Cardiol 1991; 68:187–92.

30. National Heart, Lung and Blood Institute. Eating to lower your high blood cholesterol. USDHHS publ. no. (NIH) 89–2920, 1989.

31. National Cancer Institute. Cancer control objectives for the nation — 1985–2000. NCI Monograph no. 2, Bethesda, Md.: National Cancer Institute, 1986.

32. Kottke TE, Foels JK, et al. Perceived palatability of the prudent diet: results of a dietary demonstration for physicians. Prev Med 1983; 12:588–93.

33. Grundy SM. Cholesterol and coronary heart disease: a new era. JAMA 1986; 256:2849–58.

34. Keys A, Anderson JT, Grande F. Serum cholesterol responses to change in the diet. IV. Particular saturated fatty acids in the diet. Metabolism 1965; 14:776–87.

35. Hegsted DM, McGandy RB, Myers ML, Stare FJ. Quantitative effects of dietary fat on serum cholesterol in man. Am J Clin Nutr 1965; 17:281–95.

35a. Klurfeld DM. Tropical oil turmoil. J Am Coll Nutr 1991; 10:575–6.

35b. Park YMK, Yetley EA. Trend changes in use and current intakes of tropical oils in the United States. Am J Clin Nutr 1990; 51:738–48.

36. Grundy SM. Comparison of monounsaturated

fatty acids and carbohydrates for plasma cholesterol lowering. N Engl J Med 1986; 314:745–8.

37. Bonanome A, Grundy SM. Effect of dietary stearic acid on plasma cholesterol and lipoprotein levels. N Engl J Med 1986; 318:1244–8.

38. Small DM, Oliva C, Tercyak A. Chemistry in the kitchen: making ground meat more healthful. N Engl J Med 1991; 324:73–7.

39. Willett W, Sacks FM. Chewing the fat: how much and what kind. N Engl J Med 1991; 324:121–3.

40. Connor SL, Gustafson JR, Artaud-Wild SM, et al. The cholesterol/saturated fat index: an indication of the hypercholesterolaemic and atherogenic potential of food. Lancet 1986; 1:1229–32.

41. Connor SL, Connor WE. The new American diet. New York: Simon and Schuster, 1986.

42. Grundy SM. Cholesterol and coronary heart disease: future directions. JAMA 1990; 264:3053–9.

43. Anderson JW, Spencer DB, Hamilton CC, et al. Oat bran cereal lowers serum total and LDL cholesterol in hypercholesterolemic men. Am J Clin Nutr 1990; 52:495–9.

44. Kestin M, Moss R, Clifton PM, Nestel PJ. Comparative effects of three cereal brans on plasma lipids, blood pressure, and glucose metabolism in mildly hypercholesterolemic men. Am J Clin Nutr 1990; 52:661–6.

45. National Institutes of Health. Consensus Development Conference statement. Health implications of obesity. Ann Int Med 1984; 103:1073–7.

46. Follick MJ, Abrams, DB, Smith TW, et al. Contrasting short- and long-term effects of weight loss on lipoprotein levels. Arch Intern Med 1984; 144:1571–4.

47. Hellerstedt WL, Jeffrey RM, Murray DM. The association between alcohol intake and adiposity in the general population. Am J Epid 1990; 132:594–611.

48. Kozarevic D, Demirovic J, Gordon T, et al. Drinking habits and coronary heart disease: the Yugoslavia cardiovascular disease study. Am J Epid 1982; 116:748–58.

49. Stampfer MJ, Colditz GA, Willett WC, et al. A prospective study of moderate alcohol consumption and the risk of coronary disease and stroke in women. N Engl J Med 1988; 319:267–73.

50. Savolainen MJ. How does alcohol raise HDL-cholesterol concentration? Ann Int Med 1990; 22:141–2.

51. Grobbee DE, Rimm EB, Giovannucci E, et al. Coffee, caffeine, and cardiovascular disease in men. N Engl J Med 1990; 323:1026–32.

52. Wilson PWF, Garrison RJ, Kannel WB, et al. Is coffee consumption a contributor to cardiovascular disease? Arch Int Med 1989; 149:1169–72.

52a. Vandusseldorp M, Katan MB, Vanvliet T, et al. Cholesterol-raising factor from boiled coffee does not pass a paper filter. Arteriosclerosis and Thrombosis 1991; 11:586–93.

52b. Vandusseldorp M, Katan MB, Demacker PNM. Effect of decaffeinated versus regular coffee on serum lipoproteins - a 12-week double-blind trial. Amer J Epidemiol 1990; 132:33–40.

53. Puccio EM, McPhillips JB, Barrett-Connor E, et al. Clustering of atherogenic behaviors in coffee drinkers. Am J Publ Health 1990; 80:1310–3.

54. Morabia A, and Wynder EL. Dietary habits of smokers, people who never smoked, and ex-smokers. Am J Clin Nutr 1990; 52:933–7.

55. Langford HG, Blaufox MD, Oberman A, et al. Dietary therapy slows the return of hypertension after stopping prolonged medication. JAMA 1985; 253:657–64.

56. Guidelines for the treatment of mild hypertension: memorandum from WHO/ISH meeting. Hypertension 1983; 5:394–7.

57. Alderman MH, Lamport B. Moderate sodium restriction: do the benefits justify the hazards? Amer J Hypertension 1990; 3:499–504.

58. Barnard RJ. Effects of life-style modification on serum lipids. Arch Int Med 1991; 151:1389–94.

59. Ornish DM. Dr. Dean Ornish's program for reversing heart disease. New York: Random House, 1990.

60. Bierman EL, Chait A. Nutrition and diet in relation to hyperlipidemia and atherosclerosis. In: Shils ME, Young VR, eds. Modern nutrition in health and disease. 7th ed. Philadelphia: Lea & Febiger, 1988; 1283–97.

61. Beaton GH. Criteria of an adequate diet. In: Shils ME, Young VR, eds. Modern nutrition in health and disease. 7th ed. Philadelphia: Lea & Febiger, 1988; 649–65.

62. Glanz K. The cholesterol controversy and health education: a response to the critics. Pat Educ Couns 1990; 16:89–95.

63. Glanz K. Nutrition education for risk factor reduction and patient education: a review. Prev Med 1985; 14:721–52.

64. Carmody TP, Matarazzo JD, Istvan JA. Promoting adherence to heart-healthy diets: a review of the literature. J Compl Health Care 1987; 2:105–23.

65. Hochbaum GH. Strategies and their rationale for changing people's eating habits. J Nutr Educ 1981; 13:Suppl:59–65.

66. Stunkard AJ. The social environment and the control of obesity. In: Stunkard AJ, ed. Obesity. Philadelphia: Saunders, 1980.
67. McQueen D, Sigerist J. Social factors in the etiology of chronic disease: an overview. Soc Sci Med 1982; 16:353–67.
68. Marmot MG, Syme SL, Kagan A, et al. Epidemiologic studies of coronary heart disease and stroke in Japanese men living in Japan, Hawaii and California: prevalence of coronary and hypertensive heart disease and associated risk factors. Am J Epidemiol 1975; 102:514–25.
69. Glanz K, Mullis RM. Environmental interventions to promote healthy eating: a review of models, programs and evidence. Health Educ Qtly 1988; 15:395–415.
70. Glaser S. How America eats. Editorial Research Reports, Congressional Qtly 1988; (April 29):218–31.
71. Levy AS, Ostrove N, Guthrie T, Heimbach JT. Recent trends in beliefs about diet/disease relationships: results of the 1979–1988 Health and Diet surveys. Paper presented at the FDA/USDA Food Editor Conference, Dec. 1–2, 1988.
72. Food Marketing Institute. Trends 1989: consumer attitudes and the supermarket. Washington, D.C.: Food Marketing Institute, 1989.
73. National Restaurant Association and Gallup Organization. Changes in consumer eating habits. Washington, D.C.: NRA, 1986.
74. Heimbach JT. Cardiovascular disease and diet: the public view. Publ Health Rep 1985; 100:1–12.
75. Sloan AE. Educating a nutrition-wise public. J Nutr Educ 1987; 19:303–5.
76. Rudd J, Glanz K. How individuals use information for health action: consumer information processing. In: Glanz K, Lewis FM, Rimer BK, eds. Health behavior and health education: theory, research, and practice. San Francisco: Jossey-Bass, 1990; 115–39.
77. Snetselaar LG. Nutrition counseling skills: assessment, treatment, and evaluation. 2nd ed. Rockville, Md.: Aspen Publishers, 1989.
78. Rosenstock IM. The health belief model: explaining health behavior through expectancies. In: Glanz K, Lewis FM, Rimer BK, eds. Health behavior and health education: theory, research, and practice. San Francisco: Jossey-Bass, 1990; 39–62.
79. Contento IR, Murphy BM. Psycho-social factors differentiating people who reported making desirable changes in their diets from those who did not. J Nutr Educ 1990; 22:6–14.
80. Glanz K. Compliance with dietary regimens: its magnitude, measurement and determinants. Prev Med 1980; 9:787–904.
81. Glanz K. Strategies for changing dietary behavior to reduce cardiac risk. In: Kris-Etherton PM, ed. Cardiovascular disease: nutrition for prevention and treatment. Chicago: The American Dietetic Association, 1990; 224–37.
82. Bandura A. Social foundations of thought and action: a social cognitive theory. Englewood Cliffs, NJ: Prentice-Hall, Inc., 1986.
83. Brownell KD. The psychology and physiology of obesity: implications for screening and treatment. J Amer Diet Assoc 1984; 84:406–14.
84. Bandura A. Self-efficacy mechanism in human agency. Amer Psychol 1982; 37:122–47.
85. Strecher VJ, DeVellis BM, Becker MH, Rosenstock IM. The role of self-efficacy in achieving health behavior change. Health Educ Qtly 1986; 13:73–91.
86. Bowen D, Tomoyusu N, Curry S et al. Measuring the process of changing to a low fat diet. Presented at Annual Meeting of American Public Health Association, New York, October 1990.
87. DiClemente C, Prochaska JO. Self-change and therapy change of smoking behavior: a comparison of change in cessation and maintenance. Addict Behav 1982; 7:133–42.
88. Prochaska JO, DiClemente C. Transtheoretical therapy: toward a more integrative model of change. Psychotherapy: Theory Research and Practice 1982; 19:276–88.
89. Marlatt GA, Gordon JR. Relapse prevention. New York: Guilford Press, 1985.
90. Ockene JK. Physician-delivered interventions for smoking cessation: strategies for increasing effectiveness. Prev Med 1987; 16:723–37.
91. Raab C, Tillotson JL, eds. Heart to heart: a manual on nutrition counseling for the reduction of cardiovascular disease risk factors. Bethesda, Md.: USDHHS publ. no. (NIH) 83–1528, 1983.
92. Kris-Etherton PM, ed. Cardiovascular disease: nutrition for prevention and treatment. Chicago: The American Dietetic Association, 1990.
93. Palumbo PJ. Cholesterol lowering for all: a closer look. JAMA 1989; 262:91–2.
94. Dwyer JT. Assessment of dietary intake. In: Shils ME, Young VR, eds. Modern nutrition in health and disease. 7th ed. Philadelphia: Lea & Febiger, 1988; 887–905.
95. Burk M, Pao E. Methodology for large scale surveys of household and individual diets. Home Econ research report 40. Washington, D.C.: U.S. Department of Agriculture, 1976.
96. Mojonnier L, Hall Y. The National Diet-Heart Study: assessment of adherence. J Amer Diet Assoc 1968; 52:288–92.
97. Fidanza F. Controlled experiments in human

nutrition: contemporary problems. Prev Med 1983; 12:100–2.

98. Glanz K. Dietitians' effectiveness and patient compliance with dietary regimens. J Amer Diet Assoc 1979; 74:631–6.

99. Remmell PS, Benfari RC. Assessing dietary adherence in the Multiple Risk Factor Intervention Trial. II. Food record rating as an indicator of compliance. J Amer Diet Assoc 1980; 76:357–60.

100. Remmell PS, Gorder DD, Hall Y, Tillotson JL. Assessing dietary adherence in the Multiple Risk Factor Intervention Trial. I. Use of a dietary monitoring tool. J Amer Diet Assoc 1980; 76:351–6.

101. Heller RF, Tunstall-Pedoe HD, Rose G. A simple method of assessing the effect of dietary advice to reduce plasma cholesterol. Prev Med 1981; 10:364–70.

102. Hunninghake DB, Quiter ES, Brekke ML, et al. Reliability testing of a self-administered eating pattern assessment tool. Presented at the First National Cholesterol Conference, Alexandria, Va., November 1988.

103. Mullis RM, Hunninghake DB, Brekke ML, et al. Validity testing of an eating pattern assessment tool. Presented at the First National Cholesterol Conference, Alexandria, Va., November 1988.

104. Ammerman AS, Haines PS, DeVellis RF, et al. A brief dietary assessment to guide cholesterol reduction in low income individuals — design and validation. J Am Diet Assoc 1991; 91:1385–90.

105. Ammerman AS. A physician-based dietary intervention to reduce cholesterol in low-income patients. Chapel Hill, NC: Univ of North Carolina; 1990. Dissertation.

105a. Ockene, IS, Hebert J, Ockene JK. The Worcester-Area Trial for Counseling in Hyperlipidemia (WATCH) protocol. Unpublished.

106. Block G, Clifford C, Naughton MD, et al. A brief dietary screen for high fat intake. J Nutr Educ 1989; 21:199–207.

107. Kristal AR, Shattuck AL, Henry HJ, Fowler AS. Rapid assessment of dietary intake of fat, fiber, and saturated fat: validity of an instrument suitable for community intervention research and nutritional surveillance. Amer J Health Promo 1990; 4:288–95.

107a. Hebert JR, Ockene IS, Botelho L, et al. Development and validation of a seven-day diet recall (7DDR). APHA 120th Annual Meeting, Washington, DC. November, 1992.

108. Glanz K. Strategies for nutrition counseling. J Amer Diet Assoc 1979; 74:431–7.

109. Ferguson JM. Learning to eat: behavior modification for weight control. Palo Alto, Cal.: Bull Publishing, 1975.

110. Dolecek TA, Milas NC, VanHorn LV, et al. A long-term nutrition intervention experience: lipid responses and dietary adherence patterns in the Multiple Risk Factor Intervention Trial (MRFIT). J Amer Diet Assoc 1986; 86: 752–8.

111. McCann BS, Retzlaff BM, Dowdy AA, et al. Promoting adherence to low-fat, low-cholesterol diets: review and recommendations. J Amer Diet Assoc 1990; 90:1408–14.

112. Ley P. Cognitive variables and noncompliance. J Compl Health Care 1987; 1:171–88.

113. McCabe BJ, Tysinger JW, Kreger M, Currwin AC. A strategy for designing effective patient education materials. J Amer Diet Assoc 1989; 89:1290–92.

114. Glanz K, Rudd J. Readability and content analysis of print cholesterol education materials. Pat Educ Couns 1990; 16:109–18.

115. Kanfer FH, Goldstein AP, eds. Helping people change: a textbook of methods. 3rd ed. New York: Pergamon, 1986.

116. Kanfer FH, Schefft BK. Guiding the process of therapeutic change. Champaign, IL: Research Press, 1988.

117. Carmody TP, Istvan J, Matarazzo JD, et al. Applications of social learning theory in the promotion of heart-healthy diets: the Family Heart Study dietary intervention model. Health Educ Res 1986; 1:13–27.

118. Neville JN. Position of the American Dietetic Association: nutrition services in health maintenance organizations and alternative health care delivery systems. J Amer Diet Assoc 1987; 87:1391–3.

119. Nuhlicek DR, Simpson DE, Lillich DW, Borman RJ. Teaching and funding nutrition instruction in family practice education. Acad Med 1989; 64(2):103–4.

120. Rastam L, Luepker RV, Pirie PL. Effect of screening and referral on follow-up and treatment of high blood cholesterol levels. Amer J Prev Med 1988; 4:244–8.

121. Neville JN, Gilmore CJ. President's page: a report on nutrition services payment system activities. J Amer Diet Assoc 1988; 88:953–5.

122. American Dietetic Association. Coverage and reimbursement policies for nutrition care services. Chicago, 1986.

123. American Dietetic Association. Nutrition services payment system: guidelines for implementation. Chicago, 1985.

124. Ammerman A. Personal communication, 1990.

125. Glanz K, Brekke ML, Hoffman E, et al. Patient reactions to nutrition education for cholesterol reduction. Amer J Prev Med 1990; 6:311–7.

126. Vanderschmidt HF, Koch-Weser D, Woodbury PA, eds. Handbook of clinical prevention. Baltimore: Williams & Wilkins, 1987.

127. Glanz K, Brekke ML, et al. Evaluation of implementation of a pilot cholesterol management program in physicians' offices. Health Educ Res 1992; 7, no. 2. In press.

128. Kottke TE, Solberg LI, Brekke ML. Beyond efficacy testing: Introducing preventive cardiology into primary care. Am J Prev Med 1990 VI, (suppl. I) 77–83.

129. Palmer S. Promoting desirable dietary behaviors in the population: a challenge for the future. In: Kaufman M, ed. Building support for population-based dietary change. Chapel Hill, NC: University of North Carolina, 1987; 145–58.

130. Blackburn H. Public policy and dietary recommendations to reduce population levels of blood cholesterol. Am J Prev Med 1985; 1:3–11.

131. National Cholesterol Education Program. Report of the Expert Panel on population strategies for blood cholesterol reduction. Bethesda, MD: National Heart, Lung and Blood Institute, 1990.

132. Remington RD. From preventive policy to preventive practice. Prev Med 1990; 19:105–13.

132b. Kottke TE. Clinical perspectives — the clinician's role in building support for population based dietary changes. In: Kaufman M, ed. Building support for population-based dietary change. Chapel Hill, NC: University of North Carolina, 1987; 43–8.

133. Bouchard C. Is weight fluctuation a risk factor. N Engl J Med 1991; 324:1887–9.

134. Forette B, Tortrat D, Wolmark Y. Cholesterol and mortality in the elderly. Cardiovasc Rev and Rep 1990; 11:14–6.

135. Chernoff R. Dietary assessment and management of the elderly. In: Simko MD, Cowell C, Hreha MS, eds. Practical nutrition: a quick reference for the health care practitioner. Rockville, MD: Aspen Publications, Inc. 1989; 255–68.

136. Roe DA. Nutrition assessment of the elderly. In: Simko MD, Cowell C, Hreha MS, eds. Practical nutrition: a quick reference for the health care practitioner. Rockville, MD: Aspen Publications, Inc., 1989; 237–44.

137. Austin AG. Environmental assessment of the elderly. In: Simko MD, Cowell C, Hreha MS, eds. Practical nutrition: a quick reference for the health care practitioner. Rockville, MD: Aspen Publications, Inc., 1989; 245–54.

138. Pathobiological Determinants of Atherosclerosis in Youth (PDAY) Research Group. Relationship of atherosclerosis in young men to serum lipoprotein cholesterol concentrations and smoking. JAMA 1990; 264:3018–24.

139. Lauer RM, Clarke WR. Use of cholesterol measurements in childhood for the prediction of adult hypercholesterolemia: the Muscatine Study. JAMA 1990; 264:3034–8.

140. Newman TB, Browner WS, Hulley SB. The case against childhood cholesterol screening. JAMA 1990; 264:3039–43.

10

Exercise and Exercise Intervention

ANN WARD
PAMELA ANN TAYLOR
LYNN AHLQUIST
DAVID R. BROWN
DANIEL CARLUCCI
JAMES M. RIPPE

EDITORS' INTRODUCTION

The topic of exercise is of great interest to everyone. The United States spends more money on exercise equipment and paraphernalia than any other country in the world. Yet in terms of total daily caloric expenditure we rank far down the list, as we progressively spend more time sitting in front of televisions and computer terminals, and exercise machines languish in the basement. There is increasing evidence that exercise has many beneficial effects and plays an important role in the prevention of CHD. Apart from its direct effects, the individual who exercises is likelier to eat a healthier diet, quit smoking, and be better able to cope with stress. This chapter reviews the physiology of exercise and the relationship of exercise to cardiovascular health. Then the manner in which exercise should be prescribed for patients is described in considerable detail, with attention to safety and practicality. Walking is emphasized as a particularly useful form of exercise for many individuals, and the role of the health professional underscored throughout.

Regular, dynamic physical activity can improve cardiovascular function, reduce risk factors associated with cardiovascular disease, and, consequently, be beneficial in the primary and secondary prevention of coronary heart disease (CHD). Although most people realize that exercise is important for health, 60 to 80 percent of American adults are sedentary or irregularly active [1].

In 1989 a U.S. Preventive Services Task Force (PSTF) concluded that the evidence linking exercise and health was strong enough to issue recommendations for the role of exercise counseling in clinical practice. The PSTF recommended that physicians counsel all patients "to engage in a program of regular physical activity tailored to meet their health and personal lifestyle" [2]. Physicians have an opportunity to play a major role in increasing the activity level of their patients. Recent surveys have indicated that patients cite physicians' recommendations as a significant reason for increasing their level of physical activity [3, 4]. However, another survey found that only 15 percent of internists in the United States counseled patients regarding exercise in primary prevention [5].

Physicians can help their patients increase their physical activity in several ways. First, physicians can encourage their patients to exercise by discussing the health benefits of exercise and the patient's perceived health and ability to exercise. They can determine which patients need physical examination and exercise testing before beginning an exercise program and provide medical clearance for patients wishing to start an exercise program. Physicians can prescribe exercise for patients with chronic medical problems or refer them to appropriate health care professionals for exercise counseling.

For all physicians, an understanding of exercise physiology and the health benefits of exercise is important. In addition the ability to take an accurate activity history and devise an exercise prescription is necessary for counseling patients in the type and level of exercise appropriate for their health status. This chapter examines the adaptations associated with exercise

training and the evidence linking exercise with improved cardiovascular health and the prevention of CHD. Guidelines are presented for the preexercise program evaluation and for writing an exercise prescription for healthy adults, patients at risk for developing CHD, and those with known CHD. Exercise programs for children and elderly individuals are also discussed. Guidelines for exercise prescription and the health benefits of exercise are discussed in detail in two publications by the American College of Sports Medicine [6, 7] and a series of articles by the authors (8, 9, 10, 11, 12).

Cardiovascular Responses to Exercise

Dynamic Exercise

Dynamic, or aerobic, exercise refers to activities that are rhythmic and utilize large muscle groups for a sustained period. Examples of dynamic exercise are walking, jogging, swimming, aerobic dance, and cycling. Maximal work capacity or maximal aerobic capacity is the greatest amount of sustained work that can be performed by an individual and is limited by the rate of oxygen delivery to the tissues by the cardiovascular system. This is expressed as maximal oxygen uptake (VO_2max).

VO_2max is a function of maximal cardiac output and arteriovenous oxygen difference. During progressive exercise to VO_2max, oxygen uptake increases proportionally to the work performed until maximal aerobic capacity is reached. Cardiac output increases linearly with oxygen uptake, mediated by increases in heart rate and stroke volume (Figure 10-1) [13]. Systolic blood pressure increases proportionally to the intensity of exercise, while diastolic pressure changes only slightly, due to the decline in systemic vascular resistance. Blood flow to the exercising muscles is enhanced through the increase and regional redistribution of cardiac output (Figure 10-2). The redistribution of blood is brought about by sympathetic vasoconstriction in nonexercising tissue and metabolic hyperemia in the exercising muscles [14].

In previously sedentary individuals VO_2max

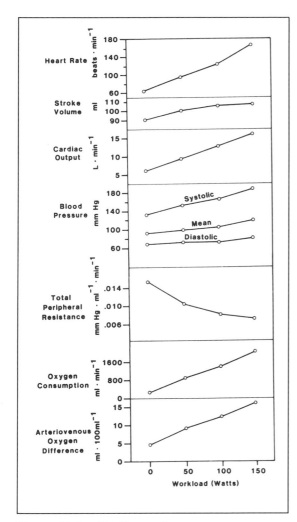

Figure 10-1. Cardiovascular responses to graded exercise. (Source: Durstine JL, Pate RR. Cardiorespiratory responses to acute exercise. In: ACSM. Resource Manual for Guidelines for Exercise Testing and Prescription, 1988; 49.)

may increase 15 to 25 percent over baseline after a few months of regular aerobic exercise when performed at 60 to 80 percent of maximum aerobic capacity for 20 to 60 minutes 3 to 5 days per week [15]. Exercise at this level results in beneficial cardiovascular changes, including decreased heart rate at rest and during submaximal exercise; increased stroke volume at rest and with submaximal and maximal exercise; and increased maximal cardiac output [16,

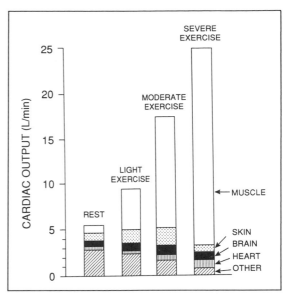

Figure 10-2. Distribution of blood flow with increasing levels of exercise. (Source: Starling, Evans. Principles of human physiology. Philadelphia: Lea & Febiger, 1968. Reprinted with permission.)

17]. The increased stroke volume and decreased heart rate with submaximal exercise result in a reduced myocardial oxygen demand. Important peripheral changes also occur, including increased systemic vascular conductance, greater number of mitochondria in muscle cells, and increases in oxidative enzymes, leading to greater oxygen extraction during exercise [17, 18]. These central and peripheral changes lead to increased oxygen transport and VO$_2$max (Figure 10-3) [19].

Resistance Exercise

Resistance exercise is characterized by a pressor response that results in a significantly greater mean arterial pressure as compared with dynamic exercise [20]. In normal individuals the marked rise in blood pressure is due to an increase in cardiac output with little or no decrease in total peripheral resistance. The magnitude of the pressor response is related to the size of muscle mass and the degree of muscular tension exerted [20].

Most of the data on the health benefits of

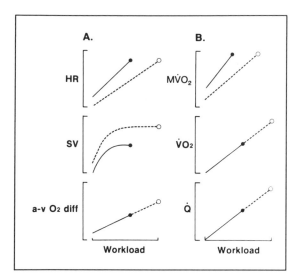

Figure 10-3. Cardiovascular responses to increasing workloads to a maximum in untrained and endurance-trained subjects. Solid line–submaximal responses in untrained subject; dashed line–submaximal responses in trained subject; Q-cardiac output; HR-heart rate; SV-stroke volume; a-VO$_2$ diff-arteriovenous oxygen difference; VO$_2$-oxygen consumption; MVO$_2$-myocardial oxygen consumption. (Source: Smith ML, Mitchell JH. Cardiorespiratory adaptations to training. In: ACSM. Resource Manual for Guidelines for Exercise Testing and Prescription. Philadelphia: Lea & Febiger, 1988. Reprinted with permission.)

exercise are based on aerobic exercise. Resistance training is gaining in popularity, but the long-term health benefits have not been evaluated. Physicians have been reluctant to prescribe resistance training for risk factor modification or cardiac rehabilitation since blood pressure increases acutely. Recent studies, however, suggest that resistance training is safe and beneficial for most persons, particularly when regimens incorporate moderate levels of resistance and high repetitions [21, 22, 23, 24, 25]. In a study of patients with CHD, training at 80 percent of maximum voluntary contraction for 30 minutes three times per week elicited no signs or symptoms of ischemia or abnormal heart rate or blood pressure responses [21]. Modest improvements in such cardiovascular risk factors as high-density lipoprotein (HDL) cholesterol [22, 23], diastolic pressure [22, 23, 24], and insulin sensitivity [22, 23, 25] have been shown with resistance training.

Effects of Physical Activity on Cardiovascular Health

Epidemiologic Evidence

No experimental study of the effect of physical activity on the primary prevention of CHD has been performed because the size, cost, and adherence problems related to such a study would make it prohibitive. However, multiple epidemiologic studies have linked physical activity to a decreased incidence of myocardial infarction (MI) and sudden death [2, 26, 27]. The early epidemiologic studies had serious limitations, including job and leisure activity changes by subjects due to changes in health status; confounding independent variables such as hypertension, obesity, hypercholesterolemia, and race; too small a gradient in physical activity within the population studied; difficulty in assessing physical activity levels; and lack of standardization and confirmation of the diagnosis of CHD [28]. In spite of these limitations, the finding of an inverse relationship between physical activity and cardiovascular disease has been consistent and provides overwhelming evidence for the benefit of exercise.

The most convincing evidence for the association between physical activity and cardiovascular health is based on four recent studies that have controlled for many of the limitations of the earlier studies. In the College Alumni Study [29] individuals who regularly expended between 500 and 3500 kcal per week in leisure time physical activity had significant reductions in cardiovascular risk and lived an average of two years longer compared to sedentary individuals. The Multiple Risk Factor Intervention Trial (MRFIT) [30] also demonstrated reduced cardiovascular risk in individuals who pursued physical activities during their leisure time. Men who averaged more than 30 minutes per day year round of moderate-intensity physical activity had one-third fewer deaths from CHD and a 20 percent lower overall mortality rate compared to less active men. A third investigation, which was an analysis of data from 43 studies, found that inactive individuals were 1.9 times more likely to develop CHD than active individuals, independent of other major risk factors [31]. To put the risk of inactivity in perspective, it is almost as high as the relative risk of smoking a pack of cigarettes per day [32]. Finally, data from the Aerobics Research Institute [33] showed that the risk of cardiovascular death for individuals in the lowest fitness quintile was eight times greater than for those in the highest fitness quintile.

The health-promoting aspects of exercise appear to be dose-related. Epidemiologic studies indicate that even light to moderate amounts of exercise (e.g., walking, stair climbing, gardening) are associated with a lower risk for CHD. In the College Alumni Study a reduced risk of CHD was demonstrated at energy expenditure levels as low as 500 kcal per week [29]. Risk became lower as the volume of exercise increased up to 2000 kcal per week (Figure 10-4). Data from the MRFIT showed that low-intensity activity, such as gardening, was associated with significant reductions in mortality from

Figure 10-4.   Age-specific mortality from all causes among 16,936 Harvard alumni, 1962 to 1978, according to physical activity levels. (Source: Paffenbarger RS, Hyde RT, Wing AL, Hsieh C. Physical activity, all cause mortality and longevity of college alumni. N Engl J Med 1986; 314:605–13. Reprinted with permission.)

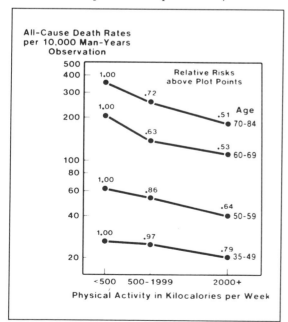

CHD [30]. On the other hand, the College Alumni Study also showed that more vigorous exercise, such as running or strenuous sports, was associated with a greater health benefit than lower-intensity exercise at the same level of energy expenditure [29]. Subjects in the College Alumni Study who participated in athletics in college but subsequently stopped exercising had levels of risk similar to those who had never exercised [29]. In the Aerobics Research Institute Study the greatest reduction in disease risk occurred between the two lowest fitness quintiles [33]. Although the optimal level of exercise to achieve improved cardiovascular health has not been precisely defined, the results of these studies suggest that physical activity should be consistent and life-long and that *moderate* levels of exercise and physical fitness, which are attainable by most adults, appear to protect against early mortality.

The exact mechanisms for the decrease in morbidity and mortality are unclear. There are, however, changes associated with exercise that may exert a favorable effect on CHD, such as decreased blood pressure [34, 35, 36], decreased obesity [37], increased HDL cholesterol [38, 39, 40], increased fibrinolytic activity in response to thrombotic stimuli [41], increased insulin sensitivity [25], and altered baroreflex function resulting in reduced susceptibility to serious ventricular arrhythmias [42]. Animal studies have shown increased size of coronary arteries, enhancement of coronary collateral circulation, and decreased vasospasm following exercise training [43, 44]. Exercise may also have an effect on lifestyle, causing behavioral changes in smoking and in diet leading to beneficial changes in obesity, cholesterol levels, and hypertension [45, 46].

Effects of Exercise in Patients with Hypertension

Epidemiologic data [47, 48] suggest that physically inactive individuals have a 35 percent to 52 percent greater risk of developing hypertension than active individuals. Data from longitudinal studies suggest that exercise is effective in reducing blood pressure by approximately 5 to 10 mm Hg in patients with essential hypertension [34, 35]. However, many of the studies of the effects of exercise on hypertension had serious methodological problems, including absence of a control group and presence of confounding variables such as weight loss [35]. A recent randomized controlled trial of an aerobic exercise regimen versus a placebo exercise regimen demonstrated a significant reduction in blood pressure (6 to 9 mm Hg) in the mildly hypertensive men who performed the aerobic exercise regimen [36]. These changes occurred after 10 weeks of training and were not associated with any potentially confounding changes in weight or urinary sodium excretion. In another recent study of hypertensive patients, a 1-hour walk three times a week was associated with a significant reduction in both systolic and diastolic blood pressure [49]. Further evidence for the blood pressure–lowering effect of exercise was provided in a crossover study by Román and colleagues [50]. In this study resting blood pressure fell significantly with training but returned to baseline levels when training was discontinued.

The mechanism for the antihypertensive effect of endurance exercise training is largely unknown. The most likely explanation is the attenuation of sympathetic nervous system activity, which may result in reduced renin-angiotensin activity, resetting of arterial baroreflexes, arterial vasodilation, and reduction in elevated peripheral vascular resistance [25, 27]. Improved insulin sensitivity and the corresponding reduction in circulating insulin may also contribute to blood pressure reduction by reducing sodium reabsorption by the renal tubules [27].

Effect of Exercise on Blood Lipids

Exercise may reduce the risk for CHD through effects on blood lipids. However, studies evaluating blood lipid changes due to exercise are confounded by changes in body mass and diet, so results are somewhat conflicting. Early cross-sectional studies indicated that habitually active individuals had lower total cholesterol levels than sedentary individuals [51]. However when habitually active men and women are compared with sedentary individuals matched for age and weight, there appears to be no difference in total cholesterol [51]. In addition, total and low-density lipoprotein (LDL) cholesterol values show little or no change with exercise training [38, 51].

Modest increases in high-density lipoprotein (HDL) cholesterol have been demonstrated with exercise training in men [38, 39, 51, 52]. The amount of exercise needed to raise HDL cholesterol is unclear, ranging from running 10 miles per week [40] to walking 5 miles per day [39]. A recent study [53] comparing men training for 30 minutes 3 days per week at either 65 percent, 75 percent, or 85 percent of maximal heart rate suggests that exercise at 75 percent of maximal heart rate is required to increase HDL cholesterol. It is unclear, however, whether HDL cholesterol increases without concomitant changes in body mass and body composition [38, 51, 54]. Men with lower levels of HDL cholesterol may benefit the most from exercise. Those who lose weight have a greater increase in HDL cholesterol [38]. Although there is little change in LDL cholesterol with exercise, an increase in HDL cholesterol leads to a decreased LDL/HDL ratio, which is related to lower CHD risk [52].

For women few well-designed studies have evaluated the effect of exercise on HDL cholesterol while also controlling for confounding factors such as menstrual status, cigarette smoking and use of female hormones. Two exercise intervention studies suggested that very high levels of exercise were necessary to increase HDL cholesterol in premenopausal women [54a, 54b]. However, in a recent study, women who walked 24 km (14.9 mi) per week had significant improvements in HDL cholesterol [54c]. In postmenopausal women, epidemiologic studies suggest a relationship between physical activity and HDL cholesterol [54d, 54e] but no effect on HDL cholesterol has been demonstrated in exercise intervention studies [55].

Exercise conditioning markedly decreases postprandial chylomicrons and triglycerides, possibly by increasing the activity of lipoprotein lipase [56, 57]. Although chylomicrons and other triglyceride-rich particles are considered atherogenic, it has not been demonstrated that their reduction results in improved health or reduced mortality.

Effects of Exercise in Patients with Diabetes Mellitus

Cerebrovascular, coronary, and peripheral arterial disease are more common in diabetics than in nondiabetics and occur at an earlier age. The Framingham Heart Study revealed an increased morbidity and mortality from all cardiovascular causes among the diabetic group, independent of the absolute level of glycemic control [58].

Diabetes mellitus is commonly classified into two major categories: insulin-dependent, or type I, diabetes and non-insulin-dependent, or type II, diabetes. Type I diabetes is caused by a lack of insulin production, whereas type II diabetes is related to cellular resistance to insulin due to either decreased insulin binding to cell receptors or to a postreceptor defect [59]. The principal precipitating factor for type II diabetes is obesity. A sedentary lifestyle appears to be another important risk factor for type II diabetes because of its relationship to obesity, and has an independent effect on insulin sensitivity [59]. An increased incidence of type II diabetes also occurs with aging, possibly as the result of the decreased physical activity and weight gain that occur as adults age [60]. Type II diabetes accounts for approximately 80 percent of all cases of the disease in our society. Recent data from the College Alumni Study indicate that increased physical activity is effective in preventing type II diabetes. This protective benefit is especially pronounced in persons at the highest risk for the disease [60a].

Exercise is associated with a variety of metabolic and endocrine responses that may benefit the diabetic patient. These include an increase in glucose uptake by skeletal muscle, a fall in serum insulin levels, and increases in levels of serum glucagon, catecholamines, and cortisol [61]. Regular exercise may also benefit the diabetic patient through improved weight man-

agement, blood lipid profile, psychosocial profile and reductions in blood pressure and platelet aggregation [59].

Effects of Exercise in Patients with CHD

Most patients with CHD can safely participate in exercise training programs [62]. As in healthy adults, patients with CHD develop an increase in VO₂max, a decrease in heart rate, and, if training intensity and duration are high enough, an increase in stroke volume [63] in response to aerobic training. Such adaptations may help CHD patients to achieve a higher functional status. Patients with angina pectoris can attain higher workloads at the same rate-pressure product following training [17, 64], typically causing a decrease in symptomatology [65].

Exercise training following MI may be associated with decreased mortality [66, 67]. Results of a meta-analysis of 22 trials that randomized patients to cardiac rehabilitation exercise programs following MI demonstrated a 20 percent reduction in overall mortality [68]. A study in which dogs exercised daily after MI demonstrated improved baroreflexes, resulting in decreased susceptibility to significant arrhythmias and sudden death [42]. Other benefits associated with cardiac rehabilitation include improvements in psychosocial characteristics, blood pressure, and lipoprotein patterns [69]. Rehabilitation programs post-MI may also improve the rate of return to work, although the data are conflicting, and return to work is heavily influenced by other factors such as psychosocial parameters [66].

Patients with decreased left ventricular function after a large MI may have more rapid progression of left ventricular dysfunction with early vigorous exercise training (70) and need close medical supervision. However, exercise has been shown to improve exercise duration and functional capacity in these patients, primarily through peripheral adaptations, including an increase in peak blood flow to exercising muscles, and increased arteriovenous oxygen difference [71, 72, 73, 74]. Improvement in functional capacity with exercise training is unrelated to baseline left ventricular function [71].

Mental Benefits of Exercise

In 1980 the National Heart, Lung and Blood Institute and the National Center for Health Care Technology held a consensus conference on coronary bypass surgery [75]. One outcome of this conference was that "despite the paucity of good data . . . the operation does improve the quality of life" of some patients. While quality of life is difficult to define, it is a construct that would seem in part to naturally encompass both physical and mental health. In this regard aerobic exercise has the potential to affect the primary and secondary prevention of CHD and the quality of life of patients. Exercise leads to reductions in anxiety and tension for many individuals [76, 77]. In one study, 40 minutes of walking reduced anxiety and tension and enhanced overall total mood state [78]. The changes were independent of walking intensity and persisted for two hours following exercise. Participation in regular aerobic activity may therefore serve to reduce stress, one of the CHD risk factors identified by the Framingham Heart Study. In addition, aerobic training has proved to be an effective treatment for some individuals suffering from mild to moderate depression [76, 77].

In summary aerobic exercise leading to physical fitness has the potential to reduce tension and alter an individual's reactivity to stressors that could theoretically precipitate a coronary event [76, 77]. It has been suggested that mental stress is a trigger mechanism leading to myocardial ischemia in CHD patients [79]. In addition, exercise may also be used to manage the anxiety and depression that many cardiac patients experience.

Little research has been done evaluating the effects of exercise on hostility or anger. To date exercise has not been found to alter the type A behavior pattern nor hostility or anger. Hostility and anger are components of the global type A behavior pattern that have been implicated as potential behavioral pathways associated with heart disease [80, 81].

Few data are available pertaining to the psy-chological benefits associated with resistance exercise. One study, however, suggests that resistance exercise increases self-esteem and has the potential to enhance mood [82].

The Overall Risk and Benefits of Exercise

The Safety of Exercise

The major risk of exercise is sudden death due to underlying cardiovascular disease. Risk of sudden death is transiently increased during exercise, but the overall risk is much lower in active men than sedentary men [83]. Appropriate medical clearance and counseling before an exercise program is begun can help reduce the risk of sudden death. Exercising with a partner and wearing an ID bracelet containing medical information are also recommended, particularly for individuals with increased risk of complications associated with exercise.

Other risks of regular exercise include musculoskeletal trauma and environmental stress. The risk of musculoskeletal injuries can be reduced by warming up gradually, exercising at moderate rather than vigorous intensities, and limiting training to 3 to 5 days per week. Participating in a variety of activities can also help decrease the chance of injury. Environmental stress can be avoided by dressing appropriately, drinking plenty of fluids, and adjusting the exercise regimen.

Economic Consequences of Physical Inactivity

Extensive automation and mechanization on the job and in the home and emphasis on television and spectator sports for leisure time activity have resulted in many Americans becoming inactive. It is difficult to estimate accurately the economic consequences of a sedentary lifestyle. To do so, one must consider two factors. The first consideration is the prevalence of sedentary behavior, estimated at 40 to 80 percent of adults in the United States. The second consideration is the prevalence of illnesses that may be at least partially prevented by regular physical activity, including CHD, hypertension, obesity, diabetes, and osteoporosis. These exceedingly common disorders probably cumulatively affect up to 50% of older Americans and make up a large part of American health care expenditure.

The high prevalence of physical inactivity and consequent serious illnesses indicates that from a public health, population-based perspective, even a small incremental increase in physical activity would have significant desirable consequences on morbidity, mortality, and health care expenditure. Interventions need not be large to result in great population benefit.

Medical Clearance for Exercise

The History and Review of Systems

The physician can determine through a baseline interview and physical examination of the patient if there are any contraindications to exercise. The cardiovascular, pulmonary, neurologic, and musculoskeletal systems should be reviewed and any symptoms explored in depth. Illnesses such as diabetes, ischemic heart disease, and peripheral vascular disease need to be identified. Chest pain, dyspnea, syncopal episodes, palpitations, claudication, and related symptoms should be evaluated in detail, since these may indicate serious medical conditions for which vigorous exercise may be contraindicated. Medications may potentially alter the physiologic response to exercise or otherwise affect the exercise prescription and should be reviewed with the patient.

The physician should also evaluate the patient's relevant social and exercise history, time available for exercise, availability and convenience of facilities, and financial resources for exercise. It is also important to assess the patient's motivation, his perception of his ability to participate in an exercise program (self-efficacy), and the support of family and friends — all are key factors in adhering to an exercise program. This information can be helpful in counseling the patient on adherence-related factors — helping him to increase his motivation, self-efficacy, and social support for exercise and helping him to find ways to fit exercise into his lifestyle. (See Chapter 7 for discussion of such counseling techniques).

The Physical Examination

The physical examination should particularly focus on detecting any abnormalities of the cardiovascular, pulmonary, and musculoskeletal systems, since the safety and tolerability of exercise may be compromised by dysfunction in these systems. The vital signs can be used to detect medical conditions that may affect exercise. Hypertension requires treatment prior to exercise since systolic blood pressure increases acutely with exercise [84]. Asymptomatic hypotension (not due to autonomic dysfunction) generally does not preclude exercise. Dysrhythmias such as atrial fibrillation are evident on examination of the pulse. Resting tachypnea may be a clue to pulmonary or cardiac dysfunction.

A careful cardiovascular examination should be done to rule out even asymptomatic abnormalities. Any cardiac murmurs suggestive of structural heart disease should be evaluated fully. Murmurs may be due to regurgitant or stenotic valvular lesions that will need further evaluation before beginning a vigorous exercise program. Murmurs may also suggest congenital cardiac abnormalities such as atrial septal defect, ventricular septal defect, or patent ductus arteriosus, which do not necessarily preclude participation in an exercise program. However, identification of these conditions prior to beginning a vigorous exercise program is mandatory. It is critical to identify potentially lethal conditions such as hypertrophic obstructive cardiomyopathy, significant aortic stenosis, or Marfan's syndrome, since these may be associated with an increased risk of sudden death during exertion.

The initial evaluation will identify some patients who will be excluded from participating in an exercise program. Exercise should not be recommended in the presence of unstable angina pectoris, untreated severe valvular regurgitation or stenosis, accelerated hypertension, ventricular pseudoaneurysm, severe aortic aneurysm, or decompensated congestive heart failure [6].

Pulmonary status must also be assessed during the preexercise program physical examination. Increased anteroposterior chest diameter, bony chest wall deformities, pursed-lip breathing, wheezing, or other abnormal auscultatory findings suggest pulmonary dysfunction, which may affect a patient's exercise capacity. If resting hypoxemia is present, exercise may cause further deterioration in oxygenation [85]. The two major determinants of aerobic capacity in healthy people are cardiac output and the ability of exercising muscles to utilize oxygen. Patients with lung disease may be unable to oxygenate blood sufficiently for the increased demands of working muscles so that pulmonary function may limit aerobic exercise.

Patients with chronic airflow obstruction, asthma, or interstitial lung disease may benefit from further pulmonary function testing to determine whether bronchodilators can improve respiratory parameters at rest or with exercise. A graded exercise tolerance test with pulse oximetry can identify patients who become hypoxemic with exertion. Supplemental oxygen during exercise may be necessary for such patients.

Neurologic and musculoskeletal examination should be directed toward detection of any focal or generalized abnormalities that may affect an exercise program. Vigorous exercise is contraindicated in active myositis, recent transient ischemic attack, or known unrepaired intracranial aneurysm. Any focal abnormalities such as severe osteoarthritis or paresis will necessitate individualization in the type of exercise prescribed.

The Exercise Tolerance Test

Because exercise increases cardiac work via increased heart rate and stroke volume, coronary artery stenoses that are not flow-limiting at rest may become flow-limiting with exercise. Insufficient coronary flow to meet required myocardial oxygen demand gives rise to regional myocardial ischemia. It is important to document both the presence of exercise-induced myocardial ischemia and the precise level of exercise at which myocardial ischemia occurs. This information may be obtained from an exercise tolerance test (ETT). The ETT also allows assessment of heart rate and blood pressure

responses to exercise. However, certain medical conditions are absolute contraindications to exercise testing; certain other complications require that exercise testing be performed only after careful evaluation by the physician (Table 10-1) [6].

Like most tests an ETT with electrocardiography (ECG) may give ambiguous or false results. When depression of ST segments occurs with exercise (particularly in a horizontal or downward sloping pattern) with or without angina, a test is considered positive for possible myocardial ischemia. When testing is performed on populations with a low prevalence of CHD, such as asymptomatic men and women, the predictive value of a positive test for significant coronary disease is low [86]. A positive electrocardiogram in this setting is frequently a false positive. This response is seen frequently in women [87]. Similarly ischemic ECG changes may not develop if the cardiac work load is below a certain threshold. If the maximum exercise heart rate is less than 85 percent of the age-predicted maximum (220 minus age), a test can only be indeterminate, not negative, since the heart may not be stressed adequately to detect ischemia. Physicians must be prepared to use their clinical judgment in determining when an ETT may be giving false positive results and must appreciate that the predictive value of a positive test in some populations is very low. A thallium ETT is often a useful adjunctive follow-up test for those patients with a possible false positive ETT. By decreasing the false positivity rate, the thallium ETT becomes a more specific test for the diagnosis of myocardial ischemia.

Physicians are commonly faced with healthy, asymptomatic people who wish to begin a vigorous exercise program. Whether these people should undergo exercise electrocardiography to detect coronary ischemia is controversial. The potential problems in using the exercise electrocardiogram to screen all patients prior to an exercise program have been reviewed by a joint task force from the American College of Cardiology and the American Heart Association [88]. The U.S. PSTF [2] has concluded that routine testing of all asymptomatic patients is un-

Table 10-1. Contraindications to exercise testing

Absolute contraindications

A recent significant change in the resting ECG suggesting infarction or other acute cardiac events
Recent complicated myocardial infarction
Unstable angina
Uncontrolled ventricular dysrhythmia
Uncontrolled atrial dysrhythmia that compromises cardiac function
Third-degree A-V block
Acute congestive heart failure
Severe aortic stenosis
Suspected or known dissecting aneurysm
Active or suspected myocarditis or pericarditis
Thrombophlebitis or intracardiac thrombi
Recent systemic or pulmonary embolus
Acute infection
Significant emotional distress (psychosis)

Relative contraindications

Resting diastolic blood pressure > 120 mm Hg or resting systolic blood pressure > 200 mm Hg
Moderate valvular heart disease
Known electrolyte abnormalities (hypokalemia, hypomagnesemia)
Fixed-rate pacemaker (rarely used)
Frequent or complex ventricular ectopy
Ventricular aneurysm
Cardiomyopathy, including hypertrophic cardiomyopathy
Uncontrolled metabolic disease (e.g., diabetes, thyrotoxicosis, or myxedema)
Chronic infectious disease (e.g., mononucleosis, hepatitis, AIDS)
Neuromuscular, musculoskeletal, or rheumatoid disorders that are exacerbated by exercise
Advanced or complicated pregnancy

Source: American College of Sports Medicine. Guidelines for exercise testing and prescription. 4th ed. Philadelphia: Lea & Febiger, 1991.

necessary. The American College of Sports Medicine (ACSM) has made recommendations for exercise testing based on the classification of patients into the following three risk categories [6]:

1. Apparently healthy: patients who are asymptomatic and apparently healthy with no more than one major coronary risk factor (hypertension, hypercholesterolemia, cigarette smoking, diabetes, or family history of CHD). These individuals can begin a *moderate*-intensity exercise program without undergoing diagnostic exercise testing regardless of age. Men over age 40 and women over age 50 should have an ETT before starting a *vigorous* exercise program.
2. Individuals at higher risk: patients who have symptoms suggestive of possible cardiopulmonary disease or metabolic disease and/or

two or more major coronary risk factors. An ETT is desirable prior to beginning a *vigorous* exercise program. An ETT may not be necessary for individuals who are asymptomatic if *moderate*-intensity exercise is undertaken gradually with appropriate guidance.
3. Individuals with disease: patients with known cardiac, pulmonary, or metabolic disease. These patients should have a diagnostic exercise test prior to beginning an exercise program.

Moderate and vigorous exercise are not defined precisely in the ACSM guidelines. We define moderate intensity as 40 to 60 percent VO_2max, or approximately 50 to 70 percent maximum heart rate (max HR) and vigorous exercise as 60 to 85 percent VO_2max, or 70 to 90 percent max HR. Above 85 percent VO_2max is severe exercise.

Exercise Prescription for the Healthy Adult

The goal of the exercise program should be determined from discussion with the patient as a way to enhance adherence. For most people the goal is to lower the risk of CAD, improve cardiorespiratory fitness, lose weight, improve body composition (ratio of lean to fat tissue), reduce stress, or strengthen certain muscle groups. Appropriate counseling for nutrition, stress reduction, smoking cessation, or other issues may also be done at this time.

Traditionally the goal of the exercise prescription has been to improve maximal aerobic capacity or fitness. The optimal prescription for exercise to improve health has not been defined. Recent research indicates that even small amounts of regular exercise without improvements in aerobic capacity may be beneficial [28, 29]. This carries important implications for patients who are not candidates for vigorous exercise or those who do not want to exercise at this level. Sedentary individuals may benefit from relatively small increases in physical activity.

Information derived from the initial evaluation of the patient, coupled with the results of any further testing, will help in placing the patient into one of two categories: the apparently healthy normal adult or the individual with medical conditions. Many of the standards of care can be reviewed in detail in guidelines developed by the ACSM [6, 7].

The exercise prescription has five components: type or mode, intensity, duration, frequency, and progression (Table 10-2).

Type of Exercise

Aerobic activities that utilize large muscle groups in rhythmic activity for a sustained period of time are recommended. Examples include running, walking, aerobic dance, bicycling, rowing, swimming, cross-country skiing, and rope skipping. These activities maximize the energy expenditure per unit time and may be performed either continuously or discontinuously to achieve a training effect.

Table 10-2. Guidelines for exercise prescription for healthy adults

Component	Guideline
Mode of activity	Aerobic or endurance exercise (jogging, swimming, cycling, aerobic dance, walking)
Intensity	50 to 85% VO_2max 50 to 85% heart rate reserve 60 to 90% max HR 12 to 16 RPE
Frequency	3 to 5 days/week
Duration	15 to 60 minutes of continuous activity (duration dependent on intensity)
Progression	as determined by the patient's response

RPE = rating of perceived exertion.

The PSTF suggests that walking may be the ideal activity for sedentary individuals and those with medical conditions, since it is simple, easily sustained, convenient, inexpensive, and appropriate for a wide range of persons [2]. Walking is associated with many of the same health benefits as other aerobic activities [89]. Furthermore, minimal risk of injuries and sudden death is associated with walking. A potential disadvantage of walking is the time required. Although fitness walking also allows achievement of a total energy cost appropriate to improvement in functional capacity, generally approximately 900 to 1500 kcal per week, this may take up to 45 minutes daily.

The ACSM recommends supplementing aerobic exercise with strength training activities two to three times per week [6]. By maintaining strength, the patient can perform leisure and occupational activities that require moving heavy objects with less physiological stress. Strength training also helps maintain lean body mass with aging. For patients with medical conditions, low-resistance, high-repetition (8 to 12 repetitions) exercises involving the major muscle groups are generally recommended. Individuals without medical complications can incorporate higher-resistance exercises.

Intensity

The prescribed intensity should be at a level that will induce a training effect without causing a metabolic load that evokes adverse symptoms or cardiovascular signs. Intensity is expressed as a percentage of maximal aerobic capacity, or VO_2max, with 50 to 85 percent as optimal [6]. For some individuals the training threshold may be less than 50 percent VO_2max.

There are several methods for monitoring exercise intensity. Since HR increases linearly with oxygen uptake in most healthy adults, it is the measurement used most frequently. If VO_2 is measured as part of the exercise tolerance test, the target heart rate (THR) at 50 to 85 percent VO_2max can be determined by plotting heart rate against VO_2.

The second method is called the Karvonen or heart rate reserve (HRR) method [90]. For this method 50 to 85 percent HRR approximates 50 to 85 percent VO_2max. The following equation is used to calculate the THR:

$$THR = \% \text{ intensity} \times (\text{max HR} - \text{resting HR}) + \text{resting HR}$$

The maximum heart rate is determined from an exercise tolerance test. For people who have not had an exercise test, the max HR can be estimated from the equation 220 minus age.

The American Heart Association uses a simplified method to determine exercise intensity [91]. The THR is calculated by multiplying maximum heart rate by the desired intensity. The percentages of max HR that correspond to 50 and 85 percent VO_2max are 60 percent and 90 percent.

These techniques rely on the patient's ability to monitor his or her own HR. HR palpation needs to be demonstrated to the patient prior to beginning the exercise program. In the early stages of the program, frequent pulse checks are necessary. After the program becomes established, the patient will be able to associate a subjective feeling of exertion with the THR. Once the patient is able to recognize this feeling, checks can be less frequent. For individuals who are unable to accurately take their pulse, electronic pulse monitors are available that range in price from $50 to $300.

The rating of perceived exertion (RPE) may also be a helpful guide for intensity for some patients. The RPE developed by Borg [92] is a 15-point scale with descriptive delimits at each odd number (Table 10-3). The scale has strong correlations with VO_2, HR, ventilation, and blood lactate concentration [93, 94]. An RPE of 12 to 13, classified as "somewhat hard," corresponds to approximately 50 percent VO_2max and is a good recommendation for initial exercise intensity for sedentary individuals. Ratings of 15 to 16 correspond to approximately 80 to 85 percent VO_2max.

Frequency

The optimal frequency of aerobic training for healthy adults is three to five times per week. Exercising only one or two sessions per week can result in modest gains in functional capacity but little change in body fat [95]. The adverse consequences of training, such as musculoskeletal problems, increase with training frequencies greater than three days per week [96]. Exercise at lower intensities (50 to 60 percent VO_2max) may be performed more frequently.

Duration

Duration and intensity are interrelated components of the exercise prescription. Exercise of

Table 10-3. Rating of perceived exertion scale

6	
7	Very, very light
8	
9	Very light
10	
11	Fairly light
12	
13	Somewhat hard
14	
15	Hard
16	
17	Very hard
18	
19	Very, very hard
20	

higher intensity is generally performed for a shorter period. The initial exercise program should include sessions of moderate duration and intensity, i.e., 15 to 20 minutes at 50 to 60 percent VO$_2$max. If no complications occur, the duration and intensity may be increased gradually. As with intensity the incidence of musculoskeletal injuries increases with longer workouts [96].

Progression

The ACSM guidelines describes three stages of progression: the initial conditioning stage, the improvement conditioning stage, and the maintenance stage [6]. The initial conditioning phase generally lasts from 4 to 6 weeks. During this time the patient may need support in making the transition from a sedentary to an active lifestyle. Patients may also need advice about how to fit exercise into their working day. The continued emotional support of the physician supplying the exercise prescription is key. During the initial conditioning stage, the patient should monitor HR regularly to ensure the exercise is of the appropriate intensity. If the HR exceeds the THR, the patient should decrease the intensity of exercise. Similarly if the HR is less than the THR, the patient should increase the exercise intensity.

Once the patient has completed the initial conditioning phase, he is ready to begin the improvement conditioning phase, in which the major physiologic adaptations to exercise occur. During the improvement conditioning phase the patient progresses in training workload at a more rapid rate. As with the initial phase, progress depends on the individual response to training.

Once a patient has reached the training goals, whether in terms of cardiorespiratory fitness, body weight, or just subjective well being, it is necessary to review those goals and establish new ones. In many cases the new goal will be maintenance of the current fitness level. To maintain a constant level of fitness, weekly caloric expenditure in exercise needs to remain constant. Patients may prefer to vary their exercise program or to try new sports that they previously felt unable to participate in, to reduce tedium and enhance motivation to maintain exercise.

Measurement of Maximal Aerobic Capacity

Knowledge of the patient's maximal aerobic capacity provides a rational basis for developing the exercise prescription and thus avoids starting patients at levels that are too difficult or too easy. Direct measurement of VO$_2$max provides the best measure of maximal aerobic capacity. However, direct measurement requires expensive equipment and specially trained personnel. If an exercise tolerance test is performed, maximal aerobic capacity can be estimated from the workload at maximal exercise or total time of the test. Equations for estimating aerobic capacity based on different test protocols are presented in the ACSM guidelines [6].

Aerobic capacity can also be estimated using submaximal exercise or field tests. The 1-mile walk test [97] is a practical field test that can be self-administered by the patient. The test is very accurate with a correlation coefficient of r = .88 between estimated and measured VO$_2$max and a standard error of estimate of 5.0 ml/kg/min. The test does however, overestimate VO$_2$max in adults taking beta blockers. The patient should be instructed to walk 1 mile on a measured track as briskly as possible, time the mile walk, and then measure HR for 15 seconds at the end of the mile. The following equation is used to estimate VO$_2$max:

$$VO_2max \ (ml/kg/min) = 132.853 - 0.0769 \ wt - 0.3877 \ age + 6.3150 \ sex - 3.2649 \ t - 0.1565 \ HR$$

where

wt	=	weight in pounds
age	=	age in years
sex	=	1 for male, 0 for female
t	=	time to walk one mile in minutes
HR	=	heart rate at the end of the mile in beats per minute

The VO$_2$max calculated from this equation can be compared with norms developed by the American Heart Association (Table 10-4) [91] to determine relative fitness levels for age and gender.

For patients who do not want to bother with calculations, a practical format has been developed to allow the rapid estimation of a patient's

Table 10-4.   Normal values of VO₂max at different ages

Age (years)	VO₂max (ml/kg/min)	
	Men	Women
20–29	43 (±22) [12 METs]	36 (±21) [10 METs]
30–39	42 (±22) [12 METs]	34 (±21) [10 METs]
40–49	40 (±22) [11METs]	32 (±21) [9 METs]
50–59	36 (±22) [10 METs]	29 (±22) [8 METs]
60–69	33 (±22) [9 METs]	27 (±22) [8 METs]
70–79	29 (±22) [8 METs]	27 (±22) [8 METs]

MET = resting metabolic equivalent (1 MET = 3.5 ml/kg/min).
Source: American Heart Association. Exercise standards. 1991. Reproduced with permission.

relative fitness level and provide a basis for exercise prescription [98]. The preceding equation has been solved for the average-weight male (170 lb) and female (125 lb) in each decade and placed in relative fitness charts based on the American Heart Association norms and exercise prescription charts. With this format all the patient must do is walk the mile briskly, record the walk time and HR at the end of the mile, and then find the appropriate age and gender charts. The relative fitness level and exercise prescription are determined by plotting the walk time and the HR.

For example, a 54–year-old woman walks the mile in 17 minutes and 15 seconds (17.25 minutes). Her HR at the end of the mile is 132 beats per minute. As indicated in Figure 10-5, she has average fitness compared with other 50- to 59-year-old women. A 20-week walking program appropriate for her level of fitness is determined by plotting her HR and walk time on the Exercise Prescription Chart (Figure 10-6). Her data place her in the Category B walking program. The 20-week Category B walking program for her level of fitness is presented in Table 10-5.

Relative fitness and exercise prescription charts and the corresponding 20-week walking programs for men and women aged 20 to over 60 are presented in Figures 10-7 through 10-11 and in Table 10-5.

Exercise Prescription for Patients at Risk for CHD

Physicians and health care professionals frequently prescribe exercise for patients with medical conditions that complicate exercise performance. Exercise training has become an important adjunct therapy in the management of medical conditions such as ischemic heart disease, hypertension, diabetes, and obesity, but it is contraindicated for other medical conditions, such as unstable angina and critical aortic stenosis. The exercise prescription for patients with medical conditions follows the same basic guidelines as for the healthy adult [8, 12]. The five components of the exercise prescription (mode, intensity, duration, frequency, and progression) are modified based on the limitations and goals of the patient.

Hypertension

Hypertension is one of the most common cardiac disorders in general practice. In addition to exercise, patients should be counseled on diet, weight management, and smoking cessation. In general, hypertensive patients should be encouraged to exercise at least four times per week, preferably daily. The duration should progress to 30 to 60 minutes per day, if possible. Exercise intensity at the low end of the scale (40 to 60 percent VO₂max) seems to be more effective in lowering resting blood pressure. High-intensity exercise and activities with a large isometric component should be minimized, since these activities can cause a large pressor response. Antihypertensive medications may affect exercise responses and are discussed in a later section.

Ischemic Heart Disease

Adequate medical evaluation is important in developing an exercise program for patients with ischemic heart disease. In addition to the exercise tolerance test to assess the ischemic response to exercise, resting left ventricular systolic function should be evaluated by two-dimensional echocardiography or radionuclide ventriculog-

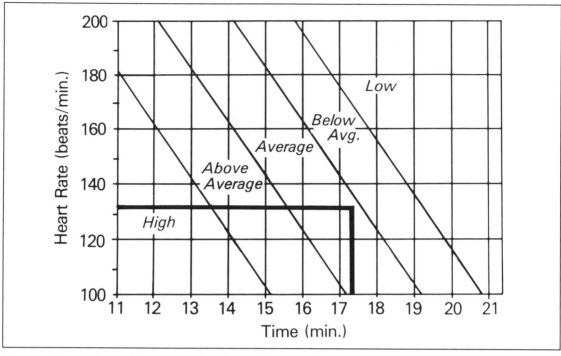

Figure 10-5. Relative fitness levels for 50- to 59-year-old women taking the 1-mile walk test. (Source: The Rockport Walking Institute, 1986.)

Figure 10-6. Determination of the appropriate exercise program for a 50- to 59-year-old woman taking the 1-mile walk test. (Source: The Rockport Walking Institute, 1986.)

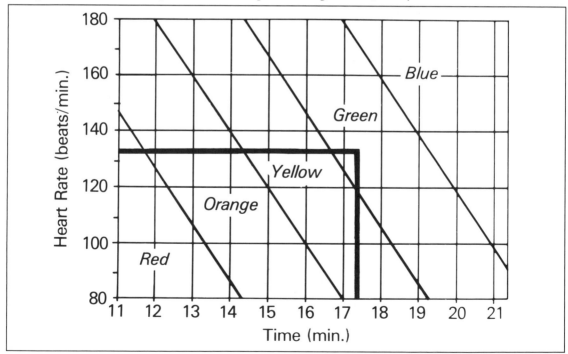

Table 10-5. Twenty-week exercise prescription programs

Category A program

Week	1–2	3–4	5	6	7–8	9	10	11	12–13	14	15–16	17–18	19–20
Warm-up (mins. before walk stretches)	5–7	5–7	5–7	5–7	5–7	5–7	5–7	5–7	5–7	5–7	5–7	5–7	5–7
Mileage	1.0	1.25	1.5	1.5	1.75	2.0	2.0	2.0	2.25	2.5	2.5	2.75	3.0
Pace (mph)	3.0	3.0	3.0	3.5	3.5	3.5	3.75	3.75	3.75	3.75	4.0	4.0	4.0
Heart rate (% of max)	60	60	60	60–70	60–70	60–70	60–70	70	70	70	70	70–80	70–80
Cooldown (mins. after walk stretches)	5–7	5–7	5–7	5–7	5–7	5–7	5–7	5–7	5–7	5–7	5–7	5–7	5–7
Frequency (times per week)	5	5	5	5	5	5	5	5	5	5	5	5	5

At the end of the 20-week fitness walking protocol, retest yourself to establish your new program.

Category B program

Week	1–2	3–4	5–6	7	8–9	10–12	13	14	15–16	17–18	19–20
Warm-up (mins. before walk stretches)	5–7	5–7	5–7	5–7	5–7	5–7	5–7	5–7	5–7	5–7	5–7
Mileage	1.5	1.75	2.0	2.0	2.25	2.5	2.75	2.75	3.0	3.25	3.5
Pace (mph)	3.0	3.0	3.0	3.5	3.5	3.5	3.5	4.0	4.0	4.0	4.0
Heart rate (% of max)	60–70	60–70	60–70	70	70	70	70	70–80	70–80	70–80	70–80
Cooldown (mins. after walk stretches)	5–7	5–7	5–7	5–7	5–7	5–7	5–7	5–7	5–7	5–7	5–7
Frequency (times per week)	5	5	5	5	5	5	5	5	5	5	5

At the end of the 20-week fitness walking protocol, retest yourself to establish your new program.

Category C program

Week	1	2	3–4	5	6–8	9–10	11–12	13–14	15	16–17	18–20
Warm-up (mins. before walk stretches)	5–7	5–7	5–7	5–7	5–7	5–7	5–7	5–7	5–7	5–7	5–7
Mileage	2.0	2.25	2.5	2.75	2.75	3.0	3.0	3.25	3.5	3.5	4.0
Pace (mph)	3.0	3.0	3.0	3.0	3.5	3.5	4.0	4.0	4.0	4.5	4.5
Heart rate (% of max)	70	70	70	70	70	70	70–80	70–80	70–80	70–80	70–80
Cooldown (mins. after walk stretches)	5–7	5–7	5–7	5–7	5–7	5–7	5–7	5–7	5–7	5–7	5–7
Frequency (times per week)	5	5	5	5	5	5	5	5	5	5	5

At the end of the 20-week fitness walking protocol, you may either retest yourself and move to a new fitness walking category or follow the Category C Maintenance Program for a lifetime of fitness walking.

Table 10-5. Twenty-week exercise prescription programs, continued

Category D program

Week	1	2	3–4	5	6	7	8	9–10	11–14	15–20
Warm-up (mins. before walk stretches)	5–7	5–7	5–7	5–7	5–7	5–7	5–7	5–7	5–7	5–7
Mileage	2.5	2.75	3.0	3.25	3.25	3.5	3.75	4.0	4.0	4.0
Pace (mph)	3.5	3.5	3.5	3.5	4.0	4.0	4.0	4.0	4.5	4.5
Incline/Weight										+
Heart rate (% of max)	70	70	70	70	70–80	70–80	70–80	70–80	70–80	70–80
Cooldown (mins. after walk stretches)	5–7	5–7	5–7	5–7	5–7	5–7	5–7	5–7	5–7	5–7
Frequency (times per week)	5	5	5	5	5	5	5	5	5	3

At the end of the 20-week fitness walking protocol follow the Category D/E Maintenance Program for a lifetime of fitness walking.

Category E Program

Week	1	2	3	4	5	6	7–20
Warm-up (mins. before walk stretches)	5–7	5–7	5–7	5–7	5–7	5–7	5–7
Mileage	3.0	3.25	3.5	3.5	3.75	4.0	4.0
Pace (mph)	4.0	4.0	4.0	4.5	4.5	4.5	4.5
Incline/Weight							+
Heart rate (% of max)	70	70	70	70–80	70–80	70–80	70–80
Cooldown (mins. after walk stretches)	5–7	5–7	5–7	5–7	5–7	5–7	5–7
Frequency (times per week)	5	5	5	5	5	5	3

At the end of the 20-week fitness walking protocol turn to the Category D/E Maintenance Program for a lifetime of fitness walking.

Category C Maintenance Program

Warm-up: 5–7 minutes before walk stretches

Aerobic Work out: mileage: 4.0 pace: 4.5 mph

Heart rate: 70–80% of maximum

Cooldown: 5–7 minutes after walk stretches

Frequency: 3–5 times per week

Weekly mileage: 12–20 miles

Category D/E Maintenance Program

Warm-up: 5–7 minutes before walk stretches

Aerobic workout: mileage: 4.0 pace: 4.5 mph weight/incline: add weights to upper body or add hill walking as needed to keep heart rate in target zone (70–80% of predicted maximum).

Heart rate: 70–80% of maximum

Cooldown: 5–7 minutes after walk stretches

Frequency: 3–5 times per week

Weekly mileage: 12–20 miles

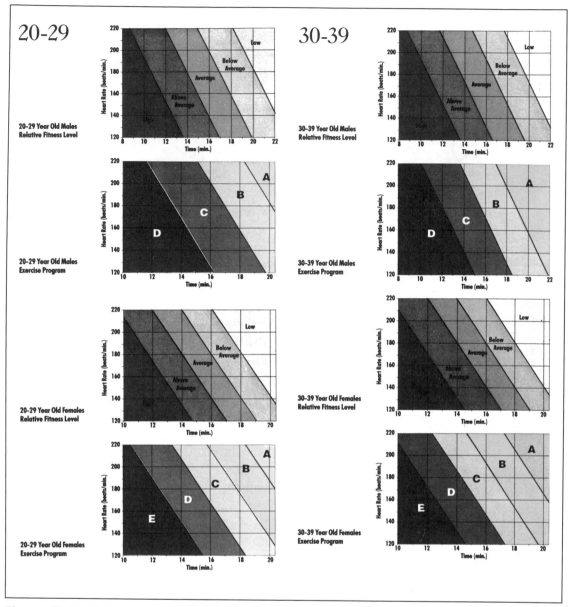

Figures 10-7 and 10-8.   Charts for relative fitness levels and exercise programs for, respectively, 20- to 29-year old males and females and 30- to 39-year old males and females. (Source: The Rockport Walking Institute, 1986.)

raphy [99]. Frequency and complexity of arrhythmias also should be assessed. Results from these tests can be used to stratify patients based on their risk for subsequent cardiac events. The exercise prescription is modified based on the degree of left ventricular dysfunction and the presence of inducible ischemia and arrhythmias.

The risk of supervised cardiac rehabilitation is very low, with one major cardiovascular complication (cardiac arrest or MI) per 81,101 patient-hours and one fatality per 783,972 patient-hours [62]. The safety of cardiac rehabil-

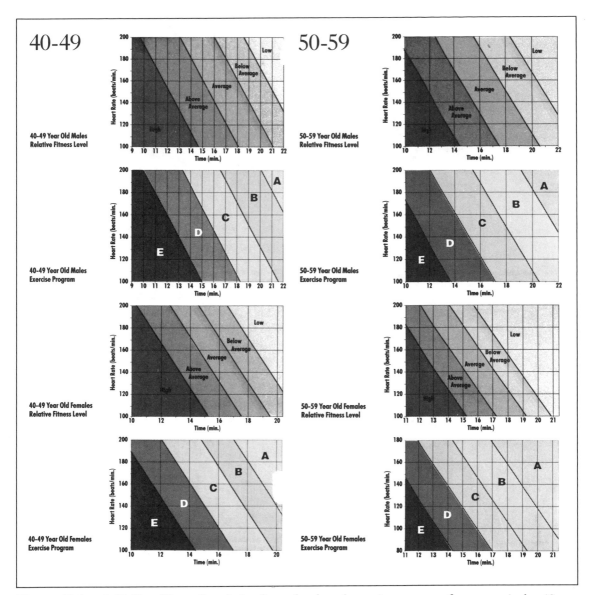

Figures 10-9 and 10-10. Charts for relative fitness levels and exercise programs for, respectively, 40- to 49-year old males and females and 50- to 59-year old males and females. (Source: The Rockport Walking Institute, 1986.)

itation results from high standards in medical screening and assessment, patient education, patient supervision, and emergency treatment.

Over 85 percent of patients with cardiac arrest reported in supervised programs have been successfully resuscitated [62]. An early study identified poor compliance to exercise prescription as a factor in cardiac arrest patients. A more recent survey [62], however, indicates that good compliance does not guarantee exercise safety. Cardiac complications were related more to degree of left ventricular dysfunction and severity of heart disease.

Patients with a recent MI, coronary artery

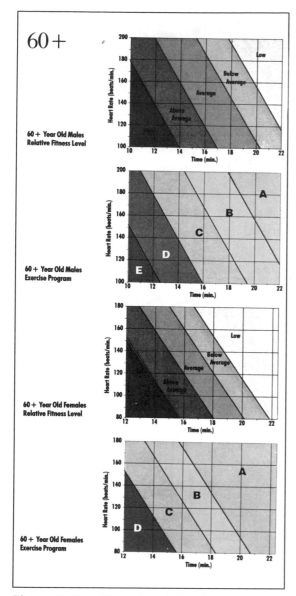

Figure 10-11. Charts for relative fitness levels and exercise programs for men and women over age 60. (Source: The Rockport Walking Institute, 1986.)

bypass surgery, or coronary angioplasty should initially participate in a supervised cardiac rehabilitation program. Selected patients who are at low risk (uncomplicated MI or bypass surgery, good left ventricular function, good functional capacity) can participate in a home

walking program. For the home program frequency should be daily. Duration should progress from 10 to 15 minutes per day up to 45 to 60 minutes per day. Intensity should be low initially and increase gradually if there are no symptoms or cardiovascular signs. While home exercise programs may be less expensive, they do not provide the important educational, emotional, and social benefits of supervised group programs.

Exercise training can be beneficial for patients with angina by increasing their functional capacity at the anginal threshold. For these patients the training HR should be set 5 to 10 beats below the ischemic threshold, or at 70 to 85 percent VO_2 at the ischemic threshold [6]. Sublingual nitroglycerin prior to exercise may allow patients with low angina thresholds to achieve higher exercise levels. Patients with unstable angina should not participate in any exercise training program.

Resistance or strength training programs may also be beneficial for patients with ischemic heart disease, particularly patients with near-normal left ventricular function. Programs that include 8 to 12 repetitions of loads corresponding to 40 to 50 percent of maximum strength appear safe for low-risk patients [100].

Concomitant Cardiac Medications

Many of the medications taken by patients with hypertension or ischemic heart disease affect cardiopulmonary or metabolic responses to exercise. An exercise tolerance test should be performed while the patient is taking his normal medications near the time of day he or she would normally exercise to determine the safety of exercise and to provide information for modifying the exercise prescription.

Beta blockers lower both HR and systolic blood pressure at any exercise intensity. Although HR is attenuated, the linear relationship between submaximal heart rate and oxygen consumption is preserved. Consequently the standard guideline for exercise intensity, 60 to 90 percent of maximal HR while on a beta blocker, is a reasonable THR, and HR may be used as a measure of intensity. RPE (12 to 15 on the Borg 20-point scale) may be used as an alternative when maximum heart rate is unavailable.

Calcium channel blockers produce vasodilation in the coronary arteries as well as in the peripheral arteries, resulting in a reduction in blood pressure. They generally attenuate HR and blood pressure responses during exercise. Normal guidelines for intensity of exercise can be used (60 to 90 percent of maximal HR), but they should be based on the HR response to an ETT. An active cool-down is important, since postexercise hypotension may occur.

Other medications such as antiarrhythmics may also modify the HR response to exercise, while antianginals such as nitrates may modify the blood pressure response. Chronic diuretic therapy may lower potassium levels and thus increase arrhythmic potential during exercise. Vasodilators may be associated with postexercise hypotension, necessitating a prolonged cool-down period. Angiotensin-converting enzyme inhibitors (ACE inhibitors) appear to have no effect on the electrocardiogram and do not require modification of the exercise prescription, although they may potentiate postexercise hypotension.

Exercise Prescription for Other Patient Populations

Peripheral Vascular Disease

Walking is the optimal exercise for patients with peripheral vascular disease, because it can improve functional capacity [101]. In addition, the relative ischemia that occurs in the calf muscles during walking may aid in the development of collateral vessels. Patients should walk to the point of claudication and then rest until the pain subsides [101]. This sequence should be repeated until the patient has completed 20 to 30 minutes of exercise. A training HR should be based on an ETT, because patients with peripheral vascular disease frequently have concomitant CAD [102]. Symptoms of claudication generally occur before attainment of a training HR. However, heart rate should be monitored and should not exceed the THR even

in the absence of symptoms. Anginal chest pain is a red flag to decrease intensity.

Diabetes Mellitus

Both type I (insulin-dependent) and type II (non-insulin-dependent) diabetics can benefit from an exercise program, and a program can be safely prescribed for most controlled diabetics. Prior to the start of any exercise program a thorough physical examination emphasizing cardiovascular risks should be conducted, since diabetics often exhibit one or more of these factors. For type I diabetics the examination should also include extensive evaluation for autonomic and sensory neuropathy and retinopathy. The exercise prescription must take into account any of these complications. Exercise testing is also recommended prior to starting an exercise program because of the high incidence of cardiovascular disease in this population.

A major concern for type I diabetics is the possible development of hypoglycemia during or after exercise, which occurs because of exercise-induced glucose uptake by skeletal muscle. The problem can be minimized by monitoring blood glucose levels and adjusting insulin dosage and carbohydrate intake. The patient will need an extensive self-management educational program along with the exercise prescription. The goal of the education program is to teach the patient to assess glucose levels before and after exercise and to judge what carbohydrate and insulin requirements are suitable for the workout. The patient will also need to learn the signs and symptoms of hypoglycemia and how to assess when changes in insulin dosage and carbohydrate intake are warranted. The physician should also emphasize proper footwear and foot hygiene and encourage the diabetic to exercise with a partner.

To help type I diabetics control their blood glucose through a regular pattern of insulin dosage and diet, the ACSM suggests having the person exercise daily at an intensity of 40 to 85 percent of functional capacity. The duration of the exercise should be lowered to 20 to 30 minutes [6].

Many type II diabetics are overweight, so the exercise prescription should be directed toward expending calories. A low-intensity (40 to 60 percent of functional capacity) program performed five times per week for 40 to 60 minutes is recommended for this population [6].

Obesity

Obesity is a major contributor to such illnesses as hypertension, hypercholesterolemia, and diabetes [103], as well as an independent risk factor for cardiovascular disease [104]. Thus, prevention or treatment of obesity is very important from a public health perspective. Although exercise alone contributes only modestly to weight loss [105], regular physical activity can reduce morbidity and mortality even in people who remain obese [33, 83].

The optimal weight loss program combines aerobic and resistance training with a moderate calorie-restricted diet [106]. The addition of exercise to a weight loss diet can increase caloric expenditure, enhance self-efficacy and a feeling of well-being, help maintain resting metabolic rate, increase fat utilization, and reduce fat stores while maintaining lean body mass [106, 107]. More importantly, people who include exercise in a weight loss program tend to keep weight off longer than those who only diet [108].

The exercise program should initially emphasize expending calories. As the patient loses weight the goal can shift toward improving cardiorespiratory fitness. Intensity should be 40 to 60 percent of VO_2max. Patients should be encouraged to work up to 50 to 60 minutes daily with the goal of expending 2000 to 3000 calories per week. The lower intensity will decrease the likelihood of injury and improve compliance. Addition of a strength training program two to three days per week can help prevent lean body mass loss and provide a well-rounded fitness program.

Patients with mild obesity (20 to 40 percent overweight) usually have few limitations to exercise. However, because the emphasis is on daily exercise, we recommend lower impact activities such as walking or stationary cycling, or interspersing vigorous activity with lower intensity activity.

Patients with moderate to severe obesity (> 40 percent overweight) may have several limitations to exercise including reduced functional capacity, heat intolerance, movement restriction, musculoskeletal pain, and poor balance [109]. Activities should be low impact. Stationary cycling or running/walking in a swimming pool provide good alternatives for these patients. Progression should be very gradual based on their tolerance to exercise.

Elderly

Osteoporosis is a common problem faced by older adults, especially postmenopausal women. More than 1.2 million fractures per year result from osteoporosis, with an estimated cost of over $6 billion [110]. Exercise, particularly participation in weight-bearing activities, has been shown to attenuate age-related bone loss in several studies [111, 112]. Moreover, Dalsky and colleagues showed that regular exercise increased vertebral density in 33 healthy postmenopausal women [113].

In addition to bone loss, aerobic capacity and strength decrease with aging while body fat increases [114]. The extent to which functional capacity decreases secondary to aging versus inactivity is controversial. Both cross-sectional and longitudinal studies, however, indicate that the rate of decline of aerobic capacity with age can be reduced by maintaining physical activity [115, 116, 117]. More important, healthy older men and women can increase aerobic capacity and strength with training in a manner similar to that seen in younger age groups [117]. Furthermore, endurance exercise of sufficient intensity can improve left ventricular systolic function in older men [118].

Exercise programs for the elderly should emphasize lower-intensity (40 to 60 percent VO_2max), low-impact activities since injuries may occur more frequently due to poor flexibility, osteoporosis, or other musculoskeletal disorders. Progression is usually slower than for younger adults.

Concomitant medical conditions and/or medications are other factors seen more frequently in the elderly population. An exercise tolerance test can help determine the safety of exercise and the patient's limitations. Healthy elderly patients may also demonstrate chronotropic incompetence or an inadequate HR response to exercise. For these patients RPE may be a better indicator of exercise intensity than HR.

Children

There is growing concern about the physical fitness of children and youth. While it is controversial whether children today have lower cardiorespiratory fitness than 20 years ago, they are definitely fatter. The National Children and Youth Fitness Study (NCYFS) [119, 120], which evaluated 4,678 first through fourth graders and 8,800 fifth through twelfth graders between 1983 and 1987, found that children and adolescents had skinfold measurements that were 2 to 3 mm greater than those of youths in a sample evaluated in the 1960s [119]. It has been suggested that the increase in fatness may be related to an increase in television viewing. The NCYFS also found that young children spend 17 hours a week watching television [120]. Another study showed that each hourly increment of television viewing by adolescents was associated with a 2 percent increase in the prevalence of obesity [121].

Other studies have shown relationships between level of physical activity and the prevalence of cardiovascular risk factors in children such as high blood pressure, obesity, and low levels of HDL-cholesterol [122, 123]. One study that followed children over a five-year period [124] related the five-year change in physical fitness to changes in CHD risk factors. In addition, some CHD risk factors appear to track over time [125, 126], so that children in the upper deciles for risk factors remain high as they become older. Exercise has also been used in the management of obesity [127] and mild hypertension [128] in children and adolescents.

Being fit as a child may not be related to health as an adult, especially if activity is not carried over into adulthood [29]. However, activity also appears to track over time [129]. Thus, active children tend to be active adults, although there is a gradual decline in physical activity and fitness during adolescence [130]. This emphasizes the need to encourage young children to be active and to teach them activities that will carry over into adulthood.

Physicians can influence school administrators and school boards to promote health-related physical education and advocate community programs and facilities for exercise and physical fitness activities. In addition, physicians should discuss physical activity with parents and children and encourage parents to exercise with their children.

Special Considerations

Warm-up/Cool-down

The exercise session should include warm-up and cool-down periods. The warm-up usually lasts 5 to 10 minutes and is designed to gradually increase exercise intensity. The warm-up can include low-intensity exercise such as walking, light jogging, stretching, and calisthenics.

The cool-down lasts 5 to 10 minutes at the end of the exercise session. Exercise intensity is gradually decreased during this period to avoid hypotension.

Environmental Conditions

Heat, cold, and altitude can impair the normal physiologic responses to exercise [131]. It is especially important for patients at high risk or with disease to modify their exercise prescription as environmental conditions change. HR and RPE can be used to maintain physiologic responses at the desired level.

HEAT STRESS

Heat stress is associated with increased sweating rate and more marked cardiorespiratory responses to submaximal exercise. HR increases independent of the exercise stress largely due to cutaneous vasodilation, which results in a redistribution of blood flow to the skin for the purpose of heat dissipation. During moderate exercise HR increases about one beat per minute for each 1°C increase in ambient temperature (20 percent humidity) when the temperature is above 25°C (75°F) [132]. The HR increase is greater during exercise of higher intensity or with higher humidity. Exercise of longer duration (more than 1 hour) may result in dehydration and cause a further increase in HR for a given workload.

When exercising in heat, patients should reduce intensity and possibly duration. Individuals, particularly cardiac patients, should monitor their HR frequently to ensure that they are exercising within safe limits. Cardiac patients should exercise in an air-conditioned area when the wet bulb temperature is above 26°C. Exercising during the cooler parts of the day (early morning or late evening) and wearing porous, light-colored, loose-fitting clothing to facilitate evaporative heat loss should be emphasized. Fluids should be ingested before, during, and after exercise.

COLD

For most healthy individuals, exercising in the cold poses few problems. Clothing that protects the head and extremities should be worn to avoid hypothermia and frostbite. Exercisers should wear layers of clothing that can be removed as they warm up.

Cardiac patients should take special precautions when exercising in cold weather. Exposure to cold can result in vasoconstriction, which causes an increased blood pressure response and increased myocardial oxygen demand. In addition, wearing extra clothing and walking or jogging on snow cause an increase in physical demand such that the patient is exercising at a greater percentage of functional capacity. Training HR should be checked frequently to ensure that the patient is exercising within safe limits. If the air temperature or windchill is below 20°F, cardiac patients should limit outdoor exposure to 30 minutes and avoid windy areas. Below 10°F patients should exercise indoors.

ALTITUDE

The partial pressure of oxygen in the atmosphere is reduced at high altitude. Consequently, oxygen transport is impaired and the cardiorespiratory response to exercise is increased. On ascent to high altitude (>1500 m), the healthy individual should decrease exercise intensity and duration and drink plenty of fluids for a few days until acclimatization occurs.

The impairment of oxygen transport presents greater risk for the cardiac patient. Brammel and colleagues [133] evaluated nine men with reproducible exercise-induced angina and/or ST depression at a residence altitude of 1600 m and a few hours after ascent to 3100 m. At 3100 m, resting HR was slightly increased, VO_2max was decreased, but peak exercise heart rate was unchanged. Rate pressure product was increased at submaximal workloads, suggesting an increased myocardial oxygen demand. HR at angina/ST depression threshold was reproducible and therefore should be a reliable guideline for activity at high altitudes. Patients with very low functional capacity or congestive heart failure should avoid travel to high altitude. Recommendations for exercise at altitude for patients with CAD are presented in Table 10-6 [8].

Compliance

Half the people who start a vigorous exercise program drop out in 6 to 12 months [134, 135, 136]. Blue-collar workers who smoke, are overweight, and have little support for their exercising from spouse or friends are at higher risk for dropping out [135] and require special attention. Physicians can play a major role in helping patients start and maintain an exercise program by discussing the benefits of exercise, helping patients develop their own goals and motivation for exercise, and providing proper guidance. Strategies to improve compliance include starting with small increases in low-intensity physical activity and gradually increasing the amount of activity. Vigorous exercise is associated with poorer adherence [137]. The physician or health care professional can help the patient choose appropriate activities and identify a convenient location and time for exercise. King et al. recently found increased compliance with a home-based exercise program compared with a group-based program [138]. The transition from fall to winter is a time when many people stop exercising because of weather conditions. For optimal health ben-

Table 10-6 Recommendations for exercise at high altitude for patients with CAD

Status	Recommendations for travel	Physical activity
Stable MI or CABG; Normal ETT; ≥ 8 METs	No restrictions	Restrict for 24–72 hours
CHD or post-MI/CABG; ETT 5 to 7 METs; ischemic ECG; or angina	Short-term exposure, <4 hours not requiring sustained activity	Restrict to slow walk, avoid alcohol or heavy meals
All cardiac patients with ETT <5 METs; CHF or angina	Travel to altitude >3000 m not advised	

ETT = exercise tolerance test; CHF = congestive heart failure.

Source: Adapted from Ward A, Malloy P, Rippe J. Exercise prescription guidelines for normal and cardiac populations. Cardiology Clinics 1987; 5:197–210.

efits it is important that exercise be performed year-round. Physicians can help their patients by recommending strategies for maintaining exercise during the winter months. Physicians can also maximize adherence by encouraging the support of the patient's family and friends and by providing positive reinforcement. Treatment should be individualized to maximize compliance.

Summary

Many health-related benefits are associated with physical activity, including decreased CHD risk, improved control of blood pressure, improved blood lipid profile, weight management, and improved mental health. In addition, regular exercise may attenuate the progression of osteoporosis and improve functional capacity following an MI, bypass surgery, or angioplasty.

The optimal amount of exercise required to achieve health-related benefits is unknown. Epidemiologic studies indicate that health benefits can be achieved with modest increases in physical activity. Despite the benefits associated with exercise most adults remain inactive or exercise infrequently.

Physicians can play a major role in encouraging patients to exercise by providing medical clearance, developing a proper exercise prescription, and counseling them on factors related to the adoption and maintenance of exercise programs. Regular rather than vigorous activities should be encouraged, since even small increases in physical activity are associated with decreased risk of morbidity and mortality.

The activity should be simple and require moderate exertion. It should not necessitate specialized facilities, equipment, or skill. Other desirable features are that the activity is conveniently and easily incorporated into daily routines, possesses minimal risk of injury, and has potential for social interaction. The U.S. PSTF recommends brisk walking as the ideal activity that can meet those requirements and serve as a first stage for increasing physical activity for most adults [2].

References

1. Stephens T, Jacobs DR Jr, White CC. A descriptive epidemiology of leisure-time physical activity. Public Health Reports 1985; 100:147–58.
2. Harris SS, Casperson CJ, DeFriese GH, Estes H Jr. Physical activity counseling for healthy adults as a primary preventive intervention in the clinical setting. Report for the U.S. Preventive Services Task Force. JAMA 1989; 261:3590–8.
3. Weaver FJ, Herrick KL, Ramirez AG, et al. Establishing a community base for a cardiovascular health education program. Health Values 1978; 2:249–56.
4. Wechsler H, Levine S, Idelson RK, et al. The physician's role in health promotion. A survey

of primary care practitioners. N Engl J Med 1983; 308:97–100.

5. Wells KB, Lewis CE, Leake B, et al. The practices of general and subspecialty internists in counseling about smoking and exercise. Am J Public Health 1986; 76:1009–13.

6. American College of Sports Medicine. Guidelines for exercise testing and prescription (4th ed.). Philadelphia: Lea & Febiger, 1991.

7. American College of Sports Medicine. In: Blair SN, Painter P, Pate RR, Smith LK, eds. Resource manual for guidelines for exercise testing and prescription. Philadelphia: Lea & Febiger, 1988.

8. Ward A, Malloy P, Rippe J. Exercise prescription guidelines for normal and cardiac populations. Cardiology Clinics 1987; 5:197–210.

9. Goldfine H, Ward A, Taylor P, et al. Exercise and coronary heart disease. Phys Sports Med 1991; 19:80–93.

10. Carlucci D, Goldfine H, Ward A, et al. The health benefits of exercise: impact on specific medical conditions. Phys Sports Med 1991; 19:46–56.

11. Taylor P, Ward A, Rippe JM. Patient evaluation and exercise prescription for the healthy person. Phys Sports Med 1991; 19:95–105.

12. Ward A, Taylor P, Rippe JM. Exercise prescription for patients with medical conditions: making modifications appropriate to individual physiology. Phys Sports Med 1991; 19:64–76.

13. Durstine JL, Pate RR. Cardiorespiratory responses to acute exercise. In: Blair SN, Painter P, Pate RR, Smith LK, eds. Resource manual for guidelines for exercise testing and prescription. Philadelphia: Lea & Febiger 1989; 48–54.

14. Smith JJ, Kampine JP. Circulatory physiology: the essentials. Baltimore: Williams & Wilkins 1980; 216.

15. American College of Sports Medicine. The recommended quantity and quality of exercise for developing and maintaining cardiorespiratory and muscular fitness in healthy adults. Med Sci Sports Exerc 1990; 22:265–74.

16. Blomqvist CG. Cardiovascular adaptations to physical training. Ann Rev Physiol 1983; 45:169–89.

17. Clausen JP. Circulatory adjustments to dynamic exercise and effect of physical training in normal subjects and in patients with coronary artery disease. Prog Cardiovasc Dis 1976; 18:459–95.

18. Saltin B, Rowell LB. Functional adaptations to physical activity and inactivity. Federation Proc 1980; 39:1506–13.

19. Smith ML, Mitchell JH. Cardiorespiratory adaptations to training. In: Blair SN, Painter P, Pate RR, Smith LK, eds. Resource manual for guidelines for exercise testing and prescription. Philadelphia: Lea & Febiger 1988; 62–5.

20. Hanson P, Nagle F. Isometric exercise. Cardiovascular responses in normal and cardiac populations. Cardiol Clin 1987; 5:157–70.

21. Ghilarducci LE, Holly RG, Amsterdam EA. Effects of high resistance training in coronary artery disease. Am J Cardiol 1989; 64:866–70.

22. Hurley BF, Hagberg JM, Goldberg AP, et al. Resistive training can reduce coronary risk factors without altering VO_2max or percent body fat. Med Sci Sports Exerc 1988; 20:150–4.

23. Hurley BF, Kokkinos PF. Effects of weight training on risk factors for coronary artery disease. Sports Med 1987; 4:231–8.

24. Harris KA, Holly RG. Physiological response to circuit weight training in borderline hypertensive subjects. Med Sci Sports Exerc 1987; 19:246–52.

25. Jennings G, Nelson L, Nestel P, et al. The effects of changes in physical activity on major cardiovascular risk factors, hemodynamics, sympathetic function, and glucose utilization in man: a controlled study of four levels of activity. Circulation 1986; 73:30–40.

26. Froelicher VF. Exercise, fitness, and coronary heart disease. In: Bouchard C, Shephard RJ, Stephens T, Sutton JR, McPherson BD, eds. Exercise, fitness and health. Champaign IL: Human Kinetics Publishers, 1990; 429–50.

27. Leon AS. Effects of exercise conditioning on physiologic precursors of coronary heart disease. J Cardiopulm Rehab 1991; 11:46–57.

28. Leon AS, Blackburn H. The relationship of physical activity to coronary heart disease and life expectancy. Ann NY Acad Sci 1977; 301:561–78.

29. Paffenbarger RS, Hyde RT, Wing AL, Hsieh C. Physical activity, all-cause mortality, and longevity of college alumni. N Engl J Med 1986; 314:605–13.

30. Leon AS, Connett J, Jacobs DR, Rauramaa R. Leisure-time physical activity levels and risk of coronary heart disease and death; the Multiple Risk Factor Intervention Trial. JAMA 1987; 258:2388–95.

31. Powell KE, Thompson PD, Caspersen CJ, Kendrick JS. Physical activity and the incidence of coronary heart disease. Ann Rev Public Health 1987; 8:253–87.

32. The Pooling Project Research Group. Relationship of blood pressure, serum cholesterol, smoking habit, relative weight, and ECG abnormalities to incidence of major coronary

events: final report of the Pooling Project. J Chron Dis 1978; 31:202–306.

33. Blair SN, Kohl HW, Paffenbarger RS, et al. Physical fitness and all-cause mortality — a prospective study of healthy men and women. JAMA 1989; 262:2395–401.

34. Blackburn H. Physical activity and hypertension. J Clin Hyperten 1986; 2:154–62.

35. Seals DR, Hagberg JM. The effect of exercise training on human hypertension: a review. Med Sci Sports Exerc 1984; 16:207–15.

36. Martin JE, Dubbert PM, Lushman WC. Controlled trial of aerobic exercise in hypertension. Circulation 1990; 81:1560–7.

37. MacMahon SW, Wilcken DEL, MacDonald GJ. The effect of weight reduction on left ventricular mass: a randomized controlled trial in young, overweight, hypertensive patients. N Engl J Med 1986; 314:334–9.

38. Superko HR, Haskell WL. The role of exercise training in the therapy of hyperlipoproteinemia. Cardiol Clin 1987; 5:285–310.

39. Cook TC, Laporte RE, Washburn RA, et al. Chronic low level physical activity as a determinant of high density lipoprotein cholesterol and subfractions. Med Sci Sports Exerc 1986; 18:653–7.

40. Williams PT, Wood PD, Haskell WL, Vranizan K. The effects of running mileage and duration on plasma lipoprotein levels. JAMA 1982; 247:2674–9.

41. Williams RS, Logue EE, Lewis J, et al. Physical conditioning augments the fibrinolytic response to venous occlusion in healthy adults. N Engl J Med 1980; 302:987–91.

42. Schwartz PJ, Stone HL. The analysis and modulation of autonomic reflexes in the prediction and prevention of sudden death. In: Zipes K, Jalif D, eds. Cardiac electrophysiology and arrhythmias. New York: Grune and Stratton, 1985.

43. Roth DM, White FC, Nichols ML, et al. Effect of long-term exercise on regional myocardial function and coronary collateral development after gradual coronary artery occlusion in pigs. Circulation 1990; 82:1778–9.

44. Bove AA, Dewey JD. Proximal coronary vasomotor reactivity after exercise training in dogs. Circulation 1985; 71:620–5.

45. Blair SN, Jacobs DR, Powell KE. Relationships between exercise or physical activity and other health behaviors. Public Health Reports 1985; 100:172–9.

46. Heyden S, Fodor GJ. Does regular exercise prolong life expectancy? Sports Med 1988; 6:63–71.

47. Paffenbarger RS Jr, Wing A, Hyde R, et al. Physical activity and incidence of hypertension in college alumni. Am J Epidemiol 1983; 117:245–56.

48. Blair S, Goodyear N, Gibbons L, et al. Physical fitness and incidence of hypertension in healthy normotensive men and women. JAMA 1984; 252:487–90.

49. Hagberg JM, Montain SJ, Martin WH, Ehsani AA. Effect of exercise training in 60 to 69 year old persons with essential hypertension. Am J Cardiol 1989; 64:348–53.

50. Román O, Camuzzi AL, Villalón E, Klenner C. Physical training program in arterial hypertension. A long-term prospective follow-up. Cardiol 1981; 67:230–43.

51. Haskell WL. The influence of exercise training on plasma lipids and lipoproteins in health and disease. Acta Med Scand 1986; 711: Suppl: 25–37.

52. Leon AS, Conrad J, Hunninghake DB, Serfass R. Effects of a vigorous walking program on body composition, and carbohydrate and lipid metabolism of obese young men. Am J Clin Nutrition 1979; 32:1776–87.

53. Stein RA, Michielli DW, Glantz MD, et al. Effects of different exercise intensities on lipoprotein cholesterol fractions in healthy middle-aged men. Am Heart J 1990; 119:277–83.

54. Wood PD, Stefanick ML, Dreon DM, et al. Changes in plasma lipids and lipoproteins in overweight men during weight loss through dieting as compared with exercise. N Engl J Med 1988; 319:1173–9.

54a. Rotkis TC, Boyden TW, Stanforth PR, Parmenter RW, Wilmore JH. Increased high-density lipoprotein cholesterol and lean weight in endurance-trained women runners. J Cardiac Rehabil 1984;4:62–6.

54b. Goodyear LJ, Fronsoe MS, Van Houten DR, et al. Increased HDL-cholesterol following eight weeks of progressive endurance training in female runners. Ann Sports Med 1986; 3:33–8.

54c. Duncan JJ, Gordon NF, Scott CB. Women walking for health and fitness. How much is enough? JAMA 1991; 266: 3295–9.

54d. Cauley JA, Laporte RE, Kuller LH, Black-Sandler R. The epidemiology of high-density lipoprotein cholesterol levels in postmenopausal women. J Gerontology 1982; 37:10–5.

54e. Cauley JA, Laporte RE, Sandler RB, et al. The relationship of physical activity to high-density lipoprotein cholesterol in postmenopausal women. J Chron Dis 1986; 39:687–97.

55. Boyden TW, Parmenter RW, Rotkis TC, et al. Effects of exercise training on plasma cholesterol, high-density lipoprotein cholesterol, and sex steroid concentrations in women. In: Eaker

ED, Packard B, Wenger NK, Clarkson TB, Tyroler HA, eds. Coronary heart disease in women. New York: Haymarket Doyma, 1987; 158–63.

56. Weintraub MS, Rosen Y, Otto R, et al. Physical exercise conditioning in the absence of weight loss reduces fasting and postprandial triglyceride-rich lipoprotein levels. Circulation 1989; 79:1007–14.

57. Thompson PD, Cullinane EM, Sady SP. Modest changes in high-density lipoprotein concentration and metabolism with prolonged exercise training. Circulation 1988; 78:25–34.

58. Garcia MJ, McNamara PM, Gordon T, Kannel WB. Morbidity and mortality in diabetics in the Framingham population. Diabetes 1974; 23:105–11.

59. Leon AS. Patients with diabetes mellitus. In BA Franklin, S. Gordon, G C Timmis, eds. Exercise in modern medicine. Baltimore: Williams & Wilkins, 1989; 118–45.

60. Kanj H, Schneider SH, Ruderman NB. Exercise and diabetes mellitus. In: Horton ES and Terjung RL, eds. Exercise, nutrition and energy metabolism. New York: Macmillan Publishing Company, 1988; 228–41.

60a. Helmrich SP, Ragland DR, Leung RW, Paffenbarger RS Jr. Physical activity and reduced occurrence of non-insulin-dependent diabetes mellitus. N Engl J Med 1991; 325:147–52.

61. Wasserman DH, Abumrad NN. Physiological bases for the treatment of the physically active individual with diabetes. Sports Med 1989; 7:376–92.

62. Van Camp SP. The safety of cardiac rehabilitation. J Cardiopulm Rehab 1991; 11:64–70.

63. Paterson DH, Shephard RJ, Cunningham D, et al. Effects of physical training on cardiovascular function following myocardial infarction. J Appl Physiol 1979; 47:482–9.

64. Bruce RA, Hossack KF. Rationale of physical training in patients with angina pectoris. Adv Cardiol 1982; 31:186–90.

65. Shephard RJ. Exercise therapy in patients with angina pectoris. Adv Cardiol 1982; 31:191–8.

66. Shaw LW. The National Exercise and Heart Disease Project: effects of a prescribed supervised exercise program on mortality and cardiovascular morbidity in patients after a myocardial infarction. Am J Cardiol 1981; 48:39–46.

67. Kallio V. Results of rehabilitation in coronary patients. Adv Cardiol 1978; 24:153–63.

68. O'Connor GT, Buring JE, Yusuf S, et al. An overview of randomized trials of rehabilitation with exercise after myocardial infarction. Circulation 1989; 80:234–44.

69. Leon AS, Certo C, Comoss P, et al. Scientific evidence of the value of cardiac rehabilitation services with emphasis on patients following myocardial infarction — section I: exercise conditioning component. J Cardiopulm Rehab 1990; 10:79–87.

70. Jugdutt BI, Michorowski BL, Kappagoda CT. Exercise training after anterior Q wave myocardial infarction: importance of regional left ventricular function and topography. J Am Coll Cardiol 1988; 12:362–72.

71. Sullivan MJ, Higginbotham MB, Cobb, FR. Exercise training in patients with severe left ventricular dysfunction: hemodynamic and metabolic effects. Circulation 1988; 78:506–15.

72. Ehsani AA, Biello DR, Schultz J. Improvement of left ventricular contractile function by exercise training in patients with coronary artery disease. Circulation 1986; 74:350–8.

73. Williams RS, McKinnis RA, Cobb FR, et al. Effects of physical conditioning on left ventricular ejection fraction in patients with coronary artery disease. Circulation 1984; 70:69–75.

74. Cobb FR, Williams RS, McEwan P, et al. Effects of exercise training on ventricular function in patients with recent myocardial infarction. Circulation 1982; 66:100–8.

75. Kalata GB. Consensus on bypass surgery. Science 1981; 211:42–3.

76. Brown DR. Exercise, fitness and mental health. In: Bouchard C, Shephard RJ, Stephens T, et al., eds. Exercise, fitness and health. Champaign, IL: Human Kinetics Publishers, 1990; 607–33.

77. Morgan WP, Goldstein SE, eds. Exercise and mental health. Washington, DC: Hemisphere Publishing, 1987.

78. Porcari JP, Ward A, Morgan W, et al. Effect of walking on state anxiety and blood pressure (abstract). Med Sci Sports Exerc 1988; 20:S85.

79. Rozanski A, Bairey CN, Krantz DS, et al. Mental stress and the induction of silent myocardial ischemia in patients with coronary artery disease. N Engl J Med 1988; 318:118–45.

80. Shekelle RB, Gale M, Ostfeld AM, Paul O. Hostility, risk of coronary heart disease and mortality. Psychosom Med 1983; 45:109–14.

81. Barefoot JC, Dahlstrom WG, Williams RB. Hostility, CHD incidence, and total mortality: a 25-year follow-up study of 255 physicians. Psychosom Med 1983; 45:59–63.

82. Brown D, Wang Y, Hinkle R, et al. The effects of four strength training programs on body cathexis, physical estimation, self esteem and mood. In preparation.

83. Siscovick DS, Weiss NS, Fletcher RH, Lasky T. The incidence of primary cardiac arrest during vigorous exercise. N Engl J Med 1984; 311:874–7.

84. Frohlich ED, Lowenthal DT, Miller HS, et al. Task Force IV: systemic arterial hypertension. J Am Coll Cardiol 1985; 6:1218–21.

85. Belman MJ. Exercise in chronic obstructive pulmonary disease. In: Franklin BA, Gordon S, Timmis GC, eds. Exercise in modern medicine. Baltimore: Williams & Wilkins, 1989; 175–92.

86. Diamond GA, Forrester JS. Analysis of probability as an aid in the clinical diagnosis of coronary artery disease. N Engl J Med 1979; 300:1350–8.

87. Guiteras VP, Chaitman BR, Waters DD, et al. Diagnostic accuracy of exercise ECG lead systems in clinical subsets of women. Circulation 1982; 65:1465–74.

88. Fisch C, DeSanctis RW, Dodge HT, et al. Guidelines for exercise testing. Circulation 1986; 74:653A–67A.

89. Rippe JM, Ward A, Porcari JP, Freedson PS. Walking for health and fitness. JAMA 1988; 259:2720–4.

90. Karvonen M, Kentala K, Mustala O. The effect of training on heart rate: a longitudinal study. Ann Med Exper Biol Fenn 1957; 35:307–15.

91. American Heart Association. Exercise standards: a statement for health professionals. Dallas: American Heart Association, 1991.

92. Borg GA. Psychophysical basis of perceived exertion. Med Sci Sports Exerc 1982; 14:377–81.

93. Skinner JS, Hustler R, Bergsteinova V, et al. Perception of effort during different types of exercise and under different environmental conditions. Med Sci Sports Exerc 1973; 5:110–5.

94. Skinner JS, Hutsler R, Bergsteinova V, et al. The validity and reliability of a rating scale of perceived exertion. Med Sci Sports Exerc 1973; 5:94–6.

95. Pollock ML, Miller HS, Linnerud AC, et al. Frequency of training as a determinant for improvement in cardiovascular function and body composition for middle-aged men. Arch Phys Med Rehabil 1975; 58:141–5.

96. Pollock ML, Gettman LR, Milesis CA, et al. Effects of frequency and duration of training on attrition and incidence of injury. Med Sci Sports Exerc 1977; 69:31–6.

97. Kline GM, Porcari JP, Hintermeister R, et al. Estimation of VO$_2$max from a one-mile track walk, gender, age, and body weight. Med Sci Sports Exerc 1987; 19:153–9.

98. The Rockport Walking Institute. The Rockport guide to fitness walking. Marlboro, MA.: Rockport Walking Institute, 1989.

99. Epstein SE, Blomqvist CG, Buja LM, et al. Task Force V: ischemic heart disease. J Am Coll Cardiol 1985; 6:1222–4.

100. Butler RM, Beierwaltes WH, Rogers FJ. The cardiovascular response to circuit weight training in patients with cardiac disease. J Cardiopulm Rehab 1987; 7:402–9.

101. Barnard RJ, Hall JA. Patients with peripheral vascular disease. In: Franklin BA, Gordon S, Timmis GC, eds. Exercise and modern medicine. Baltimore: Williams & Wilkins, 1989; 107–17.

102. Arous E, Baum PL, Cutler BS. The ischemic exercise test in patients with peripheral vascular disease. Implications for management. Arch Surg 1984; 119:780–3.

103. National Institutes of Health. Consensus Development Conference statement. Health implications of obesity. February 11–13, 1985. Ann Intern Med 1985; 103:981–1077.

104. Hubert HB, Feinleib M, McNamara PM, et al. Obesity as an independent risk factor for cardiovascular disease: a 26-year follow-up of participants in the Framingham Study. Circulation 1983; 67:968–77.

105. Pacy PJ, Webster J, Garrow JS. Exercise and obesity. Sports Medicine 1986; 3:89–113.

106. Segal KR, Pi-Sunyer FX. Exercise and obesity. Med Clin N Amer 1989; 73:217–36.

107. Thompson JK, Jarvie GJ, Lahey BB, Cureton KJ. Exercise and obesity: etiology, physiology, and intervention. Psychol Bull 1982; 91:55–79.

108. Dahlkoetter J, Callahan EJ, Linton J. Obesity and the unbalanced energy equation: exercise versus eating habit change. J Consult Clin Psych 1979; 47:898–905.

109. Foss ML. Exercise concerns and precautions for the obese. In: Storlie J, Jordan HA, eds. Nutrition and exercise in obesity management. New York: Spectrum Publications, Inc., 1984; 123–48.

110. Riggs BL, Melton LJ. Involutional osteoporosis. N Engl J Med 1986; 314:1676–86.

111. Smith EL, Gilligan C, McAdam M, et al. Deterring bone loss by exercise intervention in premenopausal and postmenopausal women. Calcif Tissue Int 1989; 44:312–21.

112. Sinaki M. Exercise and osteoporosis. Arch Phys Med Rehab 1989; 70:220–9.

113. Dalsky GP, Stocke KS, Ehsani HM, et al. Weight-bearing exercise training and lumbar bone mineral content in postmenopausal women. Ann Intern Med 1988; 108:824–8.

114. Buskirk ER, Hodgson JL. Age and aerobic power: the rate of change in men and women. Fed Proc 1987; 46:1824–9.

115. Dehn MM, Bruce RA. Longitudinal variations in maximal oxygen intake with age and activity. J Appl Physiol 1972; 33:805–7.

116. Kasch FW, Wallace JP, Van Camp SP. Effects of 18 years of endurance exercise on the physical

work capacity of older men. J Cardiac Rehabil 1985; 5:308–12.

117. Hagberg JM. Effect of training on the decline of VO₂max with aging. Fed Proc 1987; 46:1830–3.

118. Ehsani AA, Ogawa T, Miller TR, et al. Exercise training improves left ventricular systolic function in older men. Circulation 1991; 83:96–103.

119. Ross JG, Gilbert GG. The National Children and Youth Fitness Study: a summary of findings. J Phys Ed Rec and Dance 1985; 56:45–50.

120. Ross JG, Pate RR. The National Children and Youth Fitness Study. II. A summary of findings. J Phys Ed Rec and Dance 1987; 58:51–6.

121. Dietz WH Jr, Gortmaker SL. Do we fatten our children at the television set? Obesity and television viewing in children and adolescents. Pediatrics 1985; 75:807–12.

122. Sallis JF, Patterson TL, Buono MJ, Nadu PR. Relation of cardiovascular fitness and physical activity to cardiovascular disease risk factors in children and adults. Am J Epidemiol 1988; 127:933–41.

123. Treiber FA, Strong WB, Arensman FW, Gruber M. Relationships between habitual physical activity and cardiovascular responses to exercise in young children. In: Oseid SC, Carlson K-H, eds. Children and exercise XIII. Champaign IL: Human Kinetics Publishers, 1989; 285–94.

124. Hofman A, Walter HJ. The association between physical fitness and cardiovascular disease risk factors in children in a five-year follow-up study. Int J Epidemiol 1989; 18:830–5.

125. Freedman DS, Shear CL, Srinivasan SR, et al. Tracking of serum lipids and lipoproteins in children over an 8-year period: the Bogalusa Heart Study. Prev Med 1985; 14:203–16.

126. Lauer RM, Lee J, Clarke WR. Factors affecting the relationship between childhood and adult cholesterol levels: the Muscatine Study. Pediatrics 1989; 82:309–18.

127. Dietz WH Jr. Childhood obesity: susceptibility, cause, and management. J Pediatr 1987; 103:676–86.

128. Hagberg JM, Ehsani AA, Goldring B, et al. Effect of weight training on blood pressure and hemodynamics in hypertensive adolescents. J Pediatr 1984; 104:147–51.

129. Dennison BA, Straus JH, Mellits ED, Charney E. Childhood physical fitness tests: predictor of adult physical activity levels. Pediatrics 1988; 82:324–30.

130. Krahenbuhl GS, Skinner JS, Kohrt WM. Developmental aspects of maximal aerobic power in children. Exerc Sport Sci Rev 1985; 13:503–38.

131. Vogel JA, Jones BH, Rock PB. Environmental considerations in exercise testing and training. In: Blair SN, Painter P, Pate RR, Smith LK, eds. Resource m•nual for guidelines for exercise testing and prescription. Philadelphia: Lea & Febiger, 1988; 90–7.

132. Pandolf KB, Cafarelli E, Noble BJ, et al. Hyperthermia: effects on exercise prescription. Arch Phys Med Rehabil 1975; 56:524–6.

133. Brammel HL, Morgan BJ, Niccoli SA, et al. Exercise tolerance is reduced at altitude in patients with coronary artery disease. Circulation 1982; 66:II–371.

134. Martin JE, Dubbert PM. Adherence to exercise. Exercise and Sports Science Reviews 1985; 13:137–67.

135. Oldridge NB, Stoedefalke KG. Compliance and motivation in cardiac exercise programs. Clinics in Sports Medicine 1984; 3(2):443–54.

136. Dishman RK. Exercise compliance: a new view for public health. Physician Sports Med 1986; 14:127–45.

137. Sallis JF, Haskell WL, Fortmann SP, et al. Predictors of adoption and maintenance of physical activity in a community sample. Prev Med 1986; 15:331–41.

138. King AC, Haskell WL, Taylor CB, et al. Group vs. home-based exercise training in healthy older men and women. JAMA 1991; 266:1535–42.

Psychosocial Factors: Their Importance and Management

JON KABAT-ZINN

EDITORS' INTRODUCTION

The concept that there is an interrelationship between the emotions and cardiac disease is deeply rooted in folklore, but it is only recently that a substantial body of evidence has been amassed linking psychosocial factors to CHD. In this chapter Dr. Kabat-Zinn reviews the epidemiologic and laboratory studies that provide the basis for our understanding of this connection and then examines the fascinating and still controversial connection between type A behavior/hostility and disease. Several studies specifically directed at lowering CHD risk by psychosocial intervention are discussed in depth. Finally Dr. Kabat-Zinn gives us his own unique insights into physician-patient communication and suggests interesting and practical approaches whereby the physician can assess psychosocial factors and intervene for the patient's benefit. He shows how such an approach can be not only useful but also gratifying, leading to enhanced physician-patient rapport, which also improves care in areas unrelated to CHD.

There is much to be optimistic about with regard to counseling for the prevention of coronary heart disease (CHD). This optimism stems from the recent demonstration that CHD can be reversed in human beings through lifestyle changes alone, without the use of drugs or surgery; from increasingly convincing evidence that psychosocial and behavioral factors are involved in the etiology and progression of CHD; and from evidence that these factors can be modified both to reduce risk of CHD and to promote rehabilitation from CHD. Moreover, psychosocial as well as behavioral factors have been shown to be important not only in CHD morbidity and mortality, but in illness in general. Thus, the physician with knowledge and skills in this area is in an excellent position to influence patients through education, counseling, and personal modeling, as well as by referral to specialized services, thereby potentially contributing to the reduction of the incidence of CHD in our society and to the overall improvement of the health of our population.

A skills-based approach to help patients make important lifestyle and psychosocial/behavioral changes to improve health and prevent disease depends in great measure on the ability of the physician to see the patient as a whole person and establish effective interpersonal rapport. As already discussed in Chapter 7, the quality of the doctor-patient relationship is critical for counseling in the domain of psychosocial factors, where the patient's attitudes and beliefs, how he views himself and the world, and how he interacts with it can be key factors influencing clinical outcomes. The therapeutic relationship between doctor and patient is even more important for psychosocial factors than for counseling in the areas of smoking and dietary habits. The subject of psychosocial influences in heart disease thus requires that the physician understand the importance of this area to health, be personally open and sympathetic to the patient, and be prepared to tackle matters of the heart, in the metaphorical sense.

Exploration of how a patient feels about himself and others and about the major stresses in his life may touch on areas that the patient is reluctant to share with the physician or that constitute a hidden or latent agenda. These may only be revealed during the course of a skillful communication of acceptance and interest on the part of the physician, perhaps over an extended period of time. Such communication can happen only if the physician values the quality of the relationship itself and feels comfortable providing the kind of open, compassionate, nonjudgmental environment in which the patient will feel comfortable speaking about matters that may be quite personal and potentially threatening. Above all it is important for the physician to engage in active and mindful listening and to ask the kind of open-ended questions that will lead to the patient's willingness to share his own feelings and point of view.

As this chapter proceeds, we will see in more detail why this attitude is both important and effective. As an emblematic anecdote, a surgeon diagnosed as having metastatic melanoma said that he had come to realize just recently, after practicing for over 30 years, that he had never really seen his patients as people before his own illness arose, in spite of priding himself on being a sensitive and caring doctor. Rather, he confessed, he had seen them as cases. It took his own illness to awaken in him a heartfelt understanding of the suffering of others and to show him how he might use this new awareness to enhance his ability to care for his patients. It would be well if such a drastic life experience were not required to catalyze such a realization.

Physicians often express concern that inquiries into psychosocial areas may be tantamount to opening Pandora's box, an invitation to the patient to unleash emotional issues that the physician may feel neither ready nor competent to address. Such concerns, however, are largely unfounded. As we will see, such an approach has a surprisingly low cost in terms of time and energy and has major benefits. There is no need for the physician to play the role of psychiatrist or therapist nor to develop a new, potentially time-consuming and emotionally draining clinical style. Rather, what is being recommended is simply that the physician become sensitized to particular signs of psychosocial disturbance, follow through as appropriate with a brief inquiry, make appropriate referral arrangements for further work, and maintain continuity via brief follow-up inquiries as to the patient's progress.

What is most important in approaching the psychosocial domain with a patient is an awareness of that domain and an understanding of its relevance in the first place. This awareness can serve as a thread that unifies the entire clinical encounter and keeps it in human terms. Keeping psychosocial factors in mind can substantially improve the medical encounter and make for a more effective and therapeutic relationship between physician and patient.

This chapter first reviews why it is important for physicians to be aware of the metaphorical heart (a phrase used to capture the breadth of people's emotional life) when thinking of prevention and the treatment of diseases of the physical heart. It explores the accumulated epidemiologic and experimental evidence that psychological and social factors are important in the development and prevention of CHD. Then current hypotheses concerning the pathophysiology of CHD as it relates to psychosocial factors are briefly examined. (Some familiarity with epidemiologic and laboratory studies that have investigated the psychosocial influences in heart disease can be helpful in developing an adequate knowledge base for engaging in both the clinical and the counseling approaches to these problems.) The third area we review is intervention studies that suggest that it is possible to reduce the risk of CHD progression and perhaps reverse CAD itself. Finally we explore how best to intervene to help people to make the kind of psychosocial changes in their lives that will reduce their risk of CHD, help prevent its further progression, or perhaps even promote reversal of the atherosclerotic process.

Epidemiologic and Laboratory Evidence for the Role of Psychosocial and Personality Factors in CHD

Less than half of the CHD incidence in the United States is explained by the combined effect of all traditional risk factors [1, 2]. (See Chapter 1.) Numerous efforts have been directed toward identifying probable psychosocial and behavioral factors that may also contribute to the development of heart disease. The most likely candidates have been recognized anecdotally, if not scientifically, for a long time, including the observed connection between high emotional arousal and sudden cardiac death [3], the effect of poverty [4] and disruption of social ties on disease [5], a relationship between major life events and illness [6], and the observation that personality factors such as the so-called coronary-prone personality appear to be associated with heart disease [7].

These psychosocial factors are often lumped together under the umbrella rubric of *stress*, a term first utilized in a biological context by Walter B. Cannon in 1914 [8] and then elaborated and popularized by Hans Selye [9]. The term has generated much controversy among researchers, who seem to be in agreement that by itself, it is of little scientific value since it is broadly used to mean just about anything [10]. There is equal agreement, however, that the word *stress* has become an integral part of our language and that it can be a convenient descriptor for a vast range of different circumstances, both in the environment and within the psyche, that threaten to disrupt and overwhelm one's capacity to adapt effectively [11].

Among the first epidemiologic observations relevant to heart disease was the finding that different countries have very different rates of heart disease and that these differences cannot be completely explained by genetic differences or by traditional risk factors [12]. For example, American men in the Framingham Heart Study were found to have twice the risk of developing CHD as European men having the same standard risk factors [1]. Other studies showed a marked gradient of CHD mortality between individuals in Japan (1.8 deaths/1000), Hawaiian-Japanese (3.2 deaths/1000), and Caucasians (9.8 deaths per 1000), making a Caucasian U.S. male five times as likely to die of CHD as a Japanese male living in Japan [13]. Similar CHD mortality gradients were observed among Japanese men living in Japan, Hawaii, and California, with CHD death rates consistently and significantly lower in native Japanese than in Japanese Americans, and age-specific CHD death rates markedly lower in all three Japanese groups than in U.S. Caucasians [14].

Epidemiologic Studies of Social Influences and CHD

SOCIAL SUPPORT/COHESION

The nature of factors that might explain inter-country CHD differences has been the subject of much investigation. In an elegant accultur-ation study Marmot and Syme studied CHD in 3809 Japanese-Americans in the San Francisco Bay area, some of whom had adopted the American lifestyle and some of whom had maintained strong ties with the more traditional Japanese culture. When classified according to cultural upbringing (e.g., years spent in Japan, years spent in Japanese language school, religious environment when growing up), the group of Japanese-Americans who had had a traditional Japanese upbringing had approximately 2.5 times less CHD than those individuals who had had a nontraditional (acculturated) upbringing, independent of diet, smoking, serum triglycerides, serum cholesterol, blood pressure, relative weight, and serum glucose (Figure 11-1). Furthermore, when they were

Figure 11-1. Acculturation and coronary heart disease among Japanese-Americans living in California. (Reprinted with permission from Syme SL. Sociocultural factors and disease etiology. In Gentry WD (ed). Handbook of Behavioral Medicine. Guilford, New York, 1984, pp. 13–37.)

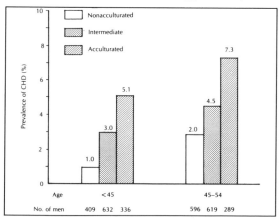

classified according to cultural upbringing *and* the degree to which they were disassociated from the Japanese ethnic group (the ethnicity of their doctor or dentist, friends, coworkers and employer, and the importance of religion), a fivefold difference in CHD between the most and the least acculturated groups was seen, again a difference not explained by genetics or by differences in traditional coronary risk factors, including diet. In both analyses the strongest effects of acculturation on CHD were found in the younger cohorts (less than 45 years of age) [15].

Marmot and others have interpreted these findings as suggesting that the social and cultural cohesiveness characteristic of the traditional Japanese way of life may be protective against the negative health effects of potentially disruptive life changes and the adopting of a different diet and work life. Childrearing practices, which favor emotional and physical contact and support over discipline, and a strong view of the individual person as embedded within the larger social fabric in both family and work are thought to be important factors. Williams [16] notes, in discussing hostility and cynicism as the toxic components of type A behavior (examined later in this chapter) that "in contrast to Western attitudes and practices, in Japan the child is regarded as basically good and free from bad or evil intentions; frequent close physical contact between mother and child is the norm. . . . the preliminary evidence of lower hostility scale scores among Japanese (in Japan) may be the direct result of these childrearing practices." The evidence from the Japanese acculturation studies certainly suggests that strong social ties and meaningful social interconnectedness/cohesiveness might be a source of significant protective benefits for individuals in Western societies as well and thus be an important factor in the prevention of CHD.

A naturalistic case study of the Pennsylvania town of Roseto [17, 18] has also been interpreted by some investigators as showing the importance of social cohesiveness in preventing CHD, although the validity of this study has been disputed [19, 20]. In the 1950s Roseto was characterized as a close-knit, traditional Italian-American community. Most of its inhabitants had emigrated from the town of Roseto in southern Italy and were exclusively Roman Catholic. Family life was described as cohesive and patriarchal. An unusually low death rate from myocardial infarction (MI) was reported in Roseto between 1955 and 1961. This rate was half the coronary death rate of Bangor, a town the same size a mile away whose population consisted of an ethnic mixture of English, German Protestants, and Italians. In Bangor male and female roles overlapped to a larger extent than in the traditional family life of the people of Roseto. The difference in mortality rates between the two towns was not explainable on the basis of diet. Analysis showed that 41 percent of the Roseto diet came from fat, and that both men and women were about 20 pounds overweight compared with the U.S. average [21].

The investigators in the Roseto/Bangor study attributed the difference in rates of MI between the two towns to the marked psychosocial differences between them in the 1950s. Attention focused on the reinforcement of mutual trust and cohesion that the people of Roseto experienced upon arrival from Italy. "Perceiving themselves as culturally isolated in an alien land, they reinforced those elements of their traditional culture that gave them a sense of security and self-appreciation [22]." Bianco [23] characterized the residents of Roseto as antagonistic toward the chief values and symbols of American society and retaining their highly traditional attitudes toward family, education, work, law, and authority.

Since that time, the patterns of culture in Roseto have gradually shifted toward the mainstream of American life under the combined influence of the mass media and education at the high school and college levels. Wolf [24] predicted that the CHD mortality rate would rise as a consequence. Over a 25-year period, as the community became more Americanized and less cohesive, the incidence of CHD rose to approximate that of the surrounding towns [25,

26]. This naturalistic experiment lends further support to the hypothesis that social cohesiveness might be an important protective factor in CHD.

To explore the role of social support networks in health and disease, Berkman and Syme [27] conducted a prospective study in 1965 of a large ($n = 4775$) population of American adults aged 30 to 69 in Alameda County, California. Data were gathered to assess the presence and the extent of four types of social connections: marriage, contacts with extended family and friends, church membership, and other formal and informal group affiliations. Mortality was assessed 9 years later. It was found that each type of social relationship by itself weakly predicted mortality over the succeeding 9 years. A combined social network rating that incorporated all four types of social connections showed that persons who scored low on the social network index were more than twice as likely to die in those 9 years as persons who scored high. This was true not only for CHD deaths, but for all causes of death, after controlling for other factors such as age, race, physical activity, obesity, socioeconomic status, and self-reported health status. Other studies have produced similar findings [28]. Measures of social integration predicted mortality in both men and women in the majority of these studies, although the associations were less strong for black Americans in the one such study reported [29].

Eliot [30] points out that one reason why the recognized risk factors of cigarette smoking, high blood pressure, and elevated serum cholesterol account for only half the incidence of CHD may be that 90 percent of people are protected by other factors related to social support and cohesion. He interprets Syme's results as suggesting that life changes are important primarily when they disrupt social *relationships,* such as would happen with a job change, a residential move, divorce, or the loss of a loved one. Even the differences between male and female risks of CHD may be at least in part related to social support. In the Alameda County study [27] men reported fewer close relationships and intimate ties than did women.

Socioeconomic Factors

Socioeconomic status is also correlated with health. For example, in the Oslo study of CHD [31], CHD risk factors, especially smoking and high serum cholesterol, were higher among lower socioeconomic classes, such that the total CHD risk in the lowest education and income class was about 2.5 times that of the highest class. Mortality from CHD and from other causes followed the same pattern. In the Alameda County study, a poverty area was compared with a more affluent area. The incidence of hypertension was 50 percent higher in the poverty area, even after controlling for social interaction, medical care, smoking, and other risk factors. Among a subgroup of more affluent people living in the poverty area, the pattern of hypertension reflected the pattern of the poverty area as a whole rather than that of the similar income group in the affluent area. Interviews revealed fears of robbery and violence. The study showed that the distribution of hypertension in the community correlated with the density of police and fire department calls [32].

Other studies have also noted an apparent relation between socioeconomic factors and disease. Harburg and colleagues [33] demonstrated that blacks who lived in areas of Detroit with low ecologic stress had less hypertension that those living in high-stress areas. However, this pilot study did not control for other CHD risk factors. Although some studies have suggested that there is a lower incidence of hypertension among rural Zulus in South Africa than among their urban counterparts [34, 35], Gampel and colleagues [36] found that the urban Zulus who were hypertensive tended to be those who had recently moved from rural areas. They proposed that the emotional stress associated with urbanization and its ensuing social disruption may have been responsible for the increased incidence of hypertension observed. However, this study too did not control for risk factors other than sex and obesity.

Two recent studies of migrant populations have added to our understanding of the risk factor changes that may accompany the transition to urban life. Poulter and colleagues [36a] studied 325 members of the Luo tribe who had migrated to Nairobi and compared them with a control group of 267 individuals who had remained in their native villages. The mean systolic pressure of the migrants was significantly higher than that of the nonmigrants throughout the study; the migrants also had higher urinary sodium:potassium ratios and pulse rates, and were significantly more obese. Zevallos and colleagues [36b] carried out a cross-sectional study comparing Indians living in a rural area of Ecuador with their first degree relatives who had migrated to the capital city, Quito. The percentage of calories taken in as fat rose from 21.6 percent in the rural area to 26.4 percent in the city (p< .0001). Although individuals in the migrant group were younger, they had significantly higher skinfold thicknesses and blood pressures. Blood pressure increased with age in the migrant group, whereas in the rural group it did not increase with age. Migrant women demonstrated higher body mass indices and a marked increase in smoking rates. Cholesterol levels were higher in migrants, although the difference was statistically significant only among women. The authors suggest that these changes are at least in part related to the stress and social disruption of the urbanization process.

Work Stress

Work-related factors also come into play as important predictors of CHD in human populations [37]. Architectural layout, excessive noise, and exposure to danger may have a significant impact on stress and health in individual cases [38]. Stressors such as unrealistic time pressures among assembly line workers; high levels of responsibility for the safety of others, as with air traffic controllers; nonsupportive superiors; and work overload have all been associated with increased incidences of hypertension, MIs, and other illnesses [38].

Central to the problem of job stress is the issue of control [39, 40]. In studies in Sweden and the United States [41, 42] a two-dimensional model of job stress has been shown to be associated with both psychological stress and CHD risk. This model proposes that work stress (which these investigators refer to as *strain*) is the result of an interaction between the psychological demands of the work situation and the decision-making latitude (job control) associated with task organization or skill usage [41].

In a study of MI prevalence in two large surveys of male American workers [the Health Examination Survey (HES) 1960 and 1961, $n = 2409$, and the Health and Nutrition Examination Survey (HANES), 1971 to 1975, $n = 2424$] Karasek and colleagues [42] found an elevated prevalence of MI in high-strain occupations. The relative risk for MI for someone in the top decile of job strain compared to someone in the lowest decile was 3.8 in the HES and 4.79 in the HANES. The authors comment that this is of the same order of magnitude as the relative risk found in other studies for smoking or for serum cholesterol. An earlier prospective study of a large random sample of the Swedish national male work force showed that over a 6-year study period, job strain predicted CHD self-reports in a population of 1461 male workers, indicating that job strain is predictive of future CHD in an asymptomatic population, independent of other risk factors [41].

Animal Studies of Social Influences and CHD

In addition to the lines of epidemiologic evidence that point toward a role for psychosocial factors in the etiology of human CHD, there is a considerable body of knowledge concerning the role of similar factors in the development of CHD in laboratory animals. This work also provides compelling evidence for the link between CHD events and psychosocial factors. Some salient findings are reviewed next.

SOCIAL STRESS

Animal studies have played a major role in the demonstration that social factors influence CHD. Henry and Stephens [22] reviewed numerous studies published up to 1977 that linked stress and the social environment. Perhaps the best recent evidence for a causal relationship between emotional stress and CHD comes from a study of social stress and atherosclerosis in male cynomolgus monkeys maintained on an atherogenic diet [43]. Aggressive, dominant monkeys were kept in an unstable social situation over a period of 22 months by periodically reshuffling the members of the social groupings. The dominant males were thus obliged to constantly reestablish their preeminence as the groupings changed. To further increase competition among the male monkeys, an estrogen-implanted ovariectomized female was occasionally placed in the cage. Under these study conditions dominant monkeys showed more extensive atherosclerosis (more than twice the degree of blockage) than equally dominant animals living in stable (unstressed) social settings. The dominant animals in the unstable state also had twice as much disease as subordinate animals in the same social condition. These psychosocial effects were independent of total plasma cholesterol and high-density cholesterol (HDL) levels and blood pressure.

In a similar series of studies, but this time with the monkeys kept on the equivalent of the American Heart Association (AHA) prudent diet (30 percent fat, 100 mg cholesterol/day), much less atherosclerosis was present, yet a strong effect of the psychosocial stress was still observed [43a]. Monkeys in the disrupted, stressed condition showed more disease than those in the stable condition. Furthermore, those monkeys with excessive pulse rate elevation in response to the stress had more disease, consistent with the hypothesis that recurrent stimulation of the sympathetic nervous system may promote arterial lesions by causing hemodynamic or hormonal disruptions.

In other experiments female monkeys were found to have significantly less atherosclerosis than male monkeys under identical conditions of diet and stress. However, low-status females had more atherosclerosis than high-status females, and almost as much as dominant male monkeys. They also had lower HDL levels and evidence of impaired ovarian function. Ovariectomy had a similar atherogenic effect [43b].

A recent study [43c, 43d] from the same laboratory has demonstrated that social disruption among male cynomolgus monkeys, in addition to causing atherosclerotic changes, also leads to changes in the ability of the coronary arteries to respond normally (vasodilation) to the administration of the muscarinic agonist acetylcholine. In the socially disrupted condition, monkeys showed a paradoxical *vasoconstrictive* response to the intracoronary infusion of acetylcholine, even under conditions of a low-cholesterol diet. This finding may have important implications for stress-induced coronary vasospasm in humans. It suggests that social stress can alter the parasympathetic regulation of sympathetic arousal in an unfavorable direction. A low-fat diet by itself may not protect against such vasomotor disregulation.

Weber and Van der Walt [44] reported that cardiomyopathy and death from cardiac failure occurred in New Zealand white rabbits subjected to cycles of crowding. Animals were placed four to a small cage for 1 week, then housed singly for 1 week, then crowded again. This continued over a 10-month period, by which time 35 of 48 animals had died, 10 having died in the first week and 10 more during the first month. The authors concluded that the cause of death was not wounding or starvation but a chronic cardiomyopathy, brought on in response to the stress, which ultimately resulted in cardiac failure.

STUDIES OF POSITIVE SOCIAL CONTACT/SUPPORT

Nerem and colleagues [45] found that rabbits that were fed a highly atherogenic diet but that were regularly petted and stroked by their handlers showed 60 percent less aortic atherosclerosis than genetically identical rabbits on the same diet that were not touched. Many other studies on the physiological effects of intra- and interspecies grooming, petting, and touching have been conducted [46]. In a recent study [47] cited by Williams [48], it was found that rat pups separated from their mothers showed stunted growth (and decreased synthesis of new proteins throughout their bodies), due not to lack of nourishment but from a lack of sensory stimulation of the pups by the mother. As Wil-

liams put it, "The mother's 'tender loving care' in the form of licking her pups was necessary to maintain sufficient levels of the hormones needed for growth" [48].

Many experimental studies using a yoked escape-avoidance design have also demonstrated the importance of psychological factors in stress-induced diseases in animals. In a classic series of studies, Weiss [49] demonstrated that rats subjected to random chronic electric shocks developed gastric lesions. Animals who could exercise control over the shocks by turning a wheel at one end of their cage had far less disease than yoked animals who received the identical shocks but were unable to control them. The latter rapidly exhibited withdrawal and unresponsiveness to the shocks, a behavior which has been termed *learned helplessness*. As Weiss pointed out, "control" in this experiment meant that the wheel-turning responses to the shocks on the part of the animals in the control-avoidance condition resulted in *relevant feedback*, that is, their wheel-turning response had direct, stimulus-associated consequences, the temporary shutting off of the shock. Attempts at wheel turning by the yoked animals were met with no relevant feedback, and the same degree of shock led to a state of helplessness.

These studies graphically illustrate that it was not the shocks per se that were responsible for the majority of the pathology observed, but the lack of control over the stressor in the helpless condition. Thus, *the psychological factor of "control" was demonstrated to be important in resistance to a stress-induced breakdown of health, even in animals.* Other escape-avoidance studies have shown that psychological control also affects the development of cardiac disease, in particular, cardiac myopathy in monkeys [50]. The concept of relevant feedback in these animal experiments sheds some light on the construct of job decision latitude in human beings, which as we have seen is important in protecting against work-related CHD [41]. It is likely that such latitude would be of value in reducing the negative health effects of job stress only if work-related decisions gave rise to relevant feedback, which promotes an overall sense of control.

The Effects of Type A Behavior and Hostility on CHD

In addition to the external social influences that can play a role in the development and progression of CHD in human beings, it has been thought for some time that inner psychological and personality factors and their associated behavioral expressions might also predispose some individuals to a greater risk of CHD. These inner characteristics are sometimes spoken of collectively as the coronary-prone personality. The so-called type A behavior pattern has been the major focus of research in this field since the early observations of Friedman and Rosenman [51] that their cardiac patients seemed to share many behavioral characteristics, notably, (1) almost obsessive attempts to achieve many poorly defined goals, (2) love of competition, (3) a strong need for recognition and advancement, (4) a consistent preoccupation with time and the need to get things done in a hurry, (5) intense concentration and alertness, and (6) high levels of "free-floating hostility." Eventually Friedman and Rosenman formulated the hypothesis that this constellation of traits, which they termed the type A behavior pattern, is a risk factor for CHD. Those who did not show this pattern were termed type Bs. The standard measures for determining type A behavior are a structured interview [52], which requires trained personnel to perform, and the Jenkins Activity Survey (JAS) [53], a self-administered, computer-scored questionnaire, which has correlated highly with the structured interview in a number of studies.

The Western Collaborative Group Study (WCGS) [54] was the first large epidemiologic study designed to identify a causal link between a behavior pattern (type A) and the subsequent development of a chronic disease (CHD). Begun in the early 1960s, it followed 3154 working men in California between the ages of 39 and 59. At the time the study started, all subjects were free of any evidence of CHD and were generally healthy. They were followed carefully for 8½ years. Structured interviews conducted at the start of the study showed that approximately half of the men were type A.

In addition to confirming the CHD risk factors identified in the Framingham Study, the results of this study showed that by 8½ years, the type A men were about twice as likely as the type Bs to have developed some manifestation of CHD. In every specific category — overt MIs, silent MIs, angina, CHD fatalities, and second MIs among those who had had a first MI during the study — the type As were found to have from 1.7 to 4.5 times the risk of the type B men [55]. The effect of type A behavior was independent of other risk factors for CHD and compounded the risk attributable to them, as would be expected of a bona fide risk factor. Other studies showed that type A behavior was strongly associated with the degree of coronary artery blockage in patients undergoing coronary angiography [56, 57, 58]. On the basis of this and other evidence, a National Institutes of Health (NIH) panel concluded in 1981 that there was sufficient evidence to designate type A behavior as a risk factor for CHD [59].

However, a number of more recent well-executed studies have been unable to reproduce the association between the type A behavior pattern and the development of CHD. No association between type A behavior and CHD was found in the type A ancillary study of the Multiple Risk Factor Intervention Trial (MRFIT), which followed approximately 3000 high-risk (i.e., in the top 10 percent of risk for CHD) healthy men over a 9-year period [60]. This negative finding was particularly surprising since the study used both the structured interview and the JAS questionnaire as measures of type A behavior and obtained the personal input of Dr. Rosenman in those cases where assessment of an individual case was problematic. The Aspirin Myocardial Infarction Study (AMIS) [61] failed as well to find an association between risk of reinfarction and type A behavior assessed with the JAS. A 22-year follow-up of CHD mortality among the 3154 subjects in the WCGS [62] also failed to show a significant association between type A behavior and CHD mortality. Furthermore, attempts to reproduce the earlier associations observed between type A behavior and the severity of CAD in patients undergoing coronary angiography were also unsuccessful [63].

The weight of the evidence suggested that something was wrong with the type A concept itself. The original formulation contained at least six separate behavioral categories. These may have been weighted differently in different studies in arriving at the characterization of type A in individual cases. Perhaps these different behavioral elements did not contribute equally to a proneness to coronary disease. In fact, recent work by Williams and his colleagues and by others probing this dilemma has shown that, indeed, not all of the original elements of the type A behavior pattern are related to CHD and that it is the elements of hostility and cynicism that constitute the so-called toxic core of the original type A description in regard to CHD [64].

Hostility and cynicism are typically measured in these studies using the Ho (for hostility) subscale of the Minnesota Multiphasic Personality Inventory (MMPI) [65]. In one study 424 patients undergoing coronary angiography were given the type A structured interview and the Ho scale. Both type A and hostility scores were significantly associated with CHD, but hostility showed a stronger relationship [65]. The relationship was found to be as strong for women as for men, and women who scored high on both scales had 3.6 times the risk of having CHD present on angiography as did their low-scoring counterparts.

Shekelle and collaborators reanalyzed health outcomes in the Western Electric Study (WES) as a function of hostility scores on the Ho scale of the MMPI [66]. The WES was a prospective epidemiologic study in which 1877 middle-aged male (ages 40 to 55) employees at Western Electric's Hawthorne Works plant in Chicago were followed from 1957 to 1978. Hostility scores, independent of other risk factors, predicted both 10-year incidence of major CHD events (MI and death) and 20-year mortality not only from CHD but from all other causes as well. After adjustment for other risk factors, a difference of 23 points on the Ho scale (the difference between the means of the highest and the lowest quintiles) was associated with a 42 percent increase in risk of death [66, 67].

Barefoot and colleagues [68] showed that hostility expressed early in life has predictable health consequences later in life. In an elegant and compelling follow-up study of 255 physicians who had taken the MMPI when they were students at the University of North Carolina Medical School, they showed that 25 years later, those physicians who had scored in the highest quintile of hostility as students were four to five times more likely to have developed CHD than those whose Ho scores were in the lowest quintile. The impact on mortality was even more striking. Those physicians with high Ho scores at age 25 were nearly seven times more likely to die by age 50 (of all causes of death, not just CHD) than those with low Ho scores (Figure 11-2). This is a substantially larger effect than the finding in the WES and is probably due to the difference in the ages of the subjects (about 25 years) when the studies were initiated. It is likely that the high-hostility middle-aged WES workers already had experienced some differ-

Figure 11-2. Differential survival rates at five-year intervals among men with Ho scores above the median as compared to those with Ho scores below the median. (Reprinted with permission from Barefoot JC, Dahlstrom WG, and Williams RB. Hostility, CHD incidence, and total mortality: A 25-year followup study of 255 physicians. Psychosom Med 1983; 45:59–63.)

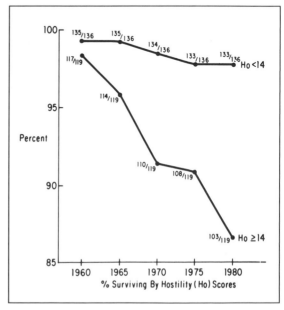

ential mortality before the study was initiated [69].

In a subsequent study of lawyers, Barefoot and colleagues [70] analyzed the items on the Ho scale and found that a subgrouping of 27 of the original 50 items predicted increased mortality far more reliably and strongly than did the entire Ho scale. This apparent distillate of the Ho scale and of the original type A pattern has been described as "a cynical and untrusting view of humankind, the frequent experience of negative emotions when dealing with others, and the frequent expression of overt anger and aggression when faced with frustration or problems [71]." Williams speculates that this hostility-cynicism factor may be inversely related to social support.

Other investigations have broken down the hostility-cynicism factor even further. Hostility can reflect two basic dimensions of personality, according to Dembroski and colleagues [72]. One is neuroticism, which refers to the tendency to experience distressing emotions, such as anger, irritability, resentment, and suspicion. Neuroticism does not prospectively predict CHD outcomes such as MI and CHD mortality [73]. The other is antagonistic hostility. This refers to a style of interpersonal interaction that is disagreeable and/or uncooperative, including expressions of arrogance, argumentativeness, condescension, surliness, and rudeness [72]. In a case-control analysis of MRFIT data Dembroski and colleagues [72] showed that only antagonistic hostility was related to CHD events after correcting for other risk factors and only in younger men (47 years old or younger). Thus, it seems that it may be the overt expression of hostility in terms of antagonism and disagreeableness that underlies the hostility-CHD relationship.

Spielberger and colleagues also view hostility as part of a more complex behavioral pattern involving anger and aggression, which they have dubbed the AHA! (anger, hostility, aggression) syndrome [74]. They postulate that the concept of anger subsumes phenomena that are both more fundamental and, in many ways, simpler than the phenomena of hostility and aggression. Thus, anger is seen as the core of the constellation. Spielberger and colleagues define anger and its relationship to hostility and aggression as follows:

Anger is generally considered to be a simpler concept than hostility or aggression. The concept of anger usually refers to an emotional state that consists of feelings that vary in intensity, from mild irritation or annoyance to fury and rage. Although hostility usually involves angry feelings, this concept has the connotation of a complex set of attitudes that motivate aggressive behaviors directed toward destroying objects or injuring other people [74].

People tend to vary widely in their habitual ways of dealing with their angry feelings. Some characteristically tend to hold anger inside and not display it outwardly (termed anger-in), whereas others vent it readily (anger-out). A number of studies have suggested that people who tend to suppress their anger have high systolic and diastolic blood pressure levels [75, 76, 77]. Dembroski and colleagues [78] found that high ratings of both potential for hostility and anger-in were significantly and positively associated with angiographically documented severity of CHD and that this effect was most pronounced in younger subjects. Spielberger and colleagues [74] showed that among 1114 high school students, systolic blood pressure was substantially higher in both males and females in the high anger-in groupings (although males always had higher readings than females at all levels of anger expression). Diastolic BP showed a similar increase with the degree of anger in this study, but, surprisingly, the females were consistently higher than the males.

Further analyses showed that anger-in scores were a better predictor of systolic and diastolic BP than any other measure for white males and for black males and females [74]. Spielberger describes hypertensives as particularly prone to react angrily in unfair or embarrassing situations. Yet a recent report of a 35-year follow-up of 126 former Harvard College students failed to show an association of either anger-in or anger-out with any chronic disease outcome, but it did find an association between severe anxiety and both CHD and all forms of illness. This anxiety was frequently "linked to marked conflict about hostile impulses" [79]. It is possible that the differences between the results of this and other studies of anger-in may be due to limitations in the instruments used 35 years ago to measure anger expression compared to what is available today, as well as the small number of subjects in the Harvard College study.

Other recent work has looked at the relationship between emotional arousability and sudden cardiac death [80]. In an 8½-year study of 929 post-MI men emotional arousability was an independent predictor of sudden cardiac death (relative risk [RR] = 2.13). The effect was stronger in younger men (less than 54 years of age) (RR = 3.19) and in men with elevations of other risk factors. Emotional arousability was determined in this study during a casual (i.e., non-structured) interview using verbal and nonverbal responses to specific questions regarding impatience, anger, and aggression (overt reactivity) and by observing a pattern of specific body movements (fast, jerky movements, tic-like facial grimaces and other facial behaviors, rapid eye blinking, and repetitive hand or leg movements) and speech characteristics (rapid speech with or without interruptions) during the interview (suppressed reactivity). Interestingly, these behavioral characteristics were part of the original type A behavior constellation and have recently been linked to hostility expression [81].

A great deal of work continues in the field of type A behavior and heart disease. Hundreds of papers were published on the subject in the past two years alone. The question of the validity of the original type A characterization has yet to be decided in full. The relationship of the type A behavior pattern to CHD is clearly not as straightforward as was originally proposed, and current evidence suggests that overt expression of hostility and cynicism is a more potent predictor of CHD.

Of course any single CHD-related behavioral component might itself be modulated by other psychosocial factors, resulting in enhanced or reduced risk. For example, a recent study from Sweden noted that social isolation was an independent mortality predictor in type A but not in type B men [82]. The 10-year mortality rate of socially isolated type A men was 69 percent, whereas that of socially integrated type A men was only 17 percent, controlling for other risk factors.

Other Indicators of an Emotion-Health Connection

Grossarth-Maticek and colleagues [83, 84] investigated the relationship between a number of psychosocial and personality factors and the incidence of and mortality from both heart disease and cancer. In a 10-year prospective epidemiologic study in Yugoslavia of approximately 1400 people, they found that an 11-item questionnaire assessing rationality-antiemotionality, or repression and denial of emotions, was the best single predictor of the subsequent development of both cancer and heart disease. The relative risk for CHD was ten times greater for those who scored high on this scale compared to those who scored lower. Rationality-antiemotionality was a stronger predictor of heart disease than the traditional CHD risk factors in this study. These results have recently been reanalyzed by Spielberger [85], who has confirmed the basic findings.

There is an entire literature related to stress, coping, and the emotions that suggests that particular attitudes, personality factors, and coping styles appear to be protective against disease in general. Among these is a construct termed *psychological hardiness*. Studies of people in stressful occupations, such as bus drivers, business executives, and lawyers, carried out by Kobasa and colleagues [86, 87], suggest that individuals who are characterized by strong feelings of confidence in their ability to control circumstances, a willingness to see life events as challenges rather than obstacles, and a strong commitment to the experiences and demands of daily living have fewer illnesses than those who are lacking in these qualities. A similar personality construct, *sense of coherence* (SOC) [88] has also been shown to differentiate between individuals who remain healthy and those who are more likely to become ill in the face of stressful life circumstances. This construct also has three major elements, comprehensibility, manageability, and meaningfulness [88]. SOC is defined as

. . . a global orientation that expresses the extent to which one has a pervasive enduring though dynamic feeling of confidence that (1) the stimuli deriving from one's internal and external environments in the course of living are structured, predictable and explicable; (2) the resources are available to one to meet the demands posed by these stimuli; and (3) these demands are challenges, worthy of investment and engagement [88].

Other psychological characteristics are also related to overall health. Bandura and colleagues have shown in numerous studies that *self-efficacy,* the belief that one is capable of mastering a particular task or behavior, predicts high performance and positive outcomes in that specific task or behavior [89, 90]. Seligman and colleagues have shown a connection between optimism and health, as well as the converse, a connection between pessimism and illness [91]. McClelland and colleagues demonstrated a positive relation between motives directed by affiliative drives (termed *affiliative trust*) and a resistance to illness, while motives directed by a strong need for power, particularly when the individual experiences stress or frustration due to resistance from others, were associated with breakdowns in health [92].

The combined thrust of this body of research suggests that it is the interaction between external and internal stressors and a person's external and internal resources for coping — including social ties, supportive and affiliative bonds, and personal attitudes and beliefs (view of the world) — that modulates the health outcomes of the individual under stress. Disease results when the internal and external resources available for coping with the demands on the organism are overwhelmed by those very demands. Thus, from the point of view of psychosocial intervention, resistance to illness might be heightened by reinforcing and strengthening those psychological attributes and qualities that may help to buffer the effects of stress, namely, stress hardiness, a strong sense of coherence, self-efficacy, optimism, and affiliative trust. These psychological qualities

modulate severe stress reactions, including the threatened or perceived loss of control, and their emotional sequelae (fear, anxiety, anger, hostility, and aggression), as well as the very different psychological consequences of an actual loss of control, namely, depression, helplessness, and hopelessness.

While the roles played by these factors have not yet been studied prospectively in heart disease, it is likely that at least some will be found to protect by providing alternative, more adaptive coping avenues for the individual, thus leading to less psychosocial distress, even under circumstances of severe social disruption or personal psychological or physical stress.

The results discussed here conform to the general hypothesis that particular patterns of emotional expression (or suppression) can contribute to the development of chronic disease. Since emotional expression is tied to our view of ourselves and of the world and is influenced by our interactions with the world, it is not surprising that our emotions function as part of our coping repertoire in the face of acute and chronic life changes and social challenges. Hostility and aggression may be functional in maintaining social status in animals and in people, but, as demonstrated in the studies of the cynomolgus monkeys [43], they can be severely maladaptive under disruptive social conditions and contribute to an accelerated progression of CHD even in the absence of large amounts of fat and cholesterol in the diet.

Coping effectively with the full range of emotions we feel as human beings may be of great importance for our health. Physicians can intervene effectively to help people become more aware of their emotions, particularly in times of great stress. One effective means is to encourage patients to develop ways of expressing and coping with their feelings that will reduce the risks associated with the suppression or denial of strong emotions, especially anger and anxiety, and with chronically hostile, aggressive, and cynical attitudes and behaviors. Interestingly the available data suggest that the suppression of anger may be associated with an increased risk of cancer (and perhaps hypertension), whereas the uncontrolled expression of anger and its ensuing aggression is related to an increase in CHD risk. Thus, a middle path in the self-regulation of emotional expression, at least regarding anger and hostility, may be the avenue of choice in terms of improving health.

The Pathophysiology of CHD-Promoting Psychosocial Behaviors

As previously noted, emotional stress due to psychosocial stimulation can induce changes in cardiovascular physiology in animals that can lead to major pathophysiology, including sudden death. At least two stress-related neuroendocrine pathways appear to be involved: the pituitary adrenal cortical system and the sympathetic adrenal medullary system [93, 94]. The former has been shown to become activated when an animal experiences a loss of control, as in a downward displacement in the social hierarchy or via the experimentally induced condition of learned helplessness. Stimulation of the pituitary adrenal cortical system is associated with depressed, withdrawn, inactive behavior and is characterized physiologically by elevations in adrenocorticotrophic hormone (ACTH) and plasma cortisone or corticosterone, a decrease in gonadotrophin levels, and enhanced vagal activity, gluconeogenesis, and pepsin production.

Stimulation of the sympathetic adrenal medullary system, on the other hand, is associated with pronounced motor activity, as in the vigorous attempts an animal makes to maintain dominant social status or control when threatened, challenged, or stressed. This is Cannon's fight-or-flight reaction [8]. Physiologically it is associated with increased secretion of catecholamines and testosterone. In primates, including humans, sympathetic arousal results in an increase in arterial pressure, cardiac output, heart rate, and skeletal muscle blood flow. Both these neuroendocrine systems are associated with pathological consequences when psychosocial stimulation is of sufficient magnitude and duration. Secretion of so-called stress hormones in both systems may occur together and these may potentiate each other.

There are basically four major mechanisms by which psychosocial stimuli might influence CHD [95]: (1) arterial injury through hemodynamic forces, such as turbulence and shear stress promoted by repeated and excessive heart rate and/or pressor responses to stress; (2) direct toxic effects on the coronary arteries by biochemical injury from an increased output of endocrine substances, such as catecholamines and corticosteroids; (3) indirect influences of catecholamines and other stress hormones on cellular functions, such as platelet aggregation and the mobilization of serum lipids; and (4) direct disruption of the central nervous system's control of the heart, leading to arrhythmic activity, lower thresholds for ventricular fibrillation, and possible sudden cardiac death.

Stress reactivity and its relation to cardiovascular disease is a rapidly growing area of interest. A great deal of recent work has explored mechanisms whereby emotional arousal and reactivity affect cardiac physiology in both animals and humans [96]. The limited scope of this chapter precludes a comprehensive discussion of pathophysiological mechanisms and pathways. We will confine ourselves to a brief discussion of the sympathetic-mediated effects of emotional reactivity and a look at some recent work on neuroendocrine responses associated with the type A behavior pattern and hostility-prone individuals.

In the studies of male cynomolgus monkeys of Clarkson and collaborators [43], a chronically unstable social situation resulted in coronary artery narrowings in the dominant monkeys that were more than twice as severe as those observed in dominant control monkeys maintained in a socially stable (unstressed) environment. BP and cholesterol levels were the same in both groups. A greater degree of CAD was found in the emotionally stressed animals under both low-fat/low-cholesterol and high-fat/high-cholesterol dietary conditions, but the degree of stenosis was much more severe in stressed animals under the high-fat/high-cholesterol condition. Other studies have shown that chronic stress increased the permeability of the monkeys' arterial walls to cholesterol and that HDL decreased in the stressed condition

[97]. Moreover, those animals in both conditions who were subsequently identified as high-heart-rate-reactive individuals on the basis of a common laboratory stressor (threat of capture) were found to have developed nearly twice the degree of CAD of their low-heart-rate-reactive counterparts [98]. This effect appeared to be independent of other variables involved in atherosclerosis, such as resting heart rate, resting BP, and serum lipid levels. One related study in humans found that diastolic reactivity to the cold pressor test significantly predicted subsequent CHD at 23-year follow-up and that this measure was more strongly predictive than the more traditional risk factors [99]. Eliot [100] has termed people who react to stress with an increase in cardiac output coupled with extreme vasoconstriction *hot reactors* and showed that they, like their monkey counterparts, are at highest risk of dying from stress reactivity.

In a study of squirrel monkeys using the yoked–escape avoidance/helplessness design, yoked helpless monkeys tended to develop severe bradycardia (the playing–dead reaction) in response to a series of tail shocks, whereas the avoidance monkeys who were able to influence the schedule of shocks developed ECG abnormalities, hypertension, and myocardial degenerative lesions. As in the escape avoidance studies of Weiss [49], mortality in the squirrel monkeys depended on their degree of relative psychological control. When the conditions were varied, mortality rates differed between the avoidance and the helpless animals depending on the degree of relative psychological control they were accorded [101].

That an animal's psychological assessment of a potentially stressful stimulus as threatening is required for a stress-related neuroendocrine response to occur was demonstrated by Mason and colleagues [102]. Fasting monkeys exposed to the sights and sounds of feeding monkeys developed marked increases in urinary cortisol excretion. However, isolated monkeys provided with nonnourishing fruit-flavored pellets showed no increase in cortisol excretion, demonstrating that the emotional arousal and not the fasting condition itself elicited the neuroendocrine response.

A large body of research has sought to classify individuals with differing behavior patterns in terms of their stress responses in the laboratory [for reviews, see 103, 104, 105, 106]. In general these studies found that individuals with the type A behavior pattern show higher levels of sympathetic reactivity (increases in BP and heart rate, secretion of epinephrine and norepinephrine; T-wave amplitude suppression) than those with the type B pattern. If this response pattern in the laboratory is typical of a type A individual's stress reactivity pattern in response to the challenges and frustrations of daily living, then repeated sympathetic hyperreactivity and chronic oversecretion of stress hormones such as epinephrine, norepinephrine, and cortisol over a long span of time might lead, via mechanisms such as endothelial injury to the coronary arteries, to increased CHD risk in type A individuals compared to type B individuals. Indeed, middle-aged type A men have recently been reported to excrete more epinephrine and norepinephrine than do type B men over a 24-hour period of normal activity [107].

Williams and colleagues [108] were able to show that in addition to other signs of sympathetic activation (such as secretion of epinephrine and norepinephrine), forearm muscle blood flow and cortisol levels were also higher in type A men than in type B men during the stress of performing mental arithmetic (serial subtractions of 13 from a large number with a prize for the winner). In response to a vigilance task (watching signals on a TV screen and pushing a button whenever a specified pattern of letters appeared), however, these same type A men showed low levels of sympathetic arousal, as did type B men, but demonstrated a larger secretion of testosterone than was seen in those with type B behavior.

When attempts were made to extend these findings to hostility, no differential effect between high- and low-hostility individuals was observed in the mental arithmetic task. However, when a realistic harassment paradigm was added to the mental arithmetic challenge to increase the likelihood that the subjects would actually overtly express irritability, anger, and hostility, those with high hostility scores did indeed show larger increases in muscle blood flow and BP than did low-hostility subjects [109]. This suggested that stressful or provocative situations in the laboratory (and presumably in daily life) have to be relevant enough to trigger the expression of hostility and anger to see physiological arousal, which otherwise remains only a potential for hostility. Thus, individuals with a high potential for hostility may be at much higher risk for CHD events from particular stressful or challenging circumstances.

Interestingly, although low hostility subjects also experienced and expressed irritability and anger when harassed, this did not lead to heightened sympathetic arousal. It may be that anger expression is particularly toxic only for individuals who have a high potential for hostility. It is possible that they differ biologically from low-hostility individuals in terms of sympathetic reactivity and also in parasympathetic regulation of sympathetic arousal. Low-hostility individuals may be protected from the negative health consequences of stress reactivity and emotional arousal via more robust parasympathetic regulation [109a].

High-hostility individuals did show higher testosterone increases than low-hostility individuals in the vigilance task [110]. The largest increases were seen in the type A men who also had high Ho scores, while the smallest responses (decreases) were found in type Bs with low Ho scores. If hostile, cynical individuals do indeed spend more time in a state of alert vigilance in the conduct of their daily lives because of their lack of trust in others, it might be expected that they would excrete more testosterone during waking hours but not during sleep (a low-vigilance state) compared to low-hostility people. Although this has not been specifically studied for hostility, type A men were found to excrete more testosterone in the urine than type Bs during waking hours but not during sleep [111]. Williams notes that testosterone levels increase during maturation in adolescent boys and are associated with lower HDL levels. Moreover, as with cortisol [112], administration of testosterone has been found to increase arteriosclerosis in animals [113]. One plausible

pathophysiologic pathway between behavior and CHD would involve hypersecretion of stress hormones and testosterone, which might individually and together contribute via increased BP and turbulent blood flow to injury to the coronary endothelium and thus lead to or accelerate the cascade of cellular events that results in CHD (see Chapter 3). Increased sympathetic arousal, unchecked by normal parasympathetic down-regulation, might also lead to a higher susceptibility to acute cardiac events, such as ventricular fibrillation, MI, and sudden cardiac death [114]. Indeed, a recent study found that an index of emotional arousability (Table 11-1) was an independent predictor of sudden cardiac death in a large cohort of post-MI men over an 8½-year period [115].

As noted several studies have found hostility to be independently associated with an increased risk of overall mortality, not just mortality associated with CHD. In the Western Electric Study [66] higher hostility levels were associated with an increased risk of cancer. There are some indications that emotional regulation and trust may also be factors in susceptibility to cancer. In a 40-year prospective study of medical students at the Johns Hopkins University School of Medicine, it was found that a lack of closeness to parents in childhood reported at the time subjects were in medical school was strongly associated with an increased risk of cancer 40 years later [116]. It is possible, as suggested by much of the evidence discussed earlier, that a lack of belief in the goodness and trustworthiness of others, perhaps exacerbated by early life experiences and relationships, could have a long-term depressive effect on immune parameters, which might lead to reduced ability to identify and reject tumor cells at an early stage [117].

Studies of Psychosocial Interventions to Reduce CHD Risk

With the rise in interest in the psychosocial elements of CHD etiology came the related question of whether particular interventions could be developed that would reduce CHD risk by

Table 11-1. Brief lines of questioning for emotional arousability

Overt emotional reactivity (usually occurs in response to specific questions)

Characteristic*	Question	Reactive response
Impatience	"How do you feel when you get stuck behind a slow driver or in an unexpectedly long bank or grocery line?"	An intense emotional reaction to any delay, e.g., "It drives me crazy!"; "I can't stand it!"
Reliving anger about the past	"Did you become mildly irritated today? Yesterday? Tell me about it."	Patient reexperiences the arousal felt in the situation upon telling the story, e.g., explosive speech, speeded-up speech, emphatic gesturing with hands or head.
Aggressive response to challenge	"When you became really angry, how did you deal with it?"	Patient uses aggression to deal with anger, e.g., is quick to take offense, is negatively judgmental, loses temper, comes to blows.

Suppressed reactivity (scan the patient during casual history taking and note presence of any of these indicators)

Characteristic	Reactive response
Fast and jerky movements	Patient *consistently* moves in a style that is fast, jerky, or characterized by frequent twitching.
Tic-like facial grimace	Tic-like drawing back of 1 or both sides of the mouth; happens as a response to holding tension in the muscles around the mouth.
Rapid eye blinking	Continuous blinking at rate of 1 per second or more, or continuous episodes of eyelid flurries.
Repetitive hand/leg movements	Knee jiggling, pill rolling noticed more than 4 times.
Rapid speech with or without interruptions	Patient speaks very fast, and interruptions are frequent. You get the feeling s/he is jumping on your questions with the answer.

*A patient who has three or more overt or suppressed characteristics is emotionally reactive.
Source: Powell, LH. Personal communication. Reprinted by permission.

modifying the factors in question, such as social isolation, inadequate coping with stress, type A behavior, stress reactivity, hostility, and cynicism. While it is often problematic to separate one element entirely from the others, the weight of accumulated evidence suggests that each of these factors can be modified by psychosocial interventions of various kinds and that CHD risk may be reduced as a consequence.

A randomized clinical trial, the Recurrent Coronary Prevention Project (RCPP), of 1000 type A men who had already suffered a heart attack showed that type A behavior was substantially reduced by a behavior modification approach focusing on time urgency and hostil-ity, compared to men undergoing a standard cardiac rehabilitation intervention [118]. Moreover, there was a 45 percent lower rate of recurrent cardiac events (fatal and nonfatal MIs) in the behavior modification group over the 3 years of the intervention period compared to those who were not trained to reduce their type A behavior [119]. Other studies have shown that a comparable degree of behavior change from the type A pattern can be accomplished in much less time [120, 121]. These interventions to reduce type A behavior explicitly target low self-esteem as the root cause of the problems of both the type A behavior pattern and of hostility and cynicism [119]. The findings of the RCPP suggest that behavior modification approaches to reduce type A behavior (and hostility) might be of benefit at the primary prevention level as well as at the level of secondary prevention. Since they tend to take place in relatively small groups and have a strong educational and social aspect [119], such interventions would serve to reduce an individual's social isolation as well as change the ways in which the person copes with stress and with the deep feelings that often drive social behaviors. It is likely that identification of individuals at risk for health problems due to hostility, emotional reactivity, suppression or denial of feelings, or social isolation and subsequent referral to educational programs oriented toward attitudinal and behavior change might have beneficial effects on reducing CHD.

One of the most interesting and important psychosocial intervention studies to date is that of Ornish and collaborators [122], who demonstrated actual regression of stenosis in a randomized group of patients (n = 28) with angiographically documented severe CAD. The intervention was multimodal, consisting of a very low-fat vegetarian diet, stress management training (consisting of biweekly yoga and meditation training in a group context, along with 1 hour daily practice by the participants) and moderate exercise (walking). Stopping smoking was also part of the intervention.

The intervention had lasted for 1 year at the time of the initial report. Stenoses were analyzed pre- and postintervention by quantitative angiography. The average percentage diameter stenosis regressed from 40.0 to 37.8 in the experimental group yet progressed from 42.7 to 46.1 in the control group (which received traditional cardiologic care and followed the dietary recommendations of the AHA). When only lesions of greater than 50 percent stenosis were analyzed, the average percentage diameter stenosis regressed from 61.1 to 55.8 in the experimental group and progressed from 61.7 to 64.4 in the control group. Overall, 82 percent of the patients in the experimental group had an average change toward regression. The degree of regression was found to be related to the overall degree of adherence to the intervention modalities among the subjects [122]. Subjects in the lifestyle intervention group also showed significant increases on Antonovsky's Sense of Coherence measure and reductions in trait anger and hostility at 1 year, while control subjects did not [123].

This is the first study to show that a nonpharmacologic intervention can result in a quantitative improvement in the degree of CHD. Marked improvements in anginal symptoms and in serum lipids were also observed prior to the documentation of reduced stenosis.

It is not possible in a multimodal intervention study of this type to separate the purely psychosocial components of the intervention from those that affect traditional risk factors (e.g., lowering cholesterol). However, in this trial great emphasis was placed on the stress management component, which was seen as the integrating modality, bringing together the dietary changes and the exercise regimen in a larger context provided by meditative awareness and the established group affiliation and social ties. Participants in the intervention group were required to practice the stress management techniques for a minimum of 1 hour per day as well as meet together twice a week to practice as a group. The stress management techniques included hatha yoga and various relaxation, visualization, and meditation practices [124]. The intervention was ambitious in scope, demanding of participants in the intervention condition a major and immediate lifestyle change in terms of both new behaviors and a significant daily time commitment. That it was at least initially successful suggests that reducing heart disease via a strictly behavioral, lifestyle modification approach may be possible if sufficient motivation and adherence to the demands of a multimodal intervention are maintained. The minimal level of intervention required to produce regression of this magnitude in this time frame is unknown and remains to be established by further study. The longer-term outcomes of this study are under current investigation.

If the results of Ornish and colleagues prove to be reproducible, they would certainly suggest that we can encourage patients to believe that heart disease may be reversible or at least retardable by making lifestyle changes, including both adopting a low-fat vegetarian diet and engaging in effective meditation-based stress management practices. Moreover, they suggest that adopting a comprehensive lifestyle regimen may prevent CHD in healthy individuals at risk for its development.

In the Ornish study the stress management component was based on participants taking time on a regular basis to cultivate and dwell in states of deep inner stillness and awareness through meditation and yoga practice. There is increasing evidence that such meditative practices may influence the reestablishing of physiological homeostasic mechanisms when they are disrupted by psychosocial stress. There is also evidence that engaging in such practices may give rise to a greater inner feeling of control and an appreciation for living with greater present moment awareness [124a, 124b, 125, 126].

Practical Issues of Assessment and Intervention for the Physician

Awareness, Knowledge, and Communication

Psychosocial factors influence not only the risk of CHD but of overall morbidity and mortality across a wide range of disorders. The physician who is knowledgeable in this area and who cultivates the simple assessment and intervention skills recommended here will be in a position to favorably affect the general health and well-being of her patients as well as reduce their risk of CHD.

For a busy medical practice, it is naive to suggest that a thorough assessment and treatment of those psychosocial factors that may place a patient at risk for illness at some future time is practicable or even desirable. Even in situations where an understanding of the patient's psychosocial background would contribute to the management of a medical problem, such an analysis usually takes a back seat to more pressing medical concerns and to inquiries and recommendations concerning better-defined and less "touchy" lifestyle risk factors such as

diet, smoking, substance abuse, and exercise. However, physicians who are aware of the importance of this area and who operate from a biopsychosocial [127, 128] rather than a purely biomedical perspective can make substantial contributions to the life and health of their patients with strategies that consume little time and energy but that can potentially produce powerful returns. Physician-performed psychosocial assessment and intervention is most appropriately interwoven into all aspects of the medical encounter, from the history and physical examination and assessment of health risk behaviors to their modification and treatment.

Most important is the quality of the relationship the clinician establishes with the patient. Physicians often bring to the clinical encounter a frame of mind in which they feel a strong need to do something immediate to fix a clearly defined problem: to act, to give drugs, to make something better. They are often reluctant to raise issues that might lead to strong emotions unless it is absolutely necessary. This may be due in part to their own discomfort, embarrassment, and feelings of helplessness in the face of the expression of feelings in general and strong emotions in particular, such as anger or grief. It may also be related in part to the fact that, until recently, little systematic attention was paid to the biopsychosocial model in medical education. A physician could complete medical training thinking that psychosocial factors were either trivial and irrelevant to the practice of medicine or relevant but far too overwhelming to approach and fraught with uncertain difficulties and obstacles.

The physician who feels such discomfort needs to remember that in probing the domain of the psychosocial, what is most important is just to be present and to listen with attentiveness and compassion. Nothing needs immediate fixing, and patients do not come with the expectation that their doctor will be able to fix such matters as unhappiness, marital strife, a history of abuse, or job stress. It is possible to help simply by inquiring about factors even the patient may not be consciously aware of or may be reluctant to talk about at first, and then by simply listening and caring. Physicians often worry that if they do inquire, they will open the proverbial Pandora's box, and the patient will go on for hours. However, patients tend to be self-limiting in this domain and usually require periodic encouragement to disclose such matters. The maintenance of equanimity and empathy by the physician in the face of expressions of emotion can lead to a greater bond with the patient as well as provide additional information for making an accurate assessment and identifying appropriate treatment options.

Sympathetic attention and inquiry also lead to greater patient satisfaction. A recent study suggests that patient satisfaction with a physician visit is more directly related to the physician's efforts to deal with the patient's psychosocial needs, such as the need for information, the need for control, and the need for support and advice regarding stressful situations than it is to the physical examination, the ordering of tests, or the recommendation of specific pharmacologic and nonpharmacologic therapies [129]. This appears to be true whether or not the patient expected to receive advice or stress counseling. Other studies have shown a significant relationship between patient satisfaction and the ability of a physician to express caring and concern in the medical encounter [130, 131, 132].

One study of medical patients identified as having psychosocial distress (anxiety, depression, stress) showed that primary care physicians who possessed relatively detailed knowledge of the patient derived from several psychosocial questionnaires filled out prior to a first medical encounter were given higher satisfaction ratings by their patients than control subjects whose physicians did not have such information [133]. The physicians who had this knowledge received patient satisfaction ratings as high as those received by physicians who had such information and also engaged in a simple single-visit stress counseling session with their patients. Having the questionnaire-based information prior to the encounter apparently led the physicians to engage in effective inquiry and informal counseling. Moreover, patients whose physicians were in possession of the information from the psychosocial questionnaires indicated

that after the medical visit, their stress had decreased more and their sense of control over that stress had increased to a greater degree than in the case of patients whose doctors were not apprised of their patients' psychosocial status before the encounter. The majority of physicians reported that they had spent less than 5 minutes counseling their patients about stress on the basis of the information from the questionnaires.

Physicians should keep in mind the following general points about the assessment and treatment of psychosocial factors that may place a patient at risk for illness:

- Successful encounters require that physicians rely on their capacity to listen and to care — they don't have to fix anything or even give advice.
- It is acceptable to inquire about a patient's feelings and stressors using brief questionnaires filled out prior to the encounter, direct inquiry, or both.
- Sometimes it is advisable to intentionally postpone discussion of psychosocial issues to a second office visit or later, when greater rapport and trust have been established.
- Ultimately, given the realities of medical practice, an assessment that indicates psychosocial risk and/or distress usually results in the need for an appropriate referral.

The next section presents the specific steps a physician can take to assess and treat psychosocial factors.

Physician-Delivered Intervention

Physician-delivered intervention to alter psychosocial risk factors follows the same general format as for the more classical CHD risk factors: (1) *assessment* to identify problem areas, i.e., high stress reactivity, hostility, social isolation, major stressors in work or family life coupled with poor coping; symptoms such as exhaustion, anxiety, depression, and functional somatic complaints; (2) *treatment/intervention,* which includes exploring the patient's commitment for change in a particular area; assessing the patient's level of confidence in his ability to change, his history of growth-enhancing experiences as well as attempts at positive behavior changes in the past; and assisting the patient to identify and undertake appropriate and practical actions for change in the present, including self-education, seeking social support, and joining a group; (3) developing and negotiating a *plan for change,* which includes goal setting by the patient and a degree of self-responsibility assumed by the patient for his health and for working toward these self-set goals; and (4) *follow-up/maintenance,* which includes assessing the results (outcomes) of actions undertaken, developing follow-up actions, and promoting maintenance and further deepening of new attitudes and behaviors. Here again, the role of the physician as a teacher-counselor-guide and a resource for support in the process of growth and change is of vital importance.

STEP 1: ASSESSMENT

Above all else the physician needs to ask, "Who is this person?" "What are the major stressors in her life?" "What are her coping resources, social supports, and beliefs about herself and her state of health?" In general patients appreciate being asked by their physicians about life stressors and their ability to handle them. It can be an invitation to disclose anxieties and problems and identify hidden agendas. Simple inquiry can lead to an assessment of how anxious, reactive, angry, hostile, or depressed a person may become under stress and, in turn, to an assessment of how confident the patient feels in his ability to cope effectively with life pressures. One can also inquire about the relationship between somatic complaints (such as chest pain, shortness of breath, palpitations, headaches, fatigue) and stressful situations. This can help the patient become more conscious of connections between particular life experiences and symptoms that may have previously gone unrecognized. Specific recommendations and referrals can then be offered as appropriate. At the very least the basis for further conversation on this subject can be established.

In assessing psychosocial and stress-related issues with the patient, it is important for the clinician to be keenly aware of the patient's ver-

bal and nonverbal responses — listening carefully not just to content but to tone of voice and rapidity of speech and noticing posture, body tension, gestures, facial expressions, and other behaviors that can provide relevant clues to the patient's level of self-esteem, comfort in the interview itself, and receptivity to suggestions for growth and change. Such observations can be used to guide the direction of the encounter and provide fruitful avenues for further inquiry. They can be made while the physician is taking the medical history, performing the physical examination or carrying out medical interventions.

Mindfulness. The key to observation is a willingness to cultivate moment-to-moment awareness, known technically as mindfulness [126], during the interview. Mindfulness can be thought of as intentional, nonjudgmental, present-moment awareness. It is cultivated by observing those instances, often frequent, when one's attention goes out of the present moment and by intentionally bringing it back to the here and now. Just keeping in mind the importance of psychosocial factors, the intention to be totally present in the presence of the patient and to be mindful of the various verbal and nonverbal exchanges occurring during the encounter can enhance the physician's effectiveness both in building rapport and in inquiring appropriately about potentially important lifestyle and emotional factors. It can also leave the physician feeling more engaged and ultimately satisfied with the encounter.

Things the physician should ask himself in attempting to cultivate mindfulness in the physician-patient encounter might include: "What is my body language saying?" "Am I keeping my distance (literally) from the patient?" "Am I hiding behind a desk?" "Are our faces at the same level or am I higher?" "Am I holding all the power here?" "Am I listening to the patient's responses or impatiently jumping ahead?"

Preservation of Hope. It is important to preserve the patient's hope and sense of control by not implying catastrophe in small and unnecessary ways. Physicians often indulge in this behavior unconsciously. There should be no place in the conscious physician-patient relationship for gratuitous physician comments such as "You can expect this to just get worse," even if it is based on knowledge of the course of disease. It is particularly important to be aware of how one frames prognostic statements, so as to not rob the patient of hope, dignity, or a sense of control.

Use of Questionnaires. It can be helpful to have the patient fill out one or more brief questionnaires prior to the encounter, to probe psychological and physical symptoms and emotional expression (e.g., anger or hostility). A quick glance at such a form can provide useful indications of problem areas as well as the areas in which the patient may have expectations of the physician. Filling out a questionnaire primes the patient to consider such areas and provides a framework for later discussion in the examination room. The patient's responses can be an effective entry point into discussion of stress reactivity, feelings, and behaviors.

Our stress reduction clinic uses a medical symptom checklist that also includes a number of psychological symptoms (see Table 11-2). If these symptoms are checked off in any great number, it provides a good basis for inquiring further about feelings such as hopelessness, nervousness, family problems, sexual difficulties, and poor concentration, all of which indicate a potential psychosocial disturbance influencing the patient's health.

An alternative to the use of questionnaires is to simply have a short list of questions that can be asked of the patient when the physician suspects that a particular psychosocial area may be of concern, such as emotional reactivity or hostility (see Table 11-1 and Table 11-3).

Awareness of Denial. Many people use denial as a way to cope with problems and feelings that threaten their sense of well-being. Patients with an increased risk of CHD often deny feeling excited, emotionally upset, or stressed in the face of contradictory evidence [134, 135]. Some cancer patients have been observed to suppress and deny strong emotions, such as

Table 11-2.   Emotional symptom questionnaire

If you have recently been bothered with these problems (in the past month) check YES.

	YES	NO
nervousness or anxiety	——	——
nervous with strangers	——	——
difficulty making decisions	——	——
lack of concentration	——	——
absentminded/loss of memory	——	——
feelings of loneliness	——	——
depression	——	——
frequent crying	——	——
hopeless outlook	——	——
difficulty relaxing	——	——
worrying a lot	——	——
frightening dreams or thoughts	——	——
feelings of desperation	——	——
feeling shy or sensitive	——	——
dislike of criticism	——	——
getting angered easily	——	——
being annoyed by little things	——	——
family problems	——	——
problems at work	——	——
sexual difficulties	——	——
change of sexual energy	——	——
thoughts of suicide	——	——
sought psychiatric help	——	——

anger [136, 137]; one study showed that cancer (malignant melanoma) patients engaged in more repressive coping than cardiovascular patients or healthy control subjects [138]. Denial, of course, is also a salient characteristic of alcoholism and other addictive disorders [139].

Although the many ways of working with a patient's unhealthy denial are beyond the scope of this chapter, the physician's gentle and skillful recommendations to a patient to pay more careful attention to particular areas in his life can often lead someone in denial to become more in touch with his problems in ways that are empowering rather than solely threatening. It is important to keep in mind that

Table 11-3. Hostility assessment

You can ask the patient to answer these three questions, by choosing from the responses *never, sometimes, often,* or *always.* Answers of *often* or *always* to two or more questions suggest a high level of hostility, which may indicate a higher risk of health problems.

1. When family members or even persons I don't know do things (or fail to do things) that hold me up or prevent me from doing something I want to do, I begin to think that they are selfish, mean, inconsiderate, and the like.

2. When strangers, friends, or members of my family do things that seem incompetent, messy, selfish, or inconsiderate, I quickly experience feelings of frustration, anger, irritation, and even rage. At the same time I become aware of these feelings, I notice unpleasant bodily sensations, like trouble getting enough breath, my heart pounding rapidly in my chest, my palms sweating, and the like.

3. When I have the thoughts, feelings, and bodily sensations just described, I am very likely to express my feelings in some way — by words, gestures, tone of voice, or facial expressions — to the other person or persons who I see as responsible for my unpleasant thoughts and feelings.

Source: Williams, RB. The trusting heart. New York: Times Books, 1989.

denial is itself a coping strategy, however unconscious, and can be of benefit to the patient in certain circumstances while problematic in others [140].

Some individuals referred by their physicians to the stress reduction clinic in our medical center intially deny or express strong doubts that stress plays a significant role in their medical complaints. Typically they enroll because of their physicians' recommendations, only to discover after a few weeks in the program that they now have a good deal of control over many of their symptoms that they thought were beyond their influence and control [141, 142]. Experiences of this kind can lead to greater understanding of the mind-body connection, increased feelings of confidence and self-esteem, and an enhanced willingness to admit to stress-related or emotional problems and to work with them more consciously and effectively.

Providers can use the following assessment strategies to determine psychosocial risk factors:

- Establish good rapport with the patient to the fullest extent possible. Be aware of your own feelings toward the patient and commit yourself to being fully present for the patient in an accepting, empathetic, and nonjudgmental mode. Cultivate moment-to-moment awareness during the encounter, observing nonverbal behaviors (your own and the patient's) as well as verbal content.

- During history taking look for indications of psychosocial risk factors and/or disturbances: cultural problems; recent life changes or disruptions/dislocations in the life of the patient or family; history of abuse, abusive behaviors, or both; drug abuse (prescription and/or recreational-street); family history of alcoholism; history of aggressive behaviors; and verbal and/or nonverbal indications of anger, hostility, low self-esteem, depression, or denial of feelings, both in the patient and in the patient's family members.

- In the context of the visit ask open-ended questions about the degree and causes of stress the patient feels and his feelings of being able to cope with it. The more details that are obtained the better: What does the patient find most stressful? Most difficult to cope with? What feelings are associated with these problems? Be on the lookout for denial of any problems or emotions, especially when you would expect the presenting situation to give rise to strong feelings.

- Determine level and patterns of affect (e.g., anger, depression) through simple questionnaires (see Table 11-2 and Table 11-3), direct observation of the patient's verbal and nonverbal behaviors (Table 11-1), direct inquiry when appropriate, and review of the patient's responses to the questionnaires.

- Assess the patient's level of confidence in her ability to make changes (self-efficacy). Confidence is generally based on one's past experiences of change. Is the patient self-motivated? Is there a history of mastery in her personal life, such as stopping smoking or drinking, losing weight, controlling temper outbursts, being assertive? What were the patient's reasons for attempting such changes in the past? Does the patient believe that she is capable of making changes or getting a handle on problem areas? Does she admire or wish to emulate someone who has made major changes? What are the impediments to assuming more control? Are they internal, external, or both? Is there an identifiable place to start? Can problem areas be prioritized by the patient? ("What is bothering you the most?") Can options be identified by the patient? ("What are some of your options?")

• Inquire about the social support structure in the individual's life: immediate family network, friends, social ties to local groups (e.g., church, civic groups, support groups). How much time is spent in this network? Does it function in a supportive and accepting way in the patient's daily experience? Is the patient able to ask for help within the support network?

Step 2: Treatment/Intervention

The physician needs to take an active role in helping patients alter psychosocial factors to prevent disease. The role can range from one that is minimal and requires little time to an intervention that is more intensive and comprehensive. These roles include (1) advising the patient of the need for change and providing information about the role of psychosocial factors and disease and ways to alter them; (2) counseling the patient to help her develop a plan for change; and/or (3) referring the patient to a specialist for individual or group help. A referral of this kind requires the physician to take a few minutes to ensure that the patient understands the reason for the referral and what to expect.

Providing Brief Advice and Information. Much of what people can do to decrease psychosocial risk for disease comes out of everyday living. As with dietary habits, smoking, and a sedentary lifestyle, it can begin with awareness of one's own behaviors. A necessary first step in intervention is to educate the patient about the need to decrease her psychosocial risk for illness and to provide her with some practical infor-

mation about how to do so. This might be done, for example, by simply informing her that intentional awareness of her behavior and of the quality of her relationships can bring about changes that might positively influence physical health as well as the quality of her life. Just as mindfulness can serve the physician in making a full and skillful assessment, it can also serve the patient in making changes in her life. Intentional awareness can be effective in modulating the tendency toward overt and covert hostility, while simultaneously fostering its opposite, what Williams [143] calls the "trusting heart," the qualities of which include affiliation, intimacy, affection, acceptance, and empathy. Cultivating such awareness may mean that people make sure they make time for their spouses, children, parents, and close friends in their lives. It may mean keeping in mind the importance (within culturally defined limits, of course) of moments of eye contact, gentle and mindful touching and hugging, and listening attentively to others without impatience or domination. The physician can actually make such behavioral suggestions when appropriate and reinforce them by inquiry during subsequent visits.

Awareness of behavior as simple as one's tone of voice can be particularly important within the family in reducing expressions of anger and hostility. If, as so often happens, an individual's own momentary anxiety produces a certain harshness, hurtfulness, and hostility in tone of voice or what is said, she can be made aware of it early on, as people would learn to do in a mindfulness-based stress reduction program. The person could then learn to intentionally observe or recall the immediate negative consequences of her behavior, both for her own body and state of mind and for the harmful effects it may have on her relationships with the people she is closest to and is loved by the most.

If the patient is socially isolated, the physician can suggest the importance of efforts to develop meaningful social bonds, which might include church groups, political groups, volunteering one's services to help others in need, or enrolling in classes. Often socially isolated people are depressed and need to be encouraged to reach out. They may also be alienated or seriously estranged from their spouses or other family members. Here, too, encouragement may be appropriate to take the initiative and reach out or to develop a range of options and strategies for coping with a chronically stressful life situation that is not likely to change in the short run. Recall that the psychological buffers to illness center around feelings of control and connectedness and the belief that one is capable of (has the innate resources for) growth and change, can see demands as challenges, can meet them with confidence and a commitment to daily living, and can make sense of things. Since low self-esteem is often present, the patient may need ongoing encouragement over an extended period of time, working slowly at attempts to make and/or deepen social connections. Referral to a group program, which would provide social contact while helping build a sense of self-efficacy and greater coherence and hardiness, can be an effective catalyst in such a process.

Having a pet can make a big difference for an otherwise socially isolated individual, and may reduce the health risks of isolation and bereavement. Pets can be an important and health enhancing way of bonding, touching, feeling connected, feeling needed, opening one's own heart to another, and having something to do each day [46, 143a]. A pet can help stabilize the emotional life of a person who is socially isolated and can also serve as a first step to reaching out and connecting with other people. Inquiring in some detail about a patient's pets and/or relationship to animals can be useful for assessing the level of affiliation and affectionate expression in a person's life.

Written materials can also educate patients and help them to expand their understanding and trust of their own bodies, to know the potential effects of stress, attitudes, emotions, and behaviors on health, and to help them to believe in and develop their inner and outer resources for improving their own health and for making lifestyle and attitudinal changes. Recommending books written for the lay public can be an excellent intervention in itself as well as an effective way for the physician to broach a difficult subject with a patient. The physician can then follow up in subsequent visits to see if the patient has read a particular book or part of it, how she felt about it, and so on. Reading material that is used to help patients make attitudinal behavioral changes related to health has been given the exalted name of *bibliotherapy*.

The books listed at the end of this chapter are written by physicians and other respected health professionals and authors. Several frame health problems and solutions in ways that physicians are not exposed to during medical training and can give the physician useful ideas about how to work more effectively with patients in the psychosocial domain.

Patient-Centered Counseling. Brief patient-centered counseling can be used by the physician who wants to and is able to go beyond 2 to 3 minutes of personalized advice and information giving. This step emphasizes the importance of the patient's input in developing an effective plan for change and can be accomplished using an additional 3 to 5 minutes of a physician's time (or however much is available). It is difficult in practice to separate the assessment step from the ongoing counseling/intervention process. If skillfully done, the assessment process becomes an important part of the treatment/intervention process. Typically counseling would continue with a further exploration of the patient's motivation, resources, strengths, problems, and past experiences in relation to the behavior or problem that has been targeted. By helping the patient become more aware of her own feelings or to articulate them when awareness is already present, the physician is in effect shifting from the assessment mode to a more facilitative role and can thus use the interview as a catalyst for positive changes in health attitudes and behaviors on the part of the patient. For the physician engaging in the counseling process, advice and information are embedded in the counseling sequence.

The counseling sequence, which includes a determination of strengths, resources, and needs, eventually should lead to a plan for change, no matter how small the goals. The plan can focus on simple and immediate goals, such as becoming more aware of a specific behavior, or on more complex goals with a longer-term end point, such as decreasing feelings of hostility. Finally the counseling sequence ends with an arrangement for follow-up. The message needs to be conveyed that this topic is important enough to talk about again.

Referring Patients for Assistance. It is likely that in many instances having identified psychosocial risk factors in a patient, the physician will not have the time or expertise to work with that patient around these problems, and it will be necessary to refer the patient for help. The most likely options are (1) individual counseling, (2) a group-oriented stress reduction and relaxation/lifestyle change program; and (3) a group-oriented support/education program that targets a specific illness or condition (e.g., AIDS, cancer, heart disease, ileostomy, COPD, chronic pain, panic disorder, alcoholism), a specific life problem (e.g., divorce, bereavement, being a relative of someone with alcoholism), or a specific behavior problem (e.g., addiction, hostility, type A behavior).

Group-based generic stress reduction clinics can be a good choice for the patient who is interested in learning self-regulatory approaches involving meditation, relaxation, and enhancement of coping skills. In our medical center such a clinic serves over 200 referring physicians each year. People are referred with a wide range of diagnoses, ranging from heart disease, cancer, and AIDS to hypertension, GI disorders, headache, chronic pain, functional somatic complaints (e.g., hyperventilation and palpitations), and other symptoms of anxiety and panic [141]. Symptom reduction, improved and healthier coping, increased self-esteem, and long-term health-related lifestyle changes are reported by the majority of patients independent of diagnosis [144, 145] and in spite of (or perhaps because of) the mix of patients with widely differing medical diagnoses [126, 141]. Referral to stress reduction and relaxation training can also help the patient develop greater awareness of mind and body and their interconnectedness; awareness, acceptance, and appropriate expres-

sion of emotional states; and greater understanding about stress and its physiological and psychological consequences.

Stress reduction clinics also help reduce social isolation because they are typically conducted in groups or classes. When based on training in consciousness disciplines [146] such as meditation and yoga (as in the Ornish study [122, 123, 124]), and in generically oriented stress reduction clinics [126, 141, 144], these interventions, rather than focusing on changing negative behaviors, promote the systematic exploration of positive behaviors and states of mind. Programs using this mind/body orientation based on training in meditation often catalyze a "rotation in consciousness" in the patient not typically achieved or even conceptualized by programs targeting specific problems or illnesses or by short-term individual therapy approaches, neither of which as a rule emphasizes intensive training in meditative awareness. This change in perspective derives from the direct experience in the meditation of calmness and interconnectedness, an experience that tends to positively influence one's view of one's body, of oneself as a person, and of oneself in relationship to the world. Recent theoretical work suggests a possible relationship between a person's inner self-representation and CHD risk factors [147].

Individual short-term counseling through an outpatient behavioral medicine clinic, a health psychology service, or outpatient psychiatry is an effective and appropriate choice if the individual is in an acute emotional crisis or is not interested in the intensity of a highly structured and demanding group program. Many patients find it beneficial to engage in both the group stress reduction and the individual counseling approaches simultaneously, while others may need to pursue them sequentially.

Group interventions that target specific problems rather than a general stress reduction approach are another option. These groups are likely to be a good choice for individuals who are facing an acute health or life crisis and who require immediate knowledge and insight about their specific problem or situation. Such programs can also provide essential social and emotional support for people in similar situations in times of crisis.

Psychiatric referrals are likely to be for clinical depression or other serious psychological disorders. Differentiating those individuals who need psychiatric care from those for whom a more educational and training-based approach would be preferable is necessary. Recent evidence suggests that the generic group stress reduction approach can be appropriate and effective with people suffering from DSM-III-R defined panic disorder and general anxiety disorder [148].

Preparation of the Patient for a Referral. When making a referral, the physician needs to be sure that the patient understands the reason for the referral and what to expect, and that the physician will continue to be involved in the patient's care. When patients are referred without adequate information and preparation, they often do not follow through with the referral.

Finding appropriate referral resources in your area can be the responsibility of someone else in your office. Although the task is initially time consuming, it is eventually very time-efficient to have a list available to give to patients on request. The following suggestions for finding appropriate resources may be helpful:
STRESS REDUCTION CLINICS. It is not always easy to find a stress reduction clinic in a specific location, particularly one that is based on training in meditative awareness. However, such programs are rapidly increasing in number. Inquiries should be directed first to local hospitals, then to community groups. Often so-called holistic health centers offer programs in stress reduction, relaxation, meditation, and yoga. Although the quality may vary greatly, many of the well-known and larger centers offer excellent programs. Meditation centers of various kinds also exist in many communities and can be a good starting point for particular patients who are open to such approaches, which may be based in non-Western cultures and traditions and not necessarily framed in a health context.
OUT-PATIENT BEHAVIORAL MEDICINE CLINICS. Many hospitals now offer behavioral counseling for health promotion, risk factor reduction, and

health attitude and behavior change. Usually these clinics offer short-term, individual counseling. Sometimes they use a group format. Such clinics may offer stress reduction classes, as well as other forms of group and individual counseling on psychosocial factors in health and illness. Inquire of local hospitals for such programs and also in the community for therapists who do this work in a private practice setting. Such people often advertise in the Yellow Pages.
SUPPORT GROUPS FOR SPECIFIC PROBLEMS OR ILLNESSES. Consult local hospitals for their programs and the Yellow Pages for community groups. Local voluntary organizations such as the American Heart Association (AHA), the American Lung Association (ALA), and the American Cancer Society (ACS) may also provide information and resources.

STEP 3: PLAN FOR CHANGE

The counseling interaction should always end with a plan that has been mindfully negotiated between the physician and the patient. A referral for specialized attention or more time-consuming ongoing support is likely to be necessary for the patient with more than moderate psychosocial risk and distress; it is unlikely that the physician has the time, desire, and in many instances the skill to provide this attention or support. The choice of referral options depends, of course, on the specifics of the assessment and the needs and desires of the patient. Any approach offered to the patient must speak effectively to the patient's particular pain, specific needs and beliefs.

A plan for change should also include information on how the patient will know whether she has achieved her goal. It is important to establish realistic, achievable goals.

STEP 4: FOLLOW-UP/MONITORING

Follow-up of any psychosocial intervention is needed to help reinforce and deepen newly acquired attitudes and behaviors and to provide continued support for growth and change. Follow-up can occur in the form of a letter, a telephone call, or an in-person visit. The type of follow-up depends on the time constraints and the needs of the patient and the physician. If the message is that psychosocial risk factors are important, then some follow-up is imperative. If the patient has been referred to a specialist or a group program, then optimally there must be communication between the specialist and the physician. The physician should make this known to programs or consultants who do not provide such feedback. It is also helpful if the physician has a system that allows such feedback to be logged in the patient's record so it can be available at the next encounter.

It is a good idea to contract with the patient to review the intervention program when it is over, with the intention of determining its value and deciding on future therapeutic options. The physician needs to reinforce the ongoing work that the patient will be doing in the program. If possible, the physician should be familiar with the program: the more the physician speaks to the patient in terms of direct experience and knowledge, the more realistic any suggestions and recommendations will be. A physician's referral of a patient for education, training, and group support, when such a referral is appropriate and understood by the patient, can be a powerful catalyst for growth and behavior change.

The physician may wish to use the following summary of strategies as a guide in the treatment/intervention and follow-up of patients to facilitate psychosocial growth and change.

- On the basis of the assessment and your knowledge of the patient begin a formulation in your own mind of possible first steps (i.e., a preliminary plan) that might be offered to the patient. Evaluate areas where the patient is lacking in awareness and knowledge, and where improvement might help in making important changes.
- At the very least advise the patient of the need to alter psychosocial risk factors and provide information helpful in achieving this goal.
- Ask the patient which options she believes to be available and appropriate. Review the pluses and minuses of each. What are her expectations of treatment? If they do not seem appropriate or inclusive enough, propose additional options, which can include specific books to read; a contract to attempt one simple behavior change between now and the next visit (e.g., calling up a friend the patient hasn't talked to in a long time or being more aware of times and circumstances of impatience, anger, hostility, and anxiety); enrolling in a stress reduction program or an appropriate behavior modification or support program; or seeing a counselor, therapist, psychiatrist, or social worker for further evaluation, individual problem solving, symptom regulation, and/or social services assistance.

- Many people do not want help or even advice in the psychosocial domain. They may interpret your efforts as implying that they are not handling things in their lives as well as they might. They may also doubt that stress, isolation, or emotional patterns could play a role in their health problems or put them at risk for future illness. In such cases discussion of such topics as thoughts, feelings, emotions, stress, life changes, and their relation to health should be seen as planting seeds. When appropriate, reminders or suggestions, made gently but consistently over an extended period, can lead to a gradual change in attitude on the part of the patient, especially if circumstances change and he finds his health worsening or life stress becoming harder to cope with effectively. Eventually this may lead to actual behavioral changes.
- When referring the patient to a stress reduction program, or to a behavior modification program oriented toward a specific issue such as hostility or type A behavior, make sure the patient understands the rationale for the referral, the level of personal commitment and effort required, the concept that she can do something for herself as a complement to whatever medicine can do for her, and your intention to review the outcomes with her.
- Keep in mind that you are working on a public health level as well as on the individual level. Every person that you can influence to move toward greater health through her own efforts and commitment to awareness and change may eventually influence others through the

sharing of her experiences and through modeling new behaviors. We have found that many patients who are changed by their experiences in the stress reduction clinic often influence their relatives and friends to enroll as well, as they observe positive changes in a person they know and respect. Not everybody in need of change is ready or willing to face and work with their own psychosocial factors to improve their health. Over time the physician who is aware of the importance of this domain for health and illness and who has developed some skill in counseling and triaging patients to appropriate psychosocial services can influence many individuals, as well as contribute to an overall movement of the entire population toward greater awareness and health.

Summary

This chapter has reviewed the major psychosocial factors that affect CHD and the importance of the physician's role in helping the patient to modify those factors. The physician interested in prevention should not focus on CHD risk to the exclusion of other medical disorders, which may also be preventable or reduced in severity by attending to psychosocial factors. The approach advocated here calls for the physician to assess and then actively advise and/or counsel patients to make behavioral changes that prevent illness, allow the individual to cope more effectively with stress, and promote health in general. Having determined via psychosocial assessment that a patient has a high degree of life stress, social isolation, hostility and anger, or trouble expressing feelings, the physician can initiate appropriate intervention and referral. Many of the changes physicians want for their patients might best be initiated and reinforced by recommending participation in mind/body-oriented group stress reduction and relaxation programs, if they are available, as well as through individual health behavior counseling, behavioral medicine clinics targeting behavior modification, and/or various support groups targeting specific social situations (isolation, bereavement) or illnesses

(AIDS, heart disease, cancer, COPD). These referral resources have skills and time beyond that which can be expected of physicians delivering medical care. They are specifically structured to give the patient guidance, support, and tools for accomplishing positive psychosocial change.

Nevertheless, physicians can play a major, in fact, a crucial role in this process by advocating, initiating, and catalyzing health-enhancing psychosocial change in the context of the medical encounter itself. This is best accomplished by brief, skillful, and mindful communication with the patient. Whether the physician continues the intervention process himself or refers the patient to specialized programs, continued physician inquiry as patients try to take responsibility for changing those aspects of their lives that only they are in a position to change is a necessary element in supporting the patients in their efforts. The physician with good communication skills and knowledge of the role of psychosocial factors in health and disease can have a profound impact on the health of his patients, an impact that ultimately changes not only the lifestyles of individuals but of our society as a whole.

Suggested Readings for Patients and Providers

Borysenko, Joan. *Minding the Body, Mending the Mind*. New York: Bantam Books, 1987.

Borysenko, Joan. *Guilt is the Teacher, Love is the Lesson*. New York: Warner, 1990.

Chopra, Deepak. *Unconditional Life*. New York: Bantam Books, 1991.

Cousins, Norman. *Head First: The Biology of Hope*. New York: W. W. Norton, 1989.

Cousins, Norman. *The Healing Heart*. New York: W. W. Norton, 1983.

Eliot, Robert, and Breo, Dennis. *Is It Worth Dying For?* New York: Bantam Books, 1987.

Goleman, D. and Gurin, J. (eds.) *Healing and the Mind*, Consumer Reports Books, Yonkers, N.Y., 1992.

Hahn, Thich Nhat. *The Miracle of Mindfulness: A Manual of Meditation*. Boston: Beacon Press, 1976.

Kabat-Zinn, Jon. *Full Catastrophe Living: Using the Wisdom of Your Body and Mind to Face Stress, Pain and Illness*. New York: Delacorte/Dell, 1990.

Locke, Steven, and Colligan, Douglas. *The Healer Within*. New York: Dutton, 1986.

Lynch, James. *The Broken Heart, The Medical Consequences of Loneliness*. New York: Basic Books, 1977.

Lynch, James. *The Language of the Heart*. New York: Basic Books, 1985.

Ornish, Dean. *Stress, Diet and Your Heart*. New York: Holt, Rinehart and Winston, 1983.

Ornish, Dean. *Dr. Dean Ornish's Program for the Reversal of Heart Disease*. New York: Random House, 1990.

Seligman, Martin F. P. *Learned Optimism*. New York: Simon & Schuster, 1991.

Williams, Redford. *The Trusting Heart: Great News About Type A Behavior*. New York: Times Books, 1989.

References

1. Keys A, Aravanis C, Blackburn H, et al. Probability of middle-aged men developing coronary heart disease in five years. Circulation 1972; 45:815–28.

2. Gordon T, Kannel WB. Multiple risk functions for predicting coronary heart disease: the concept, accuracy, and application. Am Heart J 1982; 103:1031–9.

3. Lown B, DeSilva RA, Reich P, Murawski BJ. Psychophysiologic factors in sudden cardiac death. Am J Psychiatry 1980; 137:1325–35.

4. Kitagawa EM, Hauser P. Differential mortality in the United States: a study in socioeconomic epidemiology. Cambridge: Harvard University Press, 1973.

5. Syme SL. Sociocultural factors and disease etiology. In: Gentry WD, ed. Handbook of behavioral medicine. New York: Guilford, 1984.

6. Dohrenwend BS, Dohrenwend BP, eds. Stressful life events: their nature and effects. New York: Wiley, 1974.

7. Jenkins CD. The coronary-prone personality. In: Gentry WD, Williams RD, eds. Psychological aspects of myocardial infarction and coronary care. St. Louis: Mosby, 1975; 5–23.

8. Cannon WB. Emergency function of the adrenal medulla in pain and the major emotions. Am J Physiol 1914; 33:356–72; also see Cannon WB. The wisdom of the body. 2nd ed. New York: Norton, 1939.

9. Selye H. The general adaptation syndrome and the diseases of adaptation. J Clin Endocrinol 1946; 6:117–230; also see Selye H. The stress of life. Rev. ed. New York: McGraw-Hill, 1976.

10. Elliott GR, Eisdorfer C. Stress and human health. New York: Springer, 1982; 11.

11. Lazarus RS, Folkman S. Stress, appraisal, and coping. New York: Springer, 1984; 12.

12. Keys AB. Seven countries: a multivariate analysis of death and coronary artery disease. Cambridge: Harvard University Press, 1980.

13. Gordon T. Further mortality experience among Japanese–Americans. Public Health Rep 1967; 82:973–84.

14. Marmot MG, Syme SL, Kagan A, et al. Epidemiologic studies of coronary heart disease and stroke in Japanese men living in Japan, Hawaii and California: prevalence of coronary and hypertensive heart disease and associated risk factors. Am J Epidemiol 1975; 102:514–25.

15. Marmot MG, Syme SL. Acculturation and coronary heart disease in Japanese-Americans. Am J Epidemiol 1976; 104:225–47.

16. Williams RB. The trusting heart. New York: Times Books, 1989; 159.

17. Bruhn JG. An epidemiological study of myocardial infarctions in an Italian-American community: a preliminary study. J Chron Dis 1965; 18:353–65.

18. Bruhn JG, Chandler B, Miller MC, et al. Social aspects of coronary heart disease in two adjacent, ethnically different communities. Am J Public Health 1966; 56:1493–506.

19. Keys A. Arteriosclerotic heart disease in Roseto, Pennsylvania. JAMA 1966; 195:137–9.

20. Keys A. Arteriosclerotic heart disease in a favored community. J Chron Dis 1966; 19:245–54.

21. Stout C, Morrow J, Brandt EN, Wolf S. Unusually low incidence of death from myocardial infarction: study of an Italian-American community in Pennsylvania. JAMA 1964; 188:845–9.

22. Henry JP and Stephens PM. Stress, health and the social environment. New York: Springer, 1977; 191.

23. Bianco C. The two Rosetos. Bloomington: Indiana University Press, 1974.

24. Wolf S. Protective social forces that counterbalance stress. J SC Medical Assoc 1976; 72:57–9.

25. Wolf S, Grace KL, Bruhn J, et al. Roseto revisited: further data on the incidence of myocardial infarction in Roseto and neighboring Pennsylvania communities. Trans Am Clin Climatol Assoc 1973; 85:100–8.

26. Wolf S, Herrenkohl RC, Lasker J, et al. Roseto, Pennsylvania 25 years later — highlights of a medical and sociological survey. Trans Am Clin Climatol Assoc 1988; 100:57–67.

27. Berkman LF, Syme SL. Social networks, host resistance, and mortality: a nine-year follow-up study of Alameda County residents. Am J Epidemiol 1979; 109:186–204.

28. House JS, Landis KR, Umberson D. Social relationships and health. Science 1988; 241:540–5.

29. Schoenbach VJ, Kaplan BH, Fredman L, Klein-

baum DG. Social ties and mortality in Evans County, Georgia. Am J Epidemiol 1986; 123:577–91.

30. Eliot RS. Stress and the heart: mechanisms, measurements, and management. Mount Kisco, NY: Futura, 1988; 23.

31. Leren P, Helgeland A, Hjermann I, Holme I. The Oslo Study: CHD risk factors, socioeconomic influences, and intervention. Am Heart J 1983; 106:1200–6.

32. Eliot. Stress and the heart. P. 26.

33. Harburg E, Schull WJ, Erfurt JC, Schork MA. A family set method for estimating heredity and stress. I. A pilot survey of blood pressure among Negroes in high and low stress areas, Detroit, 1966–1967. J Chronic Dis 1970; 23:69–81.

34. Scotch N. A preliminary report on the relation of socio-cultural factors to hypertension among the Zulu. Ann NY Acad Sci 1960; 84:1000–9.

35. Scotch N, Campel B, Abramson JH, Slome C. Blood pressure measurements of urban Zulu adults. Amer Heart J 1961; 61:173–7.

36. Campel B, Slome C, Scotch N, Abramson JH. Urbanization and hypertension among Zulu adults. J Chronic Dis 1962; 15:67–70.

36a. Poulter NR, Khaw KT, Hopwood BE, et al. The Kenyan Luo migration study: observations on the initiation of a rise in blood pressure. Br Med J 1990; 300:967–72.

36b. Zevallos J, Ockene IS, Callay S, et al. The impact of urbanization on cardiovascular risk factors in an indigenous population of the highlands of Ecuador. Circulation 1991; 84:II-118 (abstract).

37. McLean, AA. Work stress. Reading, MA: Addison-Wesley, 1979.

38. Eliot. Stress and the heart. P. 27.

39. Kobasa SC. Stressful life events, personality, and health: an inquiry into hardiness. J Personal Soc Psychol 1979; 37:1–11.

40. Seeman M, Seeman TA. Health behavior and personal autonomy: a longitudinal study of the sense of control in illness. J Health Social Behav 1983; 24:144–60.

41. Karasek RA, Baker D, Marxer F, et al. Job decision latitude, job demands, and cardiovascular disease: a prospective study of Swedish men. Am J Public Health 1981; 71:694–705.

42. Karasek RA, Theorell T, Schwartz JE, et al. Job characteristics in relation to the prevalence of myocardial infarction in the US Health Examination Survey (HES) and the Health and Nutrition Examination Survey (HANES). Am J Public Health 1988; 78:910–18.

43. Clarkson TB. Personality, gender, and coronary artery atherosclerosis in monkeys. Arteriosclerosis 1987; 7:1–8.

43a. Kaplan JR, Manuck SB, Clarkson TB, et al. Social stress and atherosclerosis in normocholesterolemic monkeys. Science 1983; 220:733–5.

43b. Adams MR, Kaplan JR, Clarkson TB, Kovitnik DR. Ovariectomy, social status, and atherosclerosis in cynomolgus monkeys. Arteriosclerosis 1985; 5:192–200.

43c. Williams JK, Vita JA, Manuck SB, et al. Psychosocial factors impair vascular responses of coronary arteries. Circulation 1991; 84:2146–53.

43d. Dimsdale JE. A new mechanism linking stress to coronary pathophysiology? Circulation 1991; 84:2201–2.

44. Weber HW, Van der Walt JJ. Cardiomyopathy in crowded rabbits: a preliminary report. S Afr Med J 1973; 47:1591–5.

45. Nerem RM, Levesque MJ, Cornhill JF. Social environment as a factor in diet-induced aortic atherosclerosis in rabbits. Science 1980; 208:1475–6.

46. Lynch JJ. The broken heart: the medical consequences of loneliness. New York: Basic Books, 1977; 167–80.

47. Schanberg SM, Field TM. Sensory deprivation stress and supplemented stimulation in the rat pup and preterm human neonate. Child Development 1987; 58:1431–47.

48. Williams. The trusting heart. P. 112.

49. Weiss JM. Behavioral and psychological influences on gastrointestinal pathology: experimental techniques and findings. In: Gentry WD, ed. Handbook of behavioral medicine. New York: Guilford, 1984; 174–221.

50. Corley KC. Stress and cardiomyopathy. In: Smith OA, Galosy RA, Weiss SM, eds. Circulation, neurobiology and behavior. New York: Elsevier, 1982: 121–34.

51. Friedman M, Rosenman RH. Type A behavior and your heart. New York: Knopf, 1974.

52. Rosenman RH. The interview method of assessment of the coronary-prone behavior pattern. In: Dembroski TM, Weiss SM, Shields, JL, et al., eds. Coronary-prone behavior. New York: Springer, 1978; 55–70.

53. Jenkins CD, Rosenman RH, Friedman M. Development of an objective pscyhological test for the determination of the coronary-prone behavior pattern in employed men. J Chronic Dis 1967; 20:371–9.

54. Rosenman RH, Friedman M, Straus M, et al. A predictive study of coronary heart disease: the Western Collaborative Group Study. JAMA 1964; 189:15–22.

55. Rosenman RH, Brand RJ, Jenkins CD, et al. Coronary heart disease in the Western Collaborative Group Study: final follow-up ex-

perience of 8.5 years. JAMA 1975; 233:872–7.

56. Blumenthal JA, Williams RB, Kong Y, et al. Type A behavior pattern and atherosclerosis. Circulation 1978; 58:634–9.

57. Frank KA, Heller SS, Kornfeld DS, et al. Type A behavior pattern and coronary angiographic findings. JAMA 1978; 240:761–3.

58. Zyzanski SJ, Jenkins CD, Ryan TJ, et al. Psychological correlates of coronary angiographic findings. Arch Int Med 1978; 136:1234–7.

59. Review Panel on Coronary-Prone Behavior and Coronary Heart Disease. A critical review. Circulation 1981; 63:1199–215.

60. Shekelle RB, Hulley S, Neaton J, et al. The MRFIT behavior pattern study. II. Type A behavior pattern and incidence of coronary heart disease. Am J Epidemiol 1985; 122:559–70.

61. Shekelle RB, Gale M, Norusis M. Type A behavior (Jenkins Activity Survey) and risk of recurrent coronary heart disease in the Aspirin Myocardial Infarction Study. Am J Cardiol 1985; 56:221–5.

62. Ragland DR, Brand RJ. Coronary heart disease mortality in the Western Collaborative Group Study. Am J Epidemiol 1988; 127:462–75.

63. Matthews A, Haynes SG. Type A behavior pattern and coronary risk: update and critical evaluation. Am J Epidemiol 1986; 123:923–60.

64. Williams RB, Haney TL, Lee KL, et al. Type A behavior, hostility, and coronary atherosclerosis. Psychosom Med 1980; 42:539–49.

65. Cook W, Medley D. Proposed hostility and pharaisaic-virtue scales for the MMPI. J Applied Psychol 1954; 38:414–8.

66. Shekelle RB, Gale M, Ostfeld AM, Paul O. Hostility, risk of coronary disease, and mortality. Psychosom Med 1983; 45:109–14.

67. Williams RB, Barefoot JC, Shekelle RB. The health consequences of hostility. In: Chesney MA, Rosenman RH, eds. Anger and hostility in cardiovascular and behavioral disorders. Washington, DC: Hemisphere, 1985; 173–85.

68. Barefoot JC, Dahlstrom WG, Williams RB. Hostility, CHD incidence, and total mortality: a 25-year follow-up study of 255 physicians. Psychosom Med 1983; 45:59–63.

69. Williams. The trusting heart. Pp. 56, 216.

70. Barefoot JC, Dodge KA, Peterson BL, et al. The Cook-Medley hostility scale: item content and ability to predict survival. Psychosom Med 1989; 51:46–57.

71. Williams. The trusting heart. P. 69.

72. Dembroski TM, MacDougall JM, Costa PT, Grandits GA. Components of hostility as predictors of sudden death and myocardial infarction in the Multiple Risk Factor Intervention Trial. Psychosom Med 1989; 514–22.

73. Costa, PT Jr. Influence of the normal personality dimension of neuroticism on chest pain symptoms and coronary artery disease. Am J Cardiol 1987; 60:26–8.

74. Spielberger CD, Johnson EH, Russell SF, et al. The experience and expression of anger: construction and validation of an anger expression scale. In: Chesney MS, Rosenman RH, eds. Anger and hostility in cardiovascular and behavioral disorders. Washington, DC: Hemishere, 1985; 5–30.

75. Harburg E, Erfurt JC, Hauenstein LS, et al. Socio-ecological stress, suppressed hostility, skin color, and black-white male blood pressure: Detroit. Psychosom Med 1973; 35:276–96.

76. Harburg E, Blakelock EH, Roeper PJ. Resentful and reflective coping with arbitrary authority and blood pressure: Detroit. Psychosom Med 1979; 41:189–202.

77. Gentry WD, Chesney AP, Gary HE, et al. Habitual anger-coping styles. I. Effect on mean blood pressure and risk for essential hypertension. Psychosom Med 1982; 44:195–202.

78. Dembroski TM, MacDougall JM, Williams RB, et al. Components of type A, hostility, and anger-in: relationship to angiographic findings. Psychosom Med 1985; 47:219–33.

79. Russek LG, King SH, Russek SJ, Russek HI. The Harvard Mastery of Stress Study 35-year follow-up: prognostic significance of psychological arousal and adaptation. Psychosom Med 1990; 52:271–85.

80. Powell LH, Simon SR, Bartzokis T, et al. Emotional arousal predicts sudden cardiac death in post-MI men. Paper presented at the 31st Annual Conference on Cardiovascular Disease Epidemiology. Orlando, March 14–16, 1991.

81. Chesney MA, Ekman P, Friesen WV, et al. Type A behavior pattern: facial behavior and speech components. Psychosom Med 1990; 53:307–19.

82. Orth-Gomer K, Unden AL. Type A behavior, social support, and coronary risk: interaction and significance for mortality in cardiac patients. Psychosom Med 1990; 52:59–72.

83. Grossarth-Maticek R, Bastiaans J, Kanazir DT. Psychosocial factors as strong predictors of mortality from cancer, ischemic heart disease and stroke: the Yugoslav prospective study. J Psychosom Res 1985; 29:167–76.

84. Grossarth-Maticek R, Kanazir DT, Schmit P, Vetter, H. Psychosocial and organic variables as predictors of lung cancer, cardiac infarct and apoplexy: some differential predictors. Personal and Individ Diff 1985; 6:313–21.

85. Spielberger CD, van der Ploeg HM. Psychological and personality risk factors for cancer: a

re-analysis of the Grossarth-Maticek Yugoslav epidemiological studies. Paper presented at the 2nd National Conference on the Psychology of Health, Immunity and Disease. Orlando, Dec. 5, 1990; and Spielberger CD, personal communication to Jon Kabat-Zinn, May 1, 1991.

86. Kobasa SC. Stressful life events, personality, and health: an inquiry into hardiness. J Personal Social Psychol 1979; 37:1–11.

87. Kobasa SC, Maddi SR, Kahn S. Hardiness and health: a prospective study. J. Personal Social Psychol 1982; 42:168–77.

88. Antonovsky A. Unraveling the mystery of health. San Francisco: Jossey-Bass, 1987.

89. Bandura, A. Self-efficacy mechanism in human agency. Am Psychologist 1982; 37:122–47.

90. Bandura A, Damas NE, Byer J. Cognitive processes mediating behavioral change. J Personal and Social Psychol 1977; 35:125–39.

91. Peterson C, Seligman MEP. Explanatory style and illness. J Pers 1987; 55:237–65.

92. McClelland DC, Jemmott JB. Power motivation, stress, and physical illness. J. Human Stress 1980; 6:6–15.

93. Henry JP, Stephens PM. Stress, health, and the social environment. New York: Springer, 1977; 118–88.

94. Eliot RS, Buell JC. The heart and its relationship to emotional stress and environmental factors. In: Hurst JW, ed.-in-chief. The heart. 5th ed. New York: McGraw-Hill, 1982; 1637–49.

95. Manuck SB, Krantz DS. Psychophysiologic reactivity in coronary heart disease and essential hypertension. In: Matthews KA, Weiss SM, Detre T, et al., eds. Handbook of stress, reactivity, and cardiovascular disease. New York: Wiley, 1986; 16.

96. Matthews KA, Weiss SM, Detre T, et al., eds. Handbook of stress, reactivity, and cardiovascular disease. New York: Wiley, 1986.

97. Clarkson TB, Kaplan JR, Adams MR, Manuck SB. Psychosocial influences on the pathogenesis of atherosclerosis among nonhuman primates. Circulation 1987; 76:I29–40.

98. Manuck SB, Kaplan JR, Clarkson TB. Behaviorally-induced heart rate reactivity and atherosclerosis in cynomolgus monkeys. Psychosom Med 1983; 45:95–108.

99. Keys A, Taylor HL, Blackburn H, et al. Mortality and coronary heart disease among men studied for 23 years. Arch Intern Med 1971; 128:201–14.

100. Eliot RS, Long DR, Boone JL. Stress, health and physical evaluation: the Shape Program. In: Eliot RS. Stress and the heart: mechanisms, measurements, and management. Mount Kisco, NY: Futura, 1988; 66.

101. Corley C, Mauck HP, Shiel FOM. Cardiac responses associated with "yoked-chair" shock avoidance in squirrel monkeys. Psychophysiol 1975; 12:439–44.

102. Mason JW, Maher JT, Hartley LH, et al. Selectivity of corticosteroid and catecholamine responses to various natural stimuli. In: Serban G, ed. Psychopathology of human adaptation. New York: Plenum, 1976; 147–51.

103. Houston BK. Psychophysiological reactivity and the type A behavior pattern. J Res Personal 1983; 17:22–9.

104. Krantz DS, Manuck SB. Acute psychological reactivity and the risk of cardiovascular disease: a review and methodologic critique. Psychol Bull 1984; 96:435–64.

105. Williams RB. Biological mechanisms mediating the relationship between behavior and coronary heart disease. In: Siegman A, Dembroski TM, eds. In search of coronary prone behavior. Hillsdale, NJ: Lawrence Earlbaum, 1988; 195–205.

106. Matthews KA, Weiss SM, Detre T, et al. eds. Handbook of stress, reactivity, and cardiovascular disease. New York: Wiley, 1986.

107. Williams. The trusting heart. P. 92.

108. Williams RB, Lane JD, Kuhn CM, et al. Type A behavior and elevated physiological and neuroendocrine responses to cognitive tasks. Science 1982; 218:483–5.

109. Suarez EC, Williams RB. Situational determinants of cardiovascular and emotional reactivity in high and low hostile men. Psychosom Med 1989; 51:404–18.

109a. Williams. The trusting heart. P. 107.

110. Williams. The trusting heart. P. 89.

111. Zumoff B, Rosenfield RS, Friedman M, et al. Elevated day-time urinary excretion of testosterone glucuronide in men with the type A behavior pattern. Psychosom Med 1984; 46:223–6.

112. Spraque EA, Troxler RG, Peterson DF, et al. Effect of cortisol on the development of atherosclerosis in cynomolgus monkeys. In: Kalter SS, ed. The use of nonhuman primates in cardiovascular diseases. Austin: University of Texas Press, 1980.

113. Uzunova AD, Ramey ER, Ramwell PW. Gonadal hormones and pathogenesis of occlusive arterial thrombosis. Am J Physiol 1978; 234:454–9.

114. Frank C, Smith S. Stress and the heart: biobehavioral aspects of sudden cardiac death. Psychosomatics 1990; 31:255–64.

115. Powell LH, Simon SR, Bartzokis T, et al. Emotional arousability predicts sudden cardiac deaths in post-MI men (abstract). Circulation 1991; 83:722.

116. Thomas CB. Cancer and the youthful mind:

a forty-year perspective. Advances 1988; 5:42–58.

117. Williams RB, Barefoot JC, Shekelle RB. The health consequences of hostility. In: Chesney MA, Rosenman RH, eds. Anger and hostility in cardiovascular and behavioral disorders. Washington, DC: Hemisphere, 1985; 183.

118. Friedman M, Thoresen CE, Gill JJ, et al. Alteration of type A behavior and its effect on cardiac recurrences in post-myocardial infarction patients: summary results of the Recurrent Coronary Prevention Project. Am Heart J 1986; 112:653–65.

119. Powell LH, Thoresen CE. Modifying the type A behavior pattern: a small group treatment approach. In: Blumenthal JA, McKee DM, eds. Applications in behavioral medicine: a clinician's sourcebook. Vol. 1. Sarasota, FL: Professional Resource Exchange, Inc. 1987; 171–207.

120. Gill JJ, Price VA, Friedman M, et al. Reduction in type A behavior in healthy middle-aged American military officers. Am Heart J 1985; 110:503–14.

121. Seraganian P, Oseasohn R, et al. The Montreal Type A Intervention Project: Major Findings. Health Psychol 1986; 5:45–69.

122. Ornish D, Brown SE, Scherwitz LW, et al. Can lifestyle changes reverse coronary heart disease? The lifestyle heart trial. Lancet 1990; 336:129–33.

123. Scherwitz L, Ornish DM, Sparler S, Brown S. Effects of lifestyle changes on psychosocial factors in the San Francisco Lifestyle Heart Trial. Submitted to Psychosom Med.

124. Ornish DM. Dr. Dean Ornish's program for reversing heart disease. New York: Random House, 1990.

124a. Shapiro DH and Walsh RW (eds.) Meditation: contemporary and classical perspectives. New York: Aldine, 1984.

124b. Murphy M and Donovan S. The physical and psychological effects of meditation: a review of contemporary meditation research with a comprehensive bibliography 1931–1988. San Rafael, Esalen Institute, 1988.

125. Benson H. The relaxation response. New York: Morrow, 1975.

126. Kabat-Zinn J. Full catastrophe living: using the wisdom of your body and mind to face stress, pain, and illness. New York: Delacorte, 1990.

127. Engel GL. The need for a new medical model: a challenge for biomedicine. Science 1977; 196:129–36.

128. Engel GL. The clinical application of the biopsychosocial model. J Med and Philosophy 1981; 6:101–23.

129. Brody DS, Miller SM, Lerman CE, et al. The relationship between patients' satisfaction with their physicians and perceptions about interventions they desired and received. Medical Care 1989; 27:1027–35.

130. DeMatteo MR, Prince LM, Taranta A. Patients' perceptions of physicians' behavior: determinants of patient commitment to the therapeutic relationship. J Commun Health 1979; 4:280–90.

131. Eisenthal S, Koopman C, Lazare A. Process analysis of two dimensions of the negotiated approach in relation to satisfaction in the initial interview. J Nerv Ment Dis 1983; 171:49–54.

132. Buller MK, Buller DB. Physicians' communication style and patient satisfaction. J Health Soc Behav 1987; 28:375–88.

133. Brody DS, Lerman CE, Wolfson HG, Caputo GC. Improvement in physicians' counseling of patients with mental health problems. Arch Int Med 1990; 150:993–8.

134. Nixon PGF. Human functions and the heart. In: Seedhouse D, Cribb A, eds. Changing ideas in health care. Chichester, NY: Wiley & Sons, Ltd, 1989; 31–65.

135. Hackett TP, Cassem NH. Psychological management of the myocardial infarction patient. J Human Stress 1975; 1:25–38.

136. Greer S, Morris T. Psychological attributes of women who develop breast cancer: a controlled study. J Psychosom Res 1975; 19:147–53.

137. Morris T, Greer S, Pettingale KW, Watson M. Patterns of expression of anger and their psychological correlates in women with breast cancer. J Psychosom Res 1981; 25:111–7.

138. Kneier A, Temoshok L. Repressive coping reactions in patients with malignant melanoma as compared to cardiovascular patients. J Psychosom Res 1984; 28:145–55.

139. Marlatt GA, Gordon JR, eds. Relapse prevention: maintenance strategies in the treatment of addictive behaviors. New York: Guilford, 1985.

140. Lazarus RS, Folkman S. Stress, appraisal, and coping. New York: Springer, 1984; 134–8.

141. Kabat-Zinn J, Chapman-Waldrop A. Compliance with an outpatient stress reduction program: rates and predictors of completion. J Behav Med 1988; 11:333–52.

142. Kabat-Zinn J, Lipworth L, Burney R, Sellers W. Four year follow-up of a meditation-based program for the self-regulation of chronic pain: treatment outcomes and compliance. Clin J Pain 1986; 2:159–73.

143. Williams. The trusting heart.

143a. Wilson CC. The pet as an anxiolytic intervention. J Nerv Ment Dis 1991; 179:482–9.

144. Kabat-Zinn J, Lipworth L, Burney R. The clinical use of mindfulness meditation for the self-regulation of chronic pain. J Behav Med 1985; 8:163–90.

145. Kabat-Zinn J. Symptom reduction in medical patients following stress reduction training: outcome, reproducibility and two-year follow-up. Unpublished manuscript.

146. Walsh RN. The consciousness disciplines and the behavioral sciences: questions of comparison and assessment. Am J Psychiat 1980; 137:663–73.

147. Scherwitz L, Pavone R. Society, self and the soma: a theoretical framework and review of self-processes and coronary heart disease risk factors. Unpublished manuscript.

148. Kabat-Zinn J, Massion A, Kristeller J, et al. Effectiveness of a meditation-based stress reduction intervention in the treatment of anxiety disorders. Am J Psychiatry 1992; 149. In press.

12

Pharmacologic Management of Dyslipidemias

DANIEL CARLUCCI
IRA S. OCKENE

EDITORS' INTRODUCTION

Many patients with abnormal lipid profiles can be managed by diet intervention alone, and it is our belief that physician counseling and appropriate referral to dietitians will minimize the number of patients who require pharmacologic therapy. Nonetheless, drug therapy is needed for those individuals for whom dietary therapy alone is inadequate. Using such therapy appropriately requires a sound working knowledge of the pharmacology of the available agents: their indications and contraindications, potential side effects and toxicities, and the manner in which multiple agents can augment each other's effects. This chapter provides that necessary information and also covers two other topics of interest: the use of marine oils for the modification of CHD risk and the cost of using pharmacologic therapy to modify lipids.

The appropriate treatment of hyperlipidemia depends on many factors. Preexisting CHD, the presence of cardiac risk factors, age, sex, diet, medications, and lipid profile are some of the parameters that must be assessed to make an informed treatment decision. The National Cholesterol Education Program (NCEP) Expert Panel has developed a widely accepted stepped-care approach to the treatment of high blood cholesterol levels in adults 20 years of age and over [1]. (See Chapter 9 for a discussion of the NCEP guidelines.) Although dietary change is the mainstay of the initial treatment of hyperlipidemia, lipid goals are not always attained by diet alone and pharmacologic measures are then indicated.

The patient population targeted by NCEP for the initiation of pharmacologic intervention includes those who have undergone six months of intensive dietary therapy and counseling and whose LDL cholesterol level remains either at 190 mg/dl or higher without definite CHD or two or more risk factors for CHD or at 160 mg/dl or higher with definite CHD or with two or more CHD risk factors (Table 12-1) [1]. In all cases clinical judgment should be used in con-

junction with these guidelines. Drug therapy may, in fact, be indicated after a much shorter trial of dietary management. Such situations would include patients with familial hypercholesterolemia and very high baseline total cholesterol (TC) and LDL-cholesterol, patients with very low HDL levels, patients with severe and early onset CHD, patients with conditions predisposing them to a poor dietary response, and patients with situations requiring a greater urgency to lower cholesterol. If possible, however, a minimum trial of three months of dietary management is desirable to establish an adequate baseline lipid profile. Once baseline values are established, the efficacy of subsequent interventions may be more accurately assessed.

The cholesterol-lowering goals for pharmacologic intervention are identical to those of dietary management. The current NCEP recommendations are an LDL cholesterol level of 160 mg/dl or less in patients without definite CHD or two other CHD risk factors or an LDL cholesterol level of 130 mg/dl or less in patients with definite CHD or two other CHD risk factors (Table 12-2) [1]. Although these target goals are important, it is equally important to be aware that a graded reduction in CHD events exists with a reduction in total and LDL cholesterol. In general for each 1-percent reduction

Table 12-1. Treatment determinants other than LDL cholesterol

Definite CHD
  Definite prior MI
  Definite myocardial ischemia (e.g., angina pectoris)

CHD risk factors
  Male sex
  Family history of premature CHD (definite MI or sudden death in a parent or sibling before age 55)
  Smoking
  Hypertension
  Low level of HDL cholesterol (<35 mg/dl on two consecutive tests)
  Diabetes mellitus
  History of definite cerebrovascular or occlusive peripheral vascular disease
  Severe obesity (≥ 30% overweight)

Source: Report of the National Cholesterol Education Program Expert Panel. Report on detection, evaluation, and treatment of high blood cholesterol in adults.[1]

Table 12-2. Indications and goals for pharmacologic management of hyperlipidemia

Indications
  Patient has completed six months of dietary therapy and counseling *and*
  Patient has LDL cholesterol ≥190 mg/dl without definite CHD or two or more CHD risk factors
    or
  Patient has LDL cholesterol ≥160 mg/dl with definite CHD or two or more CHD risk factors
Goals
  LDL cholesterol <160 mg/dl without definite CHD or two or more CHD risk factors
  LDL cholesterol <130 mg/dl with definite CHD or two or more CHD risk factors

Source: National Cholesterol Education Program Expert Panel. Report on detection, evaluation, and treatment of high blood cholesterol in adults.[1]

in total cholesterol, a reduction on the order of 2 percent in CHD events may be expected [2, 3, 4]. No specific goals have been developed for HDL, although the role of HDL in modifying CHD risk is being increasingly recognized, and a forthcoming revision of the NCEP guidelines is expected to give greater weight to this risk factor [5, 6].

A coordinated effort among patient, physician, dietitian, and other health care specialists must take place for optimal lipid management to exist. In many cases referral to a trained, skilled dietitian is an important step during both initial dietary management and subsequent combined dietary and pharmacologic management. A team approach to the management of hyperlipidemia is essential — physicians may not always have sufficient time to devote to optimal nutritional teaching and management, or they may not be adequately skilled in this discipline. Thus, behaviorists, exercise specialists, and other health specialists can play a significant role in optimal care.

The purpose of this chapter is to review the pharmacologic agents currently used in the management of hyperlipidemia. Each agent is profiled with respect to its mechanism of action, major clinical indications, contraindications, side effects, and corresponding major clinical trials. The interaction of lipid-lowering drugs with commonly used medications is also addressed. The use of marine oils for the therapy of lipid abnormalities is discussed, and an overview of cost considerations is presented. A summary of lipid-altering medications is presented in Table 12-3.

Bile Acid Sequestrants

Mechanism of Action

The bile acid sequestrants cholestyramine and colestipol have been extensively studied and characterized. Their mechanism of action may be considered nonsystemic in that they bind bile acids in the intestinal lumen, interrupt the enterohepatic circulation of cholesterol, and thus promote the excretion of cholesterol in the stool. The bile acid sequestrants affect three key enzyme systems. As summarized by Shepherd, these systems include phosphatidic acid phosphatase, cholesterol 7 alpha-hydroxylase, and 3-hydroxy-3-methylglutaryl coenzyme A (HMG CoA) reductase [7].

Phosphatidic acid phosphatase is an hepatic enzyme that, when activated, cleaves the phosphate group from phosphatidic acid, thereby promoting its conversion to triglyceride (TG). This enzyme is normally suppressed with a fully functional, intact, enterohepatic circulation. When phosphatidic acid phosphatase is suppressed, the enzymatic pathway favors conversion of alpha-glycerol phosphate to a variety of phospholipids. Bile acid sequestrants, by interrupting the normal enterohepatic circulation, activate phosphatidic acid phosphatase, which ultimately results in increased synthesis of triglyceride (Figure 12-1) [7]. Recognition of the triglyceride-raising effect of bile acid sequestrants is important in the appropriate prescription of these medications, since hypertriglyceridemia (TG > 300 mg/dl) is a relative contraindication for their use [8].

Cholesterol 7 alpha-hydroxylase is the rate-limiting enzyme in bile acid synthesis. Increased activity of this enzyme promotes increased hepatic synthesis of bile acids, thus depleting hepatocyte stores of cholesterol. Under normal circumstances of intact hepatobiliary circulation, bile acids returning to the liver via the portal blood inhibit the activity of cholesterol 7 alpha-hydroxylase [7]. Bile acid sequestrants decrease the return of bile acids to the liver, thereby increasing the activity of cholesterol 7 alpha-hydroxylase. The increased enzymatic activity increases bile acid synthesis, decreases intrahepatic cholesterol stores, and upregulates hepatic LDL surface receptors [7]. Serum LDL cholesterol is thus reduced because of increased hepatic uptake. In addition to the upregulation of hepatic LDL receptors, diminished intrahepatic cholesterol stores also promote the synthesis of cholesterol by ultimately increasing the activity of HMG CoA reductase (Figure 12-2). This mechanism provides the rationale for effectively using the combination of bile acid sequestrants and HMG CoA reductase inhibi-

Table 12-3. Summary of lipid-altering medications

Drug	Dose	Total cholesterol	LDL cholesterol	HDL cholesterol	Triglycerides	Side effects	Drug interactions	Other
Cholestyramine	4 g bid to tid up to 24 g per day	Reduced 10 to 20%	Reduced 10 to 20%	Increased 4 to 6%	Increased 10 to 15%	Constipation, gastrointestinal complaints	Reduced serum concentrations of thyroxine, phenobarbitol, tetracycline	Decreased incidence of CHD events
Colestipol	5 g bid to tid							
Gemfibrozil	600 mg bid	Reduced 10 to 20%	Reduced 9 to 18%	Increased 10 to 25%	Reduced 20 to 60%	Gastrointestinal complaints, hepatotoxicity	Increased incidence of myositis and rhabdomyolysis if used with HMG CoA reductase inhibitors	Decreased incidence of CHD events
Nicotinic acid	1 to 6 g per day in divided doses	Reduced 10 to 30%	Reduced 20 to 33%	Increased 10 to 25%	Reduced 20 to 50%	Flushing, pruritis, warmth, gastrointestinal complaints, gout, glucose intolerance, postural hypotension, hepatotoxicity	Increased incidence of myositis and rhabdomyolysis if used with HMG CoA reductase inhibitors	Decreased incidence of recurrent MI; atherosclerotic regression in combination regimens
Lovastatin	10 to 80 mg per day	Reduced 15 to 40%	Reduced 20 to 45%	Increased 6 to 12%	Reduced 10 to 19%	Gastrointestinal complaints, headache, fatigue, myalgias, rash, myositis, rhabdomyolysis, hepatotoxicity,	Increased incidence of myositis when used with niacin gemfibrozil, or immunosuppressive drugs	Preliminary reports of atherosclerotic regression
Pravastatin and Simvastatin	10 to 40 mg per day in divided doses							
Probucol	500 mg bid	Reduced 10 to 20%	Reduced 10 to 20%	Reduced 20 to 30%	Variable	Gastrointestinal complaints, increased QTc interval		Regression of tendinous and cutaneous xanthomas
Omega-3 fatty acids	1 g per day and up	Variable	Variable	Variable	Reduced 30 to 50%			

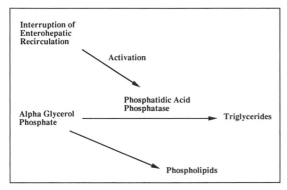

Figure 12-1. Effect of phosphatidic acid phosphatase activation resulting from interruption of the enterohepatic recirculation of cholesterol. (Adapted with permission from Shepherd J. Mechanism of action of bile acid sequestrants and other lipid lowering drugs. Cardiol 1989; 76:65–74.)

tors in hypercholesterolemic patients. These medications have, in fact, been used and studied in combination, and an additive lipid-lowering effect has been observed [9, 10, 11].

In addition to the lowering of total cholesterol and LDL cholesterol by bile acid sequestrants, several large trials have shown modest increases in HDL cholesterol [12, 13]. The HDL increase is generally on the order of 5 percent [14] and is specifically observed in the HDL 2 subfraction [7, 12]. The mechanism by which HDL is increased is not clear; however, there may be a relationship between HDL increase and increases in apolipoprotein AI (and the apolipoprotein AI:AII ratio)[7].

Clinical Indications and Rationale

The bile acid sequestrants, cholestyramine and colestipol, are first-line lipid-lowering agents whose most appropriate use is in the treatment of high LDL cholesterol. They are both powders that are mixed with water or fruit juice. The typical starting dose is 4 g of cholestyramine or 5 g of colestipol taken twice, occasionally three times, daily an hour before meals. Decreases in LDL cholesterol of 10 to 15 percent may be achieved with the initial starting dose [1]. Further reductions in LDL cholesterol may be achieved with gradual increases in resin dosage and reductions of 15 to 30 percent have

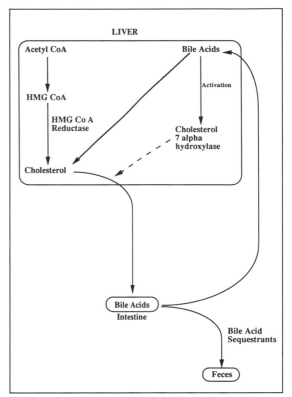

Figure 12-2. Cholesterol-altering mechanisms. (Adapted with permission from Shepherd J. Mechanism of action of bile acid sequestrants and other lipid lowering drugs. Cardiol 1989; 76:65–74.)

been achieved with dosages of 16 to 24 g per day of cholestyramine [1, 2, 12].

Several studies have shown a relationship between the lipid-lowering effects of bile acid sequestrants and reduction in the incidence of CHD and angiographic progression of coronary atherosclerosis. The Lipid Research Clinics Coronary Primary Prevention Trial (LRC-CPPT), a large, multicenter, randomized, double-blind trial, tested the efficacy of cholesterol lowering in reducing the risk of CHD. Over 3800 hypercholesterolemic men, aged 35 to 59 years, were randomized to receive cholestyramine (24 g/day) or placebo. Subjects were followed for an average of 7.4 years, primary end points being defined as definite CHD death or definite nonfatal MI. The cholestyramine group experienced additional reductions of 8.5

percent and 12.6 percent in total and LDL cholesterol levels, respectively, as compared to placebo, with a 19 percent reduction for the combined endpoint of CHD death or nonfatal MI [2].

The National Heart, Lung and Blood Institute (NHLBI) Type II Coronary Intervention Study assessed the relationship between lipid changes resulting from cholestyramine treatment and the progression of CHD as assessed angiographically. TC and LDL cholesterol were significantly decreased in the cholestyramine group, while HDL cholesterol and the ratios of HDL:TC and HDL:LDL cholesterol were significantly increased. Those subjects whose ratio of HDL:TC or HDL:LDL cholesterol increased (independent of treatment with cholestyramine) were more likely to show stabilization of atherosclerotic lesions and lack of disease progression [13].

Although causality is difficult to prove, these studies, as well as several others, provide strong evidence for a relationship between pharmacologic improvement in lipid profiles and the subsequent slowing of development of CHD events or the rate of progression of coronary atherosclerosis.

Side Effects

As might be expected from a medication that is not metabolized in or absorbed from the GI tract, the major side effects of the bile acid sequestrants are gastrointestinal in nature. The LRC-CPPT reported that constipation, flatulence, belching, bloating, and heartburn were the most frequently observed side effects in response to cholestyramine treatment [2]. These side effects are dose dependent. In general the benefits of doses greater than 16 gm of cholestyramine per day (or an equivalent dose of colestipol) are offset by reduced patient compliance and a greater incidence of gastrointestinal side effects [1]. Gastrointestinal side effects encountered in the LRC-CPPT study typically were most apparent during the initial stages of treatment and gradually resolved as the trial progressed. Symptomatic treatment or dosage reduction are frequently all that is necessary to resolve these side effects.

Systemic side effects are uncommon due to the lack of absorption of the bile resins. The resins may, however, concomitantly bind to other therapeutic medications and effectively decrease their absorption and subsequent serum concentration. A partial list of possible medication interactions includes warfarin, digitalis preparations, thiazide diuretics, thyroxine, phenobarbital, phenylbutazone, and tetracycline. Fluctuations in serum drug concentrations can be minimized if the bile acid sequestrant is given approximately one hour before a meal and the other active medications are given one hour after the same meal. Given the possibility of significant fluctuations in serum concentrations of therapeutic medications, serum drug levels should be monitored whenever possible. Particular caution is necessary in anticoagulated patients — prothrombin times may vary widely, and bile acid sequestrant agents should be used in combination with oral anticoagulants only if absolutely necessary and then with the utmost caution.

Fibric Acid Derivatives

Mechanism of Action

The fibric acid derivatives are a class of hypolipidemic medications that reduce serum triglyceride concentrations, increase serum HDL cholesterol concentrations, and, to a lesser extent, decrease serum total and LDL cholesterol levels. To date a variety of drugs have been developed in this class. All are structurally distinct and demonstrate considerable variation in their effects [15, 16]. The agents available and commonly used in the United States and Canada are gemfibrozil and clofibrate. Other fibric acid derivatives available in western European countries and Australia (benzafibrate, ciprofibrate, and fenofibrate) have been shown to lower total and LDL cholesterol levels to a greater extent than gemfibrozil and clofibrate [16, 17, 18, 19, 20]. All, however, have been shown to markedly lower serum triglyceride levels.

Although not yet fully elucidated, the lipid-altering effects of the fibrates appear to be produced by several different mechanisms. Experimental data suggest that the fibrates increase the activity of lipoprotein lipase, enhance the rate of catabolism of LDL cholesterol, and reduce the rate of VLDL synthesis, thus reducing the serum triglyceride level and decreasing both LDL and total serum cholesterol levels (see Figure 3-4) [15, 16]. The ability of fibric acid derivatives to lower total and LDL cholesterol levels has been shown to be dependent on initial serum triglyceride levels. Gemfibrozil has been shown to lower LDL cholesterol in subjects with relatively low baseline serum triglycerides while slightly increasing LDL cholesterol in subjects with initial hypertriglyceridemia [21, 22]. Grundy and Vega have proposed a potential mechanism whereby total and LDL cholesterol would be preferentially lowered in states of relatively lower serum triglyceride levels and unchanged or increased in patients with hypertriglyceridemia. Enhanced lipolysis, as a result of fibric acid treatment, would significantly increase levels of VLDL remnants in hypertriglyceridemic patients. Increased levels of VLDL remnants would then interfere with the removal of LDL cholesterol at the level of the hepatic LDL receptor. This would ultimately result in a lesser degree of LDL reduction in patients with increased levels of hypertriglyceridemia [21, 22].

The precise mechanism whereby fibric acid derivatives increase serum HDL cholesterol levels is not entirely understood. Both healthy and dyslipidemic patients have been shown to have increased concentrations of apolipoproteins AI and AII, the major apolipoproteins of HDL, in response to gemfibrozil treatment [15]. The increased apolipoprotein levels appear to be the result of increased synthesis rather than decreased catabolism [15]. The exact mechanism of increased apolipoprotein biosynthesis and its relationship to elevated HDL cholesterol levels has yet to be established. More studies are necessary to determine the effects of the fibric acid derivatives on HDL metabolism at the molecular level.

Clinical Indications and Rationale

The fibric acid derivatives gemfibrozil and clofibrate are indicated for and approved by the FDA primarily as adjunctive therapy to diet in the treatment of patients with elevated serum triglycerides. The recommended dosage of gemfibrozil is 600 mg orally given twice daily, 30 minutes before the morning and evening meals. Some patients may respond to 900 mg daily. A few individuals may show additional benefits from an increase in dosage to 1500 mg per day [23]. The equivalent starting dose of clofibrate is 1000 mg orally twice daily.

Patients with greatly elevated serum triglycerides (> 1000 mg/dl) are at an increased risk for the development of pancreatitis. The fibrates are strongly indicated in such conditions. A recent trial of the effects of gemfibrozil in patients with severe hypertriglyceridemia (type V hyperlipidemia) showed a dramatic (nearly 75-percent) reduction in serum triglyceride levels [24]. Other trials have shown serum triglyceride reductions ranging from 21 to 60 percent, depending on baseline serum lipid profiles [15, 24, 25]. Efficacy in the treatment of types IIa, IIb, III, and IV hyperlipidemia with gemfibrozil has also been established [24, 26, 27]. Patients with modestly elevated serum triglyceride levels are commonly treated with fibric acid derivatives. Currently, the benefits of reducing moderately elevated serum triglyceride levels are debatable, and the ultimate long-term effects of such interventions are not yet well established.

The strongest data in support of the use of gemfibrozil in other hyperlipidemic states come from the Helsinki Heart Study [27]. This placebo-controlled, double-blind primary prevention trial included 4081 middle-aged asymptomatic men with baseline non–HDL cholesterol levels equal to or greater than 200 mg/dl. Compared with the placebo-treated group, the gemfibrozil-treated group (600 mg twice daily) showed mean decreases of 11 percent in LDL cholesterol and 35 percent in triglycerides and a mean increase of 11 percent in HDL cholesterol over the 5-year trial period. With this change, the gemfibrozil-treated group demonstrated a significant 34 percent reduction in the incidence of CHD events (56 versus 84) [25]. LDL and total cholesterol reductions were greatest for type IIa hyperlipidemics and smallest for type IIb hyperlipidemics [25]. In contrast a greater reduction in coronary events was seen in the type IIb group than in the type IIa phenotype [26]. Further examination of the data showed that baseline HDL cholesterol levels were more predictive of coronary events than baseline LDL cholesterol levels, and the greatest benefit was seen in the high-triglyceride, low-HDL cholesterol group [28]. In addition, Q-wave MIs were significantly reduced in the gemfibrozil-treated group (45-percent reduction in events), whereas no change in the incidence of non-Q wave MIs was noted.[29]

Other trials have shown similar reductions in total and LDL cholesterol, on the order of 10 to 20 percent and 9 to 18 percent, respectively, again depending on the initial serum lipid profile (type IIa patients and those with low baseline serum triglyceride levels demonstrated the greatest reductions in total and LDL cholesterol) [15, 19, 24, 30, 31]. Direct comparison of gemfibrozil with the 3-hydroxy-3-methylglutaryl coenzyme A (HMG CoA) reductase inhibitor lovastatin has shown a two- to fourfold greater reduction in LDL cholesterol with lovastatin [31, 32]. Fibric acid derivatives with increased total and LDL cholesterol–lowering effects, such as benzafibrate, ciprofibrate, and fenofibrate, may compare more favorably with the HMG CoA reductase inhibitors.

With regard to the effect of gemfibrozil on HDL cholesterol, other trials support the data from the Helsinki Heart Study showing that the use of gemfibrozil may induce increases in serum HDL levels of 11 to 25 percent [15, 23, 25, 33, 34]. The importance of increasing serum HDL cholesterol levels was also addressed in the Helsinki Heart Study, where it was observed that increased serum HDL cholesterol levels were independently related to a reduced incidence of CHD [25]. The results of the Helsinki Heart Study were compared to those of other epidemiologic and primary prevention trials [2, 3, 12]. In these previous studies, a 1-percent reduction in total cholesterol corresponded to an approximate 2-percent reduction

in CHD event rates [2, 12]. In the Helsinki Heart Study an 11-percent reduction in total cholesterol was associated with a 34-percent decrease in the incidence of CHD. The greater reduction in coronary heart disease in the Helsinki Study was believed to be the result of gemfibrozil-induced increases in levels of HDL cholesterol [25].

Side Effects

Gemfibrozil is generally well tolerated, and relatively few patients are withdrawn from treatment as a result of side effects [15]. A review of the cumulative incidence of reported side effects in patients treated with gemfibrozil, clofibrate, and placebo showed that side effects were largely comparable in frequency [15]. Only gastrointestinal complaints (including abdominal pain, epigastric pain, and nausea) and rash were slightly more prevalent in the gemfibrozil-treated group. Both clofibrate and gemfibrozil have been shown to increase the lithogenic index of bile by increasing cholesterol secretion and decreasing bile acid formation [15]. However, 1 percent of gemfibrozil-treated patients developed gallstones over a 2-year period; this incidence is similar to that of an untreated population over the same time frame [35]. It is also important to note that the concomitant use of gemfibrozil and the HMG CoA reductase inhibitor lovastatin has been associated with acute rhabdomyolysis, myopathy, myoglobinuria, and acute renal failure [36, 37]. Although the incidence of such complications is low, the use of lovastatin in combination with gemfibrozil should be discouraged [36]; if the combination is necessary, it must be accompanied by a program of close supervision.

Clofibrate itself is little used today because of concerns raised by a study conducted by the World Health Organization (WHO). The WHO Cooperative Trial examined the effect of clofibrate on rates of CHD in a sample of over 10,000 hypercholesterolemic men who randomly received either clofibrate or placebo [38]. Serum cholesterol levels were reduced by 9 percent in the clofibrate group, compared to placebo, and the incidence of nonfatal CHD was decreased by 25 percent in the clofibrate group.

There was, however, no signficant reduction in CHD mortality. Of most concern was the statistically significant increase in mortality from all causes seen in the clofibrate-treated group, largely related to an excess of gastrointestinal and hepatic cancers. This excess of cancer deaths was not seen in later follow-up studies after the drug had been stopped. Primarily as a result of these studies, clofibrate is little used today, having been largely replaced by gemfibrozil, an agent that has not been associated with any excess incidence of cancers.

In summary, although the primary approved indication for the use of fibric acid derivatives is hypertriglyceridemia, there are several other potential benefits to be derived from the use of these agents. In conjunction with diet, these medications can be used selectively in the treatment of hypercholesterolemia, although they are felt to be first-line agents only in those patients whose lipid profile includes hypertriglyceridemia. Because of the concomitant HDL-elevating and LDL-lowering effects, however, these agents may be considered to be first-line drugs in the treatment of patients with a combination of moderately elevated LDL and decreased HDL cholesterol levels. The fibric acid derivatives are generally well tolerated with a low incidence of side effects and a high degree of compliance.

Nicotinic Acid

Mechanism of Action

Nicotinic acid (niacin) is a water-soluble B vitamin that when used to treat hyperlipidemia is given in dosages far exceeding those required for its action as a vitamin. Typical therapeutic doses range from 1 to 6 g per day. Nicotinic acid is an effective first-line hypolipidemic agent that lowers serum levels of total cholesterol, LDL cholesterol, and triglycerides, while simultaneously elevating serum HDL cholesterol levels. The lipid-lowering effects of nicotinic acid were first recognized in the 1950s by Altschul and colleagues [39, 40]. It was initially observed that certain processes that increase tissue oxidation, such as oxygen inhalation [41] and ultraviolet irradiation [42], were associated with reduced serum cholesterol levels. Altschul hypothesized that nicotinic acid, by stimulating oxidative metabolism, might have a similar effect on lipids [39]. The actual lipid-lowering effects of nicotinic acid were then demonstrated in experiments involving healthy medical students and patients with various diseases [39].

Although the significant lipid-lowering effects of nicotinic acid have been verified by numerous trials, the actual biochemical mechanisms producing these effects have not yet been fully elucidated. In hypertriglyceridemic states, VLDL particles are larger and more triglyceride-rich. Nicotinic acid has been shown to decrease the hepatic synthesis of VLDL, the size of the individual VLDL particles, and the serum concentration of triglycerides [43]. The typical action of catecholamines to stimulate lipolysis in peripheral adipose tissue (resulting in the liberation of free fatty acids) is inhibited by nicotinic acid, thus decreasing the hepatic substrate necessary to produce serum triglycerides [40, 44]. LDL cholesterol reduction may also result from the diminished number of VLDL particles synthesized, since VLDL is metabolized indirectly to LDL. Other possible mechanisms responsible for the reduction in total and LDL cholesterol levels include increased clearance of VLDL remnants and decreased synthesis of LDL cholesterol [43]. Reductions in total and LDL cholesterol are somewhat dependent on initial serum triglyceride levels. Patients whose lipid profiles show relatively high baseline serum triglycerides have proportionately smaller decreases in serum cholesterol after treatment with nicotinic acid [45]. The triglyceride-dependent cholesterol-lowering effect of nicotinic acid is analogous to that seen with the fibric acid derivatives [21, 22, 45].

One of the more attractive features of nicotinic acid treatment is the ability of this medication to significantly increase serum HDL cholesterol concentrations. Shepherd and colleagues demonstrated a 23-percent increase in HDL cholesterol levels after treatment with nicotinic acid at a dose of 3 g per day. In addition, this study showed a 7-percent increase in apoprotein A1 levels, a relative transfer of apoprotein A1 from HDL3 to HDL2 subfractions, and an increased ratio of HDL2:HDL3 [46]. These alterations may further potentiate the transfer of esterified cholesterol from HDL to VLDL or to chylomicrons, thus favoring the removal and clearance of cholesterol from peripheral stores (see Chapter 3). Other clinical trials have also shown significant increases in serum HDL cholesterol levels after treatment with nicotinic acid [40, 43, 47, 48]. As will be described next, further evidence correlates nicotinic acid treatment (or combination regimens) with a reduction in the rate of fatal and nonfatal MI [45, 49] and with regression of coronary atherosclerotic lesions [47, 48]. The combined actions of HDL cholesterol elevation, alteration in HDL composition, total and LDL cholesterol reduction, and triglyceride reduction are likely to be responsible for these outcomes.

Clinical Indications and Rationale

Nicotinic acid may be used as a first-line medication in the treatment of hypercholesterolemia and hypertriglyceridemia. Typical starting dosages range from 100 to 500 mg daily with food. If tolerated, this may be progressively increased to a maintenance dose in the range of 1.5 to 6 g per day taken in divided doses. The dosage may be increased at intervals of one to two weeks until a therapeutic maintenance dose is obtained. The medication is rapidly absorbed and maximal lipid-altering effects are seen within approximately two months [50]. When used in doses of 3 to 6 g per day, nicotinic acid reduces plasma concentrations of total cholesterol, LDL cholesterol, and triglycerides on the order of 10 to 30 percent, 20 to 33 percent, and 20 to 50 percent, respectively [16, 40, 43, 46]. Concomitant elevations in serum HDL cholesterol levels have been observed to be on the order of 10 to 25 percent [16, 40, 46] and may be increased to 30 to 37 percent with combinations of nicotinic acid and other lipid-altering medications [47, 48].

Some compelling evidence in support of the use of nicotinic acid, alone or in combination, comes from the Coronary Drug Project, first reported in 1975 and with a 15-year follow-up reported in 1986, and from the Cholesterol-Lowering Atherosclerosis Study (CLAS), first reported in 1987 and with a follow-up in 1990. The Coronary Drug Project was conducted between 1966 and 1975. Over 8000 male survivors of MIs were enrolled and randomized to receive one of five lipid-altering drugs, including niacin (3 g per day) [45]. The initial report showed that the niacin-treated patients had a modest decrease in the incidence of definite nonfatal recurrent MI but no significant decrease in total mortality. The 15-year follow-up study showed a significant (11-percent decrease compared to placebo) reduction in total mortality in the niacin-treated group [49]. This late effect was felt to result from the long-term cholesterol-lowering effect of niacin.

The CLAS study was a randomized, placebo-controlled, angiographic trial that evaluated a combination colestipol-niacin regimen versus placebo [47]. The initial group consisted of 162 men, aged 40 to 59 years, who had undergone previous coronary bypass surgery. The 2-year report showed both regression and decreased progression of coronary atherosclerosis in the drug-treated group. The 4-year follow-up confirmed these findings, demonstrated a reduced incidence in the development of new, native coronary lesions, and showed that regression can continue for 4 years [48]. Although these studies address the efficacy of nicotinic acid in secondary prevention, it can be inferred from other primary prevention drug trials that the lipid-lowering effects of niacin are likely to be of long-term benefit.

Side Effects and Interactions

Perhaps the greatest drawback to the use of nicotinic acid in the treatment of hyperlipidemia is the incidence of side effects. Dermatological side effects are frequent, with flushing, pruritis, and warmth being most prominent. The Coronary Drug Project reported incidences of flushing and pruritis of 92 percent and 49 percent, respectively [45]. There is, however, a significant reduction in the occurrence of symptoms over time. The CLAS data showed a reduction in the reported incidence of flushing and itching from 77 to 12 percent and 29 to 4 percent, respectively, over the course of 2 years [48]. Repeated dosing at a steady state over several days may significantly diminish the incidence of these side effects. Since flushing is mediated by prostaglandin release, its frequency and severity may be reduced by the administration of aspirin on a daily basis [40, 51, 52] or indomethacin [53] 1 hour prior to taking the drug. Symptoms may also be diminished if the medication is taken with meals, the dosage is slowly increased, and sustained-release [54] preparations are used. Ethanol and hot drinks should be avoided since these may potentiate the flushing effects of nicotinic acid. Persistent pruritis can be treated with antihistamines as needed.

Gastrointestinal distress, gout, postural hypotension, and atrial fibrillation have also been shown to be associated with the use of nicotinic acid [45], and glucose intolerance may be exacerbated [55, 56]. Although the incidence of flushing may diminish with the use of the sustained-release form of nicotinic acid, nausea, vomiting, and diarrhea may become more frequent. Hepatic enzymes may also become elevated as a result of nicotinic acid treatment. Elevations in liver enzymes are more commonly reported in patients whose dosages are greater than 3 g per day [40, 57] and are also more common when the sustained-release form of nicotinic acid is used [58]. It is advisable, then, to obtain a baseline serum chemistry panel and to periodically follow glucose, uric acid, and liver function tests approximately 1 month after the initiation of treatment and every 3 to 6 months thereafter [40].

Overall the use of nicotinic acid is often limited by these side effects. However, niacin's LDL- and triglyceride-lowering and HDL-increasing effects are quite potent and very beneficial. It has been our experience that attention to the details described here — cautious dosage increases, ensuring that the drug is always taken after meals, and the use of concomitant aspirin therapy — lead to tolerance in the great majority of patients.

One other curious feature of this agent is its status as a food supplement, which does not require a physician's prescription. It can therefore be found in supermarkets and health food stores in a wide variety of dosages and forms

and is not as closely regulated as are prescription drugs. We have found that various preparations have differing potencies and side effects. To be able to treat our patients rationally we have adopted the scheme of recommending a few brands that we know to be effective. Physicians should become familiar with one or two effective agents in a given geographic area and then preferentially recommend their use.

HMG CoA Reductase Inhibitors

Mechanism of Action

The endogenous synthesis of cholesterol accounts for as much as two-thirds of total body cholesterol [59]. With this in mind, attempts at lowering serum cholesterol have been directed at blocking its endogenous hepatic synthesis. More than 25 separate enzymatic reactions take place in the biosynthesis of cholesterol (Figure 12-3). Initially 3-hydroxy-3-methylglutaryl coenzyme A (HMG CoA) is synthesized after three successive condensations of acetyl-CoA. HMG CoA is then reduced to mevalonate, which, after a series of enzymatic steps, is eventually metabolized to cholesterol [59]. Early attempts at blocking this pathway utilized agents that inhibited enzymatic steps occurring later in the biosynthetic sequence. However, agents that blocked these later enzymatic stages resulted in the accumulation of cholesterol precursors both in the serum and in cellular membranes [59]. Initial use of triparanol, an agent of this type, resulted in serious side effects, including cataracts in both animal and human models [60, 61].

Recognition of the side effects resulting from the accumulation of cholesterol precursors then led to an effort to decrease cholesterol synthesis by blocking an earlier enzymatic step in the synthetic pathway. The conversion of HMG CoA to mevalonic acid is an early and major rate-limiting step in the synthesis of cholesterol, catalyzed by HMG CoA reductase. Since HMG CoA is a water-soluble molecule that can be readily metabolized and eliminated, the accumulation of HMG CoA (resulting from inhibition of HMG CoA reductase) should in theory not result in detrimental side effects. This ra-

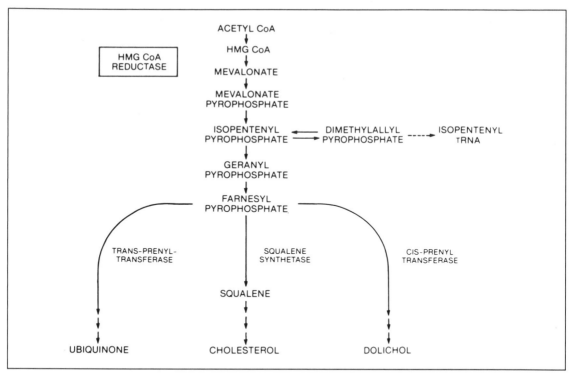

Figure 12-3.   Sequence of hepatic cholesterol synthesis. (Reprinted with permission from Alberts AW. Discovery, biochemistry and biology of lovastatin. Amer J Cardiol 1988; 62:10J–15J.)

tionale led to the discovery by Endo and colleagues of ML-236B (compactin, mevastatin), a fungal metabolite and potent inhibitor of HMG CoA reductase [62, 63]. Subsequent efforts were directed at developing other naturally occurring HMG CoA reductase inhibitors. The fungal metabolite lovastatin was first isolated by Endo and colleagues from cultures of Monascus ruber in 1979 [64, 65], then from a strain of Aspergillus terreus in Madrid, Spain, by Alberts and colleagues in 1980 [59, 66]. It was found to be an extremely potent inhibitor of HMG CoA reductase when converted enzymatically from its prodrug lactone form to the dihydroxy open-acid active metabolite [59]. As a consequence of decreased hepatic cholesterol synthesis, hepatic LDL receptor activity is augmented, resulting in a further reduction in serum LDL cholesterol [59]. There are currently three HMG CoA reductase inhibitors approved in the United States. These include lovastatin, pravastatin, and simvastatin.

The benefits of treatment with a prodrug versus an active agent were further explored as newer HMG CoA reductase inhibitors were discovered and synthesized. Two of the newer agents, pravastatin and simvastatin, have recently been approved for use in the United States. Pravastatin is the active 6-hydroxy open-acid analog of mevastatin (ML-236B), while simvastatin is a semisynthetic HMG CoA reductase inhibitor derived from lovastatin [59]. Since the enzymatic conversion of prodrug to active metabolite takes place in the liver, the target organ of cholesterol synthesis, use of prodrugs such as lovastatin or simvastatin would theoretically be beneficial, because the active moiety would be concentrated at its site of action. As a result, one might also expect lower concentrations of active drug in peripheral tissues and potentially fewer side effects. In vitro and in vivo data in support of this concept are not conclusive. In a direct comparison of the concentrations of lovastatin, simvastatin, and pravastatin in male rats, Germershausen and colleagues showed that the hydrophobic prodrugs were more concentrated in the liver, while pravastatin was relatively more concentrated in peripheral tissue [67]. In contrast, other studies addressing actual cholesterol synthesis have shown that the inhibitory effects of pravastatin were more tissue selective (specifically hepatoselective) than those of lovastatin or simvastatin [68]. The relevance of such studies will not be apparent until clinical comparisons of these agents with respect to cholesterol-lowering efficacy and side effect profiles are available.

Clinical Indications and Rationale

HMG CoA reductase inhibitors are indicated as adjuncts to diet in the treatment of individuals with elevated total and LDL serum cholesterol levels. Although these agents may be useful in the treatment of combined elevations of serum cholesterol and triglycerides, they are not typically considered first-line single agents for the management of this lipid pattern.

The usual starting dose of lovastatin is 20 mg orally per day typically given with the evening meal. For patients with markedly elevated serum cholesterol levels (TC ≥ 300 mg/dl) lovastatin therapy may be initiated at a dose of 40 mg per day. Doses as high as 80 mg per day may be used, and twice-daily divided-dose regimens are optional. Lovastatin is available in 10-, 20-, and 40-mg tablets. Dosage adjustments should be made at intervals of 4 or more weeks, since maximal cholesterol-lowering effects are seen within 4 to 6 weeks [65, 69]. Significant cholesterol-lowering effects, however, may be seen within 2 weeks [65]. Pravastatin is available in 10 and 20 mg tablets while simvastatin is available in 5, 10, 20, and 40 mg tablets. The usual starting doses of these two drugs are 10 to 20 mg per day with a maximal recommended dose of 40 mg per day given in the evening. Peak effects are achieved within a similar time frame as observed with lovastatin [71a, 71b].

Comparable doses for the three HMG CoA reductase inhibitors have not yet been established. The modest available literature suggests that lovastatin and pravastatin are comparable in potency, while simvastatin is somewhat more potent than either of the other two agents.

Cholesterol reduction with HMG CoA reductase inhibitors is dose dependent. Graded effects are observed as dosages of lovastatin increase from 10 to 80 mg per day and dosages of pravastatin and simvastatin are increased from 10 to 40 mg per day [65, 70, 71a, 71b]. Mean reductions in total and LDL cholesterol have been reported to be in the range of 15 to 40 percent and 20 to 45 percent, respectively, for all three agents [65, 71, 71a, 71b, 71c, 71d].

Patients with both familial and nonfamilial forms of hypercholesterolemia may benefit from treatment with HMG CoA reductase inhibitors [65]. Although all patients should be treated with a low-fat, low-cholesterol diet prior to beginning a lipid-lowering drug, a recent trial has shown that lovastatin produces comparable improvement in plasma lipoprotein profiles regardless of diet. Although an additive effect is observed when the combination of diet and drug is used, no further synergistic effect was noted (there was no diet-drug interaction) [72]. The LDL-lowering effects of lovastatin are somewhat greater than those of nicotinic acid [16, 40, 43, 46, 65, 71]. Lovastatin produces a more effective reduction in total cholesterol, LDL cholesterol, apolipoprotein-B concentration, and LDL/HDL cholesterol ratio than does the fibric acid derivative gemfibrozil [31].

While some studies of lovastatin have shown significant increases in serum HDL cholesterol of as much as 16 to 18 percent [71, 73, 74], others have shown either minimal or insignificant changes [75, 76]. In general it may be reasonable to expect modest increases in serum HDL cholesterol concentrations on the order of 6 to 12 percent with 20 to 80 mg of lovastatin or 10 to 40 mg of pravastatin or simvastatin per day [71a, 71b, 71c, 71d]. Both niacin and the fibric acid derivatives tend to increase serum HDL cholesterol to a greater extent than do the HMG CoA reductase inhibitors. Direct comparisons of gemfibrozil and lovastatin have shown gemfibrozil to be one and a half to three times more effective in increasing HDL [31], while indirect comparisons of lovastatin to nicotinic acid suggest an approximate twofold increased benefit with the use of niacin [16, 40, 46].

Lovastin and the newer HMG CoA reductase inhibitors have been shown to decrease serum triglyceride levels to a modest extent, on the order of 10 to 19 percent [31, 65, 70, 77]. Both niacin and the fibric acid derivatives are more potent agents in this respect. A direct comparison of lovastatin and gemfibrozil by Tikkanen and colleagues has shown triglyceride reductions on the order of 13 percent with lovastatin and 40 to 45 percent with gemfibrozil [31]. In comparison nicotinic acid produces serum triglyceride reductions on the order of 20 to 50 percent [16, 40, 43].

Although the HMG CoA reductase inhibitors are typically indicated for the treatment of significant primary hypercholesterolemia, they may also be beneficial in the treatment of patients with other forms of dyslipidemia, including secondary dyslipidemias. Grundy and colleagues have shown the HMG CoA reductase inhibitors to be effective in the treatment of mixed hyperlipidemia, diabetic dyslipidemia, nephrotic hyperlipidemia, and primary hypoalphalipoproteinemia [78]. Studies addressing the long-term benefits of treating secondary dyslipidemias with HMG CoA reductase inhibitors are not yet available.

Although no published studies to date have shown a definitive relationship between cholesterol lowering by an HMG CoA reductase inhibitor (as a single agent) and the regression of coronary atherosclerosis, there is substantial indirect evidence in support of this relationship. Kane and colleagues have shown that diet and a variety of lipid-lowering drugs, including lovastatin, may induce coronary atherosclerotic regression in both men and women [79]. In addition a preliminary report by Zhao and colleagues suggests that a combination lovastatin-colestipol regimen may promote coronary atherosclerotic regression in native coronary arteries and retard restenosis in vessels after percutaneous transluminal coronary angioplasty (PTCA) [80]. At least two regression trials studying the effects of pravastatin on coronary atherosclerosis are under way (PLAC I

and REGRESS), while a large Scandinavian trial, the Simvastatin Survival Study, will attempt to determine the effect of simvastatin over a 3-year period on 4000 subjects with ischemic heart disease and hypercholesterolemia [81, 82, 83]. The Expanded Clinical Evaluation of Lovastatin (EXCEL) trial has recently been completed, and the 5-year Air Force Coronary Atherosclerosis Prevention Study (AFCAPS) is under way. These large (8000 + subjects), randomized, placebo-controlled, double-blind, primary prevention trials will help to establish the long-term efficacy, morbidity, mortality, and side effects of lovastatin [70, 83, 84]. And finally, the Monitored Atherosclerosis Regression Study (MARS), carried out by Dr. David Blankenhorn's group, has accumulated data (not yet published) showing both slowing of progression and evidence of regression of atherosclerosis in patients with CHD being treated with lovastatin. (See Chapter 15 for further discussion of this study and the topic of regression of CHD.)

Side Effects

Since its approval in 1987 lovastatin has been found to be a very well tolerated hypolipidemic agent with a relatively low incidence of clinical and biological side effects. The most frequently reported clinical symptoms associated with lovastatin use include gastrointestinal disturbances (flatulence, nausea, diarrhea, and constipation), headache, fatigue, myalgias, and rash [65]. In addition to these clinical symptoms, the use of the HMG CoA reductase inhibitors has led to concerns over potential hepatotoxicity, myositis, and lens opacities. These are discussed separately below.

Fewer than 2 percent of patients discontinue lovastatin treatment as a result of any of the above complications [65, 70, 85, 86]. The rates and reasons for drug discontinuation are as follows: transaminase elevation, 1.3 percent; rash, .3 percent; gastrointestinal symptoms, .3 percent; myopathy, .1 percent; and insomnia, .1 percent [85]. Incidences of side effects and of drug discontinuation are highly correlated with drug dosage [70, 85]. A resolution of side effects is nearly always observed with discontinuation of the medication [70, 85]. A similar incidence of transaminase elevation has been reported by the manufacturers of both simvastatin and pravastatin [71d, 86a].

The EXCEL study of 8240 patients has shown a graded increase in transaminase elevation with doses of lovastatin ranging from 20 mg to 80 mg per day [70]. While the incidence of transaminase elevation (defined as greater than three times normal levels) was comparable in the 20-mg-per-day lovastatin group and the placebo group, the rates of transaminase elevations were significantly higher in the 40-mg-per-day and 80-mg-per-day groups. Since increases in transaminase elevations occurred unpredictably throughout the 48 weeks of observation, it is advisable to monitor transaminase levels initially on a monthly basis and subsequently on a regular periodic basis at least throughout the first year of therapy. Transaminase levels reverted toward baseline in nearly all patients on discontinuation of lovastatin. Concomitant ethanol use should be limited and use with other potentially hepatotoxic medications should be avoided.

The incidence of myositis is quite low in patients who have no other potential exacerbating factors and are taking lovastatin as a single agent. The EXCEL group found similar rates of creatine kinase (CK) elevations among all dosage groups [70]. The reported incidence of muscle symptoms was also quite similar between groups. The incidence of myositis, however, clearly increases when lovastatin is used in combination with gemfibrozil or immunosuppressive therapy. This has been especially noted in patients post organ transplantation, where cyclosporine is commonly used [87]. Sepsis and possibly the use of antibiotics in combination with lovastatin may also exacerbate the development of myositis. The serious complications of rhabdomyolysis, myoglobinuria, and renal failure have been reported in patients receiving these combined regimens, particularly when patients are septic or immunosuppressed [85]. It is, therefore, advisable to use combination treatment with great care, to avoid the use of HMG CoA reductase inhibitors in patients receiving immunosuppressive drugs, and to discontinue the use of those agents in patients who are seriously infected or septic.

Use of such earlier agents as triparanol, which blocked the hepatic synthesis of cholesterol at a distal site in the synthetic pathway, was found to be correlated with the development of lens opacities. The incidence of cataract development with the use of lovastatin has since been followed quite closely. The evidence to date suggests that there is no increased incidence of cataract development with lovastatin use [85].

Lovastatin may be used concomitantly with digoxin, beta blockers, and coumadin. There have been a few reported cases of increased prothrombin times (PT) in patients taking lovastatin and coumadin; therefore, it is recommended that a baseline PT be assessed prior to starting lovastatin and periodically thereafter until stabilization is achieved.

In summary lovastatin and the newer HMG CoA reductase inhibitors are effective agents for lowering serum total and LDL cholesterol levels that are well-tolerated and have a low incidence of significant side effects.

Probucol

Mechanism of Action

Probucol is a lipid-regulating agent with physical and biochemical properties quite distinct from those of other lipid-altering drugs. Chemically it is a lipophilic bis-phenol compound that is slowly absorbed from the gastrointestinal tract [88]. It is then transported by chylomicrons and VLDL and distributed among VLDL, LDL, and HDL particles. Probucol slowly accumulates in adipose tissue and may take several months to be eliminated after discontinuation of the drug [88]. Plasma drug concentrations increase gradually, and steady-state concentrations may not be reached for several months.

The major observed effects of probucol on lipid metabolism and atherogenesis are three-fold. First, probucol has been shown to significantly decrease both total and LDL cholesterol levels. Second, the use of probucol has been found to concomitantly decrease HDL cholesterol levels. Finally, this agent has antioxidant effects that may potentially block the oxidation of LDL and possibly diminish atherogenesis (see below). The various biochemical processes responsible for these effects remain unclear.

Reduction of LDL cholesterol levels is believed to result from probucol-induced alterations in the metabolic properties of LDL. Probucol has been shown to increase the catabolic rate and clearance of LDL [89]. The increased clearance of LDL is not believed to be related to LDL receptor changes since both human (patients with homozygous familial hypercholesterolemia) [90, 91] and animal (Watanabe heritable hyperlipidemic rabbits) [92, 93] models suggest that the lack or absence of LDL receptors does not alter the magnitude of LDL reduction seen with probucol. In addition, radiolabeled LDL transferred from probucol-treated rabbits to untreated rabbits is catabolized at a more rapid rate than LDL originating from animals not treated with probucol [93, 94]. The precise metabolic alteration accounting for this increased clearance has not yet been definitively established. The antioxidant effect of probucol may in some way be contributory.

Probucol may also decrease cholesterol levels by increasing the production of bile acids (human subjects) [95, 96, 97] or by decreasing the gastrointestinal absorption of cholesterol (animal models) [95]. No effects have been observed on triglyceride or VLDL metabolism [95].

The most problematic effect of probucol on lipid metabolism is its propensity to significantly lower HDL cholesterol levels. Given the large body of evidence showing a correlation between increased levels of HDL cholesterol and decreased incidence of CHD, many physicians have been reluctant to use an agent that almost uniformly lowers serum HDL levels. Nevertheless, there is substantial laboratory, animal, and human evidence to suggest that probucol may have a place in the lipid-modification armamentarium. Both the LDL-lowering effect and the postulated antioxidant action of probucol may contribute to its efficacy. In addition, probucol's effect on HDL may be more complex than a simple lower-HDL equals higher-risk relationship. Probucol-modified HDL particles have been postulated either to be responsible for more effective reverse cholesterol transport or to represent the end products of augmented reverse cholesterol transport.

Probucol treatment has been shown to decrease the size of HDL particles [98]. In addition, both HDL2 and HDL3 subfractions have been found to be lowered by probucol treatment.

Increased reverse cholesterol transport is thought to be a consequence of probucol treatment. Investigators have shown increased transfer of cholesterol ester from HDL to LDL after administration of probucol [99, 100]. Although the mechanism responsible for this has not been clearly established, possibilities include increases in the quantity or action of cholesterol ester transfer protein (CETP), altered binding of CETP to lipoproteins, changes in the ratio of acceptor to donor lipoproteins, or an effect on plasma inhibitors of CETP (see Figure 3-5) [99]. The end result is the enhancement of cholesterol transport from peripheral stores to LDL particles, which may then either bind to hepatic reporters and potentially remove cholesterol from the serum or again deposit cholesterol in peripheral tissues (see Chapter 3).

It has been postulated that atherogenesis may, in part, be due to oxidative modification of LDL. Oxidized LDL may be directly toxic and more avidly taken up by endothelial cells, enhance the generation of foam cells, and promote the entrapment of macrophages in developing atherosclerotic lesions (see Figure 3-8) [93, 101]. Antioxidant agents may prevent these detrimental effects. Probucol has been shown to be an active antioxidant that can block the oxidative modification of LDL particles in vitro [102]. In addition, since probucol may be transported via LDL particles, it has been suggested that the antioxidant effect on LDL may be an important antiatherogenic property of this agent. Although this possibility is of great potential importance, supporting in vivo data are still limited.

Clinical Indications and Rationale

Probucol was introduced in the 1970s as a hypocholesterolemic agent with no significant effects on triglyceride reduction. Its use became limited as its HDL-lowering effects became recognized and as concern arose over possible cardiotoxicity (QT prolongation) [103, 104]. A renewed interest in the medication has developed over the past several years because of its role as a potential antioxidant and because of a better understanding of the effects of probucol on HDL metabolism. It is currently indicated for treatment of individuals with type IIa or IIb hyperlipidemia and has been shown to be effective in polygenic, homozygous familial and heterozygous familial primary hyperlidemias [88]. Its significant effects on homozygous familial hyperlipidemia are notable since other classes of hypolipidemic medications may not be efficacious in this situation. In addition, it has been beneficial in the treatment of patients with hyperlipidemias secondary to diabetes mellitus [105] and the nephrotic syndrome [106]. Probucol has also been shown to be safe and beneficial in treating elderly patients with familial hypercholesterolemia [107].

Much of the initial interest in this agent was generated by the observation of regression of tendinous and cutaneous xanthomas, with many lesions showing dramatic and rapid regression after probucol treatment [90, 98]. Since these observations could not easily be explained by probucol's cholesterol-lowering effects alone, attention was directed at other potential antiatherogenic properties (i.e., the reverse cholesterol transport and antioxidant effects described above).

The recommended starting dose of probucol is 500 mg given twice daily with the morning and evening meals. It is available in both 250- and 500-mg tablets. A review by Buckley et al. of the many in vivo trials using probucol has shown reported reductions in total and LDL cholesterol levels in the range of 10 to 20 percent each [88]. Serum HDL cholesterol may be reduced on the order of 20 to 30 percent, with variable effects reported on serum triglyceride and VLDL levels. Because of its significant HDL-lowering effect, probucol is generally not used in patients with low baseline HDL cholesterol levels. The ultimate long-term effects of probucol treatment with respect to morbidity and mortality have not yet been established. Several human trials of this agent are currently in progress and should help to establish its proper place as a therapeutic agent.

Side Effects

Probucol is generally quite well tolerated. Gastrointestinal complaints are most frequent, with diarrhea being more common than constipation [108, 109]. Side effects usually diminish over time [109], and the overall reported discontinuation rate due to adverse side effects is in the range of 3 to 8 percent [108, 110].

Early animal studies suggested an increased incidence of ventricular dysrhythmias, including ventricular fibrillation and sudden death in probucol-treated dogs [108]. Although an increased incidence of dysrhythmias has not been seen in human subjects treated with probucol, many investigators have documented a slight prolongation in the QT interval. Troendle et al. observed increases in QTc intervals of 5 to 31 msec [104]. Conflicting data exist as to whether increased prolongations are dose (or serum concentration) related, duration related, or both [88]. The QT interval should, therefore, be closely monitored if probucol is to be used with other agents capable of causing QT prolongation, and such combinations should be used only if absolutely necessary.

In summary, probucol is a moderately effective agent in reducing total and LDL cholesterol. It is effective in treating patients with homozygous familial hypercholesterolemia, and it possesses interesting antiatherogenic properties. Both its antioxidant properties and its effects on HDL cholesterol metabolism have generated renewed interest. Probucol is generally well tolerated with few significant side effects. At present, except for patients with homozygous familial hypercholesterolemia and refractory tendinous xanthomas, probucol is not generally considered to be a first-line lipid-altering drug. Its ultimate role and efficacy as an antiatherogenic agent have yet to be determined.

Marine Oils

Interest in the possible beneficial role of marine oils originated in the early 1970s when Bang and Dyerberg noticed that Greenland Eskimos had lower plasma concentrations of triglycerides, total cholesterol, and low density lipoprotein, as well as a lower incidence of coronary heart disease, compared to mainland Danes. They also found higher plasma levels of the omega-3 fatty acid eicosapentaenoic acid (EPA) [111]. These Eskimos consume marine animal products that contain substantial quantities of omega-3 fatty acids, and it was postulated that such a diet may contribute to a beneficial lipid profile and a lower incidence of CHD [112].

More recently a number of studies have addressed the possible mechanisms by which a diet high in omega-3 fatty acids might be beneficial. In addition to lipid-altering effects, possible effects on other atherogenic factors, including hypertension, diabetes, fibrinogenesis, and platelet function, have been examined.

The primary serum lipid alteration resulting from an increased intake of omega-3 fatty acids is a reduction of serum triglycerides on the order of 30 to 50 percent [113, 114, 115, 116, 117] (although TG reductions have been observed to be greater than 60 percent by some investigators) [118]. Effects on total, LDL, and HDL cholesterol have been variable [115, 116, 117, 118]. The dosages of omega-3 fatty acids typically studied have been high, frequently over 4 g per day. Lower, more clinically practical omega-3 fatty acid doses on the order of 1 to 2 g per day may not be as efficacious in lowering TG and may possibly be associated with increases in serum LDL concentrations [119].

With regard to the effects of omega-3 fatty acids on other mechanisms related to CHD, some investigators have shown a lowering of diastolic blood pressure with high doses [114], while other preliminary studies have found little or no change in blood pressure [120]. Fasting glucose levels of diabetic individuals may be increased by omega-3 fatty acids [115]. Fibrinogen levels may be decreased [118, 119], while the effect on platelet aggregation remains unclear [114, 120].

Omega-3 fatty acid preparations are commercially available in a variety of forms and dosage strengths. As with niacin these medications are considered to be food supplements and do not require a prescription. They may be used as second or possibly third-line agents in the treatment of hypertriglyceridemia. Interest in the potential uses of these preparations remains high, but the ultimate role of omega-3 fatty acids in the lipid-altering armamentarium remains to be determined.

While the use of marine-oil supplements has only very limited indications at the present, patients asking about the use of such agents should be told that the best way to increase one's intake of these oils is to eat more fish, a dietary change that also lowers saturated fat intake.

Cost

In a patient who requires pharmacologic lipid management, the primary consideration is the efficacy and safety of a drug regimen. The cost of these agents also needs to be considered, since therapy for hyperlipidemia may need to be lifelong and the population receiving pharmacologic therapy is potentially very large.

The cost of a certain intervention properly includes not only the monetary cost per unit dose, but also the cost of side effects, physician visits, and necessary blood tests. The benefit of the intervention with regard to changes in morbidity and mortality, frequency of physician visits, hospitalizations and diagnostic procedures, and productivity should also be considered. These issues are discussed in greater detail in Chapter 21.

Schulman et al. conducted a cost-effectiveness analysis for the treatment of hypercholesterolemia [121]. Models were designed using cholestyramine, colestipol, gemfibrozil, lovastatin, niacin, and probucol. Attempts were made to incorporate all potential costs of therapy, including physician visits, laboratory studies, necessary screening tests, interventions used

Table 12-4.   Costs of commonly prescribed hypolipidemic medications

Drug	Size	Price	Annual cost
Cholestyramine	1 packet 4 g	$1.30	$949/1 packet bid
Colestipol	1 packet 5 g	$1.31	$957/1 packet bid
Gemfibrozil	600 mg	$0.99	$723/1 tab bid
Nicotinic acid (Slo-niacin)	500 mg	$0.09	$66/1 tab bid
Lovastatin	20 mg	$1.82	$666/1 tab qd
	40 mg	$3.24	$1182/1 tab qd
Pravastatin	10 mg	$1.74	$636/1 tab qd
	20 mg	$1.84	$672/1 tab qd
Simvastatin	10 mg	$1.65	$602/1 tab qd
	20 mg	$3.00	$1095/1 tab qd
Probucol	500 mg	$1.21	$884/1 tab bid

*As of the time of publication pharmacy pricing for simvastatin was not yet available.
Source: Local pharmaceutical chain, Worcester, MA. Retail prices as of February 1992.

to manage side effects, costs of side effects in terms of hospitalizations and procedures, and comedication costs. Annual medication costs ranged from $327 (niacin) to $1881 (lovastatin, 80 mg/day). Niacin was the most efficient agent for reducing LDL cholesterol levels, averaging $139 per percent reduction in LDL cholesterol. Lovastatin was also efficient at $177 per percent reduction, while cholestyramine was least efficient at $347. Niacin and gemfibrozil were determined to be most cost efficient in terms of HDL cholesterol elevation, while niacin and lovastatin were most efficient in reducing the LDL:HDL cholesterol ratio. Studies of this type are limited by their retrospective nature and the many assumptions used in formulating the model, but they are of value in pointing out the many factors that must be considered in a true cost-benefit calculation.

In practice it is useful for physicians to be aware of the costs per dose of the medications they prescribe. Monetary cost certainly plays a role in patient compliance and may indirectly affect the utility of the drug. Table 12-4 lists the cost per dose and annual costs of the medications reviewed in this chapter. Prices shown were obtained from a local pharmaceutical chain in Worcester, Massachusetts, and reflect retail prices as of February 1992.

Summary

This chapter reviewed the pharmacologic management of dyslipidemias. Several different classes of medications were discussed, each with unique lipid-altering mechanisms, indications, side effects, and outcomes. Epidemiologic, clinical, and physiologic data support the premise that cholesterol reduction in the hypercholesterolemic patient is beneficial. Therefore, it is important for the clinician to recognize those patients who should be treated pharmacologically and to be knowledgeable at selecting the optimal treatment modality. Pharmacologic therapy of lipid abnormalities is only one part of the total therapeutic plan and should always be considered in the context of the other treatment modalities discussed in this book.

References

1. The Expert Panel. Report of the National Cholesterol Education Program Expert Panel on detection, evaluation, and treatment of high blood cholesterol in adults. Arch Intern Med 1988; 148:36–69.
2. The Lipid Research Clinics Program. The Lipid Research Clinics Coronary Primary Prevention Trial Results. I. Reduction in incidence of coronary heart disease. JAMA 1984; 251:351–64.
3. Castelli WP, Garrison RJ, Wilson PWF, et al. Incidence of coronary heart disease and lipoprotein cholesterol levels. JAMA 1986; 256:2835–8.
4. Stamler J, Wentworth D, Neaton JD. Is relationship between serum cholesterol and risk of premature death from coronary heart disease continuous and graded? Findings in 356,222 primary screenees of the multiple risk factor intervention trial (MRFIT). JAMA 1986; 256:2823–8.
5. Genest JJ, Mcnamara JR, Salem DN, et al. Prevalence of risk factors in men with premature coronary artery disease. Am J Cardiol 1991; 67:1185–9.
6. Ginsburg GS, Safran C, Pasternak RC. Frequency of low serum high-density lipoprotein cholesterol levels in hospitalized patients with

"desirable" total cholesterol levels. Am J Cardiol 1991; 68:187–92.

7. Shepherd J. Mechanism of action of bile acid sequestrants and other lipid lowering drugs. Cardiol 1989; 76:65–74.

8. Crouse JR. Hypertriglyceridemia: a contraindication to the use of bile acid binding resins. Am J Med 1987; 83:243–8.

9. Mabuchi H, Haba T, Tatami R, et al. Effects of an inhibitor of 3-hydroxy-3-methylglutaryl coenzyme A reductase on serum lipoproteins and ubiquinone-10 levels in patients with familial hypercholesterolemia. N Engl J Med 1981; 305:478–82.

10. Illingworth DR. Mevinolin plus colestipol in therapy for severe heterozygous familial hypercholesterolemia. Ann Intern Med 1984; 101:598–604.

11. Grundy SM, Vega GL, Bilheimer DW. Influence of combined therapy with mevinolin and interruption of bile-acid reabsorption on low density lipoproteins in heterozygous familial hypercholesterolemia. Ann Intern Med 1985; 103:339–43.

12. The Lipid Research Clinics Program. The Lipid Research Clinics Coronary Primary Prevention Trial results. II. The relationship of reduction in incidence of coronary heart disease to cholesterol lowering. JAMA 1984; 251:365–74.

13. Levy RI, Brensike JF, Epstein SE, et al. The influence of changes in lipid values induced by cholestyramine and diet on progression of coronary artery disease. Results of the NHLBI type II coronary intervention study. Circulation 1984; 69:325–37.

14. LaRosa J. Review of clinical studies of bile acid sequestrants for lowering plasma lipid levels. Cardiol 1989; 76:55–64.

15. Todd PA, Ward A. Gemfibrozil. A review of its pharmacodynamic and pharmacokinetic properties, and therapeutic use in dyslipidaemia. Drugs 1988; 314–39.

16. Illingworth DR. An overview of lipid lowering drugs. Drugs 1988; 36:Suppl. 3:63–71.

17. Illingworth DR, Olsen DG, Cook SF, et al. Ciprofibrate in the therapy of type II hypercholesterolemia. A double blind trial. Atherosclerosis 1982; 44:211–21.

18. Rouffy J, Chanu B, Bakir R, et al. Comparative evaluation of the effects of ciprofibrate and fenofibrate on lipids, lipoproteins and apoproteins A and B. Atherosclerosis 1985; 54:273–81.

19. Weisweiler P, Merck W, Janetschek P, et al. Effect of fenofibrate on serum lipoproteins in subjects with familial hypercholesterolemia and combined hyperlipidemia. Atherosclerosis 1984; 53:321–5.

20. Weisweiler P. Effect of benzafibrate and gemfibrozil on serum lipoproteins in primary hypercholesterolemia. Arzneimittel-Forschung 1988; 38:925–7.

21. Manttari M, Koskinen P, Manninen V, et al. Effect of gemfibrozil on the concentration and composition of serum lipoproteins. A controlled study with special reference to initial triglyceride levels. Atherosclerosis 1990; 81:11–7.

22. Grundy SM, Vega GL. Fibric acids: effects on lipids and lipoprotein metabolism. Amer J Med 1987; 83:9.

23. Lewis JE. Clinical use of gemfibrozil: a controlled multicenter trial. Practical Cardiology 1983; 9:99–118.

24. Leaf DA, Connor WE, Illingworth DR, et al. The hypolipidemic effects of gemfibrozil in type V hyperlipidemia. JAMA 1989; 262:3154–60.

25. Huttunen JK, Frick MH, Heinonen OP, et al. Helsinki Heart Study. New perspectives in the prevention of coronary heart disease. Drugs 1988; 36:32–6.

26. Manninen V, Huttunen JK, Heininen OP, et al. Relation between baseline lipid and lipoprotein values and the incidence of coronary heart disease in the Helsinki Heart Study. Amer J Cardiol 1989; 63:42H–7H.

27. Frick MH, Elo O, Haapa K, et al. Helsinki Heart Study: Primary-prevention trial with gemfibrozil in middle-aged men with dyslipidemia: safety of treatment, changes in risk factors, and incidence of coronary heart disease. N Engl J Med 1987; 317:1237–45.

28. Manninen V, Koskinen P, Manttari M, et al. Predictive value for coronary heart disease of baseline high-density and low-density lipoprotein cholesterol among Fredrickson type IIa subjects in the Helsinki Heart Study. Am J Cardiol 1990; 66:A24–7.

29. Manttari M, Romo M, Manninen V, et al. Reduction in Q wave myocardial infarctions with gemfibrozil in the Helsinki Heart Study. Am Heart J 1990; 119:991–5.

30. Illingworth DR, Bacon S. Treatment of heterozygous familial hypercholesterolemia with lipid-lowering drugs. Arteriosclerosis 1989; 9:121–34.

31. Tikkanen MJ, Helve E, Jaattela A, et al. Comparison between lovastatin and gemfibrozil in the treatment of primary hypercholesterolemia: the Finnish Multicenter Study. Am J Cardiol 1988; 62:35J–43J.

32. Vega GL, Grundy SM. Comparison of lovastatin and gemfibrozil in normolipidemic patients with hypoalphalipoproteinemia. JAMA 1989; 262:3148–53.

33. Samuel P. Efficacy of gemfibrozil as a lipid regulator in a patient population in the United States. Vasc Med 1984; 2:8–15.

34. Kaukola S, Manninen V, Malkonen M, et al. Gemfibrozil in the treatment of dyslipidaemias in middle-aged male survivors of myocardial infarction. Acta Med Scand 1981; 209:69–73.

35. Hodges RM, Marcus EL. Safety of gemfibrozil (Lopid) in clinical use. Research and Clinical Forums 1982; 4:37–42.

36. Pierce LR, Wysowski DK, Gross TP. Myopathy and rhabdomyolysis associated with lovastatin-gemfibrozil combination therapy. JAMA 1990; 264:71–5.

37. Kogan AD, Orenstein S. Lovastatin-induced acute rhabdomyolysis. Postgrad Med J 1990; 66:294–6.

38. Committee of Principal Investigators. Report on a WHO cooperative trial on primary prevention of ischaemic heart disease using clofibrate to lower serum cholesterol — mortality follow up. Lancet 1980; 2:379–85.

39. Altschul R, Hoffer A, Stephen JD. Influence of nicotinic acid on serum cholesterol in man. Arch Biochem Biophys 1955; 51:308–9.

40. Figge HL, Figge J, Souney PF, et al. Nicotinic acid: a review of its clinical use in the treatment of lipid disorders. Pharmacotherapy 1988; 8(5):287–94.

41. Altschul R, Herman IH. Influence of oxygen inhalation on cholesterol metabolism. Arch Biochem Biophys 1954; 51:308–9.

42. Altschul R. Inhibition of experimental cholesterol arteriosclerosis by ultraviolet iradiation. N Engl J Med 1953; 249:96–9.

43. Grundy SM, Mok HYI, Zech L, et al. Influence of nicotinic acid on metabolism of cholesterol and triglycerides in man. J Lipid Res 1981; 22:24–36.

44. Carlson LA. Studies on the effect of nicotinic acid on catecholamine stimulated lipolysis in adipose tissue in vitro. Acta Med Scand 1963; 172:641–5.

45. The Coronary Drug Project Research Group. Clofibrate and niacin in coronary heart disease. JAMA 1975; 231:360–81.

46. Shepherd J, Packard CJ, Patsch JR, et al. Effects of nicotinic acid therapy on plasma high density lipoprotein subfraction distribution and composition and on apolipoprotein A metabolism. J Clin Invest 1979; 63:858–67.

47. Blankenhorn DH, Nessim SA, Johnson RL, et al. Beneficial effects of combined colestipol-niacin therapy on coronary atherosclerosis and coronary venous bypass grafts. JAMA 1987; 257:3233–40.

48. Cashin-Hemphill L, Mack WJ, Pogoda JM, et al. Beneficial effects of colestipol-niacin on coronary atherosclerosis. JAMA 1990; 264:3013–7.

49. Canner PL, Berge KG, Wenger NK, et al. Fifteen year mortality in coronary drug project patients: long-term benefit with niacin. J Am Coll Cardiol 1986; 8:1245–55.

50. Knopp RH, Ginsberg J, Albers JJ, et al. Contrasting effects of unmodified and time-release forms of niacin on lipoproteins in hyperlipidemic subjects: clues to mechanism of action of niacin. Metabolism 1985; 34:642–50.

51. Olsson AG, Carlson LA, Anggard E, et al. Prostaglandin production augmented in the short term by nicotinic acid. Lancet 1983; 2:565–7.

52. Hoeg JM, Gregg RE, Brewer HB. An approach to the management of hyperlipoproteinemia. JAMA 1986; 255:512–21.

53. Svedmyr N, Heggelund A, Aberg G. Influence of indomethacin on flush induced by nicotinic acid in man. Acta Pharmacol Toxicol 1977; 41:397–400.

54. Knopp RH, Ginsberg J, Alberts JJ, et al. Contrasting effects of unmodified and time-release forms of niacin on lipoproteins in hyperlipidemic subjects: clues to mechanism of action of niacin. Metabolism 1985; 34:642–50.

55. Garg A, Grundy SM. Nicotinic acid may not be first line therapy for dyslipidemia in non-insulin-dependent diabetes mellitus (NIDDM) (abstract). Clin Res 1989; 37:449A.

56. Molnar GD, Berg KG, Rosevear JW, et al. The effect of nicotinic acid in diabetes mellitus. Metabolism 1964; 13:181–9.

57. Patterson DJ, Dew EW, Gyorkey F, et al. Niacin hepatitis. South Med J 1983; 107:324–9.

58. Henkin Y, Johnson KC, Segrest JP. Rechallenge with crystalline niacin after drug-induced hepatitis from sustained-release niacin. JAMA 1990; 264:241–3.

59. Alberts AW. Discovery, biochemistry and biology of lovastatin. Am J Cardiol 1988; 62:10J–15J.

60. Steinberg D, Avigan J, Feigelson EB. Effects of triparanol (MER-29) on cholesterol biosynthesis and on blood sterol levels in man. J Clin Invest 1961; 40:884–93.

61. Kirby TJ. Cataracts produced by triparanol. Trans Am Ophthal Soc 1967; 65:494–543.

62. Endo A, Kuroda M, Tsujita Y. ML-236A, ML-236B, and ML-236C, new inhibitors of colesterogenesis produced by Penicillium citrinum. J Antibiot 1976; 29:1346–8.

63. Endo A, Tsujita Y, Kuroda M, et al. Inhibition of cholesterol synthesis in vitro and in vivo by ML-236A and ML-236B, competitive inhibitors of 3-hydroxy-3-methylglutaryl coenzyme A reductase. Eur J Biochem 1977; 77:31–6.

64. Endo A. Monacolin K, a new hypocholesterolemic agent produced by a Monascus species. J Antibiot 1979; 32:852–4.

65. Henwood JM, Heel RC. Lovastatin. A preliminary review of its pharmacodynamic properties and therapeutic use in hyperlipidaemia. Drugs 1988; 36:429–54.

66. Alberts AW, Chen J, Kuron G, et al. Mevinolin: a highly-potent competitive inhibitor of hydroxymethylglutaryl-coenzyme A reductase and a cholesterol-lowering agent. Proc Natl Acad Sci USA 1980; 77:3957–61.

67. Germershausen JI, Hunt VM, Bostedor RG, et al. Tissue selectivity of the cholesterol-lowering agents lovastatin, simvastatin and pravastatin in rats in vivo. Biochem Biophys Res Comm 1989; 158:667–75.

68. Koga T, Shimada Y, Kuroda M, et al. Tissue-selective inhibition of cholesterol synthesis in vivo by pravastatin sodium, a 3-hydroxy-3-methylglutaryl coenzyme A reductase inhibitor. Biochem Biophys Acta 1990; 1045:115–20.

69. Kannel WB, D'Agostino RB, Stepanians M, et al. Efficacy and tolerability of lovastatin in a six-month study: analysis by gender, age and hypertensive status. Am J Cardiol 1990; 66:1B–10B.

70. Bradford RH, Shear CL, Chremos AN, et al. Expanded Clinical Evaluation of Lovastatin (EXCEL) Study results. I. Efficacy in modifying plasma lipoproteins and adverse event profile in 8245 patients with moderate hypercholesterolemia. Arch Int Med 1991; 151:43–9.

71. Lovastatin Study Group II. Therapeutic response to lovastatin (mevinolin) in nonfamilial hyprcholesterolaemia. JAMA 1986; 256:2829–34.

71a. Pan HY, DeVault AR, Swites BJ, et al. Pharmacokinetics and pharmacodynamics of pravastatin alone and with cholestyramine in hypercholesterolemia. Clin Pharmacol Ther 1990; 48(2):201–7.

71b. Walker JF. Simvastatin: the clinical profile. Am J Med 1989; 87(4A):44S–6S.

71c. Crepaldi G, Baggio G, Arca M, et al. Pravastatin vs. gemfibrozil in the treatment of primary hypercholesterolemia. Arch Intern Med 1991; 151(1):146–52.

71d. Stein E, Kreisberg R, Miller V, et al. Effects of simvastatin and cholestyramine in familial and nonfamilial hypercholesterolemia. Arch Intern Med 1990; 150(2):341–5.

72. Cobb MM, Teitelbaum HS, Breslow JL. Lovastatin efficacy in reducing low density lipoprotein cholesterol levels on high- vs low-fat diets. JAMA 1991; 265:997–1001.

73. Havel RJ, Hunninghake DB, Illingworth DR, et al. Lovastatin (mevinolin) in the treatment of heterozygous familial hypercholesterolemia. Ann Int Med 1987; 107:609–15.

74. Hoeg JM, Maher MB, Bailey KR, et al. The effects of mevinolin and neomycin alone and in combination on plasma lipid and lipoprotein concentrations in type II hyperlipoproteinemia. Atherosclerosis 1986; 57:933–9.

75. Illingworth DR. Comparative efficacy of once versus twice daily mevinolin in the therapy of familial hypercholesterolaemia. Clin Pharm Therap 1986; 40:338–43.

76. Illingworth DR, Sexton GJ. Hypocholesterolemic effects of mevinolin in patients with heterozygous familial hypercholesterolaemia. J Clin Invest 1984; 74:1972–8.

77. Hirano T, Komura F, Furukawa S, et al. Effect of pravastatin sodium, a new inhibitor of 3-hydroxy-3-methylglutaryl coenzyme A reductase, on very-low-density lipoprotein composition and kinetics in hyperlipidemia associated with experimental nephrosis. Metabolism: Clin and Exper 1990; 39:605–9.

78. Grundy SM, Lena Vega G, Garg A. Use of 3-hydroxy-3-methylglutaryl coenzyme A reductase inhibitors in various forms of dyslipidemia. Am J Cardiol 1990; 66:31B–8B.

79. Kane JP, Malloy MJ, Ports TA, et al. Regression of coronary atherosclerosis during treatment of familial hypercholesterolemia with combined drug regimens. JAMA 1990; 264:3007–12.

80. Zhao X-Q, Flygenring BP, Stewart DK, et al. Increased potential for regression of post-PTCA restenosis using intensive lipid-altering therapy: comparison with matched non-PTCA lesions (abstract). J Amer Coll Cardiol 1991; 17:230A.

81. Pitt B, Ellis SG, Mancini GBJ, et al. Pravastatin limitation of atherosclerosis in the coronary arteries (PLAC I): design features and recruitment statistics of a U.S. multicenter quantitative angiographic trial of lipid-lowering (abstract). J Amer Coll Cardiol 1991; 17:37A.

82. Barth JD, Meester GT, Meijler FL, et al. "REGRESS." A trial to assess the lipid lowering effects of pravastatin in "normocholesterolemic" men with myocardial ischemia (abstract). J Amer Coll Cardiol 1991; 17:69A.

83. Jones PH. Lovastatin and simvastatin prevention studies. Am J Cardiol 1990; 66:39B–43B.

84. Bradford RH, Shear CL, Chremos AN, et al. Expanded Clinical Evaluation of Lovastatin (EXCEL) Study: design and patient characteristics of a double-blind, placebo-controlled study in patients with moderate hypercholesterolemia. Am J Cardiol 1990; 66:44B–55B.

85. Mantell G, Burke MT, Staggers J. Extended clinical safety profile of lovastatin. Am J Cardiol 1990; 66:11B–5B.

86. Tobert JA. Efficacy and long-term adverse effect pattern of lovastatin. Am J Cardiol 1988; 62:28J–34J.

86a. Physicians Desk Reference, Publisher Edward R. Barnhart, Medical Economics Data, NJ. 1992.

87. Butman SM. Hyperlipidemia after cardiac transplantation — be aware and possibly wary of drug therapy for lowering of serum lipids. Am Heart J 1991; 121:1585–90.

88. Buckley MMT, Goa KL, Price AH, et al. Probucol. A reappraisal of its pharmacological properties and therapeutic use in hypercholesterolaemia. Drugs 1989; 37:761–800.

89. Kesaniemi YA, Grundy SM. Influence of probucol on cholesterol and lipoprotein metabolism in man. J Lipid Res 1984; 25:780–90.

90. Baker SG, Joffe BI, Mendelsohn D, et al. Treatment of homozygous familial hypercholesterolaemia with probucol. S Afr Med J 1982; 62:7–11.

91. Yamamoto A, Matsuzawa Y, Kishino B, et al. Effects of probucol on homozygous cases of hypercholesterolemia. Atherosclerosis 1983; 48:157–66.

92. Naruszewicz M, Carew TE, Pittman RC, et al. A novel mechanism by which probucol lowers low density lipoprotein levels demonstrated in the LDL receptor-deficient rabbit. J Lipid Res 1984; 25:1206–13.

93. Steinberg D. Studies on the mechanism of action of probucol. Am J Cardiol 1986; 57:16H–21H.

94. Beynen AC. Discrepancies between the outcome of animal and human studies on the mode of action of probucol. Atherosclerosis 1986; 61:249–51.

95. Strandberg TE, Vanhanen H, Miettinen TA. Probucol in long-term treatment of hypercholesterolemia. Gen Pharmacol 1988; 19:317–20.

96. Miettinen TA. Mode of action of a new hypocholesterolemic drug. Atherosclerosis 1972; 15:163–76.

97. Nestel PJ, Billington T. Effects of probucol on low density lipoprotein removal and high density lipoprotein synthesis. Atherosclerosis 1981; 38:203–9.

98. Yamamoto A, Matsuzawa Y, Yokoyama S, et al. Effects of probucol on xanthoma regression in familial hypercholesterolemia. Am J Cardiol 1986; 57:29H–35H.

99. Francechini G, Sirtori M, Vaccarino V, et al. Mechanisms of HDL reduction after probucol. Changes in HDL subfractions and increased reverse cholesterol ester transfer. Arteriosclerosis 1989; 9:462–9.

100. Matsuzawa Y, Yamashita S, Funahashi T, et al. Selective reduction of cholesterol in HDL2 fraction by probucol in familial hypercholesterolemia and hyper HDL2 cholesterolemia with abnormal cholesterol ester transfer. Am Jour Cardiol 1988; 62:66B–72B.

101. Steinberg D, Parthasarathy S, Carew TE, et al. Beyond cholesterol: modifications of low-density lipoprotein that increase its atherogenicity. N Engl J Med 1989; 320:915–24.

102. Parthasarathy S, Young SG, Witztum JL, et al. Probucol inhibits oxidative modification of low density lipoprotein. J Clin Invest 1986; 77:641–4.

103. Klein L. QT-interval prolongation produced by probucol. Arch Intern Med 1981; 141: 1102–3.

104. Troendle G, Gueriguian J, Sobel S, et al. Probucol and the QT interval. Lancet 1982; I:1179.

105. Hattori M, Tsuda K, Taminato T, et al. Effect of probucol on serum lipids and apoproteins in patients with non-insulin-dependent diabetes mellitus. Curr Therapeut Res 1987; 42:967–73.

106. Iida H, Izumino K, Asaka M, et al. Effect of probucol on hyperlipidemia in patients with nephrotic syndrome. Nephron 1987; 47:280–3.

107. Morisaki N, Mori S, Kobayashi J, et al. Effects of long-term treatment with probucol on serum lipoproteins in cases of familial hypercholesterolemia in the elderly. J Amer Geriat Soc 1990; 38:15–8.

108. Heel RC, Brogden RN, Speight TM, et al. Probucol: a review of its pharmacological properties and therapeutic use in patients with hypercholesterolaemia. Drugs 1978; 15:409–28.

109. Tedeschi RE, Martz BL, Taylor HA, et al. Safety and effectiveness of probucol as a cholesterol lowering agent. Artery 1982; 10:22–34.

110. Miettinen TA, Huttunen JK, Naukkarinen V, et al. Long-term use of probucol in the multifactorial primary prevention of vascular disease. Amer J Cardiol 1986; 57:49H–54H.

111. Bang HO, Dyerberg J. Plasma lipids and lipoproteins in Greenlandic west coast Eskimos. Acta Med Scand 1972; 192:85–94.

112. Bang HO, Dyerberg J, Sinclair HM. The composition of the Eskimo food in north western Greenland. Am J Clin Nutr 1980; 33:2657–61.

113. Reis GJ, Silverman DI, Boucher TM, et al. Effects of two types of fish oil supplements on serum lipids and plasma phospholipid fatty acids in coronary artery disease. Amer J Cardiol 1990; 66:1171–5.

114. Levinson PD, Iosiphidis AH, Saritelli AL, et al. Effects of n-3 fatty acids in essential hypertension. Amer J Hyperten 1990; 3:754–60.

115. Hendra TJ, Britton ME, Roper DR, et al. Effects of fish oil supplements in NIDDM subjects. Controlled study. Diabet Care 1990; 13:821–9.

116. Dart AM, Riemersma RA, Oliver MF. Effects
     of Maxepa on serum lipids in hypercholester-
     oleaemic subjects. Atherosclerosis 1989;
     80:119–24.
117. Harris WS, Rothrock DW, Fanning A, et al.
     Fish oils in hypertriglyceridemia: a dose-re-
     sponse study. Amer J Clin Nutr 1990; 51:399–
     406.
118. Haglund O, Wallin R, Luostarinen R, et al.
     Effects of a new fluid fish oil concentrate, ES-
     KIMO-3, on triglycerides, cholesterol, fibri-
     nogen, and blood pressure. J Int Med 1990;
     227:347–53.

119. Radack KL, Deck CC, Huster GA. n-3 fatty
     acid effects on lipids, lipoproteins, and apoli-
     poproteins at very low doses: results of a ran-
     domized controlled trial in hypertrigly-
     ceridemic subjects. Am J Clin Nutr 1990;
     51:599–605.
120. Landgraf-Leurs MM, Drummer C, Froschi H,
     et al. Pilot study on omega-3 fatty acids in type
     I diabetes mellitus. Diabetes 1990; 39:69–375.
121. Schulman KA, Kinosian B, Jacobson TA, et al.
     Reducing high blood cholesterol level with
     drugs. JAMA 1990; 264:3025–33.

13

Intervention for Control of Hypertension

BRIAN F. JOHNSON

EDITORS' INTRODUCTION

Multiple studies have convincingly shown that hypertension is an important independent risk factor for CHD. Treatment of elevated blood pressure clearly reduces the incidence of cardiovascular complications such as congestive heart failure and stroke. Yet it has been much harder to provide definitive evidence that the long-term treatment of hypertension is of benefit in the prevention of CHD. In this chapter Dr. Brian Johnson reviews the data pertinent to this interesting topic, points out the weaknesses of some of the studies in this area, and looks particularly at some questions that have been raised about the use of specific agents such as the thiazide diuretics. He also reviews the possibility that overly aggressive treatment of hypertension may lead to deleterious effects, the so-called "J-shaped curve." He then looks at the value of ambulatory blood pressure monitoring and provides comprehensive recommendations for treatment, including the use of various nonpharmacologic modalities.

There is overwhelming evidence that many types of cardiovascular disease, including CAD, stroke, claudication, and heart failure, are more frequent in persons with untreated hypertension (Figure 13-1). The Framingham Heart Study [1, 2] established that high blood pressure is an independent risk factor for cardiovascular disease. Further, as shown in Figure 13-2, in both men and women higher blood pressure levels have been associated with progressively increasing risks of CHD. These conclusions have been confirmed in other prospective studies, perhaps most convincingly demonstrated in the Pooling Project, in which 7000 white men, aged 40 to 59, were followed for 10 years in five different locations in the United States [3].

Evidence from life insurance companies is also compelling, despite limitations in the methods used to measure baseline blood pressure. In the Build and Blood Pressure Study [4], over four million subjects followed for up to 20 years demonstrated a stepwise increase in mortality with increasing systolic or diastolic blood pressure. These studies all concluded that hypertensive women have lower risks than comparable men for cardiovascular complications and that blacks have somewhat higher levels of blood pressure and increased mortality when compared to whites. In the Multiple Risk Factor Intervention Trial (MRFIT) [5], when data from over 23,000 black men were compared to those from more than 325,000 white men, hypertensive blacks had somewhat lower mortality rates from CHD but a higher mortality rate from stroke.

By tradition diastolic blood pressure has been used to establish and define the severity of hypertension. However, data from the Framingham and other studies indicate that systolic blood pressure is more predictive of risk of cardiovascular complications. This is particularly true in the elderly, in whom isolated elevation of systolic blood pressure is common [6]. Isolated systolic hypertension in the elderly is associated with increased risks of all cardiovascular complications, but most dramatically with the risk of stroke.

Hypertension interacts powerfully with other independent cardiovascular risk factors. An in-

dividual's overall cardiovascular risk status can be calculated if the full range of these risk factors is known. For example, using the 18-year follow-up data from the Framingham Study, relative risk can be calculated based on age, sex, systolic blood pressure, serum total cholesterol and HDL cholesterol, history of cigarette smoking, level of glucose tolerance, and electrocardiographic evidence of left ventricular hypertrophy (LVH). Figure 13-3 illustrates the interaction of some of these factors. The prediction of CHD risk is more fully described in chapter 4 [7].

The coexistence of independent risk factors is more frequent than would be expected by chance alone. It is well known that diabetes mellitus is more common in hypertensives than in the general population. More recently it has become apparent that a plasma lipid abnormality is about four times more common in hypertensives than in the general population. A new syndrome of familial dyslipidemic hypertension has been defined as the presence of both hypertension and abnormal blood lipids in two or more siblings. With dyslipidemia defined as either LDL cholesterol or triglycerides above the ninetieth percentile or HDL cholesterol below the tenth percentile for the general population, it has been estimated that at least 48 percent of hypertensive sibling pairs diagnosed before the age of 60 years fall within the criteria of this syndrome [8].

Many of the cardiovascular complications of hypertension are almost exclusively related to the enhanced development of atherosclerosis. In larger arteries smooth-muscle cells and cholesterol ester accumulate in the intima to form the characteristic atherosclerotic plaque. In smaller arteries hypertrophy, hyperplasia, and fibrosis of the tunica media are the basic processes by which obstruction occurs. Manifestations of CHD, ischemic strokes, and nephrosclerosis may follow the development of obstructive lesions in the coronary, extra- or intracranial, or renal arteries.

These complications are simply more common in hypertensives. Some cardiovascular complications, however, are almost specific for hypertensives. Intracerebral bleeds are due to

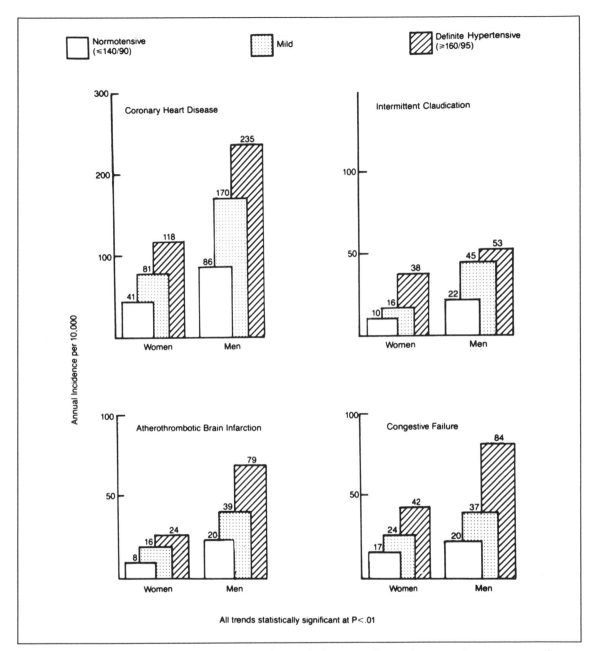

Figure 13-1. Age-adjusted risk of cardiovascular morbidity according to hypertensive status at each biennial examination over 26-year follow-up of the men and women aged 35 to 84 in the Framingham cohort. (Source: Kannel WB, In: Kaplan NM. Clinical hypertension. Baltimore: Williams & Wilkins, 1986.)

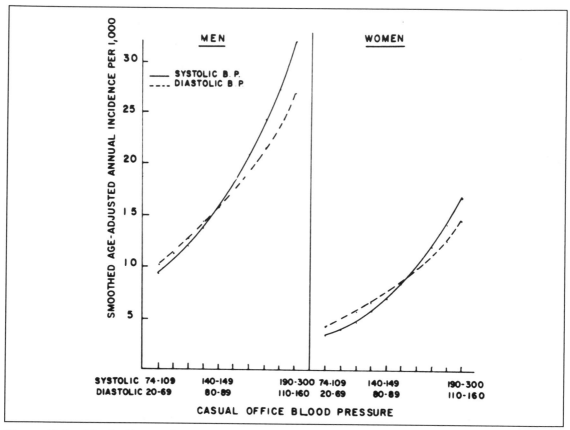

Figure 13-2. The incidence of CHD according to systolic versus diastolic blood pressure in men and women aged 45 to 74 in the Framingham study over a 20-year follow-up. (Source: Castelli WP. In: Kaplan NM. Clinical hypertension. Baltimore: Williams & Wilkins, 1986.)

rupture of Charcot-Bouchard aneurysms of small cerebral penetrating arterioles. Degenerative changes in the media of the aorta lead to an increased risk of aortic dissection in hypertensives. Further, very high levels of blood pressure may cause extensive fibrinoid necrosis in small arteries throughout the body. This accelerated malignant phase of hypertension may rapidly damage the kidneys, exacerbate the severity of hypertension, and precipitate other complications. Finally, left ventricular hypertrophy, once believed to represent a compensatory response to the increased cardiac workload associated with hypertension, is now recognized to be an indicator of increased risk of morbidity and mortality. In addition to an increased risk of congestive cardiac failure, patients with left ventricular hypertrophy have a

high risk of sudden cardiac death, which may be related to the higher incidence of ventricular dysrhythmias seen in such patients [9]. Essentially all of the complications shown in Table 13-1 result from abnormalities in arteries or the myocardium.

In recent years intriguing new data have been reported that suggest that hypertension may hasten the development of atheromatous and other cardiac diseases independent of the degree of blood pressure elevation. Peripheral resistance to the action of insulin is increased in hypertension, and although possibly secondary to decreased skeletal muscle blood supply [9a], this finding has not been seen in secondary hypertension [9b]. In essential hypertension the consequent increase in plasma insulin concentration may potentiate both plasma lipid ab-

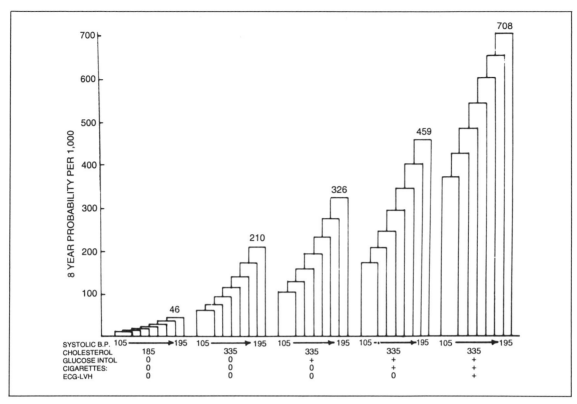

Figure 13-3. The 8-year risk of cardiovascular disease for 40-year-old men in Framingham according to progressively higher systolic blood pressure at specified levels of other risk factors. (Source: Kannel WB. In: Kaplan NM. Clinical hypertension. Baltimore, Williams & Wilkins, 1986.)

normalities and vascular smooth-muscle hypertrophy [10, 11]. Further, children of hypertensive parents may show signs of left ventricular hypertrophy and diastolic dysfunction before demonstrating any evidence of blood pressure elevation.

The Value of Blood Pressure Reduction

The rationale for reducing elevated levels of blood pressure is that the associated complications can be prevented. The evidence that the natural history of hypertension can be favorably altered is incontrovertible. Prevention of cardiovascular complications in hypertension may be considered one of the major success stories in recent medical history. However, the benefits have not been uniform. In particular, dramatic inhibition of the risks of stroke has been pro-

duced but the apparent impact of antihypertensive therapy on coronary artery disease has been much more modest.

Despite the established benefits of the treatment of hypertension, it seems unlikely that risks can be totally prevented. In several studies patients taking antihypertensive drugs have been shown to have higher morbidity and mortality rates than people whose blood pressure level did not require treatment, despite reduction of blood pressure to comparable levels. A 10-year follow-up study of 7610 Japanese men in Hawaii showed higher age-adjusted mortality from both CHD and stroke for men on medication than for untreated subjects with comparable blood pressure levels [12].

In the last 30 years there has been a steady decline in mortality rates due to cardiovascular disease. Most analyses have concluded that the treatment of hypertension has been responsible

Table 13-1. Cardiovascular complications of hypertension

Hypertensive
  Cerebral hemorrhage
  Aortic dissection
  Renal insufficiency
  Encephalopathy or retinopathy grade III or IV
  Malignant or accelerated hypertension
  Cardiac enlargement
  Left ventricular hypertrophy
Atherosclerotic
  Cerebral thrombosis
  Myocardial infarction
  Coronary insufficiency
    Angina pectoris
    Electrocardiographic abnormality: ischemia, arrhythmias, and conduction disturbances
Claudication syndromes

Source: Smith WM. Treatment of mild hypertension: results of a ten-year intervention trial. Circ Res 40:Suppl 1:I-98, 1977, and by permission of the American Heart Association.

for only a small part of this effect. It appears that morbidity rates for both MI and stroke were already declining well before effective control of hypertension was being widely applied to the population [13]. Goldman and Cook [14] concluded that about half of the observed fall in CHD mortality rates could be accounted for by decreased cigarette smoking and lifestyle changes that reduced plasma lipid levels. These authors concluded that antihypertensive treatment accounted for about 8.5 percent of the fall in the incidence of CHD mortality between 1968 and 1976.

The most important evidence that antihypertensive therapy prevents cardiovascular complications comes from clinical trials conducted over the last 30 years. The landmark studies were conducted by the Veterans Administration Cooperative Study Group. In 1967, this group reported [15] that within 1½ years, treatment with hydrochlorothiazide, reserpine, and hydralazine significantly reduced the rate of hypertensive complications in 73 men with diastolic blood pressures between 115 and 129 mm Hg. Table 13-2 compares the mortality and morbidity of the treatment and placebo groups. In the severe hypertensives who were untreated,

almost 40 percent developed serious complications of their hypertension in less than 3 years.

The second report of the Veterans Administration Cooperative Study Group [16] showed that antihypertensive therapy was also beneficial in men with more moderate hypertension: diastolic blood pressures between 90 and 114 mm Hg. Not surprisingly, larger numbers of hypertensives and longer periods of therapy were required to demonstrate significant differences between the treatment and placebo groups. In 380 men, after an average period of treatment of 3.3 years, the placebo group had more than twice the mortality and serious morbidity from hypertensive complications. Differences between the treated and the placebo groups are shown in Table 13-3. More detailed analysis showed that differences in morbidity were highly significant for those patients with diastolic blood pressures between 105 and 114 mm Hg but only compatible with a nonsignificant trend in those with diastolic blood pressure readings between 90 and 104 mm Hg [17]. Furthermore, this report provided a basis for concern that therapy might have less benefit against risks of MI than of stroke.

Subsequent studies [18, 19, 20, 21, 22, 23, 24, 25] have predictably shown less dramatic results than the Veterans Administration studies, which did not exclude patients with evidence of previous cardiovascular disease and which concentrated largely on patients with moderately severe or severe hypertension. However, studies of milder degrees of hypertension are of great importance because of the much greater prevalence of this level of blood pressure elevation. Almost 60 percent of the increased risk of mortality in hypertensives occurs among those with diastolic blood pressure levels between 90 and 104 mm Hg. Table 13-4 provides information about the major trials that have been completed in the area of mild-to-moderate hypertension. These studies varied widely in design, reflecting differing opinions about the relative importance of the ethical and scientific considerations involved. For example, in the Hypertension Detection and Follow Up Program Cooperative Group Study [23] and the MRFIT Research Group Study [24] there were

Table 13-2. Mortality and morbidity in patients with diastolic blood pressure between 115 and 129 mm Hg

	Group receiving placebo	Group receiving antihypertensive drug
Number in study	70	73
Deaths	4	0
Complications	23	2
Accelerated hypertension	12	0
Cerebrovascular accident	4	1
Coronary artery disease	2	0
Congestive heart failure	2	0
Renal damage	2	0
Treatment failure	1	1

Source: Veterans Administration Cooperative Study Group on Antihypertensive Agents. In: Kaplan NM. Clinical hypertension. Baltimore: Williams & Wilkins, 1986.

Table 13-3. Mortality and morbidity in patients with diastolic blood pressure between 90 and 114 mm Hg

Diagnosis	Placebo group (n = 194)		Antihypertensive drug group (n = 186)	
	Fatal	Nonfatal	Fatal	Nonfatal
Cerebrovascular accident	7	13	1	4
Coronary artery disease	11*	2	6	5
Congestive heart failure	0	11	0	0
Accelerated hypertension	0	4	0	0
Renal damage	0	3	0	0
Aortic aneurysm rupture	1	1	1	0
Other	0	3	0	5
Total	19	37	8	14

*Includes sudden deaths.

Source: Veterans Administration Cooperative Study Group on Antihypertensive Agents: In: Kaplan NM. Clinical hypertension. Baltimore: Williams & Wilkins, 1986.

no true placebo control groups, so that comparisons were made primarily between groups given intensive standardized care and those referred to the care of their regular community physicians. These studies have been criticized as being "as much a trial of medical care as of antihypertensive drugs" [21].

Statistical techniques have been developed to pool the results of trials with different entry criteria and treatment regimens [26]. Table 13-5 lists the results of all placebo-controlled trials of antihypertensive therapy used in such an analysis carried out by Dollery [27]. Altogether, a total of 11,284 patients in these trials received active treatment and 11,237 patients received placebo. In the placebo group there were 208 fatal and nonfatal strokes; there were 96 fewer strokes in the group receiving active treatment. The results for prevention of MI, however, are much less impressive. Whereas 348 patients developed either fatal or nonfatal MI during placebo treatment, there were only 24 fewer occurrences in the active treatment group. The reduction in the number of strokes was as anticipated from the observed reduction in blood pressure, but the 7 percent reduction in the rate of MI fell far short of the effect that would have been expected. Somewhat better results were

Table 13-4.   Major trials in mild to moderate hypertension

Study	Number of patients	% Male	Duration (years)	Initial DBP range (mm)	Group DBP difference (mm)
VA[a][16]	380	100	3.3	90–114	19
USPHS[a][18]	389	80	7	90–114	10
ANBP[a][19]	3,427	80	4	95–109	6
Oslo[a][20]	785	100	5.5	90–109	10
MRC[a][21]	17,354	52	5.5	95–109	6
EWPHE[a][22]	840	30	4.7	90–119	10
HDFP[b][23]	7,825	54	5	90–104	4
MRFIT[b][24]	8,012	100	7	90–114	4
IPPPSH[b][25]	6,357	50	4	100–125	1

[a]Control group received placebo or no treatment.
[b]Control group received less treatment.

Table 13-5.   Differences in incidence of stroke and MI in placebo-controlled trials

Study	% difference in stroke	% difference in MI
Veterans Administration 1 [18]	−67	—
Veterans Administration 2 [15]	−75	+40
US Public Health Service [16]	−83	−7
Australian Therapeutic Trial [19]	−41	0
Medical Research Council [21]	−45	−5
European Working Party [22]	−33	−18
Total	−46	−7

— = too few myocardial infarctions for meaningful comparison.

reported from subsequent meta-analysis of 14 randomized trials involving over 37,000 patients treated for a mean duration of 5 years and with a mean diastolic BP reduction of 5 to 6 mm Hg. A significant 14 percent reduction in CHD deaths and non-fatal MIs was reported [27a], but again this was well below the anticipated level of benefit.

Because the incidence of stroke and MI is declining spontaneously in many countries, it is difficult to interpret the conclusions of trials conducted without a placebo control group. The study of the Medical Research Council Working Party [28] had the great advantages of a large sample size, a placebo control group, and two active drug treatment groups (a thiazide diuretic and the beta blocker propranolol). Unfortunately about 20 percent of the study entrants were withdrawn because of adverse re-

actions to therapy or excessive rise in blood-pressure; another 20 percent simply "lapsed from follow-up". Despite the high dropout rate, the strengths of this study have aided acceptance of its main conclusions. Although total mortality rate was hardly affected by either type of active drug therapy, the rate of development of strokes was significantly reduced, particularly in those patients receiving the thiazide diuretic. No overall impact of either active drug on coronary events was seen, though benefit was apparent in nonsmoking men who took propranolol. The investigators concluded that 850 mildly hypertensive patients were required to be treated for a year to prevent one stroke.

Several explanations for the relative failure of antihypertensive therapy to reduce the incidence of manifestations of CHD have been put forward. It is conceivable that there is no direct link between the level of blood pressure and changes in the coronary arteries. If so, coronary and cerebral arteries must differ in some important but unknown way. A second hypothesis is that antihypertensive treatment is usually delayed until irreversible changes in the coronary vessels have occurred. However, comparable clinical trials of hypolipidemic therapy have shown reduced risks of clinical CHD within a 5-year period. A further argument is that antihypertensive therapy does not produce consistent control of blood pressure and that average results incorporate subgroups of both poorly controlled and overcontrolled patients. It is easy to understand that poorly controlled hypertensives would not benefit; more recently there have been concerns about a so-called J-shaped relationship between mortality and blood pressure level in treated hypertensives. Although controversial, it appears that the trend for mortality to be progressively reduced with increasing control of hypertension may be reversed in those patients showing the greatest fall in blood pressure. It has been reported that risk of death increases for some patients whose diastolic blood pressure is lowered below 85 mm Hg [29, 30]. It is possible that such patients have preexisting though undetected CAD with myocardial perfusion critically dependent on a diastolic blood pressure level in the 80 mm Hg range. Finally, it has been suggested that some commonly used drugs may themselves have negative effects that partially offset the benefits of blood pressure reduction [31].

In almost all of the major trials of antihypertensive therapy, a thiazide diuretic was the first active drug to be administered. In three of the trials, subsequent analysis of morbidity or mortality raised concerns that hypertensives with ECG abnormalities have higher risks of CHD, particularly sudden death, if treated with thiazides. Originally suggested in the MRFIT [24], similar nonsignificant trends were subsequently found in the Hypertension Detection and Follow-Up Program Study [23] and in a trial conducted in Oslo, Norway [20]. Although these results were inconclusive [32], suspicions that

thiazide diuretics could have specific risks have greatly reduced their popularity as first-line treatment for hypertensives.

Only one study has suggested that CHD might be better prevented with beta-blocking treatment than with thiazide diuretics. Unfortunately, the Metoprolol Atherosclerosis Prevention in Hypertensives (MAPHY) trial was an extension study of a patient sample that had completed an earlier trial in which patients could receive either metoprolol or atenolol. The differing conclusions of the original trial and the extension trial have greatly limited acceptance of the claim that metoprolol has special value in preventing CHD [33].

Detection and Evaluation

In the last decade it has become more common for blood pressure to be measured routinely by almost all health care professionals. The importance of hypertension has been extensively reported in the media, and a high proportion of people now want to know their own blood pressure levels. Unfortunately, as it becomes less common for hypertension to remain undiagnosed, large numbers of people may be inappropriately labeled as hypertensive on the basis of inadequate information. In particular, the extent to which blood pressure responds to such factors as an unaccustomed clinical environment is not appreciated by all physicians.

Criteria for diagnosis have been established by the Joint National Committee on Detection, Evaluation and Treatment of High Blood Pressure [34]. It is important to average the results of multiple readings on a minimum of two visits, after measuring blood pressure with the appropriately sized sphygmomanometer cuff after the patient has been sitting quietly for 5 minutes. Table 13-6 lists the classifications appropriate for adults based on an average of multiple blood pressure readings. Decisions about treating elevated blood pressure should usually be deferred until hypertension has been confirmed and its severity established. More rapid institution of treatment is recommended, however,

Table 13-6. Classification of blood pressure in adults age 18 years or older

Range (mm Hg)	Category*
Diastolic	
<85	Normal blood pressure
85–89	High normal blood pressure
90–104	Mild hypertension
105–114	Moderate hypertension
≥115	Severe hypertension
Systolic, when diastolic blood pressure is <90	
<140	Normal blood pressure
140–159	Borderline isolated systolic hypertension
≥160	Isolated systolic hypertension

Classification based on the average of two or more readings on two or more occasions.

*A classification of borderline isolated systolic hypertension (SBP 140–159 mm Hg) or isolated systolic hypertension (SBP ≥160 mm Hg) takes precedence over high normal blood pressure (diastolic blood pressure, 85–89 mm Hg) when both occur in the same person. High normal blood pressure (DBP 85 to 89 mm Hg) takes precedence over a classification of normal blood pressure (SBP <140 mm Hg) when both occur in the same person.
Source: National High Blood Pressure Education Program. The 1988 report of the Joint National Committee on Detection, Evaluation, and Treatment of High Blood Pressure. U.S. Department of Health and Human Services, National Institutes of Health. USDHHS publ. no. (NIH) 88-1088, May 1988.

if diastolic blood pressure is greater than 115 mm Hg on two visits or greater than 130 on any visit.

The evaluation of an individual presenting with consistent elevation of blood pressure is aimed at answering three major questions:

• Does the patient have the common inherited form of essential hypertension or a much rarer and potentially curable secondary form of hypertension?
• Is there evidence that the hypertension may have already produced complications?
• Are other risk factors for cardiovascular disease present?

Secondary causes of hypertension should be expected in children or young adults with hypertension, in subjects in whom hypertension has suddenly appeared or suddenly worsened,

in hypertensives in whom the family history is clearly negative, or in patients refractory to various drug treatments. Hyperaldosteronism may be suggested by muscle cramps or weakness and most commonly by the detection of hypokalemia. Pheochromocytoma often presents with attacks of sweating, palpitations, flushing, and headache, and the patient may also have a tendency to orthostatic hypotension. During the physical examination abdominal bruits should suggest renal artery stenosis, and delayed or absent femoral pulses indicate the likelihood of arotic coarctation.

The second and third questions are particularly important in borderline and mild hypertensives because they provide information relevant to the risk of future cardiovascular complications. Control of relatively minor levels of blood pressure elevation is important in hypertensives who have concurrent diabetes or who have already suffered a complication such as a stroke. Table 13-7 lists the most important factors a physician should elicit during the evaluation of the typical patient.

It has been shown that left ventricular hypertrophy is a better predictor of cardiovascular mortality in hypertension than the level of blood pressure itself. Echocardiographic determination of left ventricular mass detects seven to ten times more patients with left ventricular hypertrophy than electrocardiography [35]. Whereas about 4 percent of hypertensives have left ventricular hypertrophy according to ECG criteria, echocardiographic studies have determined its presence in 20 to 50 percent of hypertensives. Echocardiographic measurements of left ventricular mass are correlated with increased risks of cardiovascular complications, cardiovascular mortality, and overall mortality [36]. These observations have raised questions about the advisability of routine echocardiographic screening of hypertensives and of subsequent follow-up to determine reversal of left ventricular hypertrophy. There is, however, a clear need to standardize echocardiographic methods. Clinical trials are needed to determine whether the different capacities of antihypertensive agents to reverse left ventricular hyper-

Table 13-7. Major factors in the evaluation of essential hypertension

History of:	Any complications (see Table 13-1)
	Smoking
Physical examination findings of:	
	Cardiac dilatation with added heart sound
	Congestive cardiac failure
	Retinal arteriovenous compression
	Retinal exudates, hemorrhages, or papilledema
	Diminished carotid or pedal pulses
	Carotid or femoral bruit
Laboratory evaluation showing:	
	Renal function impairment
	Left ventricular hypertrophy detected by ECG
	Diabetes mellitus
	Plasma lipid abnormality

trophy are related to comparable benefits in reduction of morbidity and mortality rates. Currently echocardiographic assessment should probably be used selectively, focusing on patients with severe or drug-resistant hypertension.

Whereas all experts agree that patients with moderately or severely elevated levels of blood pressure require treatment, there are differing opinions about mild hypertension. Various authorities have recommended that therapy should be instituted with persistent diastolic blood pressure measurements above levels of 90, 95, or 100 mm Hg. Within the diastolic blood pressure range of 90 to 100 mm Hg, treatment should more readily be initiated in patients who are black, male, or exhibiting any of the factors listed in Table 13-7.

Isolated systolic hypertension may rarely be found in younger adults, in whom it may be the first manifestation of the prehypertensive state. However, the incidence of this finding rises exponentially with age. Although the pathogenesis remains somewhat controversial, it is a separate entity from essential hypertension and is not caused by atherosclerosis. The available evidence suggests that decreased compliance of large arteries renders them less able to absorb systolic pressure and to recoil effectively during diastole. Heart rate, stroke volume, and left ventricular ejection rate are usually within normal limits. Although the mechanism of elevation of systolic pressure is different in this disorder from that of essential hypertension, isolated systolic hypertension is equally associated with increased risks of cardiovascular morbidity and mortality [37].

Despite the clear risk associated with isolated systolic hypertension, until recently there was no definite evidence that treatment of this condition was of value. There are now two studies, however (Swedish Trial in Old Patients with Hypertension; Systolic Hypertension in the Elderly Program (SHEP)) that have shown important and significant reductions in morbidity and mortality from cardiovascular disease and stroke resulting from treatment of elderly patients with hypertension [37a, 37b]. In the SHEP study the relative risk (RR) of stroke was .64 in the treatment group; the RR for clinical nonfatal myocardial infarction plus coronary death was .73. Therapy in this study was stepped-care drug treatment, beginning with low-dose chlorthalidone.

In addition to diuretics it has been suggested that calcium channel blockers and angiotensin-converting enzyme (ACE) inhibitors may have special value in reducing isolated systolic hypertension. Because the elderly are at greater risk for electrolyte imbalance, drowsiness, or mental confusion as side effects of some antihypertensive agents, extra care in selecting the appropriate drug is required.

The Relevance of Ambulatory Blood Pressure Measurement

As methods of recording ambulatory blood pressure have become more reliable and less expensive, interesting new information has been presented about the relationship between ambulatory blood pressure and the incidence of complications and about the temporal relationship between circadian variations in blood pressure and the incidence of cardiovascular disease.

The great variability of blood pressure in any given individual was first demonstrated by pioneering work at Oxford, England, in which an intra-arterial catheter, pump, pressure transducer, and recording device were worn by volunteers for many hours [38]. The development of automated sphygmomanometer methods has permitted reasonably frequent blood pressure measurements to be obtained in patients in a much less invasive manner. Such determinations have exposed the relative weaknesses of the customary office or outpatient clinic methods of determining blood pressure. In many subjects a clinic determination is higher than representative values during normal activity. More important the differences between clinic and ambulatory levels vary strikingly between patients, and repeated clinic measurements are less consistent than repeated determinations of ambulatory blood pressure, probably due to variability in individual patients' alerting, or "white-coat," responses to the clinical environment. It is believed that between 10 and 25 percent of subjects have been misdiagnosed as hypertensive on the basis of office or outpatient clinic readings. It may be argued that the association between hypertension and cardiovascular risk has been established using outpatient clinic measurements, and the latter therefore represent the validated method of blood pressure determination. However, several studies have demonstrated a better correlation between left ventricular hypertrophy and ambulatory blood pressure than with clinic determinations [39, 40]. Further, the only reasonably sized study comparing blood pressure methods concluded that ambulatory determinations are a better predictor than clinic blood pressure of the future incidence of cardiovascular complications [41].

There may also be an important link between circadian changes in blood pressure and the similar rhythms in incidence of cardiovascular diseases. As shown in Figure 13-4, mean values of blood pressure and heart rate show a circadian rhythm, with the lowest values occurring during sleep. Blood pressure begins to rise about two hours before waking and continues to rise to reach a peak value by about 10 a.m. [42]. This period of 4 to 6 hours is associated with a similar rise in heart rate and is termed the *acceleration phase*. The potential importance of this phase is that it coincides with the time of maximal incidence of episodes of angina pectoris, MI, sudden cardiac death, and stroke [43]. Figure 13-5 shows that in 24 patients with symptomatic angina documented by positive exercise tests the frequency of ischemic episodes detected by ambulatory ECG monitoring began to increase at 6 a.m. and reached a peak at about 9 a.m. During this period of the day plasma concentrations of catecholamines and platelet aggregability increase, and blood fibrinolytic activity decreases [44]. The concurrent increase in vascular resistance (determined by forearm plethysmography) can be reversed by alpha-adrenergic blockade [44a]. Circadian changes in autonomic nervous system activity are the probable underlying mechanism for some of these changes, which could have a causative role in precipitating cardiovascular events. Possible mechanisms include increased left ventricular work and oxygen requirement, increased blood coagulability, and rupture of atherosclerotic plaques by the increasing pressure of blood both in the lumen of the artery and in the proliferating vasa vasorum that are known to surround a plaque [45]. If a causative relationship exists between the acceleration phase and increased risk of cardiovascular complications, therapeutic programs aimed at modifying circadian changes in blood pressure and heart rate might have promise. By inference treatments that reduce overall liability during waking hours could have special value.

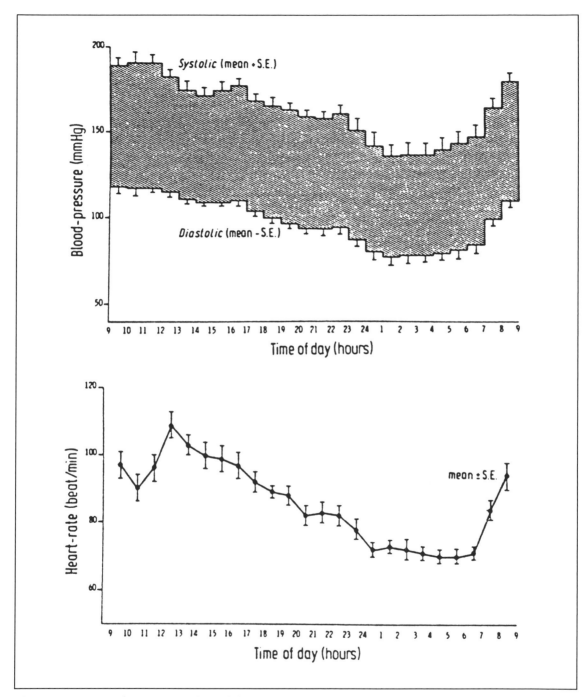

Figure 13-4.   Hourly mean systolic and diastolic blood pressures and heart rates throughout 24 hours in 20 untreated hypertensive patients. (Source: Millar-Craig MW, Bishop CN, Raftery EB. Circadian variation of blood-pressure. Lancet 1978; 1:795–7.)

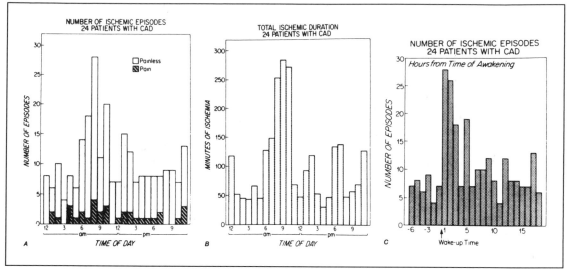

Figure 13-5.   Hourly distribution of number of episodes (*A*) and total minutes of ischemic duration (*B*) in 24 patients with ischemic ST segment depression. There is a significant peak of ischemic activity between 6 a.m. and 12 noon. When the number of episodes is corrected for the time of waking (*C*), the peak density of ischemic activity occurs immediately upon rising. (Source: Rocco MB, Barry BA, Campbell S, et al. Circadian variation of transient myocardial ischemia in patients with coronary artery disease. Circulation 1987; 75:395, and by permission of the American Heart Association.)

Nonpharmacologic Therapy of Hypertension

Although most patients with significant hypertension require drug therapy, nonpharmacologic forms of therapy should be considered for all. In general such therapy is less reliable than drug treatment and usually produces relatively modest blood pressure reduction. Of course efficacy is greatest in those patients who are appropriately instructed and motivated. As with other changes in lifestyle, it is counterproductive to prescribe too many therapies initially. The following methods have a rational basis for their efficacy and are listed in decreasing order of recommended priority.

1. Alcohol restriction. There is a clear relation between excessive alcohol intake and hypertension [46]. Although opinions differ as to the minimal daily level of alcohol ingestion required to raise blood pressure, patients should be strongly encouraged to lower their consumption to two drinks per day, assuming an alcohol content of 8–10g per drink.

2. Weight reduction. There is a clear correlation between body weight and blood pressure, and reduction in weight may be associated with a fall in blood pressure in obese hypertensives. Vigorous attempts to promote weight control are indicated, despite the realization that weight loss is difficult to achieve in most patients and there is a high rate of recidivism. Even modest amounts of weight loss, on the order of 10 pounds, are sometimes associated with significant decreases in BP [46a].

3. Exercise. Aerobic exercises such as walking, bicycling, and swimming are clearly preferable to isometric efforts such as weightlifting, which have an excessive blood pressure-increasing effect. Exercise programs should be initiated gradually at levels appropriate for the general health status of the individual patient. A minimal program should include at least 30 minutes of exercise at least 3 days per week.

4. Sodium-restricted diet. There is no doubt that excessively high sodium intake is important in maintaining high blood pressure

in some patients and in inhibiting the effectiveness of drug therapy. However, only a proportion of patients have blood pressure levels sensitive to the effects of moderate sodium restriction, i.e., daily allowances of 70 mEq of sodium, equivalent to 4 g of salt, and opinions differ as to whether blood pressure can be significantly reduced in this manner [47, 47a]. Currently, there is no simple way of recognizing whether a patient is salt-sensitive or -insensitive [48]. It seems reasonable to assess the effect of reduced salt intake in all patients and continue it in those showing measurable benefit. Although improved labeling of the sodium content of processed foods may prove helpful, most patients require dietary counseling to achieve adequate sodium restriction.

It is important to point out that while the value of salt restriction in the individual patient with hypertension appears to be relatively modest, there is increasing evidence that lowering the population dietary intake of salt would be of considerable value. The INTERSALT study showed a clear relationship between salt intake and mean population blood pressure [48a], and other analyses of population-based data have come to similar conclusions [48b].

Furthermore, the recently reported phase I results of the Trials of Hypertension Prevention [48c] showed significant reductions of both systolic and diastolic blood pressure with salt-reduced diets in individuals with high normal levels of blood pressure, suggesting that reduction of salt intake may be of special value in preventing the onset of hypertension.

5. Other dietary changes. Evidence regarding other dietary modifications appears inconclusive. An increase in potassium intake to above 80 mEq per day can produce moderate reduction in blood pressure [49]. A high potassium diet should not be recommended for patients with impaired renal function or for those taking potassium-sparing diuretics or ACE inhibitors. The role of other modifications is even more controversial, including the great attention that has been given to dietary calcium. Despite the possible direct relationship between serum ionized calcium concentration and blood pressure, dietary calcium supplementation has unreliable effects on blood pressure in hypertensives. There is also conflicting evidence concerning the value of increasing the polyunsaturated component of dietary fat in lowering blood pressure, although this change should reduce the risk of CHD in hypertensives with hypercholesterolemia. Finally, there are unconfirmed reports that increasing the fiber content of the diet can lower blood pressure to a modest extent in some patients.

6. Biofeedback and relaxation. Programs of biofeedback and relaxation therapy have shown promising results in selected groups of hypertensives [50]. A combination of the two techniques may have preferable results, but well-designed clinical trials are still needed to assess the definitive place of such programs in antihypertensive therapy. As with most other nonpharmacologic treatments, careful training and follow-up to ensure long-term patient compliance are needed if any lasting benefit is to be obtained.

Although drinking caffeine-containing beverages and smoking can both acutely raise blood pressure, it appears that tolerance to hemodynamic effects develops so that there is no increased frequency of hypertension in smokers or those consuming excessive amounts of caffeine. All hypertensives must be strongly encouraged to stop smoking, not because blood pressure will be reduced but because of the greatly increased risks of cardiovascular disease in such patients.

General Principles of Antihypertensive Drug Therapy

The aim of antihypertensive drug therapy should be to consistently lower the resting level of systolic blood pressure to below 140 mm Hg and the resting level of diastolic blood pressure to below 90 mm Hg. Because few patients have complaints before treatment begins, the long-term objective must be to prevent increased morbidity and mortality without reducing the quality of the patient's life. In most situations therapy should be chosen in an unhurried manner after full evaluation of the patient during multiple clinic visits. Immediate therapy is required only for those rare patients who have developed life-threatening complications, such as encephalopathy. Although less urgent, there should be no delay in initiating treatment in patients with retinal hemorrhages or exudates, or diastolic blood pressure levels that remain above 130 mm Hg after resting for at least 30 minutes.

Selection of an Appropriate Drug

Unfortunately no clinical trials have been performed to compare the effects on morbidity or mortality of beginning therapy with representative drugs from the major groups available. This is a serious deficiency, because it follows that there is no solid basis for preferring any specific drug. The Joint National Committee on Detection, Evaluation and Treatment of High Blood Pressure [34] recommends that initial drug treatment be selected from one of four classes: diuretics, beta blockers, calcium channel antagonists, and ACE inhibitors. A reasonable case can be made for the use of members of any of these drug classes, since they are uncommonly associated with severe adverse effects and are each capable of effectively reducing blood pressure in 60 to 70 percent of unselected groups of patients.

The traditional way to increase therapy is to maintain the ineffective drug, while adding a second one, i.e., step care [34]. In practice most physicians now prefer to replace an ineffective drug with the second one to be tried, although adding a second agent to a partially-effective first agent is also very reasonable. If a representative agent from each of the four first-line drug groups is utilized and no single agent is effective, combinations of previously used agents may provide adequate control.

It has been assumed that drugs equally effective in lowering blood pressure probably also have equal benefits. This may be a naive view in light of the different pharmacologic actions of the drugs and their different effects on other predictors of the risk of CHD.

In the absence of data on comparative long-term effects on morbidity or mortality, the factors that should be considered when choosing an antihypertensive drug are listed in Table 13-8. In general beta blockers and ACE inhibitors are less effective than diuretics in lowering blood pressure in blacks or the elderly. Tables 13-9 through 13-12 list the more common adverse effects of antihypertensive drugs. If minimizing cost of therapy is crucial, either generic propranolol or a diuretic should be considered first. Diuretics or ACE inhibitors may have added value in a hypertensive patient with signs of congestive heart failure; similarly a beta blocker or calcium antagonist may be the most efficient therapy for a hypertensive patient with angina or migraine headaches. Patients are more likely to take their prescribed medication consistently if it is effective when conveniently taken once a day.

Other selection criteria reflect the varying effects of drugs on cardiovascular risk factors, with the reasonable inference that they will have different effects on morbidity and mortality. Thiazide diuretics are of particular concern. As previously noted, they have been associated with higher risks of sudden death in certain subgroups of hypertensives, possibly because dysrhythmia may be precipitated by potassium loss in patients with high preexisting risk levels. Thiazide diuretics should not be the drug of first choice in a patient with electrocardiographic abnormalities suggestive of CHD, left ventricular hypertrophy, or ventricular dysrhythmia. Thia-

Table 13-8. Factors physicians should consider when choosing an antihypertensive drug

Efficacy in relation to age and race
Frequency of adverse symptoms
Cost
Value in concurrent illness
Convenience/compliance
Change in cardiovascular risk profile
Reversal of left ventricular hypertrophy

Table 13-9. Common adverse effects of thiazide diuretics

Typical regimens	*More common adverse effects*
Hydrochlorothiazide, 25–50 mg once daily Methoclothiazide, 2.5–10 mg once daily Chlorthalidone, 25–50 mg once daily Hydrochlorothiazide, 50 mg plus triamterene 75 mg (Maxzide) once daily	Hypokalemia (muscle weakness or pains) Gout precipitated Worsening of diabetes Hyperlipidemia
Hydrochlorothiazide, 25 mg plus triamterene 50 mg (Dyazide) once or twice daily	All of the above except hypokalemia

Table 13-10. Common adverse effects of beta-blockers

Typical regimens	*More common adverse effects*

Nonselective
  Propranolol (long acting), 80–240 mg daily
  Nadolol, 40–160 mg once daily
	
	Bronchospasm
	Slowed cardiac conduction

Cardioselective
  Metoprolol, 50–200 mg twice daily
  Atenolol, 50–100 mg once daily
  Betaxolol, 10–20 mg once daily
	
	Bradycardia
	Fatigue/lethargy
	Cold hands and feet

Table 13-11. Common adverse effects of ACE inhibitors

Typical regimens	*More common adverse effects*
Captopril, 25–100 mg twice daily	Dry cough
Enalapril, 5–40 mg once daily Lisinopril, 5–40 mg once daily	Rash Loss of taste Orthostatic faintness

Table 13-12. Common adverse effects of calcium channel blockers

Typical regimens	*More common adverse effects*
Nifedipine (sustained action), 60–90 mg once daily	Ankle swelling Palpitations Headache Dizziness
Verapamil (sustained release), 240 mg once daily	Constipation Slowed cardiac conduction Raised serum digoxin level
Diltiazem (sustained release), 90–180 mg twice daily	Any of above, but all less frequent

zide diuretics also worsen glucose tolerance, probably by inducing tissue resistance to the effects of circulating insulin. This is a particular concern in hypertension, in view of the known enhanced risk of vascular disease in conditions in which resistance to plasma insulin is a feature (e.g., obesity and non–insulin-dependent diabetes).

Another area of concern is the potentially detrimental effect of some antihypertensive agents on plasma lipoprotein profiles [51]. Table 13-13 provides calculated approximations of the effects of antihypertensive agents on plasma lipids. It is clear that thiazides have the potential to elevate both cholesterol and triglyceride levels. With the exception of agents like pindolol, which have intrinsic sympathomimetic activity, almost all beta blockers have an equally worrying propensity to lower HDL cholesterol levels. Calcium channel blockers and ACE inhibitors generally do not affect plasma lipoprotein profiles.

If patients fail to respond appropriately to any of the four first-line drugs, two alternatives are of particular interest. Alpha-1 blockers like prazosin (1 to 10 mg twice daily) and terazosin (1 to 10 mg once daily) produce potentially beneficial changes in the lipid profile by improving the ratio of HDL to LDL cholesterol. Limited information suggests that the alpha-2 stimulant group of drugs, which includes guanabenz (4 to 8 mg twice daily) and clonidine (.1 to .3 mg twice daily), may also lower total cholesterol in hypertensives. In general, the use of thiazide diuretics and most of the beta blockers should be avoided in hypertensive patients with lipid abnormalities. In such patients it is reasonable to use a lipid-neutral agent (calcium channel blocker or ACE inhibitor). It is also appropriate to consider one of the agents that has potentially beneficial effects. However these agents are more likely to cause side effects: first-dose fainting, dizziness, headache, palpitations, or ankle swelling with alpha-1 blockers; and dry mouth, drowsiness, or risk of withdrawal-rebound effects with alpha-2 stimulants.

Finally, because left ventricular hypertrophy is a major independent risk factor for cardiac dysrhythmia and sudden death [52], it is reasonable to favor therapy that is most effective in restoring thickened myocardium to normal size. All four first-line drugs may reverse hypertrophy, but thiazide diuretics are much slower and less effective in this regard. They also do not reduce ventricular ectopy, at least not within 2 to 3 months of observation [53]. Direct-acting vasodilators such as minoxidil and hydralazine have been shown to worsen left ventricular hypertrophy.

Thiazide diuretics are implicated in most of the areas of concern in relation to cardiovascular risk. A suitable alternative for hypertensives in whom a diuretic seems essential is indapamide, which has less tendency to cause hypokalemia, does not worsen hyperlipidemia or glucose tolerance, and may reverse left ven-

Table 13-13. Calculated approximations of the extent of antihypertensive-drug effect on plasma lipids

Drug	TC	TG	HDLC	LDLC
Thiazides	+7%	+14%	+ 2%	+10%
Propranolol	0	+16%	−11%	− 3%
Atenolol	0	+15%	− 7%	− 2%
Pindolol	− 1%	+ 7%	− 2%	− 3%
Alpha-1 blockers	− 4%	− 8%	+ 5%	−13%
Alpha-1 stimulants	− 7%	—	—	—
Calcium channel blockers	0	0	0	0
ACE inhibitors	0	0	0	0

TC = total cholesterol; TG = triglycerides; HDLC = high-density lipoprotein cholesterol; LDLC = low-density lipoprotein cholesterol.

Source: Adapted from Johnson BF, Danylchuk MA. The relevance of plasma lipid changes with cardiovascular drug therapy. Med Clinics of NA 1989; 73(2):449.

tricular hypertrophy more rapidly than a thiazide diuretic. It is, however, considerably more expensive.

Possible Direct Effects of Antihypertensive Drugs Against Atherosclerosis

Increasing evidence from animal studies suggests that at least some antihypertensive agents may have the capacity to inhibit atherosclerosis. Hypertension produces altered morphology and permeability of the arterial endothelium, permitting entry of leukocytes into the subendothelium with accumulation of smooth-muscle cells and macrophages. However, abnormal plasma lipids are required for these changes to progress to lesions typical of atherosclerosis. Therefore, most studies have been performed in cholesterol-fed normotensive rabbits, Watanabe heritable hyperlipidemic (WHHL) rabbits that have defective LDL receptors, or rats with balloon-catheter carotid artery injury. Antihypertensive drugs have been reported to have varied effects on the development of lesions in these models [54]. Propranolol was seen to have an inhibitory effect in several models, possibly due to inhibition of endothelial permeability. There has been a great deal of interest in the observation that various calcium channel blockers can inhibit lesions in cholesterol-fed rabbits, possibly by altering hemodynamics or by affecting cell migration, growth-regulatory substances, or the binding of oxidized LDL cholesterol to subintimal extracellular materials [54a]. More recent studies have shown that the ACE inhibitor captopril is effective in the WHHL rabbit model, in which other agents are usually ineffective.

These studies have raised the possibility that some antihypertensive agents may have important beneficial effects apart from their potential for lowering blood pressure. Important concerns include the variability of response in different animal models and the probability that dosages used in experiments are considerably higher than relevant dosages of the drugs used clinically.

Regardless of their limitations, the animal studies have stimulated several important clinical trials. In the International Nifedipine Trial on Antiatherosclerotic Therapy (INTACT) [55] progress of CHD was assessed in 348 patients over 3 years by coronary arteriography. There was no difference in rate of progression or regression of existing lesions, but the group receiving 80 mg of nifedipine daily showed a 28-percent reduction in the number of new coronary lesions. It has been suggested that the nifedipine analogue isradipine may be unique in being effective in animal models at doses comparable to those prescribed clinically. The Multi-Center Isradipine Diuretic Atherosclerosis Study (MIDAS) is a large-scale clinical trial comparing isradipine with hydrochlorothiazide [56]. A goal of this study is to compare the effects of the two drugs on the wall thickness of carotid arteries using ultrasonography.

Hypertension That Responds Poorly to Treatment

A minority of patients fail to obtain adequate control of blood pressure despite receiving combination therapy with full doses of at least three agents. In these situations it is first necessary to confirm that the blood pressure is truly elevated persistently. Lack of clinical evidence of hypertensive complications should raise the suspicion that clinic blood pressure determinations are not representative of the patient's normal levels. In particular, left ventricular hypertrophy should be demonstrable by echocardiography in patients with long-standing hypertension of any severity. Ambulatory blood pressure monitoring may demonstrate that the clinic readings are always considerably higher than average waking-period levels. Sphygmomanometer cuff readings may also produce artifactual elevations in elderly patients with rigid, poorly compressible arteries (pseudohypertension).

Once it is established that hypertension is truly refractory to prescribed medication, the following causes should be evaluated:

• Poor compliance. Failure of the patient to take the prescribed medication is the most common reason for poor control of high blood pressure. Combinations of strategies to improve compliance [57] include fully involving patients in the plan to reach agreed blood pressure targets, encouragement of home blood pressure determinations, education of both the patient and selected relatives, use of once-daily regimens, and demonstration that the physician will rapidly respond to a reported drug side effect.

- Drug interactions. The effectiveness of antihypertensives may be reduced by concurrent administration of other drugs that include sympathomimetic agents used as nasal decongestants or appetite suppressants, steroids, nonsteroid anti-inflammatory agents, and tricyclic antidepressants.
- Secondary hypertension. Secondary forms of hypertension are frequently refractory to drug treatment. Endocrine and renal causes of hypertension should be considered, with atherosclerotic renal artery stenosis being a particular consideration in a patient in whom previously well-controlled hypertension has become resistant.
- Fluid retention. In patients who retain excessive quantities of sodium and water, drug refractory hypertension is common. This may occur with various types of renal disease and is also a feature of some types of antihypertensive agents. Fortunately this has become a much less common problem with the increased use of agents from the recommended four first-line drug groups.

In the small percentage of patients who are refractory for some reason other than the above listed causes, it is recommended that powerful drugs with higher risks of adverse side effects be considered. For men minoxidil should be given in conjunction with a diuretic and a beta blocker. For women it may be preferable to use guanethidine with a diuretic, to avoid the side effect of hirsutism seen with minoxidil.

Summary

Although most types of vascular disease are more frequent in untreated hypertension, treatment does not produce consistent benefit. Sustained control of hypertension radically reduces the risk of stroke, but there is relatively modest evidence of a major beneficial effect to prevent MIs and other manifestations of CHD. Since the latter are now the most common complications of hypertension, this relative failure has been disappointing. Various explanations have been proposed, including the possibility that some of the effects of thiazide diuretics and beta-blocking drugs may be detrimental.

A patient with an apparent elevation of blood pressure should be fully evaluated before the physician decides whether to treat. If diastolic blood pressure levels are below 100 mm Hg, evidence of existing complications or other vascular risk factors must be considered. For a sizable minority of subjects, blood pressure levels obtained at home or with ambulatory methods are substantially lower than clinic blood pressure levels, which suggests that some subjects are being treated unnecessarily.

Nonpharmacologic therapy is less reliable than drug treatment, but it should be part of the care of all hypertensives and should be the initial treatment for patients with mild hypertension. In the absence of information about the relative effects on morbidity or mortality of antihypertensive drugs, there is little basis for recommending that any specific drug should be generally preferred for treating a new hypertensive patient. Diuretics, beta blockers, calcium antagonists, and ACE inhibitors are each well-accepted and usually effective in about two-thirds of the patients who receive them. Drug selection is frequently based on the patient's age and race, the cost of the agent, concurrent illness that may respond to a specific agent, interaction with other CHD risk factors, and convenience in administration. The agents differ in their impact on factors believed predictive of risk of CHD and/or sudden death, and may have different effects upon the incidence of these complications. In particular there are concerns that thiazide diuretics could be less beneficial than other agents and might increase cardiovascular risk in some patients. There is a clear need for a major trial to compare the relative effects of thiazide diuretics, beta blockers, calcium antagonists, and the ACE inhibitors on cardiovascular morbidity and mortality. Only after such a trial has been conducted will it be possible to select a particular therapy as optimal.

References

1. Kannel WB, Doyle JT, Ostfeld AM, et al. Optimal resources for primary prevention of atherosclerotic disease. Circulation 1984; 70:157A–205A.
2. Castelli WP. Epidemiology of coronary heart disease: the Framingham study. Amer J Med 1984; 76:4–12.
3. The Pooling Project Research Group. Relationship of blood pressure, serum cholesterol, smoking habit, relative weight and ECG abnormalities to incidence of major coronary events: final report of the Pooling Project. J Chron Dis 1978; 31:201–306.
4. Society of Actuaries and Association of Life Insurance Medical Directors of America. Blood pressure study, 1979 and 1980.
5. Neaton JD, Kuller LH, Wentworth D, Borhani NO. Total and cardiovascular mortality in relation to cigarette smoking, serum cholesterol concentration, and diastolic blood pressure among black and white males followed up for five years. Am Heart J 1984; 108:759–69.
6. Curb JD, Borhani NO, Entwisle G, et al. Isolated systolic hypertension in 14 communities. Am J Epidemiol 1985; 121:362–70.
7. Kannel WB, Wolf PA. Putting it all together: changing the cardiovascular outlook. Am Heart J 1992; 123:264–7.
8. Williams RR, Hopkins PN, Hunt SC, et al. Population-based frequency of dyslipidemia syndromes in coronary-prone families in Utah. Arch Intern Med 1990; 150:582–8.
9. Messerli FH, Ventura HO, Elizardi DJ, et al. Hypertension and sudden death: increased ventricular ectopic activity in left ventricular hypertrophy. Am J Med 1984; 77:18–22.
9a. Julius S, Gudbrandsson T, Jamerson J, et al. The hemodynamic link between insulin resistance and hypertension. J Hypertension 1991; 9:983–6.
9b. Shamiss A, Carroll J, Rosenthal T. Insulin resistance in secondary hypertension. Amer J Hypertension 1992; 5:26–8.
10. Falkner B, Hulman S, Tannenbaum J, Kushner H. Insulin resistance and blood pressure in young black men. Hypertension 1990; 16:706–11.
11. Zavaroni I, Bonora E, Pagliara P, et al. Risk factors for coronary artery disease in healthy persons with hyperinsulinemia and normal glucose tolerance. N Engl J Med 1989; 320:702–6.
12. Yano K, McGee D, Reed DM. The impact of elevated blood pressure upon 10-year mortality among Japanese men in Hawaii: the Honolulu heart program. J Chron Dis 1983; 36:569–79.
13. Garraway WM, Whisnant JP, Drury I. The continuing decline in the incidence of stroke. Mayo Clin Proc 1983; 58:520–3.
14. Goldman L, Cook EF. The decline in ischemic heart disease mortality rates. An analysis of the comparative effects of medical interventions and changes in lifestyle. Ann Intern Med 1984; 101:825–36.
15. Veterans Administration Cooperative Study Group on Antihypertensive Agents. Effects of treatment on morbidity in hypertension. Results in patients with diastolic blood pressures averaging 115 through 129 mm Hg. JAMA 1967; 202:116–22.
16. Veterans Administration Cooperative Study Group on Antihypertensive Agents. Effects of treatment on morbidity in hypertension. II. Results in patients with diastolic blood pressure averaging 90 through 114 mm Hg. JAMA 1970; 213:1143–52.
17. Veterans Administration Cooperative Study Group on Antihypertensive Agents. Effects of treatment on morbidity in hypertension. III. Influence of age, diastolic pressure, and prior cardiovascular disease; further analysis of side effects. Circulation 1972; 45:991–1004.
18. Smith WM. Treatment of mild hypertension. Results of a ten-year intervention trial. U.S. Public Health Service Hospitals Cooperative Study Group. Circ Res 1977; 40:I-98–105.
19. Report by the Management Committee. The Australian therapeutic trial in mild hypertension. The Lancet 1980; 1261–7.
20. Holme I, Helgeland A, Hjermann I, et al. Treatment of mild hypertension with diuretics. The importance of ECG abnormalities in the Oslo Study and in MRFIT. JAMA 1984; 251:1298–9.
21. Peart WS, Miall WE. MRC. mild hypertension trial. The Lancet 1980; 1:104–5.
22. Amery A, Brixko P, Clement D, et al. Mortality and morbidity results from the European Working Party on high blood pressure in the elderly trial. The Lancet 1985; 1349–54.
23. Hypertension Detection and Follow-up Program Cooperative Group. Five-year findings of the hypertension detection and follow-up program. III. Reduction in stroke incidence among persons with high blood pressure. JAMA 1982; 247:633–8.
24. Multiple Risk Factor Intervention Trial Research Group. Baseline rest electrocardiographic abnormalities, antihypertensive treatment, and mortality in the Multiple Risk Factor Intervention Trial. Am J Cardiol 1985; 55:1–15.
25. The IPPPSH Collaborative Group. Cardiovascular risk and risk factors in a randomized trial of treatment based on the beta-blocker oxprenolol: the International Prospective Primary Pre-

vention Study in Hypertension (IPPPSH). J Hypertension 1985; 3:379–92.

26. Yusuf S, Peto R, Lewis J, et al. Beta blockade during and after myocardial infarction: an overview of the randomized trials. Prog Cardiovasc Dis 1985; 27:335–71.

27. Dollery CT. Risk predictors, risk indicators, and benefit factors in hypertension. Am J Med 1987; 82:Suppl 1A:2–8.

27a. Collins R, Peto R, MacMahon S, et al. Blood pressure, stroke and coronary heart disease. II: short-term reductions in blood pressure: overview of randomized drug trials in their epidemiological context. Lancet 1990; 335:827–38.

28. Medical Research Council Working Party. MRC trial of treatment of mild hypertension: principal results. Br Med J 1985; 291:97–104.

29. Samuelsson OG, Wilhelmsen LW, Pennert KM, et al. The J-shaped relationship between coronary heart disease and achieved blood pressure level in treated hypertension: further analyses of 12 years of follow-up of treated hypertensives in the Primary Prevention Trial in Gothenburg, Sweden. J Hypertension 1990; 8:547–55.

30. Farnett L, Mulrow CD, Linn WD, et al. The J-curve phenomenon and the treatment of hypertension. Is there a point beyond which pressure reduction is dangerous? JAMA 1991; 265:489–95.

31. Johnson BF. The emerging problem of plasma lipid changes during antihypertensive therapy. J Cardiovasc Pharmacol 1982; 4:Suppl 2:S213–21.

32. Freis ED. Critique of the clinical importance of diuretic-induced hypokalemia and elevated cholesterol level. Arch Intern Med 1989; 149:2640–8.

33. Kaplan NM. Critical comments on recent literature. SCRAAPHY about MAPHY from HAPPHY. Am J Hyper 1988; 1:428–30.

34. The Joint National Committee. The 1988 report of the Joint National Committee on detection, evaluation, and treatment of high blood pressure. Arch Intern Med 1988; 148:1023–38.

35. Pfeffer MA, Pfeffer JM. Reversing cardiac hypertrophy in hypertension. N Engl J Med 1990; 322:1388–90.

36. Levy D, Garrison RJ, Savage DD, et al. Prognostic implications of echocardiographically determined left ventricular mass in the Framingham Heart Study. N Engl J Med 1990; 322:1561–6.

37. Staessen J, Amery A, Fagard R. Isolated systolic hypertension in the elderly (editorial review). J Hypertension 1990; 8:393–405.

37a. Dahlöf B, Lindholm LH, Hansson L, et al. Morbidity and mortality in the Swedish Trial in Old Patients with Hypertension (STOP-Hypertension). Lancet 1991; 338:1281–5.

37b. SHEP Cooperative Research Group. Prevention of stroke by antihypertensive drug treatment in older persons with isolated systolic hypertension: final results of the Systolic Hypertension in the Elderly Program (SHEP). JAMA 1991; 265:3255–64.

38. Bevan AT, Honour AJ, Stott FH. Direct arterial pressure recording in unrestricted man. Clin Sci 1969; 36:329–44.

39. Pickering TG, Harshfield GA, Devereux RB, Laragh JH. What is the role of ambulatory blood pressure monitoring in the management of hypertensive patients? Hypertension 1985; 7:171–7.

40. White WB, Schulman P, McCabe EJ, Dey HM. Average daily blood pressure, not office blood pressure, determines cardiac function in patients with hypertension. JAMA 1989; 261:873–7.

41. Perloff D, Sokolow M, Cowan R. The prognostic value of ambulatory blood pressure. JAMA 1983; 249:2792–8.

42. Millar-Craig MW, Bishop CN, Raftery EB. Circadian variation of blood-pressure. The Lancet 1978; 795–7.

43. Rocco MB, Barry J, Campbell S, et al. Circadian variation of transient myocardial ischemia in patients with coronary artery disease. Circulation 1987; 75:395–400.

44. Rocco MB, Nabel EG, Selwyn AP. Circadian rhythms and coronary artery disease. Am J Cardiol 1987; 59:13C–17C.

44a. Panza JA, Epstein SE, Quyyumi AA. Circadian variation in vascular tone and its relation to α-sympathetic vasoconstrictor activity. N Engl J Med 1991; 325; 968–90.

45. Muller JE, Tofler GH, Stone PH. Circadian variation and triggers of onset of acute cardiovascular disease. Circulation 1989; 79:733–43.

46. MacMahon SW, Norton RN. Alcohol and hypertension: implications for prevention and treatment. Ann Intern Med 1986; 105:124–6.

46a. Beilin LJ. Diet and lifestyle in hypertension — changing perspectives. J Cardiovasc Pharmacol 1990; 16:562–6.

47. Kaplan, NM. New evidence on the role of sodium in hypertension. The Intersalt Study. Am J Hypertension 1990; 3:168–9.

47a. Krakoff LR. Is reduction of dietary salt a treatment for hypertension? Amer J Hyperten 1991; 4:481–2.

48. Dustan HP, Kirk KA. Corcoran lecture: the case for or against salt in hypertension. Hypertension 1989; 13:696–705.

48a. Stamler J, Rose G, Stamler R, et al. INTERSALT study findings. Public health and medical care implications. Hypertension 1989; 14:570–7.

48b. Law MR, Frost CD, Wald NJ. By how much does dietary salt reduction lower blood pressure? I: analysis of observational data among populations. Br Med J 1991; 302:811–5.

48c. The Trials of Hypertension Prevention Collaborative Research Group. The effects of non-pharmacologic interventions on blood pressure of persons with high normal levels: results of the Trials of Hypertension Prevention, Phase I. JAMA 1992; 267:1213–20.

49. MacGregor GA, Smith SJ, Markandu ND, et al. Moderate potassium supplementation in essential hypertension. The Lancet 1982; 567–70.

50. Health and Public Policy Committee, American College of Physicians. Biofeedback for hypertension. Ann Intern Med 1985; 102:709–15.

51. Johnson BF, Danylchuk MA. The relevance of plasma lipid changes with cardiovascular drug therapy. Med Clin North Amer 1989; 73:449–73.

52. Frolich ED. Cardiac hypertrophy in hypertension. N Engl J Med 1987; 317:831–3.

53. Messerli FH, Nunez BD, Nunez MM, et al. Hypertension and sudden death. Disparate effects of calcium entry blocker and diuretic therapy on cardiac dysrhythmias. Arch Intern Med 1989; 149:1263–7.

54. Chobanian AV. 1989 Corcoran Lecture: adaptive and maladaptive responses of the arterial wall to hypertension. Hypertension 1990; 15:666–74.

54a. Atkinson JB, Swift LL. Nifedipine reduces atherogenesis in cholesterol-fed heterozygous WHHL rabbits. Atherosclerosis 1990; 84:195–201.

55. Lichtlen PR, Hugenholtz PG, Rafflebeul W, et al. Retardation of angiographic progression of coronary artery disease by nifedipine. Results of the International Nifedipine Trial on Antiatherosclerotic Therapy (INTACT). Lancet 1990; 335:1109–13.

56. Furberg CD, Byington RP, Borhani NA. Multicenter Isradipine Diuretic Atherosclerosis Study (MIDAS). Design features. The Midas Research Group. Am J Med 1989; 86:Suppl 4A:37–9.

57. Haynes RB, Dantes R. Patient compliance and the conduct and interpretation of therapeutic trials. Controlled Clinical Trials 1987; 8:12–19.

14

Intervention for the Prevention of Coronary Heart Disease in Diabetes

TREVOR J. ORCHARD

EDITORS' INTRODUCTION

Diabetes is a fascinating and enigmatic disorder. The mechanism linking diabetes to an increased risk of atherosclerosis is not yet fully clarified, and in this chapter Dr. Trevor Orchard takes us through the accumulated evidence and possible mechanisms for this relationship. He also discusses the concept of insulin resistance and the association of diabetes with numerous alterations of hemostatic function. Although it has not yet been shown with certainty that the treatment of diabetes will lead to reduced risk for CHD, Dr. Orchard makes a compelling argument that such treatment is likely to be beneficial. He then recommends practical methodologies for the treatment of elevated blood sugar levels and also pays particular attention to the other risk factors, such as hypertension and hyperlipidemia, commonly associated with diabetes. There is a need for further investigation in this area, but the information and advice given here will assist the practitioner in preventing the development or progression of CHD in these high-risk patients.

Although it has been recognized for many years that individuals with diabetes have an increased risk of developing and dying from cardiovascular disease (CVD), the reasons underlying that increased risk remain obscure. There are multiple mechanisms by which diabetes and an increased risk of heart disease may be linked. It has even been suggested that it may be more appropriate to think of diabetes as a complication of a metabolic derangement that primarily leads to heart disease and also, in a subset, to diabetes, rather than to consider diabetes itself as a risk factor for heart disease [1]. The importance of these two diseases in public health terms is underscored by the high prevalence of both conditions. Over a million Americans suffer heart attacks annually [2], while over 10 million Americans have diabetes and a further 7 million have impaired glucose tolerance (IGT) [3], a condition also thought to increase cardiovascular risk.

In this chapter, after defining diabetes and describing its diagnosis, we discuss from an epidemiologic viewpoint the overall associations between diabetes, glucose intolerance, insulin, and cardiovascular disease. We then consider, in more depth, the pathophysiology of diabetes and how it relates to the various cardiovascular risk factors, including the potential role of insulin as a common mediator of the two disease entities. Finally, we discuss the management of patients with diabetes and IGT in terms of prevention of heart disease from general diabetic, nutritional, and pharmacologic viewpoints.

Definition and Diagnosis of Diabetes

The term *diabetes* covers a heterogeneous group of conditions that share the common features of decreased insulin action and high blood sugar. These include insulin-dependent diabetes mellitus (IDDM), an autoimmune disease that leads to complete insulin deficiency; various degrees of glucose intolerance often associated with obesity and hyperinsulinemia; and the most common form, non-insulin-dependent diabetes mellitus (NIDDM), which accounts for over 80 percent of all cases of diabetes. These

latter patients may have high, normal, or low insulin concentrations. It is, therefore, a mixed bag of conditions, and unfortunately many studies (understandably) have examined mixed populations, which adds further confusion to the study of diabetes and CVD. As discussed later, there is considerable doubt as to the exact mechanism whereby diabetes increases CVD risk. Nonetheless, the concept of peripheral insulin resistance, which also leads to a compensatory increase in insulin levels in the circulation, underlies much of our current understanding of the relationship between diabetes and CVD. (In advanced NIDDM, failure to secrete enough insulin to overcome this resistance may lead to hypoinsulinemia.) IDDM patients, who all require systemic insulin, are also often exposed to high circulating insulin concentrations. Thus, the diabetic may have to cope not only with the problem of peripheral insulin resistance (and the relative lack of insulin action) but also with high circulating levels of insulin, which may directly promote atherosclerosis (Figure 14-1).

The diagnosis of insulin-dependent diabetes is fairly straightforward in that these patients are usually symptomatic and present with polyuria and weight loss. They often have extremely high blood sugar levels, and consequently little formal testing is needed to diagnose this state. However, diagnosing older individuals, particularly with NIDDM, which constitutes about 80 to 85 percent of all diabetic subjects, is more problematic, as is identifying individuals likely to have IGT. The practitioner needs to be aware that IGT or diabetes is a common finding in any individual with manifestations of cardiovascular disease, and it is strongly recommended that at least a fasting blood sugar (and preferably a postprandial blood sugar) be measured. The National Diabetes Data Group (NDDG) [4] and World Health Organization (WHO) [5] criteria both state that a repeated fasting plasma sugar greater than 140 mg/dl constitutes clear evidence of diabetes.

A more formal approach to the diagnosis of diabetes is the conduct of an oral glucose tolerance test. It is critical to recognize that over 80 percent of those subjects who have diabetes

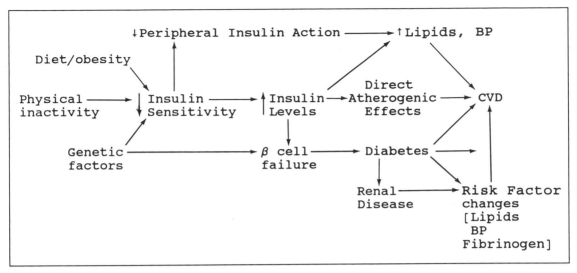

Figure 14-1. Glucose intolerance, insulin, and CVD.

but are unaware of it have a fasting blood sugar less than 140 mg/dl and consequently require formal testing to be diagnosed [6, 7]. This is traditionally done in a fasting state. The patient drinks a standard dose (now almost universally agreed to be 75 g) of glucose and has blood glucose measures made, preferably half-hourly, for 2 hours afterward. The key measurement after the glucose tolerance test is the 2-hour value, which in both the WHO and the NDDG classification systems should be above 200 mg/dl to diagnose diabetes. A patient with a 2-hour value of 140 to 200 mg/dl is classified as having IGT. One important difference does exist between the two sets of criteria. The NDDG [4] criteria require an intervening value to be above 200 mg/dl to label an individual as having glucose intolerance, while the WHO criteria do not [5]. This has the effect of doubling the prevalence of IGT in the WHO system compared to that of the NDDG. Because this would involve millions of people in the United States alone, it is a very important and still hotly debated issue. In round figures, approximately 3.2 percent of the population has known diabetes, and this figure can be doubled if one takes into account individuals who have diabetes but are not currently aware of it. Thus, more than 6 percent of Americans have diabetes. If we also include individuals with IGT (4.6 percent), the total fig-

ure further increases, so that nearly 11 percent of the adult population has some form of disturbed glucose tolerance [4].

While the practice is not universally accepted, this author recommends that further testing, either as indicated above or possibly carried out by obtaining a glycohemoglobin level (a measure of long-term blood sugar elevation), should be performed in any patient at high risk for diabetes, which includes those with CVD. The measurement of glycohemoglobin has a relatively low sensitivity and specificity for detection of diabetes in the general population [8], but as a simple test it helps to confirm in many clinical situations whether a patient has significant hyperglycemia and therefore is likely to be hyperinsulinemic and at risk for diabetic and cardiovascular complications. It is one of those curiosities of clinical practice that diabetes, an endocrine disease associated with a deficiency of insulin action, is not usually diagnosed on the basis of insulin concentration. With the increasing recognition of hyperinsulinemia as a cardiovascular risk factor, this may well change in the future and it is hoped that proper normal ranges for insulin concentrations will become more routinely accepted.

One of the problems in the diagnosis of diabetes is the variability of tests such as the oral glucose tolerance test. The body strives to maintain glucose homeostasis at the expense of increasing insulin secretion in an attempt to overcome peripheral insulin resistance. This may result in a situation where individuals with the same blood sugar level may have widely different insulin concentrations. Initially this increased insulin output is seen only postchallenge, but eventually it is also seen in the fasting state. As indicated earlier, when this need to produce excess insulin continues over a prolonged period of time, insulin secretion may eventually fail and hypoinsulinemia and gross hyperglycemia result. This sequence of events has been nicely demonstrated in the Pima Indian population [9], where a great excess of diabetes is associated with obesity. Although routine screening for diabetes is not generally recommended (primarily because we do not yet have good evidence that rigorously treating asymptomatic patients with glucose intolerance is beneficial), a substantial proportion of the scientific community does recommend screening, particularly in high-risk situations [10]. These would include patients with disorders likely to be complications of diabetes, including all manifestations of atherosclerotic disease, and also hypertensives, patients with families with a strong family history of diabetes, the obese, and patients with proteinuria.

Epidemiology of Diabetes, Insulin, and CVD Risk

It is reflective of the more advanced state of cardiovascular epidemiology that the most convincing prospective evidence of the association between diabetes and cardiovascular disease comes from cardiovascular, not diabetic, cohort studies. Many reviews have been published evaluating the association between atherosclerosis and diabetes [1, 11, 12]; in this section we will only highlight some of the major findings of the studies that have been conducted. Many of the large prospective studies, such as the Framingham Heart Study [13], have demonstrated that people with diabetes (because of the unique definition used in Framingham, a preferable term in this study would be glucose intolerance) have a greatly increased risk of cardiovascular

disease. This excess relative risk is comparable in magnitude to that of the other standard risk factors [13] (elevated serum cholesterol, smoking, high blood pressure) and in some groups (e.g., women and young adults) greatly exceeds that of the standard risk factors [11, 13, 14, 15]. In young males (35 to 44 years old), diabetes is a very potent risk factor and accounts for much of the early excess cardiovascular mortality experienced in this age group [16]. The following summary is based on a number of studies — the Framingham [13, 17, 18], Evans County [19], Whitehall [20], Rancho Bernardo [14], and Paris Heart [21] studies — all of which substantiate the high risk of cardiovascular disease in people with diabetes. This section discusses some of the more important epidemiologic findings.

The association of diabetes and atherosclerosis is not limited to the manifestations of CHD alone, since increased rates of cerebrovascular and peripheral (lower limb) vascular disease are also seen [11, 17]. In the majority of these studies, however, diabetes is particularly associated with coronary heart disease mortality and also with the prevalence of peripheral vascular disease [11, 17]. Indeed, individuals who have to undergo amputation for peripheral vascular disease generally fall into one of two categories: they have diabetes or are heavy smokers. Diabetes accounts for nearly half of all amputations for arterial disease [22].

Another important finding is that the occurrence of cardiovascular disease in diabetes appears to be associated with the other traditional cardiovascular risk factors in much the same way as it is in the general population. Cholesterol, blood pressure, and smoking all increase risk in approximately the same proportion in those with diabetes as in those without [18]. Some of the multivariate analyses from the Framingham Study have even gone so far as to suggest that if one takes into account all the other risk factors, then in men diabetes may not be an additional risk factor at all [18]. This would lead one to suppose that the mechanism by which diabetes enhances cardiovascular risk is only by causing a greater prevalence or severity of other cardiovascular risk factors, and there is nothing unique about the role of diabetes in exacerbating the atherosclerotic process. While this has been the case for NIDDM in men in some studies (Framingham [18], Evans County [19]), the lipoprotein profile and blood pressures of individuals with NIDDM do not often show major differences from the general population [11, 23, 24]. In the case of IDDM, little difference was seen in one study comparing cases with sibling controls [25]. Thus, the extent of the difference between diabetic and nondiabetic CVD risk profiles is not as great as would be needed to explain the enhanced CVD risk in diabetes, especially for women, who in virtually all studies suffer a great excess of CHD events even after accounting for the other risk factors [11, 17, 18, 19, 23].

Recent data from the enormous study of screenees for the MRFIT trial suggest that the diabetics among the 360,000 screened men had an increased risk of cardiovascular death compared to nondiabetics at all levels of cholesterol. The relative risk among diabetics rose with increasing cholesterol in a similar manner to that of nondiabetics, although there was a somewhat less consistent pattern in the lower quintiles. However, those with diabetes were at two to five times greater risk than those with normal glucose tolerance at each level of cholesterol [26]. These data, therefore, support the hypothesis that cholesterol is an important cardiovascular risk factor among individuals in the diabetic population, but do not explain their increased risk. Similar findings from this study are seen for blood pressure and, to a lesser extent, smoking. Thus, it appears that the standard risk factors are operative within diabetic populations with a similar strength to that seen in the general population, but that diabetics have a greatly increased risk at any level of blood pressure or cholesterol.

Another potential explanation for the increased risk of cardiovascular disease in diabetes might be that individuals with diabetes are more likely to have multiple cardiovascular risk factors than are those in the nondiabetic population. This possibility was explored in some depth by Elizabeth Barrett-Connor in the Rancho Bernardo Study, and indeed it appeared that

patients with diabetes were more likely to have multiple risk factors [27]. Nonetheless, even this explanation is unlikely to totally explain their greatly increased risk.

It is well known that in the general population men are at considerable excess risk for cardiovascular disease compared to women. One of the striking features of the effect of diabetes on cardiovascular disease is the reduction and even total elimination of this sex differential, as seen in many studies. Data from the Evans County Study [19], as well as Framingham [18] and others [11] support this concept. However, a recent analysis of individuals followed up after the first National Health and Nutritional Examination Survey shows that men with diabetes still have a greater risk of CVD death compared to women [28]. Even more recent data from the London cohort of the WHO multinational study of vascular disease in diabetes [29] suggest that the reduction in the sex differential of CVD mortality is largely limited to those with IDDM. Therefore, the evidence does not totally suggest an elimination of the sex differential, although these latter studies are possibly biased because the definition of diabetes was based on history alone [28], which may result in a more complete capture of those at risk among females than among males because of a higher rate of contact with the medical system among the female population [29].

It has been proposed that one of the major reasons for the reduction in diabetics of the normal sex differential for CHD, whether IDDM or NIDDM, is the loss of the normally greater insulin sensitivity seen in the female nondiabetic population, with its attendant better lipoprotein profile and blood pressure [11, 31, 32]. When insulin is not being produced, as in IDDM, or there is resistance to its action, as in NIDDM, this advantage may be lost; consequently, women and men are placed on a more equal footing. Of interest the Rancho Bernardo Study [33] suggests that there is a threshold effect in women above which blood glucose becomes important, while in men the risk appears more linearly related.

Another mechanism that might lead to increased cardiovascular mortality in persons with diabetes is an increased case fatality rate related to the concomitant metabolic derangement. While there is evidence that the survival of diabetic patients, particularly female, is reduced after a cardiac event [11, 34], this would not appear to be a full explanation; nonfatal events are also increased in diabetes. Attention has also been recently directed to the role of renal disease or proteinuria. This role has been demonstrated most clearly by the Steno Group in Denmark, who have shown that in IDDM the macrovascular risk and, indeed, most of the excess total mortality is limited to the subgroup of patients who develop renal disease (proteinuria) as a complication of diabetes [35]. While renal disease is not as prevalent in the NIDDM population and many NIDDM patients develop cardiovascular disease without concomitant renal disease, recent data have nonetheless suggested that proteinuria is also a CVD risk factor in NIDDM [36]. These data are even more intriguing in the light of the striking inverse relationship seen between serum albumin and subsequent mortality from a whole range of diseases, including CVD [37]. How proteinuria and renal disease increase CVD risk in diabetes is not fully understood, although it is likely to reflect, at least in part, the marked elevations of blood pressure and lipids that occur in renal disease [38, 39]. A further hypothesis suggests that IDDM subjects who develop renal disease have a genetic impairment in heparin sulphate metabolism, which may also lead to CVD by interfering with lipoprotein lipase activity [40]. It has also been proposed on the basis of some autopsy and coronary angiography studies [41, 42] that patients with diabetes have more diffuse and extensive atherosclerosis than is seen in nondiabetics, but other studies have not reached this conclusion [11, 43].

If diabetes itself is a strong risk factor for CHD, one would suppose that the longer one has diabetes (i.e., the greater the duration) the greater the risk of heart disease. While a relationship with duration is seen in IDDM [11, 44, 45], this has not generally been the case in NIDDM, where little association with duration is seen after controlling for age in most [11, 45, 46] but not all [47] studies. In both diseases the

concomitant increase of age with increasing duration confounds the issue, as does the subsequent development of renal disease, which has profound effects on lipoprotein concentrations, blood pressure, and a whole range of other cardiovascular risk factors [38, 39].

This lack of a marked duration effect has led Jarrett to propose that diabetes itself is not truly a cardiovascular risk factor, but rather that there is an underlying metabolic disorder that predisposes certain individuals to both heart disease and diabetes [1]. This theory is further supported by a number of other findings:

- Cardiovascular risk factors such as lipoprotein concentrations and blood pressure predict the subsequent development of diabetes [48, 49].
- IGT predicts both subsequent diabetes [50, 51] and CHD, as shown by the Paris Heart [52], Whitehall [53], and Bedford studies [15] (although blood sugar concentration itself has not been shown in many populations to be an independent risk factor [54]).
- Offspring of NIDDM patients have abnormal lipoprotein patterns [55].

One potential mechanism whereby individuals may be at increased risk both for cardiovascular disease and diabetes is insulin resistance. High insulin concentrations have been shown to be a risk factor for cardiovascular disease independent of other risk factors in three prospective studies in men [56, 57, 58], although the data from the only study that evaluated the issue in women are less convincing [58]. The data from that study reported from Busselton, Australia are more difficult to interpret because, in contrast to the other two studies, a smaller glucose challenge was used (50 g) and subjects were not fasted.

The importance of insulin is further underscored by the finding in the Paris Heart Study that insulin, as opposed to glucose level or diabetic status, was the strongest predictor of subsequent CHD [21]. Further analysis of the Paris Heart Study shows that hyperinsulinemia is particularly powerful as a predictor in the subset of obese patients [59]. As described below, the proper action of insulin is important in lipoprotein metabolism and probably has a role in essential hypertension. A further component of the insulin hypothesis is that central adiposity, often measured as an increased waist/hip ratio (a characteristic of men compared to women) has been shown to be associated with insulin resistance [60] and with both an increased risk of cardiovascular disease [61] and the subsequent development of diabetes [62, 63]. High insulin concentrations in the blood resulting from insulin resistance may also lead to direct stimulation of the atherogenic process by stimulating smooth-muscle cell proliferation and the synthesis of cholesterol in vascular cells [64].

There is, therefore, a considerable body of evidence that insulin resistance leading to hyperinsulinemia may be a metabolic derangement that leads to both diabetes and cardiovascular disease. The clinical implication of these concepts in managing patients with diabetes or IGT is that interventions that improve insulin sensitivity (e.g., weight loss and physical exercise) may very well be valuable from a preventive cardiologic viewpoint. This possibility is strengthened by a recent Australian study of urban aboriginal diabetics who, after returning to a traditional lifestyle of increased activity and a low-fat diet, showed a dramatic improvement in insulin sensitivity and triglyceride levels [65]. As discussed earlier, hyperinsulinemia is an important concern for IDDM patients as well as for those with NIDDM. Although insulin resistance is not such a marked feature of IDDM, since insulin has to be administered systemically, IDDM patients are exposed to high circulating levels of insulin and are consequently placed in a hyperinsulinemic state. Such patients should be treated with adequate, but not excessive, insulin doses, as will be discussed later.

It has been suggested that specific risk factors beyond the big three already discussed — cholesterol, smoking, and blood pressure — are of importance in increasing the risk of cardiovascular disease in diabetics. Many studies have suggested that serum triglycerides are particularly powerful as a predictor of macrovascular disease. For example, although the WHO multinational study showed increased levels of serum cholesterol to be significantly associated with Q-wave abnormalities on the ECG, in a subgroup of diabetics in whom fasting triglycerides were measured triglycerides were the predominant predictor [66]. Likewise, the Paris Heart Study has reported that in subjects with diabetes or IGT, triglycerides were the strongest lipid predictor of CHD mortality, especially in those with high fasting insulin concentrations [67]. Both of these studies primarily involved patients with NIDDM, as did an earlier study by Santen [68]; however, the same pattern of macrovascular complications was seen in IDDM in the prospective Schwabing study in Germany [45]. In another IDDM study triglycerides were strong, cross-sectional univariate correlates of all manifestations of large-vessel disease (calcification of peripheral arteries, lower-extremity arterial disease, and coronary disease), and triglyceride/ApoA$_1$ ratio was a multivariate predictor of arterial calcification [69].

Lp(a) concentrations, though reported to be increased in diabetes [70, 71], have not yet been clearly associated with cardiovascular complications; indeed the case control study in IDDM showed no cross-sectional association, mean concentrations being 17 mg/dl in both CHD cases and controls. The various lipoprotein compositional changes seen in diabetes likewise have yet to be clearly associated with macrovascular disease. However, like Lp(a) concentrations they may still show important effects in prospective studies. Beyond lipoproteins, diabetes is associated with altered platelet function [72], increased platelet aggregability [73, 74], increased fibrinogen concentration [75, 76], and decreased fibrinolytic activity [75], changes seen particularly in those with renal disease [76].

In conclusion, extensive evidence exists demonstrating that diabetes, IGT, and insulin resistance are associated with increased cardiovascular risk. Indeed the strength of this association is perhaps further underscored by the observation that in populations that have a low prevalence of CVD generally, e.g., Pima Indians [77], Chinese [78], and Japanese [79, 80] diabetics still have an increased risk of mortality from CVD. Indeed in the Pimas cardiovascular mortality appears almost totally limited to those with diabetes [77]. Thus, as Pyörälä concludes in his review [12], although CVD rates vary by geographic and ethnic groups among diabetics in the same way as they do in the general population [80], diabetics in virtually all populations have an increased risk.

Pathophysiology of Cardiovascular Risk in Diabetes

Lipoprotein Metabolism

As we have seen, diabetes is characterized by a deficiency of insulin action, although the two major types of diabetes, IDDM and NIDDM, differ in the way such deficiency arises, i.e., lack of insulin production in the former and resistance to its action (primarily at the postreceptor level) [81] in the latter. These differences underlie the different lipid abnormalities seen in the two types of diabetes. The situation, however, is further complicated in IDDM by the variable doses of insulin used and in NIDDM by the recognition that while many patients have increased insulin concentrations, others have a deficiency in insulin response after allowing for obesity [81]. This has been underscored recently by the development of more specific insulin assays, which suggest that previous measures may have overestimated true insulin levels [82].

The types of disturbances that occur in lipoprotein metabolism in diabetes are listed in Table 14-1. Postheparin lipoprotein lipase (LPL) is the key enzyme for the catabolism of chylomicrons and VLDL particles, enabling them to form remnants that are cleared by the E (chylomicron remnant) and B/E (LDL) receptors in the liver. Since LPL is an insulin-dependent enzyme [83], a decrease in insulin action (as seen in poorly controlled IDDM and NIDDM) leads to increased triglyceride levels (VLDL). If the deficiency is considerable, chylomicron clearance is also impaired, leading to classic diabetic lipemia. Because of the relationship between VLDL clearance and HDL cholesterol (especially HDL_2 cholesterol) [84], the latter is also decreased in insulin deficiency. The impaired

VLDL clearance seen as a result of decreased LPL activity [85] can lead to increased remnant concentrations, which are thought to be atherogenic [86]. Diminished hepatic triglyceride lipase (HTL) activity, which is also thought to be insulin-sensitive [86a], may also contribute to impaired remnant clearance.

In addition to decreased catabolism and removal of triglyceride-rich lipoproteins, the hyperinsulinism often seen in NIDDM is associated with increased hepatic VLDL secretion [87]. This may result from an increased supply of nonesterified fatty acids reaching the liver, as a result of increased lipolysis [88]. It also appears that insulin has an inhibitory effect on VLDL secretion, which is receptor-mediated [89]. In addition apo B production does not seem to be increased as much in NIDDM as are VLDL triglycerides, which leads, it is thought, to an altered VLDL particle with relative triglyceride enrichment [90].

Diabetes is also thought to affect another aspect of lipoprotein metabolism, namely, the transfer of esterified cholesterol from HDL to VLDL and LDL [91]. This process, commonly referred to as reverse cholesterol transport, provides a mechanism for removal of cholesterol from the peripheral tissues.

The clearance of LDL particles, which is largely mediated by LDL receptors, is also affected by insulin, which has been shown to partially regulate LDL receptor binding [92] and internalization [93], resulting in decreased LDL catabolism and a rise in plasma LDL cholesterol concentration in the insulin-deficient state seen in diabetes.

Another abnormality that occurs in diabetes and interferes with LDL clearance is nonenzymatic glycosylation of apoprotein B (the major protein in diabetes) [94]. Glycosylation can also occur in collagen, causing products to be formed that can trap LDL, thus potentially accelerating lipid accumulation in damaged vascular endothelium [95]. Another effect of glycosylation of LDL may be an enhanced uptake of LDL cholesterol by macrophages, via low-affinity mechanisms, thus promoting the atherogenic process still further [96].

The delayed clearance of LDL that may occur

Table 14-1.   Alterations in lipoprotein metabolism in diabetes

Alteration	Lipoprotein effect
↓ Lipoprotein lipase (LPL)	↑ TG, ↓ HDL, chylomicronemia,* remnants*
↓ Hepatic triglyceride lipase (HTL)	↑ Remnants* ↑ HDL
↓ Lecithin cholesterol acyltransferase (LCAT)	Altered composition
Altered lipid transfer	Altered composition
↓ LDL receptor activity	↑ LDL
↑ VLDL production/secretion	↑ TG
Glycosylation of lipoproteins, especially LDL	? ↑ LDL
Oxidation of LDL	? ↑ LDL

*If severe.

in diabetes may also lead to a relative increase in oxidized LDL, the presence of which is thought to lead to preferential uptake by macrophages in the developing atheromatous plaque [97]. With regard to HDL metabolism, HDL concentrations, especially HDL$_2$, are reported to be lowered in NIDDM as a result of decreased lipolytic clearance of VLDL and elevated hepatic lipase activity, which is thought to be involved in HDL catabolism [86].

In conclusion, it is clear that multiple disturbances of lipoprotein metabolism occur in diabetes (Figure 14-2). The effects of these vary between IDDM and NIDDM and also as a function of glycemic control and the relative degree of insulin resistance and dosage (particularly in IDDM). In addition to these disturbances, the practitioner should also be aware that the concentrations of lipoproteins, our usual means of monitoring therapy, may not reveal the whole story, because compositional changes in the lipoprotein profile may further enhance the atherogenic process [98]. It should also be remembered that individuals with diabetes are just as likely to suffer from the monogenic (and polygenic) lipid disorders as are members of the general population.

Blood Pressure

The importance of blood pressure elevation in diabetes is highlighted by the fact that 2.5 million Americans have both conditions [99]. For further details on the relationship between diabetes and blood pressure, particularly management of the latter, the reader is referred to the Final Report of the Working Group on Hypertension in Diabetes [99]. The links between insulin and blood pressure have also been reviewed recently [100]. As with lipids, there are multiple reasons why blood pressure is increased in diabetes. These are summarized in Table 14-2.

As in the general population, the most common type of hypertension seen in diabetes is essential hypertension. However, essential hypertension may itself be related to the linked factors of obesity, central adiposity, and insulin resistance. As has already been mentioned, central adiposity is related to both cardiovascular risk and diabetes. Blood pressure is also related to central adiposity [101, 102]. One likely explanation for much of the association between obesity and fat distribution type with blood pressure is insulin resistance and hyperinsulinemia [100]. The Paris Heart Study suggests that the association of increased fasting plasma insulin levels with an increased prevalence of high blood pressure is limited to those in the overweight group [103].

The two most likely mechanisms responsible for insulin's links with blood pressure are postulated to be increased sympathetic activity and sodium retention. The former hypothesis is supported by evidence that plasma insulin and sympathetic activity are linked [104] and that increased catecholamine concentrations are seen

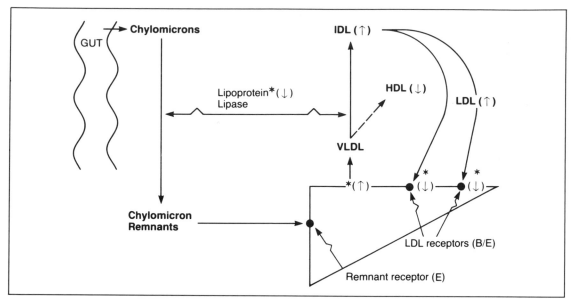

Figure 14-2.   The major effects of diabetes on lipoprotein metabolism. Asterisk (*) indicates effect of diabetes. Arrows indicate direction of effect.

Table 14-2.   Blood pressure and glucose intolerance: underlying links

Obesity
Central adiposity
Hyperinsulinemia/insulin resistance
  Sodium retention
  ↑ Sympathetic activity
Renal disease
  Diabetic nephropathy
  Renovascular hypertension
Secondary causes of diabetes

in hypertensive subjects [105]. Defronzo has shown that insulin enhances sodium transport in the kidney [106] and suggests that the resulting sodium retention leads to hypertension. Recent studies suggest there may be a further link between insulin and sodium-lithium countertransport, a genetically determined correlate of hypertension [107].

That renal disease is associated with increased blood pressure is well known. In the diabetic this link is particularly common, since renal disease is a common complication of diabetes and, after 30 years of IDDM, affects over 45 percent of subjects [44]. In addition to diabetic nephropathy, diabetics also have an increased frequency of renal artery stenosis (and thereby hypertension) because of their increased tendency toward generalized vascular atherosclerosis [99]. Finally hypertension occasionally occurs in patients whose diabetes or glucose intolerance is secondary to hormonal excesses related to pheochromocytoma, Cushing's syndrome, or primary aldosteronism, disorders that themselves cause elevated blood pressure.

Other Risk Factors

Extensive reference has been made in the preceding sections to the influence of diabetes and insulin resistance on other cardiovascular risk factors. These include the exacerbation of lipid, blood pressure, and fibrinogen abnormalities as renal disease develops. The interested reader is referred to the literature cited in those discussions. Similarly, the effects of diabetes on platelet function and the clotting system and the possible direct atherogenic effects of diabetes are not discussed further, but the reader is referred to reviews of those areas [72, 108, 109, 110].

Practical Cardiovascular Risk Reduction in Diabetes/Glucose Intolerance

General Management

Recognizing that a patient who is at risk for or already has cardiovascular disease has a problem with glucose tolerance is important for a number of reasons. First of all, although definitive evidence is lacking, it is likely that improvement of blood sugar levels would be beneficial, since the methodologies used to control elevated blood sugar levels, particularly weight loss (and, if clearly diabetic, tight glucose control with insulin or oral agents) often result in improved lipoprotein concentrations [65, 111], blood pressure [112], and other concomitant risks.

Second, from a psychological viewpoint, patients may be more likely to adopt appropriate preventive measures if they know that they are also at increased risk for diabetes complications as well as subsequent cardiovascular disease. As already discussed, one complication of diabetes, renal disease, has specific cardiovascular relevance in part because of its association with disturbed lipoprotein and fibrinogen concentrations and increased blood pressure.

Third, because the diabetic state is associated with a whole range of other cardiovascular risks and disturbances, it would seem advisable to take into account these added risks that a diabetic experiences. Some of these factors, such as altered platelet function leading to increased platelet aggregation, may relate to both increased macrovascular and microvascular disease and further compromise the coronary microvascular circulation, exacerbating the effect of large epicardial coronary artery stenoses. It is thus recommended that the practitioner screen all patients with CVD for diabetes along the lines discussed earlier in this chapter. Although a fasting blood sugar is not a sensitive measure, if combined with a glycohemoglobin in suspicious cases it provides a reasonably practical and quick way to check for any major glucose tolerance problem.

From the foregoing discussions, it is clear that patients with diabetes have an increased risk of cardiovascular disease and that the standard risk factors that are seen in the general population are also operative in diabetes. It therefore follows that all the principles outlined elsewhere in this book for the management of cardiovascular risk in the general population apply equally well to those with diabetes. However, a number of special problems in practicing preventive cardiology in the diabetic subject need to be addressed.

The first major issue to be discussed concerns the National Cholesterol Education Program (NCEP) guidelines for the detection and treatment of adults with hypercholesterolemia [113]. In this report the goal LDL cholesterol for any male with diabetes is 130 mg/dl, but for women with diabetes who do not have other risk factors the LDL cholesterol goal is 160 mg/dl. In view of the great reduction in the sex differential in cardiovascular risk seen in diabetes, we strongly believe that all persons with diabetes should have an LDL cholesterol goal of 130 mg/dl or below irrespective of gender. Indeed, we could go one step further and suggest that a goal of 100 mg/dl would be even more desirable for those with additional risk factors in addition to diabetes.

The screening and follow-up recommendations of the NCEP also need to be extended for patients with diabetes. As part of the routine care of individuals with diabetes, a fasting lipid profile should be performed at least annually. This is recommended because fluctuation in glycemic control and the development of renal disease in diabetes causes the lipid profile to be subject to much greater change than is seen in the general population. Clearly if lipoproteins are disturbed, more frequent follow-up is needed during the initial treatment phase.

It is just as important in the diabetic as in the nondiabetic to look for other causes of lipid (and to a lesser degree blood pressure) elevation. The genetic lipid disorders may present in both IDDM and NIDDM quite independently of diabetic status. Consequently a detailed family history and knowledge of the lipid profile of family members is at least as important as in the general population. Since it has been demonstrated that even mild proteinuria (i.e., microalbuminuria) is associated with alterations in blood pressure and lipoprotein profile [39], it is our opinion that part of the routine assessment of a diabetic patient from a preventive cardiology viewpoint should include annual assessments of albumin excretion. While screening for microalbuminuria in Europe has become a fairly standard part of diabetic management, it has not yet been fully accepted in clinical practice in the United States. The main reason for this is the lack of evidence from long-term, large-scale trials of benefit from treating patients with microalbuminuria in any special way.

Three interventions have been considered for microalbuminuria: tight glucose control, protein restriction, and blood pressure lowering. The hypothesis that microalbuminuric patients should be treated vigorously for hypertension at levels that in the general population would be considered normal (diastolic blood pressures in the 80s, for example) is currently under trial. Because of the ability of ACE inhibitors to decrease intraglomerular pressure and thereby hopefully reduce renal damage, interest has focused particularly on the use of these agents in mild proteinuria. While there is some evidence that irrespective of blood pressure levels, ACE inhibitors, e.g., enalapril [114] — and hypertensive treatment in general [115] — may reduce albumin excretion, the long-term benefits of such therapy are currently undemonstrated, though it is hoped that current trials will be positive. Similar arguments apply to tight glycemic control [116] and protein restriction [117], both of which show promise. The general or family practitioner, internist, cardiologist, and diabetologist should all be aware of the renal status of their diabetic patients and bring the above considerations into their deliberations when deciding on which preventive measures to advise.

The next issue of importance is the value of good glycemic control and how far one should go to achieve this. As has been discussed, the relationship between blood sugar level and cardiovascular disease both in the general population and in the diabetic population is not clear.

Indeed, in the diabetic population there is very little evidence that higher blood sugars are related to greater or more severe cardiovascular disease. Furthermore, the relationship between glycemic control and all complications of diabetes is still somewhat controversial and is the subject of a major multicenter trial (the Diabetes Control and Complications Trial) [118]. Nonetheless, as indicated earlier there are cogent reasons for considering glycemic control to be a primary focus of preventive cardiology in the diabetic patient. First of all, many of the maneuvers used to improve glycemic control in the diabetic, particularly weight loss and exercise, are associated with multiple benefits for general health. Weight loss also improves insulin sensitivity and thereby enables one to improve the lipoprotein profile and possibly blood pressure, while at the same time reducing the level of circulating insulin required, whether exogenously in IDDM or endogenously in NIDDM. As we have shown earlier, high insulin levels may have a direct atherogenic effect. Improved insulin sensitivity lowers triglyceride levels and probably raises HDL cholesterol, and these components appear to be particularly strong risk factors for cardiovascular disease in diabetes.

The second major reason for being concerned with good control of diabetes as a component of preventive cardiology is that there may well be a relationship between glycemic control and subsequent renal disease, which as we have shown before greatly increases cardiovascular risk and dramatically affects virtually all the cardiovascular risk factors. If good glycemic control is shown to delay the development of renal disease, clearly this should be considered an important part of good preventive cardiology practice. Therefore, even if the cross-sectional relationship between glycemic control and cardiovascular disease is weak, there are good reasons to promote close control of blood sugar levels in the diabetic.

The next question is how best to achieve good glycemic control. In the insulin-dependent diabetic, where insulin is given exogenously and usually via two or more injections a day, a number of general principles should be followed. First of all, insulin should be delivered in as physiological a manner as possible, that is, the dose of insulin should be timed to cover the postprandial rise in blood sugar. This is not to suggest that all IDDM patients at an increased risk for cardiovascular disease should be on an insulin pump or multiple injections a day. However, such maneuvers should be seriously considered if other parameters of cardiovascular risk, e.g., lipoprotein profile, blood pressure, and other microvascular complications, are not well controlled on the usual one or two daily insulin injections. Multiple doses of regular insulin are likely to result in a slightly lower total dose of insulin than the use of intermediate or longer-acting insulins on a less frequent basis.

It is also important to recognize that the liver is more active in producing lipoproteins at night, and therefore adequate overnight insulinization is an important component of the control of lipoproteins in the diabetic. Many hypertriglyceridemic diabetics seen in lipid clinics who appear resistant to standard approaches to control do very well when either they are put on insulin (if they have NIDDM and were hitherto treated with oral agents) or, if already treated with insulin, they have their doses changed such that they are receiving adequate doses of insulin at night. Finally, it should be appreciated that the presence of diabetes may make other genetic predispositions to lipoprotein disorders, for example, familial hypertriglyceridemia (type IV) or familial dyslipoproteinemia (type III) in those with $ApoE_2$ homozygosity, more likely to be manifest and more difficult to control. In such situations it is important to minimize the additional effects of diabetes by an improvement of blood sugar levels.

Nutritional Advice

The next component of the practice of preventive cardiology in the diabetic concerns the diet to be recommended. Clearly weight loss is fundamental to good management of most NIDDM patients and many IDDM patients to maximize insulin sensitivity. Thus, a relatively hypocaloric diet is required for most patients.

However, it must be remembered that many diabetic subjects, particularly those with IDDM, are already under significant dietary restrictions, which may become even stricter in the future as greater attention is paid to the protein content of the diet. Consequently, there is a real risk that patients will abandon dietary control altogether if recommendations become too stringent. Over the last 20 years there has been a dramatic shift away from advising patients with diabetes to consume more fat and less carbohydrate to essentially the reverse. The American Diabetes Association (ADA) recommends a diet similar [119] to that of the NCEP [113]: total fat should constitute less than 30 percent of calories, saturated fat less than 10 percent, and polyunsaturated fat 6 to 8 percent. Cholesterol intake should be less than 300 mg daily. However, there is a continuing debate as to the amount of carbohydrate that should be utilized in the diet. One school of thought suggests that a high-carbohydrate diet exacerbates insulin resistance and elevates triglyceride values, a risk factor that is already increased in diabetes [120]. Others find that a high-carbohydrate diet actually improves glucose tolerance [121].

A different approach to the problem was taken by Ullmann and colleagues [121a] who hypothesized that carbohydrate-induced hypertriglyceridemia might be related to the rapidity with which the new diet was introduced. They fed gradually increasing amounts of carbohydrates and gradually decreasing amounts of fat to volunteers, increasing carbohydrate by 5 percent of total calories and decreasing fat by 5 percent in each of four successive time periods, the final diet having 20 percent of calories as fat and 65 percent of calories as carbohydrates. With this schema they found no change in plasma TG or VLDL levels. In a second protocol they went directly to the fourth-phase, highest-carbohydrate lowest-fat diet, and now they found a prompt 47 percent increase in plasma TG levels and a 73 percent increase in plasma VLDL levels. Thus it may very well be that a high-carbohydrate diet will not raise TG levels if it is introduced gradually.

In any case, a high-fat diet tends to be a high-protein diet, and most authorities are now cautious about recommending high-protein diets in the diabetic in view of the increased risk of renal disease [122].

The net result of all these considerations is a situation with little room for maneuver if one accepts that the caloric distribution of the diet should comprise no more than 10 percent from saturated fat, 8 percent from polyunsaturated fat (it is not recommended to push polyunsaturates much above this level), 55 percent (the lower end of the ADA-recommended range) from carbohydrates, and 12 percent from protein. One is thus left with only 15 percent of calories to play with in terms of monounsaturated fat versus greater amounts of carbohydrate. Monounsaturated fat has been proposed as a valuable component of the diet, since it appears both to be safe and to have cholesterol-lowering potential [123]. It should be particularly advocated in its natural cis form (e.g., oleic acid where possible), but there are limits as to how much of an appealing regular diet can be composed of olive oil, peanut oil, and avocados — its major sources. The argument eventually comes down to whether one increases monounsaturated fat from the 10 percent recommended by the NCEP [113] to 15 percent of calories. It would seem most reasonable for the diabetic (with the help of a dietician) to use this 5 percent caloric balance in whatever split between monounsaturates and carbohydrates is wished.

Fiber intake, both insoluble (for its benefits in bowel regulation and delaying carbohydrate/sugar absorption) and soluble (for its cholesterol-lowering properties), is to be encouraged [124]. Although fish oil supplements, rich in omega-3 fatty acids, have triglyceride-lowering, hypotensive, and antiplatelet-aggregatory properties [125], their use is not recommended except for those patients with moderate or severe hypertriglyceridemia, because of the potential for raising both LDL cholesterol and blood sugar [126]. Sodium intake should be moderately restricted, as is recommended for the general population, to an intake of 1000 mg per 1000 kcal. This is especially appropriate in

view of the increased risk of hypertension in diabetes [99]. However, in those with fluid balance problems or postural hypertension, increased salt may be needed occasionally. The judicious use of artificial, noncaloric sweeteners (e.g., aspartame and saccharin) is recommended, particularly in those patients needing to lose weight. A balance of use between these two agents is recommended to reduce any potential risks [119].

Use of Hypolipidemic Drugs

When diet and improved glycemic control fail to fully correct lipid disturbances, drug therapy should be considered, especially if there are additional risk factors. Usually, at least a 3-month period is needed to assess the effects of diet changes. The choice of pharmacologic agent depends on the type of lipid disturbance present. The major indications for and adverse effects of the commonly used agents are listed in Table 14-3. A fuller discussion of lipid pharmacotherapy can be found in Chapter 12; here we address only those issues relevant to diabetes.

Bile acid resins, usually the first choice in the treatment of pure (type IIa) hypercholesterolemia (i.e., raised LDL cholesterol) when triglycerides are normal, have a useful but somewhat reduced place in diabetes. A rise in triglycerides is seen in many patients on resin therapy. It is therefore necessary to monitor triglycerides and limit the use of resins to those patients with (fasting) triglycerides below the 200- to 250-mg/dl range. The other major problem with bile acid resins is the high incidence of gastrointestinal side effects, which may be particularly troublesome in patients with autonomic neuropathy. As in the general population, it is important to build up the dose gradually.

Niacin, or nicotinic acid, would seem to be the ideal drug, because its use results in a desirable pattern of lipoprotein change (decreased total cholesterol, triglycerides, and LDL; increased HDL). Unfortunately, as Molnar et al showed some years ago [127], niacin causes a rise in blood sugar, which may require an increase in insulin dose in diabetics and can also precipitate some patients with IGT into the diabetic range. A recent study by Grundy con-

Table 14-3. Hypolipidemic drugs in diabetes: indications and concerns

Drug	Indication	Concerns
Bile acid resins (cholestyramine/colestid)	↑ LDL cholesterol	↑ Triglycerides (do not use if Triglycerides >250 mg/dl)
Niacin	↑ LDL cholesterol ↑ Triglycerides ↓ HDL cholesterol	↑ Blood sugar ↑ Uric acid
Gemfibrozil	↑ Triglycerides ↓ HDL cholesterol	LDL cholesterol lowering small and variable
Lovastatin	↑ LDL cholesterol ↑ Triglycerides	Risky in combination with gemfibrozil and/or cyclosporine; long-term effect in diabetes unknown

firmed these findings [128]. Because this side effect (whose mechanism is poorly understood) may be dose-dependent, a trial of niacin in the 1.0- to 2.5-g range may be worthwhile, particularly for the typical NIDDM patient with moderate increases of both VLDL and LDL. However, careful attention to glucose control is needed, and if significant increases in insulin dose occur, the use of this agent may need to be curtailed.

Gemfibrozil, a potent triglyceride-lowering fibric acid derivative that has been shown in men to reduce the risk of CHD events by some 34 percent (thought to be due to its HDL-raising and LDL-lowering effects), also has a place in diabetes. Garg and Grundy showed profound triglyceride-lowering effects in NIDDM [129]. In NIDDM patients without marked hypertriglyceridemia, the LDL cholesterol–lowering effect seen in the Helsinki Study was not so apparent, so its use in diabetes may be best limited to those patients with severe hypertriglyceridemia. Earlier studies had also shown a failure of gemfibrozil to lower β-lipoproteins in diabetes [130].

Fortunately lovastatatin, an HMG CoA reductase inhibitor, appears very effective in diabetes, with falls in both total cholesterol and triglycerides of over 20 percent reported [131]. Glucose levels do not appear to be disturbed, and the frequency of hepatic and myalgic problems would appear to be similar to that seen in the general population. As described in Chapter 12, caution is advised in its use in combination with gemfibrozil because of an increased risk of myositis, and great care needs to be exercised in its use with patients who are on cyclosporine post–renal transplant, since this combination may lead to rhabdomyolysis and further renal complications.

Probucol, an agent that lowers LDL cholesterol but also lowers HDL cholesterol, has not been extensively used in diabetes. However, its antioxidant properties may in the future be shown to be of value in the diabetic.

Overall, it would seem that HMG CoA reductase inhibitors are probably the most useful drugs for patients with diabetes or glucose intolerance, with the best side effect profile for most diabetic subjects. In patients with marked hypertriglyceridemia gemfibrozil is probably the agent of first choice.

Antihypertensive Medications

The management of blood pressure in the diabetic is particularly important. Not only does it remain a significant CVD risk factor in many studies, but it also relates to the development of other complications, including nephropathy [99], neuropathy [132], and retinopathy [99]. The arguments for more intensive therapy of blood pressure in the diabetic, even at levels usually considered normal, are currently under close consideration. While it may be reasonable to await the results of current trials before universally advocating the initiation of pharmacologic therapy (if weight loss and salt reduction are unsuccessful) at levels in the high normal range (e.g., above 130/85), such treatment in those with proteinuria (or microalbuminuria) would seem appropriate. The choice of agent to be used is the same as in the nondiabetic; however, because of special considerations in diabetes, as listed in Table 14-4, the working group [99] recommends certain drugs as step one medications.

Though no agents are contraindicated in diabetes, traditional drugs like thiazide diuretics and beta blockers need to be used cautiously. The thiazides pose a number of concerns. They may elevate both LDL cholesterol and triglycerides, undesirable in a high-risk population. Furthermore, they may elevate blood sugar levels. Therefore, if they are used (and they are particularly useful in those with an increased blood volume, e.g., blacks and the elderly), potassium supplementation and careful glucose and lipid monitoring are needed. Potassium-sparing diuretics can also be used, although in patients with renal disease hyperkalemia must be carefully watched for.

Beta blockers have usually been thought to be problematic in diabetes because of their aggravation and masking of hypoglycemia. This is especially likely to occur with the noncardioselective beta blockers. However, with care and appropriate warning of patients, they may be used with benefit, as in those patients with concomitant angina. The α-adrenergic blocker prazosin has the advantage of little adverse and possibly a small beneficial effect on the lipid profile with little or no disturbance of glucose tolerance.

Perhaps the most appealing drugs to use in the diabetic are the ACE inhibitors. These have the benefit of little change in glucose control or lipoprotein levels and, perhaps due to their ability to reduce intraglomerular hypertension, appear to slow the decline of renal function and reduce albuminuria [133]. Indeed, as noted earlier, potentially beneficial effects have been seen in diabetics with normal blood pressure [114]. Trials currently underway will help to determine if these are the most efficacious drugs in early renal disease in diabetes. Calcium channel blockers are a further first-line choice, although orthostatic hypotension can be a problem.

Other medications can be used in the diabetic

Table 14-4.   First-line antihypertensive medications in diabetes: specific considerations

Drug	Advantages	Concerns
Thiazides	Effective in patients with increased blood volume, sodium retention	Raise cholesterol, triglycerides Raise blood sugar Lower serum K+ Impotence
Loop diuretics	Same as thiazides; also effective in renal failure	Same as thiazides
Potassium-sparing diuretics	No potassium loss, little effect on lipids	Hyperkalemia in renal failure
Beta blockers	Useful in patients with angina or tachycardia	Raise triglycerides, lower HDL cholesterol* Aggravate hypoglycemia Mask hypoglycemic symptoms Impotence
Alpha blocker (prazosin)	No effect on glucose or insulin	
ACE inhibitors	Little effect on glucose or lipids; lowers microalbuminuria and intraglomerular hypertension	
Calcium channel blockers	Little effect on lipids	Orthostatic hypotension

*Especially noncardioselective agents.

in place of or in combination with the first-line drugs, but all have important limitations. Central and peripheral acting adrenergic inhibitors have particular problems with orthostatic hypotension, salt retention, and impotence, which limit their usefulness in many diabetics, as does the sedation and depression seen with the centrally acting group of these drugs. Vasodilators may worsen coronary disease and cause sodium retention. The management of hypertension becomes increasingly difficult with worsening renal function, and the reader is referred to the working group document for further details [99].

Other Measures

Smoking should be strongly discouraged, as in the general population [134]. In particular its role in peripheral vascular disease and, as recently reported, neuropathy [132] make the combination of diabetes and smoking a disaster that must be avoided at all costs. It is a sad reflection on our management of diabetes that most studies show diabetics to smoke as frequently as, if not more than, the general population. Although the evidence that physical activity is of direct benefit in diabetes is as yet limited, the ADA rightly advocates reasonable activity, which should be encouraged whenever appropriate [135].

Summary

Diabetes constitutes a major cardiovascular risk, especially for women, and is associated with significant changes in cardiovascular risk factors, which include blood lipids, blood pressure, fibrinogen, platelets, and insulin resistance and concentration. Many of these changes become more profound with renal disease. The clinician should be alert to these problems and should treat them vigorously by diet, improved glycemic control, and, when indicated, drug therapy. Although the evidence to date suggests that correction of lipoprotein abnormalities, raised blood pressure, and smoking are likely to be beneficial, there is sadly a paucity of direct clinical trial evidence of benefit of such maneu-

vers in diabetes, because diabetics have been systematically excluded from all the major trials. Some caution is therefore advised, particularly in terms of drug therapy. The need for primary and secondary intervention trials of virtually all potential prevention regimens for cardiovascular disease in diabetes is one of the most pressing problems in preventive cardiology.

References

1. Jarrett RJ. Type II (non-insulin dependent) diabetes mellitus and coronary heart disease — chicken, egg, or neither? Diabetologia 1984; 26:99–102.
2. American Heart Association. 1990 heart and stroke facts. Greenville, Dallas, 1990.
3. Hadden WC, Harris MI. National Center for Health Statistics. Prevalence of diagnosed diabetes, undiagnosed diabetes, and impaired glucose tolerance in adults 20–74 years of age, United States 1976–1980. Vital and Health Statistics 1987; series 11, no. 237. DHHS publ. no. (PHS) 87-1687.
4. National Diabetes Data Group. Classification and diagnosis of diabetes mellitus and other categories of glucose intolerance. Diabetes 1979; 28:1039–57.
5. World Health Organization Expert Committee. Second report on diabetes mellitus. Technical Report Series no. 646. Geneva: WHO, 1980.
6. Bennett PH, Knowler WC. Early detection and intervention in diabetes mellitus: Is it effective? J Chron Dis 1984; 37:653–66.
7. Harris MI, Hadden WC, Knowler WC, et al. International criteria for the diagnosis of diabetes and impaired glucose tolerance. Diabetes Care 1985; 8:562–7.
8. Orchard TJ, Daneman D, Becker DJ, et al. Glycosylated hemoglobin: a screening test for diabetes mellitus. J Prev Med 1982; 11:595–601.
9. Saad MF, Knowler WC, Pettitt D, et al. The natural history of impaired glucose tolerance in the Pima Indians. New Engl J Med 1988; 319:1500–6.
10. American Diabetes Association. Position statement: screening for diabetes. Diabetes Care 1989; 12:588–90.
11. Barrett-Connor E, Orchard TJ. Diabetes and heart disease. In: Harris MJ, Hamman RF, eds. Diabetes in America. Bethesda, Md.: National Institutes of Health, National Diabetes Data Group, 1985. NIH publ. no. 85-1468.
12. Pyörälä K, Laakso M, Uusitupa M. Diabetes

and atherosclerosis: an epidemiologic view. Diab Metab Rev 1987; 3:463–524.

13. Garcia MJ, McNamara PM, Gordon T, et al. Morbidity and mortality in diabetics in the Framingham population. Sixteen year follow-up study. Diabetes 1974; 23:105–11.

14. Barrett-Connor E, Wingard DL. Sex differential in ischemic heart disease mortality in diabetics: a prospective population-based study. Am J Epidemiol 1983; 118:489–96.

15. Jarrett RJ, McCartney P, Keen H. The Bedford survey: ten year mortality rates in newly diagnosed diabetics, borderline diabetics and normoglycaemic controls and risk indices for coronary heart disease in borderline diabetics. Diabetologia 1982; 22:79–84.

16. Dorman JS, LaPorte RE, Kuller LH, et al. The Pittsburgh insulin-dependent diabetes mellitus (IDDM) morbidity and mortality study. Mortality results. Diabetes 1984; 33:271–6.

17. Kannell WB, McGee DL. Diabetes and cardiovascular disease. The Framingham study. JAMA 1979; 241:2035–8.

18. Kannel WB, McGee, DL. Diabetes and glucose tolerance as risk factors for cardiovascular disease: the Framingham study. Diabetes Care 1979; 2:120–6.

19. Heyden S, Heiss G, Bartel AG, Hames CG. Sex differences in coronary mortality among diabetics in Evans County, Georgia. J Chron Dis 1980; 33:265–73.

20. Fuller JH, Shipley MJ, Rose G, et al. Mortality from coronary heart disease and stroke in relation to degree of glycaemia: the Whitehall study. Br Med J 1983; 287:867–70.

21. Eschwège E, Richard JL, Thibult N, et al. Coronary heart disease mortality in relation with diabetes, blood glucose and plasma insulin levels. The Paris prospective study, ten years later. Horm Metab Res Suppl 1985; 15:41–6.

22. Palumbo PJ, Melton LJ. Peripheral vascular disease and diabetes. In: Harris MJ, Hamman RF, eds. Diabetes in America. Bethesda, Md.: National Institutes of Health, National Diabetes Data Group, 1985. NIH publ. no. 85-1468.

23. Orchard TJ. Dyslipoproteinemia and diabetes. Endocrinology and Metab Clin of North America 1990; 19:361–80.

24. Barrett-Connor E, Grundy SM, Holdbrook MJ. Plasma lipids and diabetes mellitus in an adult community. Am J Epidemiol 1982; 115:657–63.

25. Cruickshanks KJ, Orchard TJ, Becker DJ. The cardiovascular risk profile of adolescents with insulin-dependent diabetes mellitus. Diabetes Care 1985; 8:118–24.

26. Stamler J. Epidemiology of diabetes with respect to cardiovascular diseases. Presented at Second World Conference on Diabetes Research, Monaco, March 1988.

27. Wingard DL, Barrett-Connor E, Criqui MH, et al. Clustering of heart disease risk factors in diabetic compared to nondiabetic adults. Am J Epid 1983; 117:19–26.

28. Kleinman JC, Donahue RP, Harris MI, et al. Mortality among diabetics in a national sample. Am J Epidemiol 1988; 128:389–401.

29. Morrish NJ, Stevens LK, Head J, et al. A prospective study of mortality among middle-aged diabetic patients (the London cohort of the WHO multinational study of vascular disease in diabetics). II. Causes and death rates. Diabetologia 1990; 33:538–41.

30. West KM. Epidemiology of diabetes and its vascular lesions. New York: Elsevier, 1978; 231–48.

31. Orchard TJ, Becker DJ, Bates M, et al. Plasma insulin and lipoprotein concentrations: an atherogenic association? Am J Epidemiol 1983; 118:326–37.

32. Orchard TJ, Becker DJ, Kuller LH, et al. Age and sex variations in glucose tolerance and insulin responses: parallels with cardiovascular risk. J Chron Dis 1982; 35:123–32.

33. Scheldt-Nave C, Barrett-Connor E. Gender differences in fasting glycemia as a risk factor for IHD death (abstract). Circulation 1990; 81(2):6.

34. Abbott RD, Donahue RP, Kannel WB, et al. The impact of diabetes on survival following myocardial infarction in men vs. women. The Framingham study. JAMA 1988; 260:3456–60.

35. Borch-Johnsen K, Kreiner S. Proteinuria: value as predictor of cardiovascular mortality in insulin dependent diabetes mellitus. Br Med J 1987; 294:1651–4.

36. Mattock MB, Keen H, Viberti GC, et al. Coronary heart disease and urinary albumin excretion rate in type 2 (non-insulin-dependent) diabetic patients. Diabetologia 1988; 31:82–7.

37. Phillips A, Shaper AG, Winchup PH. Association between serum albumin and mortality from cardiovascular disease, cancer and other causes. Lancet 1989; 2:1434–6.

38. Orchard TJ, Ellis D, Dorman J. Lipid and lipoprotein concentrations in IDDM controlling for renal disease: the Pittsburgh epidemiology of diabetes complications study (abstract). 23rd Int Res Symp: Diabetes, lipoproteins, and atherosclerosis. Am Diabetes Assoc, Hilton Head, SC, March 6–8, 1989.

39. Jensen T, Borch-Johnsen K, Kofoed-Enevoldsen A, et al. Coronary heart disease in young type 1 (insulin-dependent) diabetic patients with and without diabetic nephropathy; incidence and risk factors. Diabetologia 1987; 31:144–8.

40. Deckert T, Feldt-Rasmussen B, Borch-Johnsen K, et al. Albuminuria reflects widespread vascular damage. The Steno hypothesis. Diabetologia 1989; 32:219–26.

41. Robertson WB and Strong JP. Atherosclerosis in persons with hypertension and diabetes mellitus. Lab Invest 1968; 18:78–91.

42. Dortimer AC, Shenoy PN, Shiroff RA, et al. Diffuse coronary artery disease in diabetic patients. Circulation 1978; 57:133–6.

43. Waller BJ, Palumbo PJ, Lie JT, et al. Status of the coronary arteries at necropsy in diabetes mellitus with onset after age 30 years. Analysis of 229 diabetic patients with and without clinical evidence of coronary heart disease and comparison to 183 control subjects. Am J Med 1980; 69:498–506.

44. Orchard TJ, Dorman JS, Maser RE, et al. Prevalence of complications in IDDM by sex and duration. Pittsburgh epidemiology of diabetes complications study II. Diabetes 1990; 39:1116–24.

45. Janka HU. Five-year incidence of major macrovascular complications in diabetes mellitus. Horm Metab Res Suppl 1985; 15:15–19.

46. Jarrett RJ, Shipley MJ. Type 2 (non-insulin-dependent) diabetes mellitus and cardiovascular disease-putative association via common antecedents; further evidence from the Whitehall study. Diabetologia 1988; 31:737–40.

47. Nelson RG, Sievers ML, Knowler WC, et al. Low incidence of fatal coronary heart disease in Pima indians despite high prevalence of non-insulin-dependent diabetes. Circulation 1990; 81:987–95.

48. Wilson PWF, Kannel WB, Anderson KM. Lipids, glucose intolerance and vascular disease: the Framingham study Monogr. Atheroscler 1985; 13:1–11.

49. McPhillips JB, Barrett-Connor E, Wingard DL. Cardiovascular disease risk factors prior to the diagnosis of impaired glucose tolerance and non-insulin-dependent diabetes mellitus in a community of older adults. Am J Epidemiol 1990; 131:443–53.

50. Jarrett RJ, Keen H, Fuller JH, McCartney M. Worsening to diabetes in men with impaired glucose tolerance ("borderline diabetes"). Diabetologia 1979; 16:25–35.

51. Sasaki A, Suzuki T, Horiuchi N. Development of diabetes in Japanese subjects with impaired glucose tolerance: a seven-year follow-up study. Diabetologia 1982; 22:154–7.

52. Eschwège E, Ducimetière P, Papoz L, et al. Blood glucose and coronary heart disease. Lancet 1980; 2:472–3.

53. Fuller JH, Shipley MJ, Rose G, et al. Mortality from coronary heart disease and stroke in relation to degree of glycaemia: the Whitehall study. Br Med J 1983; 287:867–70.

54. Stamler J, Stamler R. Asymptomatic hyperglycemia and coronary heart disease. A series of papers by the international collaborative group, based on studies in fifteen populations. Introduction. J Chron Dis 1979; 32:683–91.

55. Ganda OP, Soeldner JS, Gleason RE. Alterations in plasma lipids in the presence of mild glucose intolerance in the offspring of two type II diabetic parents. Diabetes Care 1985; 8:254–60.

56. Ducimetière P, Eschwège E, Papoz L, et al. Relationship of plasma insulin levels to the incidence of myocardial infarction and coronary heart disease mortality in a middle-aged population. Diabetologia 1980; 19:205–10.

57. Pyörälä K. Relationship of glucose tolerance and plasma insulin in the incidence of coronary heart disease: results from two population studies in Finland. Diabetes Care 1979; 2:131–41.

58. Welborn TA, Wearne K. Coronary heart disease incidence and cardiovascular mortality in Busselton with reference to glucose and insulin concentrations. Diabetes Care 1979; 2:154–60.

59. Fontbonne A, Tchobroutsky G, Eschwège E, et al. Coronary heart disease mortality risk: plasma insulin level is a more sensitive marker than hypertension or abnormal glucose tolerance in overweight males. The Paris prospective study. Internat J Obesity 1988; 12:557–65.

60. Peiris AN, Mueller RA, Struve MF, et al. Splanchnic insulin metabolism in obesity: influence of body fat distribution. J Clin Invest 1986; 78:1648–57.

61. Lapidus L, Bengtsson C, Larsson B, et al. Distribution of adipose tissue and risk of cardiovascular disease and death: a 12 year follow-up of participants in the population study of women in Gothenburg, Sweden. Br Med J 1984; 289:1257–61.

62. Haffner SM, Stern MP, Hazuda HP, et al. Role of obesity and fat distribution in non-insulin-dependent diabetes mellitus in Mexican Americans and non-Hispanic whites. Diabetes Care 1986; 9:153–61.

63. Ohlson L-O, Larsson B, Svärdsudd K, et al. The influence of body fat distribution on the incidence of diabetes mellitus: 13.5 years of follow-up of the participants in the study of men born in 1913. Diabetes 1985; 34:1055–8.

64. Stout RW, Bierman EL, Ross R. Effect of insulin on the proliferation of cultured primate arterial smooth muscle cells. Atherosclerosis 1977; 27:271–8.

65. O'Dea K. Marked improvement in carbohydrate and lipid metabolism in diabetic Australian aborigines after temporary reversion to traditional lifestyle. Diabetes 1984; 33:596–603.

66. West KM, Ahuja MMS, Bennett PH, et al. The role of circulating glucose and triglyceride concentrations and their interactions with other "risk factors" as determinants of arterial disease in nine diabetic population samples from the WHO multinational study. Diabetes Care 1983; 6:361–9.

67. Fontbonne A, Eschwège E, Cambien F, et al. Hypertriglyceridaemia as a risk factor of coronary heart disease mortality in subjects with impaired glucose tolerance or diabetes. Results from the 11-year follow-up of the Paris prospective study. Diabetologia 1989; 32:300–4.

68. Santen RJ, Willis PW, Fajans SS. Atherosclerosis in diabetes mellitus. Arch Intern Med 1972; 130:833–43.

69. Maser RE, Wolfson SK, Ellis D, et al. Cardiovascular disease and arterial calcification in insulin dependent diabetes mellitus: interrelationships and risk factor profiles. Pittsburgh Epidemiology of Diabetes Complications Study V. Arteriosclerosis and Thrombosis 1991; 11:958–65.

70. Schernthaner G, Kostner GM, Dieplinger H, et al. Apolipoproteins (A-I, A-II, B), Lp(a) lipoprotein and lecithin: cholesterol acyltransferase activity in diabetes mellitus. Atherosclerosis 1983; 49:277–93.

71. Mertz DP, Bürvenich K. Different levels of lipoprotein Lp(a) in adult diabetic patients depending on the therapeutic regimen. Klin Wochenschr 1985; 63:648–50.

72. Colwell JA, Winocour PD, Halushka PV. Do platelets have anything to do with diabetic microvascular disease? Diabetes 1983; 32:14–19.

73. Watanabe J, Wohltmann HJ, Klein RL, et al. Enhancement of platelet aggregation by low-density lipoproteins from IDDM patients. Diabetes 1988; 37:1652–7.

74. Cho NH, Becker D, Dorman JS, et al. Spontaneous whole blood platelet aggregation in insulin-dependent diabetes mellitus: an evaluation in an epidemiologic study. Thrombosis and Haemostasis 1989; 61:127–30.

75. Fuller JH, Keen H, Jarrett RJ, et al. Haemostatic variables associated with diabetes and its complications. Br Med J 1979; 2:964–6.

76. Jensen T, Stender S, Deckert T. Abnormalities in plasma concentrations of lipoproteins and fibrinogen in type 1 (insulin-dependent) diabetic patients with increased urinary albumin excretion. Diabetologia 1988; 31:142–5.

77. Nelson RG, Sievers ML, Knowler WC, et al. Low incidence of fatal coronary heart disease in Pima indians despite high prevalence of non-insulin-dependent diabetes. Circulation 1990; 81:987–95.

78. Chi Zhi-sheng. Some aspects of diabetes in the People's Republic of China. In: Mann JI, Pyörälä K, and Teuscher A, eds. Diabetes in epidemiological perspective. Edinburgh: Churchill Livingstone, 1983; 78–86.

79. Sasaki A, Uehara M, Horiuchi N, Hasagawa K. A long-term follow-up study of Japanese diabetic patients: mortality and causes of death. Diabetologia 1983; 25:309–12.

80. Keen H, Jarrett TJ. The WHO multinational study of vascular disease in diabetes. 2. Macrovascular disease prevalence. Diabetes Care 1979; 2:187–95.

81. Olefsky JM, Kolterman OG. Mechanisms of insulin resistance in obesity and non-insulin-dependent (type II) diabetes. Am J Med 1981; 70:151–68.

82. Temple RC, Carrington CA, Luzio SD, et al. Insulin deficiency in non-insulin-dependent diabetes. Lancet 1989; 1:293–5.

83. Cryer A. Tissue lipoprotein lipase activity and its action in lipoprotein metabolism. Int J Biochem 1981; 13:525–41.

84. Eisenberg S. High density lipoprotein metabolism. J Lipid Res 1984; 25:1017–58.

85. Pfeifer MA, Brunzell JD, Best JD, et al. The response of plasma triglyceride, cholesterol and lipoprotein lipase to treatment in non-insulin-dependent subjects without familial hypertriglyceridemia. Diabetes 1983; 32:525–31.

86. Zilversmit DB. Atherogenesis: a postprandial phenomenon. Circulation 1979; 60:473–85.

86a. Harno KE, Nikkila EA, Kuusi T. Plasma HDL-cholesterol and postheparin plasma hepatic endothelial lipase activity: relationship to obesity and non-insulin-dependent diabetes. Diabetologia 1980; 19:281.

87. Bagdade JD, Bierman EL, Porte D Jr. The influence of obesity on the relationship between insulin and triglyceride levels in endogenous hypertriglyceridemia. Diabetes 1971; 20:664.

88. Reaven GM. Non-insulin-dependent diabetes mellitus, abnormal lipoprotein metabolism and atherosclerosis. Metabolism 1987; 36:1–8.

89. Patsch W, Franz S, Schonfeld G. Role of insulin in lipoprotein secretion by cultured rat hepatocytes. J Clin Invest 1983; 71:1161–74.

90. Howard BV. Lipoprotein metabolism in diabetes mellitus. J Lipid Res 1987; 28:613–28.

91. Fielding CJ, Reaven GM, Liu G, et al. Increased free cholesterol in plasma low and very low density lipoproteins in non-insulin-dependent diabetes mellitus: its role in the inhibition of cholesterol ester transfer. Proc Natl Acad Sci USA 1984; 81:2512–6.

92. Chait A, Bierman EL, Albers JJ. Low density lipoprotein receptor activity in cultured human skin fibroblasts-mechanism of insulin-induced stimulation. J Clin Invest 1979; 64:1309–19.

93. Hiramatsu K, Bierman EL, Chait A. Metabolism of low density lipoproteins from patients with diabetic hypertriglyceridemia by cultured human skin fibroblasts. Diabetes 1985; 34:8–14.

94. Steinbrecher UP, Witztum JL. Glycosylation of low-density lipoproteins to an extent comparable to that seen in diabetes slows their catabolism. Diabetes 1984; 33:130–4.

95. Brownlee M, Vlassara H, Cerami A. Nonenzymatic glycosylation products on collagen covalently trap low-density lipoprotein. Diabetes 1985; 34:938–41.

96. Witztum JL, Mahoney EM, Branks MJ, et al. Nonenzymatic glycosylation of low-density lipoprotein alters its biologic activity. Diabetes 1982;31:283–91.

97. Goldstein JL, Ho YK, Basu SK, et al. Binding site on macrophages that mediates uptake and degradation of acetylated low density lipoprotein, producing massive cholesterol deposition. Proc Natl Acad Sci 1979; 76:333–7.

98. Schonfeld G, Birge C, Miller JP, et al. Apolipoprotein B levels and altered lipoprotein composition in diabetes. Diabetes 1974; 23:827–34.

99. The working group on hypertension in diabetes: statement on hypertension in diabetes mellitus. Final report. Arch Intern Med 1987; 147:830–42.

100. Donahue RP, Skyler JS, Schneiderman N, Prineas RJ. Hyperinsulinemia and elevated blood pressure: cause, confounder, or coincidence? Am J Epidemiol 1990; 132:827–36.

101. Weinsler RL, Norris DJ, Birch R, et al. The relative contribution of body fat and fat pattern to blood pressure. Hypertension 1985; 7:578–85.

102. Blair D, Habicht JP, Sims EAH, et al. Evidence for an increased risk for hypertension with centrally located body fat and the effect of race and sex on this risk. Am J Epidemiol 1984; 119:526–40.

103. Cambien F, Warnet JM, Eschwège E, et al. Body mass, blood pressure, glucose and lipids: does plasma insulin explain their relationships? Arteriosclerosis 1987; 7:197–292.

104. Rowe JW, Young JB, Minaker KL, et al. Effect of insulin and glucose infusions on sympathetic nervous system activity in normal men. Diabetes 1981; 30:219–25.

105. Goldstein DS. Plasma catecholamines and essential hypertension: an analytic review. Hypertension 1983; 5:86–99.

106. DeFronzo RA. The effect of insulin on renal sodium metabolism. Diabetologia 1981; 21:165–71.

107. Bunker CH, Mallinger AG. Sodium-lithium countertransport, obesity, insulin, and blood pressure in healthy premenopausal women (abstract). Circulation 1985; 72:Suppl III:296.

108. Stout RW. Insulin and atheroma: 20-year perspective. Diabetes Care 1990; 13:631–54.

109. Ruderman NB, Haudenschild C. Diabetes as an atherogenic factor. Prog Cardiovasc Dis 1984; 26:373–412.

110. Porta M, La Selva M, Molinatti P, Molinatti GM. Endothelial cell function in diabetic microangiopathy (review). Diabetologia 1987; 30:601–09.

111. Lopes-Virella MF, Wohltmann HJ, Mayfield RK, et al. Effect of metabolic control on lipid, lipoprotein, and apolipoprotein levels in 55 insulin-dependent diabetic patients. A longitudinal study. Diabetes 1983; 32:20–5.

112. 1984 Joint National Committee on Detection, Evaluation, and Treatment of High Blood Pressure. Nonpharmacological approaches to the control of high blood pressure: final report of the subcommittee on nonpharmacological therapy. Hypertension 1986; 9:444–67.

113. The Expert Panel of the National Cholesterol Education Program. Report of the expert panel on detection, evaluation and treatment of high blood cholesterol in adults. Arch Intern Med 1988; 148:36–69.

114. Rudberg S, Aperia A, Freyschuss U, Persson B. Enalapril reduces microalbuminuria in young normotensive type 1 (insulin-dependent) diabetic patients irrespective of its hypotensive effect. Diabetologia 1990; 33:470–6.

115. Christensen CK, Mogensen CE. Effect of antihypertensive treatment on progression of incipient diabetic nephropathy. Hypertension 1985; 7:109–13.

116. Feldt-Rasmussen B, Mathiesen ER, Deckert T. Effect of two years strict metabolic control on the progression of incipient nephropathy in insulin-dependent diabetes. Lancet 1986; 2:1300–4.

117. Cohen D, Dodds R, Viberti G. Effect of protein restriction in insulin dependent diabetics at risk of nephropathy. Br Med J 1987; 294:795–8.

118. The DCCT Research Group. The diabetes control and complications trial (DCCT); design and methodologic considerations for the feasibility phase. Diabetes 1986; 35:530–45.

119. American Diabetes Association. Nutritional recommendations and principles for individuals with diabetes mellitus: 1986. Diabetes Care 1987; 10:126–32.

120. Liu GC, Coulston AM, Reaven GM. Effects of high-carbohydrate-low-fat diets on plasma glucose, insulin and lipid responses in hypertriglyceridemic humans. Metabolism 1983; 32:750–3.

121. Simpson RW, Mann JI, Eaton J, et al. Improved

glucose control in maturity-onset diabetes treated with high-carbohydrate modified fat diet. Br Med J 1979; 1:1753–6.

121a. Ullmann D, Connor WE, Hatcher LF, et al. Will a high-carbohydrate, low-fat diet lower plasma lipids and lipoproteins without producing hypertriglyceridemia. Arteriosclerosis and Thrombosis 1991; 11:1059–67.

122. Brenner BM, Meyer TW, Hostetter TH. Dietary protein intake and the progressive nature of kidney disease: the role of hemodynamically mediated glomerular injury in the pathogenesis of progressive glomerular sclerosis in aging, renal ablation, and intrinsic renal disease. N Engl J Med 1982; 307:652–9.

123. Garg A, Bonanome A, Grundy SM, et al. Comparison of a high-carbohydrate diet with a high-monounsaturated-fat diet in patients with non-insulin-dependent diabetes mellitus. N Engl J Med 1988; 319:829–34.

124. Savage PJ, Knowler WC. Diet therapy for type 2 (non-insulin-dependent) diabetes mellitus: can new approaches improve therapeutic results? Nutrition Abstracts and Reviews in Clinical Nutrition–Series A 1984; 54:69–87.

125. Leaf A, Weber PC. Cardiovascular effects of n-3 fatty acids. N Engl J Med 1988; 318:549–57.

126. Kasim SE, Stern B, Khilnani S, et al. Effects of omega-3 fish oils on lipid metabolism, glycemic control, and blood pressure in type II diabetic patients. J Clin Endocrinol Metab 1988; 67:1–5.

127. Molnar GD, Berge KG, Rosevear JW, et al. The effect of nicotinic acid in diabetes mellitus. Metabolism 1964; 13:181–9.

128. Garg A, Grundy SM. Nicotinic acid may not be first line therapy for dyslipidemia in non-insulin-dependent diabetes mellitus (NIDDM) (abstract). Clin Res 1989; 37:449A.

129. Garg A, Grundy SM. Gemfibrozil alone and in combination with lovastatin for treatment of hypertriglyceridemia in NIDDM. Diabetes 1989; 38:364–72.

130. Konttinen A, Kuisma I, Ralli R, et al. The effect of gemfibrozil on serum lipids in diabetic patients. Ann Clin Res 1979; 11:240–5.

131. Garg A, Grundy SM. Lovastatin for lowering cholesterol levels in non-insulin-dependent diabetes mellitus. N Engl J Med 1988; 318:81–6.

132. Maser RE, Steenkiste AR, Dorman JS, et al. Epidemiological correlates of diabetic neuropathy. Report from the Pittsburgh Epidemiology of Diabetes Complication Study. Diabetes 1989; 38:1456–61.

133. Insua A, Ribstein J, Mimran A. Comparative effect of captopril and nifedipine in normotensive patients with incipient diabetic nephropathy. Postgrad Med J 1988; 64:Suppl 3:59–62.

134. ADA Consensus Statement. Role of cardiovascular risk factors in prevention and treatment of macrovascular disease in diabetes. Diabetes Care 1989; 12:573–9.

135. ADA Position Statement. Diabetes mellitus and exercise. Diabetes Care 1990; 13:804–5.

15

Intervention for Secondary Prevention

BONNIE H. WEINER

EDITORS' INTRODUCTION

For many years achieving regression of CHD in human beings has been an elusive goal. In the last few years, however, a number of studies have shown definite regression of the atherosclerotic process in patients with clinically advanced disease. These results have been attained with methodologies varying from potent lipid-modifying drugs to pure lifestyle intervention. The common denominator in all these efforts has been a dramatic lowering of blood cholesterol and LDL levels into a range much below that which is usually considered normal. Dr. Weiner reviews these fascinating studies and the epidemiologic and animal research efforts that preceded them and then offers practical suggestions for the secondary prevention of CHD. It is now evident that modification of the course of CHD is possible even after the development of angina or MI. Progression of plaque formation can be slowed or halted, and with aggressive intervention true reversal of CHD has become realizable.

Previous chapters have extensively discussed the development of atherosclerosis and the approaches to primary prevention of coronary heart disease. This chapter reviews the pathophysiologic basis for secondary prevention, examines the animal and clinical studies that form the basis for present opinion, and recommends a clinical approach to patients who have already suffered a coronary event. The majority of studies that support risk factor intervention for secondary prevention are in the areas of smoking and hyperlipidemia; however, hypertension and diabetes are briefly discussed here as well. Other non-risk factor interventions are also described.

In discussing secondary prevention, we are referring to individuals who already have angiographically documented atherosclerosis or who have had a clinical event or developed symptoms of CHD. Ideally the goal would be to reverse the course of the disease. A goal only slightly less desirable would be to arrest the disease process at the point at which it is first encountered. This also would be likely to result in a reduction in clinical events and symptoms.

Major Coronary Risk Factors in Secondary Prevention

Hypertension

Hypertension is a major risk factor for the development of CHD. Primary prevention trials have shown beneficial effects of treatment on the incidence of cerebrovascular complications; however, the effects on cardiac morbidity and mortality have been much more modest [1, 2, 3, 4]. There are as yet no data to support a beneficial role of hypertension therapy for elevated diastolic blood pressure in the secondary prevention of CHD. It has been suggested that this may be in part explained by the potential negative effects of many of the commonly used antihypertensive agents on lipid metabolism, thereby offsetting possible positive effects [5, 6, 7].

The recently reported Systolic Hypertension in the Elderly Program (SHEP), although designed with a primary end point of evaluating the effects of treating isolated systolic hypertension on the incidence of fatal and nonfatal

stroke, included the assessment of cardiovascular events as secondary end points (8). In this trial nearly 5000 patients over the age of 60 with isolated systolic hypertension (ISH) were randomized to active treatment or placebo and followed for 5 years. Although blood pressure reduction was observed in both the active treatment and the placebo groups, the active treatment group on the average had systolic pressures 11 to 14 mmHg lower and diastolic pressures 3 to 4 mmHg lower than the placebo group at each annual evaluation. The active treatment group had significantly fewer cardiovascular events during the follow-up period (Table 15-1). The combined end point of CHD death and overall CHD, including fatal and nonfatal MI, sudden death (<1 hour), rapid death (1 to 24 hours), and revascularization, also demonstrates a reduction in risk in the active treatment arm. There was also a 13-percent reduction in overall mortality in the active treatment group which did not achieve statistical significance. The trial was not designed to have the power to demonstrate a change in overall mortality; the finding is therefore of considerable interest.

Although SHEP was designed as a primary prevention trial, it is reasonable to assume that in the age group studied, atherosclerotic disease was present in a significant percentage of the subjects. Thus, the results can be interpreted as consistent with the findings likely to be seen in a definitive secondary prevention trial and therefore suggest that therapy of systolic hypertension is beneficial in the secondary prevention of CHD (see Chapter 13 for further review of this topic).

Diabetes Mellitus

The presence of diabetes mellitus, another major risk factor for the development of CHD, has been shown to correlate with increased severity of atherosclerosis, particularly in women using oral hypoglycemic agents [9]. The effects of this systemic disease on the atherosclerotic process are multifactorial, resulting from lipid abnormalities, abnormalities of platelet function, and abnormalities in other metabolic pathways [10, 11, 12, 13, 14, 15, 16, 17].

Table 15-1. Cardiovascular events in SHEP

Event	Active treatment group (n = 2365)	Placebo group (n = 2371)	Relative risk (95% confidence interval)
Nonfatal MI	50	74	0.67 (0.47–0.96)
CABG	30	47	0.63 (0.40–1.00)
PTCA	19	22	0.86 (0.47–1.59)
CHD death	59	73	0.80 (0.57–1.13)
Sudden death	23	23	1.00 (0.56–1.78)
Rapid death	21	24	0.87 (0.48–1.56)
Fatal MI	15	26	0.57 (0.30–1.08)

There are no data that suggest that optimal control of glucose metabolism by itself has a major impact on existing atherosclerosis. However, poor control of diabetes may result in wide fluctuations in lipid values and a negative effect on cellular function. Furthermore, as described in Chapter 12, some of the primary agents used in lipid-lowering therapy must be used with caution in these patients. The primary goal of secondary prevention of CHD in a diabetic patient should be control of the other risk factors, such as smoking and hyperlipidemia, whose deleterious effect is exacerbated by diabetes. This topic is fully discussed in Chapter 14.

Cigarette Smoking

Smoking cessation has not yet been demonstrated by angiography or pathology to result in regression of atherosclerosis. Smoking cessation has, however, been shown to be of major benefit in reducing the complications of CHD. Smokers may be classified for these purposes as smokers, quitters, and never-smokers. In an early investigation, Mulcahy pointed out that never-smokers who suffered an MI had worse overall profiles for other coronary risk factors than did smokers, which emphasizes the importance of cigarette smoking as an accelerator of CHD [18]. Quitters had a better overall outcome than those who had never smoked. Those patients who quit smoking following an MI had approximately half the risk of recurrent MI or CHD death compared to those who continued to smoke. These findings are supported by several other investigations. In general there is approximately a 40- to 50-percent reduction in risk of recurrent events or death in individuals who quit smoking compared to those who continue to smoke. The long-term risk for those who quit falls rapidly and approximates the risk of those who have never smoked by about 5 years after cessation [19, 20, 21, 22, 23, 24].

In two reports, the primary benefit was observed early in the follow-up period and especially affected risk of sudden death [25, 26]. This suggests an effect of smoking cessation in this early period that is not related to changes in atherosclerosis. Since cigarette smoking is known to increase platelet aggregability and also affects other components of the clotting cascade, as well as causing endothelial injury and predisposing to coronary artery spasm, modification of these processes by cessation is a likely mechanism for the rapid favorable effect of smoking cessation [27, 28, 29, 30, 31, 32, 33, 34, 35, 36, 37, 38].

Lipid Therapy and Secondary Prevention

Rationale for the Role of Lipid Modification in Secondary Prevention

The literature strongly supports the relationship between blood cholesterol level, dietary saturated fat intake, and morbidity and mortality related to CHD [39, 40, 41, 42, 43] (see Chapters 1, 3, and 4). Furthermore, it is apparent that lowering cholesterol is of benefit even in the presence of severe disease, such as is seen in patients who have already undergone bypass surgery [44, 45]. Whether there is a differential response to therapy in different stages of plaque development remains unclear. It may be that severe, complicated, calcified atherosclerotic plaques respond more slowly and less completely, if at all, than do plaques at an earlier stage.

Two pathologic studies have reported findings consistent with this hypothesis. In a study of eight women who had died of CHD before the age of forty, the coronary artery plaques were found to have more cellular fibrous tissue and foam cells and lesser amounts of dense fibrous tissue and calcium than those seen in an older population (mean age 59) also dying of CHD [46]. The opposite findings were observed in patients 90 years of age or older [47]. The authors conclude that the lesion characteristics found in the younger patients would be more amenable to regression.

Cellular and Chemical Basis for Atherosclerosis Change

To determine the effect of lipid-lowering regimens on the plaque itself, lipid metabolism in the growing plaque must be understood. The importance and the effects of abnormalities of lipoprotein fractions are discussed in Chapter 3. There are also processes occurring within the arterial wall that may be important in placing the observations from clinical and animal trials of regression in perspective.

Small and colleagues have studied the physicochemical properties of plaque lipids during various stages of development [48, 49]. Although cholesterol esters accumulate in normal arterial intima with age, the lipid content of fatty streaks is predominantly extracellular LDL and VLDL particles, and the majority of lipids in the vascular intima of children are phospholipids [50, 51]. Foam cells develop (and therefore the fatty streak appears) when the cholesterol esters reach a sufficient level to exceed their solubility in membranes and become droplets, which are then seen within the cells. It is at this level that chemical modification of

these lipids may become an important determinant of whether the fatty streak remains quiescent or progresses to a more advanced stage [52, 53, 54]. The amount of free cholesterol in the fatty streak varies, but those with a higher free-cholesterol content (transitional or intermediate lesions) are more likely to progress, because the cholesterol is more likely to crystallize and therefore lead to the formation of a necrotic core [55].

Early investigations suggested that cholesterol turnover in the advanced plaque is slow and that plaque regression would be unlikely to occur or would proceed at an exceedingly slow rate [56, 57]. Current knowledge suggests that although this is generally the case there are differences in lipid turnover rates across the arterial wall and between the different physicochemical states of the plaque lipids [58]. Turnover is most rapid in the cholesterol ester phase near the surface of the plaque and extremely slow in the crystallized phase at the core. These findings were borne out in vivo as attempts to apply these concepts to regression were undertaken [59].

Using a standard regression design Small and colleagues evaluated these factors in a well-accepted animal model of atherosclerosis, the cynomolgus monkey [59]. Eighteen animals were assigned to one of three control groups (chow fed for either 18, 24, or 30 months). Sixty additional animals, prechallenged with a high-cholesterol diet to identify them as neither high nor low responders, were divided into five progression groups (6-, 12-, 18-, 24-, and 30-month end points) and two regression groups. The latter 20 animals were fed the atherogenic diet for 18 months and were then placed on a standard chow diet (low cholesterol) for either 6 or 12 months. The blood cholesterol values for all these groups are shown in Table 15-2.

An unexpected finding in this study was that although the animals in the progression group showed increasing amounts of atherosclerosis over time, as measured by intimal area involvement and maximal intimal thickness of the thoracic aorta, the regression group also showed continued growth of lesions after 6 months on the chow diet. This relationship was reversed

Table 15-2. Cholesterol levels–cynomolgus regression trial (mg/dl)

	Atherogenic diet	*Chow diet*
Progression group		
6-month end point	708±127	
12-month end point	733±183	
18-month end point	736±169	
24-month end point	681±99	
30-month end point	709±145	
Regression group		
18 month progression, followed by:	837±199	
2-month regression		297±126
4-month regression		168±55
6-month regression		153±52
18 month progression, followed by:	713±132	
2-month regression		223±86
4-month regression		166±67
12-month regression		127±27
Control group		
18-month end point		121±3
24-month end point		118±9
30-month end point		121±16

after 12 months of the regression protocol. After the first 6 months of a chow diet, the lesions in the regression animals demonstrated increased free cholesterol and decreased cholesterol esters. This may be due to increased cholesterol ester hydrolysis in the early regression period, which in turn may result in the production of more cholesterol crystals. This is consistent with the morphologic findings: these lesions were bigger compared to the lesions in animals after both 12 and 18 months on the atherogenic diet, and therefore it could be said that progression rather than regression had taken place, despite a marked reduction in serum cholesterol levels. By 12 months, however, the regressing plaques had lost both cholesterol ester and free cholesterol compared to both the earlier regression group and the corresponding progression group, suggesting that cholesterol crystals had disappeared and the lesion regressed. Some crystal was still present, demonstrating the slow mobilization of cholesterol from this pool. The remainder of the lesion at this time was composed primarily of collagen, calcium, and other matrix tissues.

This swelling of lesions early in the regression period raises concerns that a similar phenomenon may occur in humans, although the clinical regression trials described below have not reported such findings. Other factors, including the methods of measurement and the impact of other risk factors, may come into play in the clinical setting. It is also true that the drop in blood cholesterol levels achieved in humans, even in trials intended to produce regression, rarely exceeds 100 mg/dl, whereas the change in animal trials, such as that carried out by Small et al., may be five times as great. Lesser degrees of cholesterol lowering may not produce the early adverse changes seen in cynomolgus monkeys. This hypothesis remains to be tested.

As described in Chapter 3, oxidation products of lipoproteins may play a role in plaque growth. Antioxidant agents such as probucol and n–3 fatty acids may modify cellular function and the elaboration of chemotactic and chemoattractant molecules in a favorable manner, independent of their effects on circulating lipid levels. Cyclo-oxygenase inhibitors such as aspirin, nonsteroidal anti-inflammatory agents, and n–3 fatty acids may affect the vasomotor tone of the coronary arteries and therefore alter angiographic measurements, as well as the propensity of a noncritical plaque to rupture [60]. These factors may be more important than a small change in lesion size in modifying risk of a clinical event.

Measurement of Atherosclerosis Change

Pathology remains the gold standard for the measurement of the extent of atherosclerosis and the composition of lesions. Pathologic examination freezes the disease in time and for the evaluation of interventions in animal studies is the most appropriate technique currently available. It has the disadvantage of requiring multiple groups of animals and, therefore, larger numbers, since the individual cannot serve as its own control. In humans alternative methodologies for the measurement of atherosclerotic lesions have been developed.

The progressive development of angiography and the associated precise computer analysis of angiographic images have made angiography the current standard for interventional trials in humans. Angiography is applicable to longitudinal investigations, and the precision of the measurements provides the power to detect small changes in lumen dimensions. The use of angiography, however, is not without problems. The technique may provide incorrect information as to the state of the atherosclerotic process, since vessels tend to undergo compensatory enlargement during the development of atherosclerosis in order to maintain lumen size [61]. The intervention itself, as described below, may also change the state of vascular tone without a true change in the degree of atherosclerosis in the arterial segment. Additionally angiography is an invasive procedure, which carries risk, albeit small.

High-resolution ultrasound has been employed in the serial study of carotid atherosclerosis [62, 63, 64]. This technique has been well-standardized and has sufficient resolution to be able to detect small changes in the extent of mural disease. It also may be able to distinguish thrombus from actual lesion change. However, there is not a close correspondence between the presence and/or changes in carotid artery disease and disease observed in the coronary arteries. This technique, therefore, cannot be applied to the study of coronary artery changes, nor can it function as a surrogate end point in intervention trials aimed at the coronary vascular bed. Magnetic resonance imaging (MRI) or high-resolution cine-computerized tomography (cine-CT) hold promise for noninvasive imaging of the coronary arteries; however, the current technology does not meet the needs of ongoing clinical trials.

A new technology that may complement the angiographic assessment of lumen changes is percutaneous intravascular ultrasonic imaging (IVUS) [65, 66]. Although also still in a developmental stage, IVUS may ultimately help to address some of the limitations of angiography. Current devices have not yet been well-validated, but they hold the promise of not only being able to quantitate the extent of disease with computer assistance but also by ultrasonic characterization to differentiate between some of the plaque components. These devices, however, still have the risks associated with an invasive procedure. The ideal technique for assessing longitudinal changes in CAD noninvasively remains elusive.

Since improvement in clinical outcome is the goal of secondary prevention, physiologic testing is an important adjunct to clinical trials of intervention strategies. Standard treadmill exercise testing has been shown to predict outcome in patients with known CHD but its usefulness in asymptomatic patients is limited by low specificity and sensitivity [67, 68, 69, 70, 71, 72]. Perfusion imaging techniques add little to the utility of exercise testing in this latter group. Some investigators have suggested that positive emission tomography (PET) scanning may more effectively stratify the large population of asymptomatic patients at higher risk for the development of coronary disease [73]. This technique has been included in the evaluation of patients in the Lifestyle Intervention Trial, described below [74]. These patients, however, were all symptomatic and had significant coronary atherosclerosis. Application of this procedure to patients with less severe disease in an interventional trial has yet to be reported.

Evidence That Regression Is Possible

Early Human Evidence

Following two periods of semistarvation in Europe, investigators reported autopsy data showing less aortic atherosclerosis than would have been expected [75, 76]. Although uncontrolled, these reports suggested that dietary intervention (at least of an extreme degree) could have a favorable effect on the atherosclerotic process.

Several investigators attempted to control their observations more carefully and arrived at similar conclusions [77, 78, 79]. Wilens described the aortas and coronary arteries of patients who had died of diseases associated with a weight loss of up to 45 kg (most were cancer patients). The control group were patients who had died without a terminal weight loss. Significantly more atherosclerosis was seen in the latter group. Many of the control group patients may have died from atherosclerosis-related diseases, and therefore the differences between the two groups were probably accentuated [77]. Wanscher and colleagues, however, compared pathologic specimens from cancer patients to noncancer patients in whom major atherosclerotic complications had been excluded and arrived at similar conclusions [78].

Tuberculosis was also used as a model of a wasting disease and patients dying from this disease were compared to individuals dying from accidents and illnesses of short duration [80]. Care was taken to exclude patients with known heart disease, hypertension, or diabetes, and the investigators drew their conclusions from analyses based on age of death and age at which weight loss began. The investigators noted evidence of retardation of the atherosclerotic process during the wasting period.

These observations suggest that both cessation of progression and actual regression of disease occur during severe wasting states associated with chronic diseases or semistarvation. It cannot be concluded, however, that more modest interventions would have similar effects.

Animal Studies

There is an extensive literature on regression of atherosclerosis in animal models. Only a few of the more important studies are described here. The general consensus is that if blood cholesterol levels are lowered to those seen in free-living animals (generally below 150 mg/dl), regression of atherosclerosis can be expected.

Attempts at regression have been successful in multiple animal models with dietary intervention alone, drug therapy alone, or both. Vesselinovitch and colleagues induced aortic atherosclerosis in Rhesus monkeys by feeding them high-cholesterol, high-saturated-fat diets for either 12 or 14 months [81, 82]. The animals were then divided into five groups: I, baseline atherosclerosis control; II, atherogenic diet for an additional 14 months; III, prudent diet; IV, prudent diet plus cholestyramine; and V, atherogenic diet plus cholestyramine. The findings measured as percent of aortic intimal involvement with lesions are shown in Table 15-3.

Significant reductions in the extent of disease are seen with all the interventions. The most striking change occurred in group IV, where a lowered-fat diet was coupled with lipid-lowering therapy. Because of the relatively small sizes of these groups (five animals each), no statistically significant differences could be demonstrated between the regression groups. Although all the regression groups demonstrated lowered cholesterol levels, these levels did not return to baseline. These findings have been duplicated in other animal models, particularly swine [83, 84].

Similar trials have been reported with cholesterol levels in a more normal clinical range. Bond and colleagues demonstrated that reducing blood cholesterol levels from 300 to 200 mg/dl in monkeys resulted in regression after 24 months. The lesions were smaller and contained less lipid than those in control animals [85]. In swine moderate drug and dietary interventions also resulted in regression [86].

Evidence of regression in another nonhuman primate model (cynomolgus monkeys) has been less impressive [87]. This may represent contin-

Table 15-3.   Regression of atherosclerosis in Rhesus monkeys

Group	Percent intimal involvement
I: baseline atherosclerosis control	68± 3.9
II: atherogenic diet for 14 more months	88± 4.3
III: prudent diet	20± 8.4
IV: prudent diet plus cholestyramine	7± 2.5
V: atherogenic diet plus cholestyramine	43±12.0

ued immune complex injury to the vessel wall in the cynomolgus monkey that is not present either in other animal models or in humans except in rare circumstances. This phenomenon may contribute to transplant atherosclerosis, which appears to have a different pathologic basis than that seen in native CAD [88, 89, 90].

Although n-3 fatty acids have been shown to be of benefit in the primary prevention of atherosclerosis in several animal models [91, 92], the role of these dietary fats in secondary prevention is not clear. There appears to be a favorable effect on the aorta and coronary arteries in pigs [93]. Compared to animals sacrificed at the end of atherosclerosis induction, there was less lipid in the abdominal aorta of animals treated with n-3 fatty acids plus continued atherogenic diet for an additional period after a comparable induction phase. There was no difference in the extent of coronary luminal encroachment, but only minimal disease was present (mean percent luminal encroachment 11 to 13 percent in the left anterior descending coronary artery (LAD) and only 3 to 4 percent in the right coronary artery (RCA)). Preliminary data from other investigators suggest that rather than modifying the extent of coronary atherosclerosis, these fatty acids, because of their other metabolic effects, lead to vessel dilatation and therefore less luminal encroachment for a given amount of disease [Weiner, unpublished data].

Other risk factor interventions such as exercise and behavioral changes have been investigated in animal models [94, 95, 96]. Most of these investigations have been in primary prevention models, and little is known of the effect of these factors on secondary prevention.

Clinical Trials of Lipid Lowering and Secondary Prevention

Nonangiographic Trials

The attention of most investigators has been on the primary prevention of CHD. The Lipid Research Clinics Coronary Primary Prevention Trial (LRC-CPPT) can, however, be viewed as a secondary prevention trial from the standpoint of atherosclerosis [40, 97]. In this trial hyperlipidemic middle-aged men treated with cholestyramine had a lower follow-up coronary event rate than did a control group treated with diet advice alone. As described in Chapter 3, atherosclerosis is a process that generally begins in childhood or adolescence. As such, lipid interventions commencing in middle age, although primary interventions from a symptom standpoint, are secondary from the perspective of the disease process itself. Studies such as the LRC-CPPT cannot differentiate between a favorable outcome related to a direct effect on the degree of atherosclerosis or on the propensity of individual lesions to become unstable and therefore precipitate clinical events.

The Helsinki Heart Study can be interpreted in a similar fashion [98]. Middle-aged men who were asymptomatic at the time of study entry had lower cardiovascular mortality and morbidity if treated with gemfibrozil when compared to placebo-treated controls. The investigators concluded that the major effect responsible for the findings was the increase in HDL levels observed in the drug-treated group. Again it could be argued that gemfibrozil has effects on the arterial wall and the interaction and activity of cells involved in the atherosclerotic process in addition to any possible effect on the degree of atherosclerosis. Since angiographic data from this population are not available, no clear conclusion on this matter can be reached.

The importance of serum lipid levels in the long-term outcome after MI has been described in both epidemiologic and observational studies [42, 99, 100, 101, 102, 103]. These studies suggest that for men who already have clinical manifestations of CHD at baseline, the risk of another cardiac event is as much as three to four times higher if they continue to have a high serum cholesterol level than if the cholesterol level is in the desirable range. These studies do not address the question of whether lowering cholesterol after symptomatic disease is present has a beneficial effect on outcome. The implication, however, is clearly that this might be the case.

A number of trials designed specifically as secondary prevention studies have been reported using coronary events (fatal and nonfatal MI) as the primary end point [104, 105, 106, 107, 108]. These studies have the advantage of not having selected participants on the basis of cholesterol levels. Nonetheless, average cholesterol levels were between 244 and 296 mg/dl. Although several of these trials are positive for a favorable effect of the intervention (diet or drug) on the rate of fatal and nonfatal MI combined, the evidence becomes more convincing when the combined data from eight of these trials are subjected to a meta-analysis [109]. When the data are viewed in this manner, there are significant reductions in nonfatal (odds ratio, .75; $p < .001$), fatal (odds ratio, .84; $p < .01$), and total (odds ratio, .78; $p < .001$) MI rates. The overall relationship between the degree of cholesterol reduction and subsequent event rates was similar to that observed in the major primary prevention trials [40, 98]. In contrast to the primary prevention trials, however, this analysis also demonstrates a trend toward a reduction in overall mortality [109].

As a whole these studies may have too short a period of follow-up for a clinical end point difference such as mortality to become significant. This is exemplified in the longer follow-up of the niacin arm of the Coronary Drug Project [110]. It was not until a total follow-up time of 15 years was analyzed that a reduction in overall mortality became apparent. Similar trends are being seen in some of the primary prevention trials that have now had long follow-up results reported [39, 111, 112].

These secondary prevention trials taken together support the importance of risk factor intervention, particularly lipid lowering, in the long-term management of patients with CHD. The mechanisms of these beneficial effects cannot be deduced from these studies, but further information is now available from the angiographic studies described next.

Angiographic Trials

More recently, as we have acquired a better understanding of aggressive lipid-lowering regimens and have come to realize that lipid lowering may have a favorable effect on outcome even in the presence of established disease, several trials have been performed using angiography as the end point. These trials, because of the precision of the measurement technique, can be performed with smaller patient populations and at lower costs than the large clinical trials using death and cardiovascular events as their major end points.

The earliest angiographic trials focused on changes in femoral atherosclerosis. Ost and colleagues demonstrated favorable changes in femoral atherosclerosis during niacin treatment [113]. The patients received 3 g/day of niacin, and although the lipid changes are not described, 3 of the 31 treated patients showed angiographic evidence of improvement associated with improved symptomatology. An additional untreated 112 patients showed no progression. Barndt and colleagues described 25 patients treated with a variety of lipid-lowering agents (most of which are not currently recommended for use) who underwent serial femoral angiograms [114]. Significant regression of disease was seen in 9 of these 25 patients. A femoral angiographic trial utilizing current medications was reported by Erikson [115]. In a single-blind, placebo-controlled, nonrandomized trial, 62 patients were treated with fenofibrate and niacin, and serial angiograms were evaluated. The majority of intervention patients showed no change in femoral atherosclerosis over an 18-month period. In the Cholesterol Lowering Atherosclerosis Trial (described in more detail below), serial femoral angiograms were also obtained. These patients, half of them treated with niacin and colestipol, demonstrated a significant favorable treatment effect compared to placebo-treated controls [116].

The first risk factor intervention study to directly evaluate the coronary circulation was the Leiden Intervention Trial [117, 118]. Unlike most later investigations, this trial utilized diet alone in an attempt to intervene in the atherosclerotic process. Thirty-nine patients with stable angina and documented CAD by angiography were placed on a largely vegetarian diet for two years and then underwent repeat angiography. The diet had a P:S ratio of 2:1 and a cholesterol content of no more than 100 mg/day. There was no control group. The clinical changes in these patients over this period are shown in Table 15-4.

At 2-year angiography, progression of disease was demonstrated in 21 of the 39 patients enrolled. No progression was seen in the remaining 18 patients. In patients with total cholesterol/HDL ratio of less than 6.9 at baseline or achieved in response to the dietary intervention, the mean vessel diameter was unchanged over the 2-year study period. In contrast the patients with a total cholesterol/HDL ratio greater than 6.9 had a mean reduction in vessel diameter of .23 mm over that same interval. Although the changes in HDL were not statistically significant, the finding of differential results based on the total cholesterol/HDL ratio

suggests that this may be an important factor in modifying the progression of disease.

This trial was performed at a time when severe changes in P:S ratios were being advocated. Later data suggested that this was not desirable because of adverse effects on HDL and the possibility that cancer incidence might be increased. This was the first angiographic study, however, to suggest that the progression of coronary atherosclerosis in humans could be modified. Interpretation of the study is unfortunately limited by the absence of a control group.

The first drug intervention trial assessing the coronary circulation was reported by Nikkilä in 1984 [119]. Twenty-eight patients treated with diet and drugs (clofibrate, niacin, or both) were compared to 20 patients in another trial carried out concurrently at that center who were not receiving lipid-lowering therapy. Baseline data on the two groups were comparable, including the extent of CAD. Angiography was performed at baseline and 2 and 7 years after entry into this trial in the drug treatment group. In the control group, as part of the alternate trial, repeat angiography was performed at 5 years. To compare these data, the investigators assumed that progression of disease was linear and extrapolated the 5-year data to 7 years on this basis. This assumption may not be valid.

In the intervention group, blood cholesterol fell 18 percent, triglycerides 38 percent, and LDL 19 percent; HDL increased by 10 percent. There were no significant changes in the control-group lipids. Nine of the 24 surviving drug treatment patients showed no change in their

Table 15-4. Risk factor changes over time in the Leiden Intervention Trial ($n = 39$)

Risk factor	Baseline	2 years	P
Weight	74.5 kg	73.5 kg	<.01
Total cholesterol	267 mg/dl	240 mg/dl	<.001
HDL cholesterol	39.1 mg/dl	37.9 mg/dl	NS
Total cholesterol/HDL	7.1	6.4	<.01
Blood pressure			
Systolic	130.4 mmHg	128.3 mmHg	<.01
Diastolic	84.4 mmHg	82.1 mmHg	NS
Smoking (# pts)	18	18	NS

angiographic status at 7 years. There was progression in 12 of the 13 surviving patients in the control group at 5 years. No regression was seen in either group. Despite the difference in the protocols, the cardiac survival in the treatment group at 7 years (89 percent) was significantly better than cardiac survival in the control group at 5 years (65 percent, $p < .05$).

Detre and colleagues reported the findings of a randomized trial in type II hyperlipidemic patients with CHD that began recruitment in 1972 [120]. One hundred forty-three individuals who met the criteria for entry into this trial (LDL cholesterol level on diet therapy alone greater than ninetieth percentile based on age and documented CAD by angiography) were randomized to diet and cholestyramine therapy or diet and placebo. Although the drug-treated patients demonstrated a 17-percent reduction in total cholesterol and a 26-percent decrease in LDL cholesterol at 5 years compared to baseline values, the average LDL cholesterol in the drug-treated group remained above that which would be considered a desirable value today (mean LDL 178 mg/dl at 5 years). There were no significant changes in lipid values in the control group. The placebo group demonstrated more progression of disease than was seen in those patients treated with cholestyramine. The drug-treated individuals were also more likely to have shown no change (53 percent in the treated group versus 42 percent in the placebo group). The number of patients with regression was too small to draw meaningful conclusions.

The Lifestyle Heart Trial is a more recent nondrug intervention trial [74]. This trial utilized a selected population of patients who could commit to the extensive lifestyle changes that they might be asked to undertake. All patients at the participating institutions who had clinically indicated catheterizations, were 35 to 75 years old, and had not had an MI in the preceding 6 weeks were eligible for participation in this study if they also had significant lesions in vessels that had not been subjected to bypass grafting or to angioplasty. Ninety-four eligible patients were randomized; 48 (intervention = 28, control = 20) agreed to participate and were the subject of a 1-year progress report. The trial is intended to run for 4 years.

These 48 individuals were randomized to usual care or to a program of comprehensive lifestyle changes that included a low-fat vegetarian diet with no animal products except egg white and 1 cup of nonfat milk or yogurt per day. Ten percent of calories came from fat, and the diet contained only 5 mg of cholesterol. As a convenience, frozen dinners prepared by the study center were available for the intervention patients. No caffeine was allowed. In addition to the dietary changes the patients received stress management training and support in twice-weekly group sessions. The patients exercised at least 3 hours per week, practiced stress relaxation techniques (meditation) for 1 hour per day, and received smoking intervention. The baseline and 1-year lipid values are shown in Table 15-5.

Over the interval of this 1-year report, the intervention group reported fewer episodes of angina with the episodes being of shorter duration and lesser severity than in the control group. Eighteen patients (82 percent) of the intervention group were felt to have demonstrated regression based on the serial angiograms. The remaining four patients had progression of disease. In contrast, in the control group 53 percent of patients showed progression, while regression was seen in eight patients (42 percent), with one patient felt to be unchanged.

This study, like the Leiden Intervention Trial, suggests that diet and lifestyle changes are important in modifying the progression and regression of CAD. Both studies represent marked departures from the usual lifestyle and dietary recommendations of the AHA and the NCEP for the population as a whole. They may be applicable to highly motivated and high-risk subsets of society.

The Familial Atherosclerosis Treatment Study (FATS) extended these observations by utilizing currently available and highly effective drug regimens for lowering cholesterol [121]. One hundred forty-six men less than 62 years of age were included. All of them had documented CAD, a family history of vascular dis-

Table 15-5.   Risk factor changes in the Lifestyle Intervention Trial

Risk factor	Baseline		One year		
	Control	Intervention	Control	Intervention	P-value
Total cholesterol	245 ± 39.5	228 ± 49.9	232 ± 59.8	172 ± 44.4	<0.02
LDL cholesterol	167 ± 29.8	152 ± 48.2	158 ± 45.2	95 ± 59.8	<0.008
HDL cholesterol	52.2 ± 20.1	39 ± 10.0	51 ± 14.7	38 ± 15.4	NS
Triglycerides	217 ± 218	211 ± 112	198 ± 158	258 ± 130	NS
Weight (kg)	80.4 ± 22.8	91.1 ± 15.5	81.8 ± 25.0	81.0 ± 11.4	<0.0001

ease and an apolipoprotein B level of 125 mg/dl or more. All the patients underwent coronary angiography at baseline and 2.5 years after beginning therapy. Following dietary counseling, the patients were randomized to one of three possible drug regimens: (1) lovastatin and colestipol, (2) niacin and colestipol, or (3) placebo (patients in this group were treated with colestipol alone if the LDL cholesterol was ≥ ninetieth percentile). Nearly half of this last group (43 percent) actually received drug therapy.

The "placebo"-treated group demonstrated no significant change in their lipid profile. In contrast patients in both the lovastatin/colestipol and the niacin/colestipol groups showed marked improvement in their lipid status. The former patients had a 46-percent reduction in LDL cholesterol level and a 15-percent increase in HDL cholesterol, while the latter demonstrated a 32-percent decrease in LDL and a 43-percent increase in HDL. The absolute magnitude of these changes is shown in Table 15-6.

In overall terms 46 percent of the placebo group demonstrated progression only on their follow-up angiograms, while only 11 percent showed regression only. These findings were reversed in both drug-treated groups, with only 21 percent and 25 percent of the lovastatin/colestipol and niacin/colestipol patients, respectively, demonstrating progression only. Thirty-two percent of the former group and 39 percent of the latter showed regression only on their follow-up angiograms. Specific proximal areas of the angiograms were targeted for quantitative assessment by a standardized computer-assisted

technique. These finding are shown in Table 15-7.

Although this study was not designed to demonstrate a difference in clinical events, significant differences were seen. The placebo-treated patients had more clinical events (defined as death, documented MI, or new ischemic symptoms requiring either peripheral or coronary revascularization) than either of the other two groups (Table 15-8). This dramatic and unexpected finding in a short-duration trial with relatively modest changes in vessel morphology suggests that a leveraging effect may occur with potent lipid-lowering interventions — a favorable change in other cellular factors that contribute to spasm, thrombosis, or plaque instability.

The Program on the Surgical Control of the Hyperlipidemias (POSCH) used an approach in which patient compliance was not an issue [122]. Eight hundred thirty-eight men (90.7 percent) and women who were survivors of a first MI were studied. The average age of this population was 51 years, and they had total cholesterol levels of 220 mg/dl or more or LDL cholesterol levels of 140 mg/dl or more at the time of enrollment. All patients were placed on an AHA step 2 diet and were randomized to either partial ileal bypass or no surgery. The rationale behind this approach was that this type of surgery mimics the effect of bile acid sequestrants in interrupting the enterohepatic circulation of cholesterol and would have a similar lipid-lowering effect without the problems of patient compliance seen with these agents. It

Table 15-6.   Lipid and lipoprotein values before and during therapy in FATS (mg/dl)

	Placebo		Lovastatin-colestipol		Niacin-colestipol	
	Baseline	2.5 years	Baseline	2.5 years	Baseline	2.5 years
Total cholesterol	262.1	252.8	274.8	181.8	269.8	208.8
VLDL	47.8	50.2	45.9	35.9	42.1	23.2
LDL	174.9	162.1	196.1	106.9	189.9	128.9
HDL	37.8	40.1	35.1	40.9	39.0	54.8
Triglyceride	229.2	263.7	200.1	183.2	193.8	137.2
Lp(a)	41.1	36.4	33.4	30.1	32.6	24.2
Apo B	149	142	159	103	155	111

Table 15-7.   Angiographical results by treatment group in the FATS trial

	Percent stenosis		Vessel diameter (mm)	
Group	Baseline	2 years	Baseline	2 years
Placebo	34	36	1.91	1.86
Lovastatin/colestipol	34	33.3	1.91	2.03
Niacin/colestipol	34	33.1	1.91	2.26
		p <.03		p <.01*

*P values are for difference between placebo and either treatment group.

Table 15-8.   Clinical events in FATS*

Group	Total number of patients	Number of events
Placebo	52	10
Lovastatin/colestipol	46	3
Niacin/colestipol	48	2

*P = 0.01 for difference between placebo and either treatment group.

was felt this could be safely accomplished with little morbidity. Only 22 patients who were randomized to surgery refused the operation. These patients are included in the surgery group for analysis purposes. An additional 23 patients had the bypass reversed because of intractable side effects (5.4 percent).

In the patients who had reached the 5-year follow-up point, the surgical group had total plasma cholesterol levels 23.3 percent lower than the control group, LDL cholesterol levels 37.7 percent lower, and HDL cholesterol levels 4.3 percent higher. Overall mortality and coronary mortality were reduced in the surgical group but not significantly so. In those patients with an ejection fraction of 50 percent or more, however, the surgical subgroup had a significantly lower overall mortality. For the combined end point of death due to coronary disease and confirmed nonfatal MI, there were 35 percent fewer events in the surgical group compared to the control group (82 versus 125 events, p < .001).

Serial angiograms were evaluated by blinded reading panels and assigned global change scores based on the degree of improvement or worsening seen between the two films. At each time point the difference between the surgical and control groups was significant (p < .001) (Figure 15-1). The data for those patients with regression only are less clear. As shown in Figure 15-2, regression only is seen more frequently in the surgery group up to 7 years after randomization. Although this difference persists at 10 years, the difference is less marked; however, the difference in global change score remains significant (p = .0002).

The Cholesterol Lowering Atherosclerosis Study (CLAS-I) investigated patients presumed to have the most advanced disease, those with previous coronary bypass surgery [44]. One hundred sixty-two male nonsmokers were pretested for tolerance to large (therapeutic) doses of niacin and colestipol and were randomized to treatment with diet alone (with placebo) or diet plus the combination of these two agents. Angiography was performed at baseline and at 2 years after the initiation of therapy.

Entry cholesterol levels in this study ranged from 185 to 350 mg/dl. In the drug-treated group, total cholesterol was reduced by 26 percent, triglycerides by 22 percent, and LDL cho-

lesterol by 43 percent (Table 15-9). Diet therapy resulted in 4- to 5-percent reductions in all these measurements. HDL cholesterol increased by 37 percent in the treatment group and by only 2 percent in the diet-alone patients. There was also a significant loss of weight in the treatment group that was not observed in those treated with diet alone. This may have contributed to the marked improvement in lipid profile observed in this group over and above the drug effects.

The effect of drug therapy on global change score is demonstrated in Table 15-10. There was a significant difference in average global change score between the two groups (p < .001). These differences were found both for changes in native vessels (p < .03) and for bypass grafts (p < .03).

Even when the patients were grouped by baseline cholesterol measurement into those patients with low (185 to 240 mg/dl) and high (241 to 350 mg/dl) levels, the same findings held. There was a significant difference between the average global change scores in the drug-

Figure 15-1. Frequency of progression in POSCH.

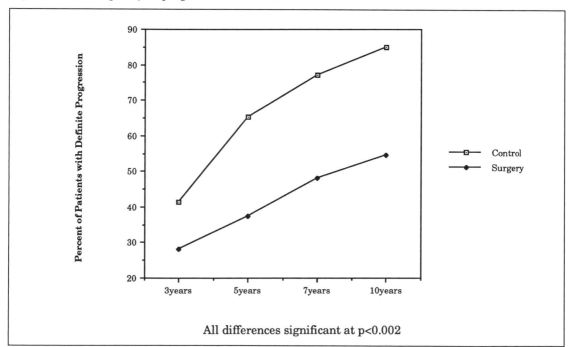

All differences significant at p<0.002

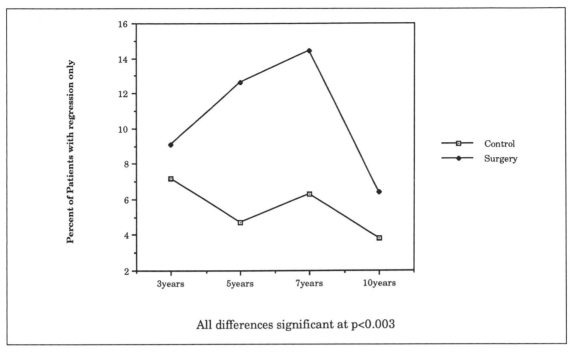

Figure 15-2. Frequency of regression only in POSCH.

Table 15-9. Lipid changes compared to baseline in the CLAS trials

| | | Percent change | | |
	Group	CLAS-I	CLAS-II	P-value*
Total cholesterol	Drug	− 26	− 25	<0.001
	Placebo	− 4	− 6	
LDL cholesterol	Drug	− 43	− 40	<.001
	Placebo	− 4	− 6	
HDL cholesterol	Drug	+ 37	+ 37	<.001
	Placebo	+ 2	+ 2	
Triglycerides	Drug	− 22	− 18	<.03
	Placebo	− 5	− 5	

*P values from Wilcoxon rank sum for differences between drug and placebo groups at four years (P values are the same in both trials).

Table 15-10. Effect of treatment on progression and regression of disease in CLAS-I

Group	Progression (percent)	No change (percent)	Regression (percent)
Drug	38.8	45	16.2
Placebo	60.0	36.6	2.4

treated and nontreated groups. This difference was, however, more marked in the higher baseline cholesterol group.

These data were further analyzed in an attempt to predict those lipid and nonlipid factors that predicted change in the serial angiograms [123]. Univariate analysis suggested that total cholesterol, non-HDL cholesterol (a measure of LDL and VLDL), diastolic blood pressure, apoliproprotein A-I, apolipoprotein B, and apolipoprotein C-III were all predictors of progression. Multivariate analysis, however, demonstrated that in the placebo group only non-HDL cholesterol predicted progression (risk ratio 1.9, 95-percent confidence interval 1.2 to 3.2). In the drug treated group only apolipoprotein C-III-HS (the amount contained in HDL) was a significant predictor. The relative risk of progression decreased with increasing Apo C-III-HS (risk ratio .6, 95-percent confidence interval .4 to .9). These data are the first in a prospective intervention trial to confirm the importance of triglyceride-rich lipoproteins in the progression and regression of atherosclerosis. This analysis also suggests that at higher cholesterol levels, the effects of LDL on progression are dominant. At lower levels, other factors become more important. Apo C-III in HDL may be a marker of the importance of increasing HDL at these levels or may be important in its own right, since shifting the distribution of this lipoprotein to HDL rather than VLDL may increase the catabolism of the atherogenic VLDL particle and decrease the catabolism of the more beneficial HDL particle, thereby increasing the likelihood of reverse cholesterol transport occurring [124, 125].

CLAS-II was intended to be the 4-year follow-up of this population [45]. One hundred and thirty-eight members of the original study group agreed to continue in the study for an additional 2 years and to undergo repeat angiography at that time. This extended portion of the study was stopped, however, when the CLAS-I data became known, since it was felt not to be appropriate to continue. At that time 103 patients had undergone their third (4-year) angiogram. The beneficial changes in lipids were again demonstrated in the CLAS-II partipants (see Table 15-9).

The angiographic effects of the lipid-lowering regimen demonstrated in CLAS-I at 2 years were more pronounced on the 4-year follow-up angiograms performed in CLAS-II. Although the drug group response was more variable at 4 years and demonstrated somewhat more progression (14.3 percent of patients with new lesions in native arteries, 16.1 percent of patients with new lesions in grafts, and 14.3 percent patients with new graft closures in CLAS-II compared to 12.5 percent, 14.3 percent, and 5.4 percent, respectively, in CLAS-I) than had been seen at 2 years, the placebo group showed marked and more consistent progression, with 87 percent of the patients showing definite to severe progression. Fewer patients in the placebo group remained angiographically stable (change score of 0) than in the treatment group. The opposite relationship was seen with regression. Eighteen percent of the drug-treated individuals showed regression, while only 7 percent of the placebo group demonstrated this finding.

A very recent study by the same group, not reported in the literature at the time of this writing, is the Monitored Atherosclerosis Regression Trial (MARS), which utilized a study design similar to CLAS [125a]. Lovastatin (80 mg/day) rather than niacin and colestipol was used as the drug intervention. At two-year follow-up lovastatin produced the expected changes in the lipid profile and was associated with less progression of disease as determined by global change score. Regression was seen more often in the drug treatment group than in the placebo group (28 patients in the lovastatin group versus 13 patients in the placebo group, $p = .05$). Again, as in CLAS, a treatment benefit ($p = .05$) was demonstrated whether the total cholesterol was greater than 240 mg/dl or not.

Although there was no significant difference in numbers of coronary events between the two groups, longer follow-up is planned. The study was not designed specifically to address this issue over the initial two years. These findings are consistent with the impression that there are multiple regimens which may be effective in modifying the progression of coronary atherosclerosis as long as the necessary changes in lipid profile occur.

The studies described here used different populations and different interventions; nonetheless, overall conclusions can be drawn. For those trials for which comparable data are available (Figure 15-3), there is a correlation between the extent of total cholesterol reduction and the percentage of the population with progression of disease, irrespective of how it is measured. The corollary is also true: the greater the reduction in total cholesterol, the greater the proportion of the population with no change or regression of disease (Figure 15-4). Of interest is the fact that the slope of this curve is similar to that shown in the LRC-CPPT trial for the relationship between cardiovascular mortality and cholesterol change. There are no clear relationships between the extent of change in

HDL and regression of disease when the data are viewed in this manner. The importance of HDL changes may be overwhelmed by the high LDL levels in many of the patients studied in these trials.

The progression of aortocoronary vein graft atherosclerosis may have a somewhat different pathophysiology. It is well-known that the pathologic characteristics of this disease differ from those of native CAD [126, 127, 128, 129, 130, 131]. Grondin et al. described the angiographic appearance of vein grafts 6 years after operation and correlated vein graft disease and closure with triglyceride levels [132]. More recent data from this same group demonstrate similar findings, confirming the relationship between elevated LDL and VLDL levels and lower HDL with the progression of vein graft atherosclerosis [133, 134, 135]. This relationship is also suggested but not specifically addressed in the further analysis of the lipids in the CLAS-I

Figure 15-3. Relationship between change in cholesterol and frequency of "progression only". (C) denotes control and (T) denotes treatment group for each study.

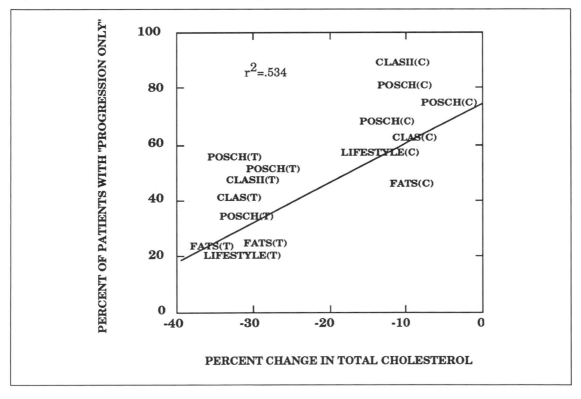

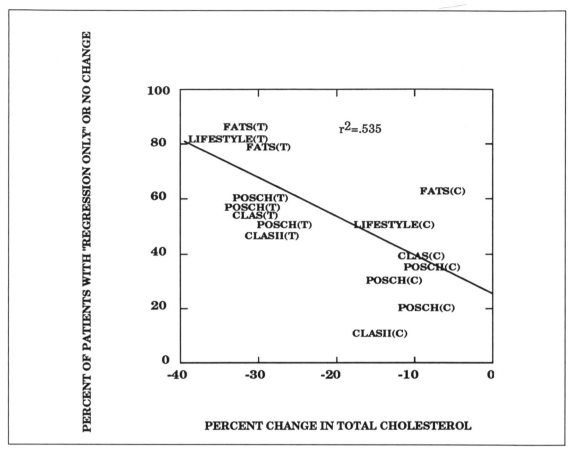

Figure 15-4. Relationship between change in cholesterol and frequency of "regression only" or no change. (C) denotes control and (T) denotes treatment group for each study.

patients [123]. Solymoss also showed that cigarette smoking following surgery has a negative impact on long-term graft patency [136]. Although there was a 17 percent difference in graft patency between those individuals who smoked following surgery and those who did not, this difference did not reach statistical significance (p = .08). In a stepwise logistic regression analysis of these data, however, smoking was the second most important factor influencing graft patency.

Platelets and interventions aimed at platelet function may be important in the long-term patency of bypass grafts. Animal studies have suggested that these agents (particularly aspirin) are important in decreasing lipid accumulation in vein grafts even in the presence of normolipidemia [137]. Clinical trials have also corroborated these findings and have resulted in the

routine use of these agents in clinical practice [138, 139, 140].

Restenosis following percutaneous transluminal coronary angioplasty (PTCA) was initially felt to be an accelerated atherosclerotic response to the vessel injury. It now appears from pathologic investigations to be more of a proliferative, primarily smooth-muscle lesion containing little lipid [141]. There have been conflicting reports on the role of risk factors in this process [142, 143, 144, 145, 146, 147]. One explanation for these findings is that the population of patients undergoing PTCA may be relatively homogeneous with regard to CHD risk factors, and therefore individual influences may not be apparent. Galan and colleagues showed that patients who continued to smoke after successful angioplasty had a higher incidence of restenosis [148]. The two groups were comparable in all other clinical respects; however, the smokers had an angiographically defined restenosis rate of 55 percent, while the quitters had a restenosis rate of only 38 percent (p = .03).

In a trial of lipid lowering with lovastatin, Sahni et al. demonstrated a reduction in restenosis [149]. Seventy-nine patients who had undergone successful dilatation were randomized in a nonblinded manner to lovastatin plus conventional therapy (aspirin, dypiridamole, calcium channel blocker) or conventional therapy alone. There were reductions in blood cholesterol levels in both groups (212±49 to 175±41 mg/dl in the lovastatin group versus 207±49 to 196±48 mg/dl in the control group). Further information on their lipid levels was not supplied. There were significant reductions in restenosis in the treatment group, as shown in Table 15-11. Fewer than half of the enrolled patients actually underwent the follow-up catheterization, with a differential rate of catheterization sharply favoring the intervention group. The data are of interest, particularly in light of evidence that suggests that lovastatin may have antiproliferative qualities in addition to its lipid-lowering effects [150, 151, 152], but require confirmation by better-designed studies.

N-3 fatty acids as potential antiproliferative agents have also been considered in the setting of restenosis. The data are variable, but this variability is largely explained by differences in study design (clinical versus angiographic end points and differences with regard to when the agents are begun relative to the angioplasty) and doses of the agents [153, 154]. In addition each of the reported trials is small. The ongoing NHLBI-sponsored Fish Oil Restenosis Trial (FORT) was designed to address these issues in a population of 500 patients, and enrollment should be complete within the next year. No preliminary data are available.

The majority of the trials described above were carried out in patients with baseline cholesterol levels outside the desirable range. Except for CLAS, which included patients with cholesterol levels as low as 185 mg/dl, the entry criteria for many of these trials excluded patients with lower levels. In this situation it is not surprising that changes in total and LDL cholesterol appear to be the major factors determining progression and regression. However, the data from FATS and CLAS in particular would suggest that HDL may play an important role in the progression and regression of disease [121]. For a given LDL level, particularly as it is reduced to a desirable level, a higher HDL level would be expected to be of benefit. This rationale suggests that the approach to secondary prevention should focus not only on LDL reduction but also on HDL improvement by either lifestyle changes, such as exercise and smoking cessation, or the use of drugs that tend to increase HDL, such as niacin and the fibrate derivatives.

Other Approaches to Secondary Prevention

Other approaches to secondary prevention of coronary atherosclerosis have also been investigated. Medications commonly used in the therapy of symptomatic CHD have been of interest in this setting.

Beta blockers, despite their potential negative effects on the lipid profile, have been extensively studied and are clearly of value [155, 156].

Table 15-11.   Effect of lovastatin on restenosis

| | Lovastatin group | | Control group | | |
	n	Restenosis	n	Restenosis	P-value
By patient	50	6 (12%)	29	13 (44.8%)	0.001
By vessel	72	9 (12.5%)	34	13 (38.2%)	0.002
By lesion	80	10 (12.5%)	36	15 (41.7%)	<0.001

Multiple trials to assess the role of beta blockers in the post-MI period have been performed and have been uniformly positive irrespective of the specific agent utilized [157, 158, 159, 160, 161, 162, 163]. In general all patients have shown improved survival, a decrease in cardiovascular events, and fewer ischemic symptoms during the first year after an MI. Late withdrawal of metoprolol therapy has been shown to have a negative impact [157]. There are no data with regard to the usefulness of these agents in patients who have undergone a revascularization procedure.

The mechanism whereby beta blockers exert their favorable effect is unclear and may be unrelated to any effect on atherosclerosis progression. There may a direct protective effect on the arterial wall due to a diminution of hemodynamic stress and possibly a reduction in vessel wall injury, particularly in hypertensive individuals [164]. The Beta Blocker Heart Attack Trial (BHAT) was not able to delineate the mechanism of improvement observed in this trial but did demonstrate that the major effect was seen in events occurring between 10 p.m. and 7 a.m. [165]. This would suggest some relationship to the circadian changes in platelet function and occurrence of unstable coronary syndromes observed by other investigators [166, 167, 168, 169, 170].

Loaldi and colleagues compared the effects of nifedipine, propranolol, and isosorbide dinitrate on serial angiograms in patients with angina performed 2 years apart [171]. All patients were untreated prior to entering the trial and were assigned to treatment groups based on their response to each therapy as documented by a standard exercise test. No antiplatelet or lipid-lowering therapy was administered. The only changes in lipids over time were seen in the propranolol-treated group, which demonstrated a 28-percent increase in triglycerides and a 25-percent decrease in HDL. Absolute values for lipid levels in all the groups are not given but are reported as being normal in all but 14 patients.

Worsening of the angiogram, as measured by progression of existing lesions or the develop-

ment of new lesions, was less common in the nifedipine-treated group than in either the propranolol or isosorbide group. However, considering the manner in which patients were assigned to treatment groups, this may be related to a problem of study design.

The beneficial effect of nifedipine may also be due to other factors such as an effect on platelet function. One may or may not be able to generalize these findings to other calcium channel blockers. Calcium channel antagonists have been demonstrated to have antiatherogenic effects in experimental models [172, 173]. Some of these beneficial effects may be due to antiplatelet activity [174, 175, 176, 177, 178, 179, 180].

The INTACT Trial (the International Nifedipine Trial on Antiatherosclerotic Therapy) also demonstrated a beneficial effect of nifedipine in a randomized study in patients with minimal CAD [181]. Although existing lesions appeared to be unaffected by this therapy, new lesions were fewer in the nifedipine-treated group. Again this may be due to an effect on cellular function.

Approach to Patients with Known CHD

The aggregate data support the contention that aggressive attention to risk factors, particularly smoking and lipids, can favorably affect the long-term outcome in patients with established disease. The approach described here is more aggressive than current recommendations of the AHA or the NCEP. We feel that these recommendations are justified because the currently available data strongly suggest that halting of progression or actual regression of CAD is possible, particularly if LDL cholesterol is effectively lowered and the HDL level is maximized, even in individuals who have already developed clinical disease. The drugs and other interventions that may be employed have been shown to be safe and effective and can be utilized with minimal side effects to accomplish these goals. To that end a reasonable approach to these patients would be as follows:

1. Characterize risk factors and stratify them as to their relative importance.
2. Identify and treat secondary causes of hyperlipidemia, such as diabetes and hypothyroidism.
3. Encourage lifestyle change to the greatest extent possible to include the following:
   a. smoking cessation
   b. a low-cholesterol, low-fat diet (as close to the AHA step 3 diet as possible), including weight reduction if appropriate
   c. regular exercise
   d. stress reduction
4. If needed, aggressive drug therapy with the most effective agent or agents with the fewest side effects aimed at the following:
   a. lowering total cholesterol below 180 mg/dl (preferably as close to 150 mg/dl or below as possible)
   b. lowering LDL cholesterol at least below 130 mg/dl, and preferably below 100 mg/dl in patients who already have clinical evidence of CHD
   c. raising HDL cholesterol to the fullest extent possible
5. Long-term beta-blockade therapy in patients who have sustained an MI but have not gone on to revascularization.

Methods for assisting patients in making these changes are discussed in previous chapters in this book.

Summary

Secondary prevention of coronary atherosclerosis is a reasonable and achievable goal with currently available therapy. Whether one measures an effect by changes in the angiogram or by clinical outcome, lipid therapy can favorably affect this process. The manner in which lipids are altered, whether by lifestyle and diet changes or by drug therapy, appears not to matter. Achieving the lowest possible LDL-cholesterol levels with the highest HDL-cholesterol levels is the aim. Balancing lifestyle changes and drug therapy in a given individual is a mutual decision reached between the health care provider and the patient. Those factors that contribute to primary prevention are equally effective in the secondary prevention of CHD, but the motivation to achieve the goals should be greater.

References

1. Helgeland A. Treatment of mild hypertension: a five-year controlled drug trial. The Oslo Study. Am J Med 1980; 69:725–32.
2. Hypertension Detection and Follow-up Program Cooperative Group. I. Reduction in mortality of persons with high blood pressure, including mild hypertension. JAMA 1979; 242:2562–71.
3. U.S. Public Health Service Hospitals Cooperative Study Group. Treatment of mild hypertension. Results of a ten-year intervention trial. Circ Res 1977; 40:Suppl I:I98–I105.
4. Veterans Administration Cooperative Study Group on Antihypertensive Agents. Effects of treatment on morbidity in hypertension. II. Results in patients with diastolic blood pressure averaging 90 through 114 mm Hg. JAMA 1970; 213:1143–52.
5. Hunninghake DB. Effects of celiprolol and other antihypertensive agents on serum lipids and lipoproteins. Am Heart J 1991; 121:696–701.
6. Hunninghake DB. The effects of cardiovascular vasodilating beta-blockers on lipids. Am Heart J 1991; 121:1029–32.
7. Middeke M, Holzgreve H. Review of major intervention studies in hypertension and hyperlipidemia: focus on coronary heart disease. Am Heart J 1988; 116:1708–12.
8. SHEP Cooperative Research Group. Prevention of stroke by antihypertensive drug treatment in older persons with isolated systolic hypertension: final results of the Systolic Hypertension in the Elderly Program (SHEP). JAMA 1991; 265:3255–64.
9. Freedman DS, Gruchow HW, Bamrah VS, et al. Diabetes mellitus and arteriographically-documented coronary artery disease. J Clin Epidemiol 1988; 41:659–68.
10. Janka HU, Ziegler AG, Standl E, Mehnert H. Daily insulin dose as a predictor of macrovascular disease in insulin treated non-insulin-dependent diabetics. Diabet Metab 1987; 13:359–64.
11. Laakso M, Pyörälä K, Voutilainen E, Marniemi J. Plasma insulin and serum lipids and lipoproteins in middle-aged non-insulin-dependent diabetic and non-diabetic subjects. Am J Epidemiol 1987; 125:611–21.
12. Lemp GF, Vander ZR, Hughes JP, et al. As-

sociation between the severity of diabetes mellitus and coronary arterial atherosclerosis. Am J Cardiol 1987; 60:1015–9.

13. Lobo RA. Lipids, clotting factors, and diabetes: endogenous risk factors for cardiovascular disease. Am J Obstet Gynecol 1988; 158:1584–91.

14. Macaulay AC, Montour LT, Adelson N. Prevalence of diabetic and atherosclerotic complications among Mohawk Indians of Kahnawake, PQ. Can Med Assoc J 1988; 139:221–4.

15. Stolar MW. Atherosclerosis in diabetes: the role of hyperinsulinemia. Metabolism 1988; 37: Suppl 1:1–9.

16. Stout RW. Insulin and atheroma. 20-yr perspective. Diabetes Care 1990; 13:631–54.

17. Raichlen JS, Healy B, Achuff SC, Pearson TA. Importance of risk factors in the angiographic progression of coronary artery disease. Am J Cardiol 1986; 57:66–70.

18. Mulcahy R. Influence of cigarette smoking on morbidity and mortality after myocardial infarction. BHJ 1983; 49:410–5.

19. Hermanson B, Omenn GS, Kronmal RA, Gersh B. Beneficial six-year outcome of smoking cessation in older men and women with coronary artery disease: results from the CASS Registry. N Engl J Med 1988; 319:1365–9.

20. Daly LE, Hickey N, Graham IM, Mulcahy R. Predictors of sudden death up to 18 years after a first attack of unstable angina or myocardial infarction. BHJ 1987; 58:567–71.

21. Mulcahy R, Hickey N, Graham IM, MacAirt J. Factors affecting the 5 year survival rate of men following acute coronary heart disease. Am Heart J 1977; 93:556–9.

22. Rønnevik P, Gundersen T, Abrahamsen A. Effect of smoking habits and timolol treatment on mortality and reinfarction in patients surviving acute myocardial infarction. BHJ 1985; 54:134–9.

23. Sparrow D, Dawber T, Colton T. The influence of cigarette smoking on prognosis after a first myocardial infarction. A report from the Framingham Study. J Chron Dis 1978; 31:425–32.

24. Vlietstra R, Kronmal RA, Oberman A, et al. Effect of cigarette smoking on survival of patients with angiographically documented coronary artery disease: report from the CASS Registry. JAMA 1986; 255:1023–7.

25. Salonen J. Stopping smoking and long-term mortality after acute myocardial infarction. BHJ 1980; 43:463–9.

26. Johansson S, Bergstrand R, Pennert KM, et al. Cessation of smoking after myocardial infarction in women. Effects on mortality and reinfarctions. Am J Epidemiol 1985; 121:823–31.

27. Albers JA, Cabana VG, Wernck GR, Hazzard WR. Lp(a) lipoprotein: relationship to smoking, pre-β lipoprotein, hyperlipoproteinemia, and apolipoprotein B. Metabolism 1975; 24:1047–54.

28. Grundy SM. Atherosclerosis: pathology, pathogenesis, and role of risk factors. Dis Mon 1983; 29:1–58.

29. Kannel WB, DAgostino RB, Belanger AJ. Fibrinogen, cigarette smoking, and risk of cardiovascular disease: insights from the Framingham Study. Am Heart J 1987; 113:1006–10.

30. Renders J, Brinkman H, Van Mourik J, De Groot P. Cigarette smoke impairs endothelial cell prostacyclin production. Arteriosclerosis 1986; 6:15–23.

31. Martin J, Wilson J, Ferraro N, et al. Acute coronary vasoconstrictive effects of cigarette smoking in coronary heart disease. Am J Cardiol 1984; 54:56–60.

32. Maouad J, Fernandez F, Barrillon A, et al. Diffuse or segmental narrowing (spasm) of the coronary arteries during smoking demonstrated on angiography. Am J Cardiol 1984; 53:354–5.

33. Folts JD, Bonebrake F. The effects of cigarette smoke and nicotine on platelet thrombus formation in stenosed dog coronary arteries: inhibition with phentolamine. Circulation 1982; 65:465–70.

34. Fitzgerald GA, Oates JA, Nowak J. Cigarette smoking and hemostatic function. Am Heart J 1988; 115:267–71.

35. Ernst E, Matrai A. Abstention from chronic cigarette smoking normalizes blood rheology. Atherosclerosis 1987; 64:75–7.

36. De Lorgeril M, Reinharz A, Busslinger B, et al. Acute influence of cigarette smoke in platelets, catecholamines and neurophysins in the normal conditions of daily life. Eur Heart J 1985; 6(12):1063–8.

37. Davis J, Shelton L, Eigenberg D, et al. Effects of tobacco and non-tobacco cigarette smoking on endothelium and platelets. Clin Pharmacol Ther 1985; 37:529–33.

38. Davis JW, Shelton L, Hartman CR, et al. Smoking-induced changes in endothelium and platelets are not affected by hydroxyethylrutosides. Brit J Exp Path 1986; 67:765–71.

39. Hjermann I, Holme I, Leren P. Oslo Study Diet and Antismoking Trial: results after 102 months. Am J Med 1986; 80:7–11.

40. Lipid Research Clinics Program. The Lipid Research Clinics Coronary Primary Prevention Trial results. I. Reduction in incidence of coronary heart disease. JAMA 1984; 251: 351–64.

41. Anderson KM, Wilson PW, Garrison RJ, Castelli WP. Longitudinal and secular trends in lipoprotein cholesterol measurements in a

general population sample. The Framingham Offspring Study. Atherosclerosis 1987; 68:59–66.

42. Wong ND, Cupples LA, Ostfeld AM, et al. Risk factors for long-term coronary prognosis after initial myocardial infarction: the Framingham Study. Am J Epidemiol 1989; 130:469–80.

43. National Cholesterol Education Program. Report of the expert panel on detection, evaluation, and treatment of high blood cholesterol in adults. Arch Intern Med 1988; 148:36–69.

44. Blankenhorn DH, Nessim SA, Johnson RL, et al. Beneficial effects of combined colestipol-niacin therapy on coronary atherosclerosis and coronary venous bypass grafts. JAMA 1987; 257:3233–40.

45. Cashin-Hemphill L, Mack WJ, Pogoda JM, et al. Beneficial effects of colestipol-niacin on coronary atherosclerosis: a four year follow-up. JAMA 1990; 264:3013–7.

46. Dollar AL, Kragel AH, Fernicola DJ, et al. Composition of atherosclerotic plaques in coronary arteries in women less-than-40 years of age with fatal coronary artery disease and implications for plaque reversibility. Am J Cardiol 1991; 67:1223–7.

47. Gertz SD, Malekzadeh S, Dollar AL, et al. Composition of atherosclerotic plaques in the four major epicardial coronary arteries in patients greater than or equal to 90 years of age. Am J Cardiol 1991; 67:1228–33.

48. Small DM, Shipley GG. Physical-chemical basis of lipid deposition in atherosclerosis. Science 1974; 185:222–9.

49. Small DM. George Lyman Duff memorial lecture. Progression and regression of atherosclerotic lesions. Insights from lipid physical biochemistry. Arteriosclerosis 1988; 8:103–29.

50. Smith EB. The influence of age and atherosclerosis on the chemistry of aortic intima. Part I. The Lipids. J Atheroscler Res 1965; 5:224–40.

51. Katz SS. The lipids of grossly normal human aortic intima from birth to old age. J Biol Chem 1981; 256:12275–90.

52. Hollander W, Paddock J, Colombo M. Lipoproteins in human atherosclerotic vessels. Exp Mol Pathol 1979; 30:144–71.

53. Hoff HF, Heideman CL, Gaubatz JW. Low density lipoproteins in the aorta. In: Gotto AM, Smith LC, Allen B, eds. Atherosclerosis. V. New York: Springer, 1980; 533–6.

54. Steinberg D, Parthasarathy S, Carew TE, et al. Beyond cholesterol: modifications of low-density lipoprotein that increase its atherogenicity. N Engl J Med 1989; 320:915–24.

55. Katz SS, Shipley GG, Small DM. Physical

chemistry of the lipids of human atherosclerotic lesions. Demonstration of a lesion intermediate between fatty streaks and advanced plaques. J Clin Invest 1976; 58:200–11.

56. Jagannathan SN, Connor WE, Baker WH, Bhattacharyya AK. The turnover of cholesterol in human atherosclerotic arteries. J Clin Invest 1974; 54:366–77.

57. Chobanian AV, Hollander W. Body cholesterol metabolism in man. I. The equilibration of serum and tissue cholesterol. J Clin Invest 1962; 41:1732–7.

58. Katz SS, Small DM, Smith FR, et al. Cholesterol turnover in lipid phases of human atherosclerotic plaque. J Lipid Res 1982; 23:733–7.

59. Small DM, Bond MG, Waugh D, et al. Physicochemical and histological changes in the arterial wall of nonhuman primates during progression and regression of atherosclerosis. J Clin Invest 1984; 73:1590–605.

60. Steering committee of the Physicians' Health Study Research Group. Final report on the aspirin component of the ongoing Physicians' Health Study. N Engl J Med 1989; 321:129–35.

61. Glagov S, Weisenberg E, Zarins CK, et al. Compensatory enlargement of human atherosclerotic coronary arteries. N Engl J Med 1987; 316:1371–5.

62. Poli A, Paoletti R. Regression of the atherosclerotic lesion in man: the impact of noninvasive techniques. Int Angiol 1987; 6:327–9.

63. Senin U, Parnetti L, Mercuri M, et al. Evolutionary trends in carotid atherosclerotic plaques: results of a two-year follow-up study using an ultrasound imaging system. Angiology 1988; 39:429–36.

64. Grotta JC, Yatsu FM, Pettigrew LC, et al. Prediction of carotid stenosis progression by lipid and hematologic measurements. Neurology 1989; 39:1325–31.

65. Hodgson JM, Graham SP, Savakus AD, et al. Clinical percutaneous imaging of coronary anatomy using an over-the-wire ultrasound catheter system. Int J Card Imaging 1989; 4:187–93.

66. Mallery JA, Tobis JM, Griffith J, et al. Assessment of normal and atherosclerotic arterial wall thickness with an intravascular ultrasound imaging catheter. Am Heart J 1990; 119:1392–1400.

67. Ellestad MH, Famularo MA, Paliwal YK. Exercise testing in the evaluation of coronary artery disease. Herz 1982; 7:76–90.

68. Froelicher VF, Duarte GM, Oakes DF, et al. The prognostic value of the exercise test. Dis Mon 1988; 34:677–735.

69. Gianrossi R, Detrano R, Mulvihill D, et al. Exercise-induced ST depression in the diagnosis

of coronary artery disease: a meta-analysis. Circulation 1989; 80:87–98.

70. Paolillo V, Marra S, Rendine S, et al. The prognostic significance of clinical history, exercise testing and ambulatory electrocardiography in patients with uncomplicated myocardial infarction. G Ital Cardiol 1985; 15:465–71.

71. Weiner DA, McCabe CH, Ryan TJ. Prognostic assessment of patients with coronary artery disease by exercise testing. Am Heart J 1983; 105:749–55.

72. Wyns W, Musschaert-Beauthier E, Van Domburg R, et al. Prognostic value of symptom limited exercise testing in men with a high prevalence of coronary artery disease. Eur Heart J 1985; 6:939–45.

73. Demer LL, Gould KL, Goldstein RA, et al. Assessment of coronary artery disease severity by positron emission tomography: comparison with quantitative arteriography in 193 patients. Circulation 1989; 79:825–35.

74. Ornish D, Brown SE, Scherwitz LW, et al. Can lifestyle changes reverse coronary heart disease? The Lifestyle Heart Trial. Lancet 1990; 336:129–33.

75. Vartianinen I, Kanerva K. Arteriosclerosis and war-time. Ann Med Intern Fenn 1947; 36:748–58.

76. Aschoff L. Atherosclerosis, Lane Lecture, San Francisco. In: Lectures in Pathology. New York: Hoeber, 1924; chapter 6.

77. Wilens SL. The resorption of arterial atheromatous deposits in wasting disease. Am J Pathol 1947; 23:793–804.

78. Wanscher O, Clemmesen J, Nielsen A. Negative correlation between atherosclerosis and carcinoma. Brit J Cancer 1951; 5:172–4.

79. Juhl S. Cancer and atherosclerosis. Acta Path Micro Scand 1957; 41:99–104.

80. Eilersen P, Faber M. The human aorta. Arch Pathol 1960; 70:103–7.

81. Vesselinovitch D, Wissler R, Hughes R, Borensztajn J. Reversal of advanced atherosclerosis in Rhesus monkeys. Atherosclerosis 1976; 23:155–76.

82. Vesselinovitch D, Wissler RW. Prevention and regression in animal models by diet and cholestyramine. In: Hauss W, Wissler R, Lehmann R, eds. International symposium: state of prevention and therapy in human arteriosclerosis and in animal models. Opladen, Germany: Westdeutscher Verlag, 1978: 127–34.

83. Fritz KE, Augustyn JM, Jarmolych J, et al. Regression of advanced atherosclerosis in swine. Chemical studies. Arch Pathol Lab Med 1976; 100:380–5.

84. Doaud AS, Jarmolych J, Augustyn JM, et al. Regression of advanced atherosclerosis in swine. Arch Pathol Lab Med 1976; 100:372–9.

85. Bond J, Bullock B, Lehner N, Clarkson T. Regression of atherosclerosis with plasma cholesterol concentrations achievable in man. In: G Schettler et al., eds. IV International Symposium on Atherosclerosis. New York: Springer, 1977; 42.

86. Augustyn J, Fritz K, Daoud A, et al. Biochemical effects of a moderate diet and clofibrate on swine atherosclerosis. Arch Pathol Lab Med 1978; 102:294–7.

87. Hollander W, Kirkpatrick B, Paddock J, et al. Studies on the progression and regression of coronary and peripheral atherosclerosis in the cynomolgus monkey. I. Effects of dipyridamole and aspirin. Exp Mol Pathol 1979; 30:55–73.

88. Foegh ML, Khirabadi BS, Chambers E, et al. Inhibition of coronary artery transplant atherosclerosis in rabbits with angiopeptin, an octapeptide. Atherosclerosis 1989; 78:229–36.

89. Gossard D, Langlais J. Transplantation and lipids. Can Med Assoc J 1991; 144:1003.

90. Otto DA, Kahn DR, Hamm MW, et al. Improved survival of heterotopic cardiac allografts in rats with dietary n-3 polyunsaturated fatty acids. Transplantation 1990; 50:193–8.

91. Davis HR, Bridenshire RT, Vesselinovitch D, Wissler RW. Fish oil inhibits development of atherosclerosis in Rhesus monkeys. Arteriosclerosis 1987; 7:441–8.

92. Weiner BH, Ockene IS, Levine PH, et al. Inhibition of atherosclerosis by cod liver oil in a hyperlipidemic swine model. N Engl J Med 1986; 315:841–6.

93. Sassen LM, Koning MM, Dekkers DH, et al. Differential effects of n-3 fatty acids on the regression of atherosclerosis in coronary arteries and the aorta of the pig. Eur Heart J 1989; 10(suppl F):173–8.

94. van Oort G, Gross DR, Spiekerman AM. Effects of eight weeks of physical conditioning on atherosclerotic plaque in swine. Am J Vet Res 1987; 48:51–5.

95. Kaplan JR, Manuck SB, Clarkson TB, et al. Social stress and atherosclerosis in normocholesterolemic monkeys. Science 1983; 220:733–5.

96. Kaplan JR, Manuck SB, Clarkson TB, et al. Social status, environment and atherosclerosis in cynomolgus monkeys. Arteriosclerosis 1982; 2:359–68.

97. Rifkind BM. The Lipid Research Clinics Coronary Primary Prevention Trial: results and implications. Monogr Atheroscler 1985; 13:74–84.

98. Frick MH, Elo O, Haapa K, et al. Helsinki Heart Study; primary-prevention trial with gemfibrozil in middle-aged men with dyslipidemia: safety of treatment, changes in risk factors, and incidence of coronary heart disease. N Engl J Med 1987; 317:1237–45.

99. Pekkanen J, Linn S, Heiss G, et al. Ten-year mortality from cardiovascular disease in relation to cholesterol level among men with and without preexisting cardiovascular disease. N Engl J Med 1990; 322:1700–7.

100. Ulvenstam G, Bergstrand R, Johansson S, et al. Prognostic importance of cholesterol levels after myocardial infarction. Prev Med 1984; 13:355–66.

101. Frost PH, Verter J, Miller D. Serum lipids and lipoproteins after myocardial infarction: associations with cardiovascular mortality and experience in the Aspirin Myocardial Infarction Study. Am Heart J 1987; 113:1356–64.

102. Heliövaara M, Karvonen MJ, Punsar S, Haapakoski J. Importance of coronary risk factors in the presence or absence of myocardial ischemia. Am J Cardiol 1982; 50:1248–52.

103. Goldbourt U, Cohen L, Neufeld HN. High density lipoprotein cholesterol: prognosis after myocardial infarction; the Israeli Ischaemic Heart Disease Study. Int J Epidemiol 1986; 15:51–5.

104. The Coronary Drug Project Research Group. Clofibrate and niacin in coronary heart disease. JAMA 1975; 231:360–81.

105. Carlson LA, Rosenhamer D. Reduction of mortality in the Stockholm Ischaemic Heart Disease Secondary Prevention Study by combined treatment with clofibrate and nicotinic acid. Acta Med Scand 1988; 223:405–18.

106. Trial of clofibrate in the treatment of ischaemic heart disease: five-year study by a group of physicians of the Newcastle upon Tyne region. Br Med J 1971; 14:767–75.

107. Ischaemic heart disease: a secondary prevention trial using clofibrate: Report by a research committee of the Scottish Society of Physicians. Br Med J 1971; 790:775–84.

108. Hanefeld M, Hora C, Schulze J, et al. Reduced incidence of cardiovascular complications and mortality in hyperlipoproteinemia (HLP) with effective lipid correction. The Dresden HLP study. Atherosclerosis 1984; 53:47–58.

109. Rossouw JE, Lewis B, Rifkind BM. The value of lowering cholesterol after myocardial infarction. N Engl J Med 1990; 323:1112–9.

110. Canner PL, Berge KG, Wenger NK, et al. Fifteen year mortality in Coronary Drug Project patients: long-term benefit with niacin. J Am Coll Cardiol 1986; 8:1245–55.

111. The Multiple Risk Factor Intervention Trial Research Group. Mortality rates after 10.5 years for participants in the Multiple Risk Factor Intervention Trial: findings related to a priori hypotheses of the trial. JAMA 1990; 263:1795–801.

112. Leren P. The Oslo Diet-Heart Study: eleven-year report. Circulation 1970; 42:935–42.

113. Öst RC, Stenson S. Regression of peripheral atherosclerosis during therapy with high doses of nicotinic acid. Scand J Clin Lab Invest 1967; 99:Suppl:241–5.

114. Barndt RJ, Blankenhorn DH, Crawford DW, et al. Regression and progression of early femoral atherosclerosis in treated hyperlipoproteinemic patients. Ann Intern Med 1977; 86:139–46.

115. Erikson U, Helmius G, Hemmingsson A, et al. Repeat femoral arteriography in hyperlipidemic patients. A study of progression and regression of atherosclerosis. Acta Radiol 1988; 29:303–9.

116. Blankenhorn DH, Azen SP, Crawford DW, et al. Effects of colestipol-niacin therapy on human femoral atherosclerosis. Circulation 1991; 83:438–47.

117. Arntzenius AC, Kromhout D, Barth JD, et al. Diet, lipoproteins, and the progression of coronary atherosclerosis: The Leiden Intervention Trial. N Engl J Med 1985; 312:805–11.

118. Arntzenius AC. Regression of atherosclerosis. Horm Metab Res 1988; 19 (Suppl):19–22.

119. Nikkilä EA, Viikinkoski P, Valle M, Frick MH. Prevention of progression of coronary atherosclerosis by treatment of hyperlipidaemia: a seven year prospective angiographic study. Br Med J 1984; 289:220–3.

120. Detre KM, Levy RI, Kelsey SF, et al. Secondary prevention and lipid lowering: results and implications. Am Heart J 1985; 110:1123–7.

121. Brown G, Albers JJ, Fisher LD, et al. Regression of coronary artery disease as a result of intensive lipid-lowering therapy in men with high levels of apolipoprotein-B. N Engl J Med 1990; 323:1289–98.

122. Buchwald H, Varco RL, Matts JP, et al. Effect of partial ileal bypass surgery on mortality and morbidity from coronary heart disease in patients with hypercholesterolemia — Report of the Program on the Surgical Control of the Hyperlipidemias (POSCH). N Engl J Med 1990; 323:946–55.

123. Blankenhorn DH, Alaupovic P, Wickham E, et al. Prediction of angiographic change in native human coronary arteries and aortocoronary bypass grafts. Lipid and nonlipid factors. Circulation 1990; 81:470–6.

124. Le NA, Gibson JC, Ginsberg HN. Independent regulation of plasma apolipoprotein C-II and C-III concentrations in very low density and high density lipoproteins: implications for the regulation of the catabolism of the lipoproteins. J Lipid Res 1988; 29:669–77.

125. Kuusi T, Saarinen P, Nikkilä EA. Evidence for the role of hepatic endothelial lipase in the me-

tabolism of plasma high density lipoprotein$_2$ in man. Atherosclerosis 1980; 36:589–93.

125a. Blankenhorn DH. Personal communication.

126. Ratliff NB, Myles JL. The pathogenesis of atherosclerosis in aortocoronary saphenous vein grafts — reply. Arch Pathol Lab Med 1989; 113:1323.

127. Kern WH. The pathogenesis of atherosclerosis in aortocoronary saphenous vein grafts. Arch Pathol Lab Med 1989; 113:1322–3.

128. Numano F, Tsukada T, Amano J, Suzuki A. Experimental studies on vein graft atherosclerosis. I. Histochemical studies using monoclonal antibodies for smooth muscle cells and macrophages. Japan Circ J 1990; 54: 1398–408.

129. Zwolak RM, Kirkman TR, Clowes AW. Atherosclerosis in rabbit vein grafts. Arteriosclerosis 1989; 9:374–9.

130. Buckley BH, Hutchins GM. Accelerated "atherosclerosis." A morphologic study of 197 saphenous vein coronary artery bypass grafts. Circulation 1977; 55:163.

131. Barboriak JJ, Batayias GE, Pintar K, Korns ME. Pathological changes in surgically removed aortocoronary vein grafts. Ann Thorac Surg 1976; 21:524.

132. Grondin CM, Campeau L, Lesperance J, et al. Atherosclerotic changes in coronary vein grafts six years after operation. Angiographic aspect in 110 patients. J Thorac Cardiovasc Surg 1979; 77:24–31.

133. Bourassa MG, Campeau L, Lesperance J, Grondin CM. Changes in grafts and coronary arteries after saphenous vein aortocoronary bypass surgery: results at repeat angiography. Circulation 1982; 65:90–7.

134. Campeau L, Enjalbert M, Lesperance J, et al. Atherosclerosis and late closure of aortocoronary saphenous vein grafts: sequential angiographic studies at 2 weeks, 1 year, 5 to 7 years, and 10 to 12 years after surgery. Circulation 1983; 68:111–17.

135. Bourassa MG. Fate of venous grafts: the past, the present and the future. J Am Coll Cardiol 1991; 17:1081–3.

136. Solymoss BC, Nadeau P, Millette D, et al. Late thrombosis of saphenous vein coronary bypass grafts related to risk factors. Circulation 1988; 78:suppl I:I-140–3.

137. Bonchek LI, Boerboom LE, Olinger GN, et al. Prevention of lipid accumulation in experimental vein bypass grafts by antiplatelet therapy. Circulation 1982; 66:338–41.

138. Chesebro JH, Clements IP, Fuster V, et al. A platelet-inhibitor-drug trial in coronary-artery bypass operations: benefit of perioperative dipyridamole and aspirin therapy on early postoperative vein-graft patency. N Engl J Med 1982; 307:73–8.

139. Chesebro JH, Fuster V, Elveback LR, et al. Effect of dipyridamole and aspirin on late vein-graft patency after coronary bypass operations. N Engl J Med 1984; 310:209–14.

140. Fuster V, Chesebro JH. Role of platelets and platelet inhibitors in aortocoronary artery vein-graft disease. Circulation 1986; 73:227–32.

141. Califf RM, Fortin DF, Frid DJ, et al. Restenosis after coronary angioplasty: an overview. J Am Coll Cardiol 1991; 17 (Suppl B):2B–13B.

142. Arora RR, Konrad K. Badhwar K, Hollman J. Restenosis after transluminal coronary angioplasty: a risk factor analysis. Cathet Cardiovasc Diagn 1990; 19:17–22.

143. Benchimol D, Benchimol H, Bonnet J, et al. Risk factors for progression of atherosclerosis six months after balloon angioplasty of coronary stenosis. Am J Cardiol 1990; 65:980–5.

144. Bonnier H, Bronzwair P, Michels R, El Gamal M. Long-term follow-up of 100 patients with left anterior descending artery lesions treated with percutaneous transluminal coronary angioplasty. Eur Heart J 1989; suppl H:49–51.

145. Fleck E, Regitz V, Lehnert A, et al. Restenosis after balloon dilatation of coronary stenosis: multivariate analysis of potential risk factors. Eur Heart J 1988; 9:Suppl C:15–8.

146. Macdonald RG, Henderson MA, Hirshfeld JWJ, et al. Patient-related variables and restenosis after percutaneous transluminal coronary angioplasty — a report from the M-HEART Group. Am J Cardiol 1990; 66:926–31.

147. Quigley PJ, Hlatky MA, Hinohara T, et al. Repeat percutaneous transluminal coronary angioplasty and predictors of recurrent restenosis. Am J Cardiol 1989; 63:409–13.

148. Galan KM, Deligonul U, Kern MJ, et al. Increased frequency of restenosis in patients continuing to smoke cigarettes after percutaneous transluminal coronary angioplasty. Am J Cardiol 1988; 61:260–3.

149. Sahni R, Maniet AR, Voci G, Banka VS. Prevention of restenosis by lovastatin after successful coronary angioplasty. Am Heart J 1991; 121:1600–8.

150. Cuthbert JA, Lipsky PE. Inhibition by 6-fluoromevalonate demonstrates that mevalonate or one of the mevalonate phosphates is necessary for lymphocyte proliferation. J Biol Chem 1990; 265:18568–75.

151. Witte LD, Fairbanks KP, Barbu V, Goodman DS. Studies on cell proliferation and mevalonic acid metabolism in cultured human fibroblasts. Ann NY Acad Sci 1985; 454:261–9.

152. el-Sayed GN, Cenedella RJ. Relationship of cholesterolgenesis to DNA synthesis and pro-

liferation by lens epithelial cells in culture. Exp Eye Res 1987; 45:443–51.

153. Milner MR, Gallino RA, Leffingwell A, et al. Usefulness of fish oil supplements in preventing clinical evidence of restenosis after percutaneous transluminal coronary angioplasty. Am J Cardiol 1989; 64:294–9.

154. Reis GJ, Boucher TM, Sipperly ME, et al. Randomised trial of fish oil for prevention of restenosis after coronary angioplasty. Lancet 1989; 2:177–81.

155. Kaplan NM. Strategies to reduce risk factors in hypertensive patients who smoke. Am Heart J 1988; 115:288–93.

156. Miller NE, Nanjee MN, Raiput-Williams J, Coltar DJ. Double-blind trial of the long term effect of acebutolol and propranolol on serum lipoproteins in patients with stable angina pectoris. Am Heart J 1987; 114:1007–10.

157. Olsson G, Oden A, Johansson L. Prognosis after withdrawal of chronic postinfarction metoprolol treatment: a 2-7 year follow-up. Eur Heart J 1988; 9:365–72.

158. Hjalmarson A. International beta-blocker review in acute and postmyocardial infarction. Am J Cardiol 1988; 61:26B–9B.

159. Hjalmarson AC. Use of beta blockers in postinfarct prophylaxis: aspects on quality of life. Am Heart J 1987; 114:245–50.

160. Decorde P. Beta-blockers in the secondary prevention of myocardial infarction: a review of clinical trials of 12 months or more duration. Pharmatherapeutica 1984; 3:515–25.

161. Boissel JP, Leizorovicz A, Picolet H, Peyrieux JC. Secondary prevention after high-risk acute myocardial infarction with low-dose acebutolol. Am J Cardiol 1990; 66:251–60.

162. Braunwald E, Muller JE, Kloner RA, Maroko PR. Role of beta-adrenergic blockade in the therapy of patients with myocardial infarction. Am J Med 1983; 74:113–23.

163. Cruickshank JM, Pennert K, Sorman AE. Low mortality from all causes, including myocardial infarction, in well-controlled hypertensives treated with a beta-blocker plus other antihypertensives. J Hypertens 1987; 5:489–98.

164. Kaplan NM. Arterial protection: a neglected but crucial therapeutic goal. Am J Cardiol 1990; 66:36C–8C.

165. Peters RW, Byington R, Arensberg D, et al. Mortality in the beta blocker heart attack trial: circumstances surrounding death. J Chronic Dis 1987; 40:75–82.

166. Muller JE, Tofler GH, Stone PH. Circadian variation and triggers of onset of acute cardiovascular disease. Circulation 1989; 79:733–43.

167. Mickley H, Pless P, Nielsen JR, Moller M. Circadian variation of transient myocardial ischemia in the early out-of-hospital period after first acute myocardial infarction. Am J Cardiol 1991; 67:927–32.

168. Stone PH. Triggers of transient myocardial ischemia — circadian variation and relation to plaque rupture and coronary thrombosis in stable coronary artery disease. Am J Cardiol 1990; 66:G32–6.

169. Thompson DR, Sutton TW, Jowett NI, Pohl JEF. Circadian variation in the frequency of onset of chest pain in acute myocardial infarction. BHJ 1991; 65:177–8.

170. Hjalmarson Å, Gilpin, EA, Nicod P, et al. Differing circadian patterns of symptom onset in subgroups of patients with acute myocardial infarction. Circulation 1989; 80:267–75.

171. Loaldi A, Polese A, Montorsi P, et al. Comparison of nifedipine, propranolol and isosorbide dinitrate on angiographic progression and regression of coronary arterial narrowings in angina pectoris. Am J Cardiol 1989; 64:433–9.

172. Henry PD. Atherogenesis, calcium, and calcium antagonists. Am J Cardiol 1990; 66:13–6.

173. Henry PD, Bently KI. Suppression of atherogenesis in cholesterol-fed rabbit treated with nifedipine. J Clin Invest 1981; 68:1366–9.

174. Sugano M, Nakashima Y, Tasaki H, et al. Effects of diltiazem on suppression and regression of experimental atherosclerosis. Br J Exp Pathol 1988; 69:515–23.

175. Mehta P, Kimura A, Lawson D. Effects of calcium channel-blocking agents on platelet-osteogenic sarcoma interaction: platelet aggregation and electron microscopic findings. J Orthop Res 1990; 8:629–34.

176. Addonizio VPJ, Fisher CA, Strauss JF III et al. Effects of verapamil and diltiazem on human platelet function. Am J Physiol 1986; 250:H366–71.

177. Edvinsson L, Ikomi KJ, Monti M. Effects of calcium entry blockers on human platelet metabolism measured by microcalorimetry. Hum Toxicol 1989; 8:131–3.

178. Ring ME, Corrigan JJ Jr, Fenster PE. Effects of oral diltiazem on platelet function: alone and in combination with "low dose" aspirin. Thromb Res 1986; 44:391–400.

179. Valone FH. Inhibition of platelet-activating factor binding to human platelets by calcium channel blockers. Thromb Res 1987; 45:427–35.

180. Vinge E, Andersson TL, Larsson B. Effects of some calcium antagonists on aggregation by adrenalin and serotonin and on alpha-adrenoceptor radioligand binding in human platelets. Acta Physiol Scand 1988; 133:407–16.

181. Lichtlen PR, Hugenholtz PG, Rafflebeul W, et al. Retardation of angiographic progression of coronary artery disease by nifedipine. Results of the International Nifedipine Trial on Antiatherosclerotic Therapy (INTACT). Lancet 1990; 335:1109–3.

16

Intervention in Childhood

CHRISTINE L. WILLIAMS

EDITORS' INTRODUCTION

There is no longer any doubt about the time course of athero-sclerotic CAD; it does not develop within a few years of the first clinical event but rather has its origins in childhood. It is also clear that CHD-promoting or -preventing lifestyle behaviors are established in childhood; once these behavior patterns are set they become increasingly difficult to change. Thus, the argument for intervention in childhood is compelling. Nonetheless, the topic is controversial, with concerns raised about unnecessary intervention, excessively restricted diets, labeling of healthy children as having a problem, and the appropriateness of childhood screening. All these issues are dealt with in this chapter, which reviews current pediatric guidelines and makes reasonable recommendations, both for routine pediatric practice and for the management of children who are at particularly high risk.

The rationale for primary prevention of CHD in childhood is based on the high prevalence of the disease among adults in most developed countries, its early insidious onset, pathologic evidence that atherosclerosis begins in childhood, and the knowledge that many of the risk factors for CHD are related to lifestyle and are thus potentially preventable.

Elevated cardiovascular risk should be preventable through population-based programs, such as school health curricula, that teach changes in risk-related behavior, including nutrition, physical activity, and cigarette smoking. Pediatric population-based interventions have the greatest potential for reducing overall CHD morbidity and mortality. Small decreases in mean serum cholesterol, mean systolic and diastolic BP, and the prevalence of cigarette smoking, if carried from childhood into adulthood, could significantly reduce CHD mortality.

High-risk approaches, such as those practiced in the physician's office or clinic, complement the population approach and are necessary to provide treatment for children with moderately severe to severe risk factor elevations. In addition physicians can incorporate general counseling in risk reduction into routine child health assessment as part of population-based prevention.

This chapter describes one approach to the clinical practice of pediatric preventive cardiology in the office setting.

Atherosclerosis in Childhood

In the past two decades it has been increasingly recognized that traditional risk factors for CHD can be easily identified in childhood and that they are largely the result of lifestyle habits (cigarette smoking, poor eating habits, and lack of regular physical activity) acquired early in life [1, 2, 3, 4, 5, 6]. This recognition has stimulated clinical initiatives in pediatric preventive cardiology practice [7, 8, 9, 10].

Evidence that the pathological process of atherosclerosis begins in childhood is also strong. Early support for this view came from autopsy studies of children killed accidentally and of young combat casualties. During the Korean conflict an autopsy study of 300 soldiers (mean age 22 years) revealed that 77 percent of these young men had evidence of coronary atherosclerosis. Fifteen percent had more than 50 percent stenosis of one or more coronary vessels [11]. Similarly during the Vietnamese conflict a study of 105 combat casualties (mean age 22 years) showed that 44 percent had evidence of coronary atherosclerosis. Remarkably 1 in 20 of these young soldiers had severe lesions [12]. These data suggest that lesions present to such an extensive degree in young men must have been progressing silently through childhood.

Additional evidence for the childhood onset of atherosclerosis came from the classic studies of Holman et al. in New Orleans published in 1958 [13]. This group systematically studied aortas fom 526 autopsies of children and young adults between the ages of 1 and 40 years. Fatty streaks were demonstrated in the aortas of all children over the age of 3 years. The percentage of intimal surface covered with fatty streaks increased slowly through the first decade of life and then more rapidly during adolescence (occurring sooner in blacks than in whites). Fibrous plaques in the aorta began to appear during adolescence but increased significantly only in the fourth decade of life. Overall there was about a 15-year lag between the development of fatty streaks and fibrous plaques, and in this case, whites had a greater extent of intimal involvement than blacks.

Strong and McGill studied both coronary and aortic lesions in 4737 children and young adults (ages 10 to 39), a subset of the International Atherosclerosis Project sample [14, 15]. Again almost all aortas had evidence of fatty-streak involvement. Coronary fatty streaks were not as frequent but were detected even in some of the 10- to 15-year-old children. Coronary fibrous plaques were rare before age 20 but increased rapidly between 20 and 40 years of age, more so in men than in women.

Stary has studied the left coronary arteries of 422 individuals who died between full-term birth and 29 years of age [16]. He describes four types of intimal lesions. The last three types (fatty streaks, preatheromas, and atheromas) began during the second decade of life, in a manner similar to the results of other studies.

The Bogalusa Heart Study recently reported on autopsy specimens from 110 children and young adults, 40 percent of whom had participated in a study of cardiovascular risk factors in childhood. In a report of 35 subjects (mean age 17.9 years) with previously measured risk factor levels these investigators found that aortic fatty streaks covered between 1 and 61 percent of the intimal surface. Coronary fatty streaks were found in almost all cases but covered only about 1 percent of the intimal surface (maximum 6.2 percent). More advanced fibrous plaques were found in 6 subjects (all male) [17].

Since all these subjects had had previous measurements of coronary risk factors, correlations between the degree of intimal surface coverage and the level of risk factors could be determined. Aortic fatty streaks were highly correlated with serum total cholesterol and serum LDL cholesterol (r = .67; P < .001). Coronary fatty streaks as well as fibrous plaques were significantly correlated with VLDL cholesterol. There was also a general positive association with all the traditional risk factors (total and LDL cholesterol, triglycerides, systolic and diastolic blood pressure, and ponderal index) as well as a negative association with HDL cholesterol [17].

Risk Factors in Children

Foremost among the modifiable risk factors for atherosclerotic cardiovascular disease are cigarette smoking, hypertension, and increased levels of plasma cholesterol. These and other contributing factors, such as obesity, inactivity, stress, and a family history of premature CHD, hypertension, or dyslipidemia, have been studied in populations of adults and children in the United States and abroad.

Most of the information on CHD risk factor prevalence has been obtained on adult populations. More recently efforts have been made to extend these observations to children. In the past two decades a great deal has been published on the distribution of CHD risk factors in several populations of children [18, 19, 20, 21, 23, 24]. In the United States the New York Know Your Body Study [19, 22], the Bogalusa Heart Study [20], the Muscatine Study [21, 23], the Cincinnati Lipid Research Clinic Study [24], and others have provided information on thousands of children. Numerous other studies have investigated similar risk factors in other countries [25, 26, 27, 28, 29, 30, 31]. Estimates of the prevalence of CHD risk factors in pediatric populations vary according to the age, sex, and ethnicity of the children studied. They also vary according to the choice of at-risk cutoff points for clinical indices such as blood pressure and cholesterol. For example, when total cholesterol levels above 175 mg/dl are considered to be an elevated risk factor, far more children are classified as being at risk than if a level of 200 mg/dl is utilized. Studies using adult cutoff points for high risk therefore have tended to underestimate the magnitude of risk status in children.

In New York a survey of 3000 11- to 14-year-old children found that 36 percent had one or more coronary risk factors exclusive of family history [22]. The most common risk factors observed in this junior high school population were elevated serum cholesterol (18 percent were above 180 mg/dl), obesity (16 percent were more than 20 percent above ideal weight for height), and cigarette smoking (8 percent were regular smokers). In a similar study of 95 first-grade students in two New York schools (mean age 6 years), 21 percent had one or more risk factors identified. In this age group, elevated serum cholesterol was common (22 percent were above 180 mg/dl). Obesity was much less prevalent among the 6-year-olds (2 percent were more than 20 percent above ideal weight for height) [32].

In Wisconsin a survey of 8- to 12-year-old boys found 46 percent with at least one risk factor for CHD and 14 percent with two or more risk factors [33].

Cardiovascular risk factors among children under age 10 are primarily hypercholesterolemia and obesity. Among older children and adolescents these risk factors are still most prevalent, but in addition cigarette smoking and hypertension become more common.

Lipids

Epidemiologic studies have established that elevated levels of serum total and LDL cholesterol (as well as decreased HDL cholesterol) accelerate atherogenesis and increase the incidence of CHD. Lipids are essential structural components of animal cells. In addition they are involved in energy metabolism, production of hormones, and development of the myelin sheath around nerves. The liver synthesizes cholesterol itself, so that at any given time about two-thirds of the cholesterol in plasma has been synthesized by the liver; the other one-third has been contributed by exogenous dietary sources [34]. The liver appears capable of synthesizing all the cholesterol required for body structure and metabolism. Excess plasma LDL cholesterol (resulting either from dietary saturated fat and cholesterol overload or from genetic abnormalities in cellular cholesterol receptors) contributes to atheromatous build-up in arteries [35, 36, 37]. Studies have now shown that reduction of plasma LDL cholesterol can result in reduction of mortality and morbidity from CHD, as well as regression of atherosclerotic plaque size [38].

During the past two decades a large body of literature has emerged describing the distribution of lipid and blood pressure levels in children and adolescents. In adults risk of CHD rises sharply at total cholesterol levels above 240 mg/dl (approximately the upper quartile of the adult population). The National Institutes of Health Consensus Committee has determined that adult total cholesterol levels between 200 and 239 mg/dl should be considered borderline high risk and levels at or above 240 mg/dl should be considered high risk [39].

In children in the United States the upper quartile of total cholesterol levels is generally about 170 mg/dl for 2- to 11-year-old children, varying somewhat by age, sex, and race [40, 41, 42, 43] (Table 16-1). Approximately 25 to 40 percent of children in various surveys have total cholesterol levels above 170 mg/dl, and between 5 to 15 percent of children over the age of 2 years have total cholesterol levels above 200 mg/dl, a level considered elevated even for adults [8]. The need to reduce cholesterol levels in these children is generally agreed upon, unless the elevation is due to high levels of protective HDL cholesterol, and the LDL cholesterol levels are normal.

Total cholesterol levels are about 70 mg/dl at birth (more than half as HDL cholesterol). Levels increase dramatically by 1 month of age and are essentially similar to those of 2- to 11-year-olds when table foods are introduced.

Table 16-1.   Selected lipid and lipoprotein concentrations in children and adolescents (mg/dl)

Age (years)	Total cholesterol		HDL cholesterol			LDL cholesterol		Triglycerides	
	Mean	95th percentile	95th percentile	Mean	95th percentile	Mean	95th percentile	Mean	95th percentile
5–9									
Male	160	203	38	56	75	93	129	56	101
Female	164	205	36	53	73	100	140	60	105
10–14									
Male	158	202	37	55	74	97	133	66	125
Female	160	201	37	52	70	97	136	75	131
15–19									
Male	150	197	30	46	63	94	130	78	148
Female	158	203	35	52	74	96	137	75	132

Source: Lipid Research Clinics. Population studies data book. I. The prevalence study. U.S. Department of Health and Human Services, National Institutes of Health, 1980. USDHHS publ. no. (NIH) 80-1527.

From 2 to 11 years of age cholesterol levels are relatively stable, followed by a small dip during puberty (more so in white males). During late adolescence, boys assume more of an adult male lipid pattern with elevated LDL cholesterol and decreased HDL cholesterol. The increasing estrogen levels in maturing girls, on the other hand, help them to maintain their more favorable lipid profile, with higher protective HDL cholesterol levels and a lower risk profile [8, 44].

Many factors influence cholesterol and lipoprotein levels in childhood, including diet, inactivity, obesity, medications, cigarette smoking, inherited conditions, and specific diseases. The majority of children with hypercholesterolemia due to elevated LDL cholesterol are those with both environmental (dietary excess, inactivity, overweight) and genetic components. It is also important to identify the smaller number of children with specific genetic dyslipoproteinemias, such as familial hypercholesterolemia (FH), which occurs in the heterozygous form in about 1 in 200 children (Table 16-2) [45, 46]. Secondary causes of elevated lipids, such as liver, kidney, and thyroid disorders, must also not be ruled out.

Blood Pressure

Elevated blood pressure has repeatedly been shown in epidemiologic studies to be a major independent risk factor for the development of atherosclerosis and subsequent cardiovascular and cerebrovascular disease. Both systolic and diastolic blood pressure elevations are related to the risk of cardiovascular disease. In addition cardiomegaly, congestive heart failure, stroke, and renal disease are major consequences of hypertension.

Blood pressure levels in children are lower than in adults and tend to increase with age at an average increment of 1.3 mm Hg systolic and .7 mm Hg diastolic per year [47, 48]. Many factors, both genetic and environmental, influence blood pressure variance in children and adolescents. Studies of blood pressure in twins, parents, offspring (both natural and adoptive), and siblings have provided evidence that genetic variation may account for 35 to 50 percent of total blood pressure variation in children [49].

Many studies have shown that larger children (both heavier and/or taller) have higher blood pressure than smaller children of the same age, and obese children have significantly higher blood pressure than lean children. This relationship between obesity and hypertension appears to be stronger among white than black children [50].

Sodium intake also appears to play a role in the etiology of hypertension, especially among sodium-sensitive individuals. The correlation of high sodium intake with hypertension between populations has been demonstrated in numerous studies. When all members of a population are ingesting very small amounts of sodium, blood pressure does not rise with age, and hypertension is virtually absent. Conversely, when all members of a population consume large amounts of sodium, a high percentage develop hypertension. Between these extremes the relationship is more difficult to quantitate, probaly because there is a wide variation in genetic susceptibility. Other factors, such as potassium, calcium, magnesium, and certain vitamins, may also play a role [51].

Errors in the technical measurement of blood pressure in children are common. Most often they are the result of using the wrong size blood pressure cuff or of trying to measure blood pressure when the child is agitated or the room is too noisy [52, 53].

Over the past two decades studies have sought to identify the prevalence of hypertension in children as well as to study the early natural history of hypertension, including the onset of target organ damage. The reported prevalence of high blood pressure in pediatric populations varies between 1.4 and 11 percent, with wide ranges of frequency of essential and secondary hypertension [23, 54, 55, 56]. The World Health Organization definition of adult borderline hypertension of 140 mm Hg systolic and 90 mm Hg diastolic has been used by many investigators as the definition of hypertension. These levels roughly correspond to the ninety-fifth-percentile values for a 10-year-old child. Kilcoyne [55] and Levine [56] reported less than

Table 16-2. The genetic hyperlipidemias

Name	DLP type and lipid levels	Genetic mechanism	Comments
Familial hypercholesterolemia	IIa LDL high Chol high TG nl Clear serum	Autosomal Dominant	High risk of early CHD. Tendinous xanthomas common. Xanthelasma common. .1–.5% population frequency. 3–6% among MI<60 population. LDL receptor defect. Homozygotes/CHD in adolescence.
Genetic hypercholesterolemia	IIa (IIb) LDL high Chol high TG nl Clear serum	Polygenic	Increased risk of early CHD. Rare xanthomas. 5% population frequency. Increased frequency among MI< 60.
Familial combined hyperlipidemia	IIa, IIb, IV Rarely V Chol high TG high VLDL high Turbid serum	Autosomal Dominant	Increased risk of early CHD. Rare xanthomas. 1–5% population frequency. 11–20% frequency among MI<60 population. ⅓ ↑ Chol; ⅓ ↑ TG. ⅓ have high Chol and TG. Multiple patterns in 1 family. VLDL overproduced in liver.
Familial hypertriglyceridemia	IV (V) VLDL high Chol nl TG high	Autosomal Dominant	Slight increased risk of CHD. No xanthomas. 1% population frequency. 5% frequency among MI<60 population. Probably heterogeneous.
Broad beta disease (remnant hyperlipidemia)	III IDL ↑ Chol high TG high Turbid serum ±creamy layer	Autosomal Recessive	Marked increase of early CHD. Frequent tuberous xanthomas on palmar creases. Rare disease in general population. 1% frequency among MI<60 population. Peripheral vascular disease. Test isolated VLDL.
Familial LPL deficiency	I Chylomicrons ↑ Chol sl ↑ TG very high Cream on serum Clear below	Autosomal Recessive	No increase in risk of CHD. Eruptive xanthomas common. Very rare disease in population. No increase among MI <60. Disease onset by 2nd decade. Abdominal pain/ pancreatitis. Lipoprotein lipase deficient.
Familial type 5 disease	V VLDL ↑ Chylomicrons ↑ Chol nl or sl ↑ TG ↑ ↑ Cream on serum Cloudy below	Autosomal Dominant	Variable increase of CHD risk. Often secondary to disease: diabetes, obesity, ethanol. May be primary genetic disease. Adult onset usual. Abdominal pain/ pancreatitis.

3 percent hypertension on repeated screening of adolescent school children using a definition of 140/90 mm Hg as elevated.

In the Muscatine Study 6622 children 5 to 18 years of age were examined 2 years apart. Forty-one (.6 percent) were found to have sustained hypertension. More than half of these children had relative weights of 120 percent or more. Secondary causes of hypertension were found for five children, all of whom were lean [57].

In a survey of 3000 New York schoolchildren 11 to 14 years of age, 43 (1 percent) were found to have systolic and/or diastolic hypertension on the basis of three measurements (averaged) taken at a single setting [58]. Although such school screenings can identify relatively large numbers of children with initially elevated blood pressure, the exact significance of this elevation is unknown since most are normal on repeated examination. However, since a single casual elevated blood pressure determination in the Framingham study was significantly associated with increased risk of future CHD, these findings in children may be more significant than we believe at present. Only longitudinal studies of children will answer these questions.

In 1977 and again in 1987 the National Heart, Lung and Blood Institute (NHLBI) convened a Task Force on Blood Pressure Control in Children and published guidelines on the measurement, interpretation, and management of blood pressure and its elevations in childhood [59, 60]. The later report utilized blood pressure data from more than 70,000 children in the United States and Great Britain. The Task Force defined normal blood pressure as systolic and diastolic blood pressures less than the ninetieth percentile for age and sex (based on their published norms). High normal blood pressure is defined as being between the ninetieth and ninety-fifth percentiles, and high blood pressure as equal to or above the ninety-fifth percentile level. These guidelines have been helpful in the clinical assessment of children's blood pressure (Tables 16-3 and 16-4).

Obesity

Although obesity does not appear to be as strong an independent risk factor for CHD as hypertension and hyperlipidemia, its relationship to the development of these risk factors as well as to the development of insulin resistance makes it an important variable in the evaluation of CHD risk status as well as in risk reduction programs. Both heredity and environment play important roles in the etiology of obesity. Studies of skinfold thickness in monozygotic and dizygotic twins estimate the heritability of adipose tissue development at .88 [61]. A child with one obese parent has been estimated to have a 40 percent likelihood of becoming obese. This increases to 80 percent if both parents are obese [62].

On the other hand, environmental causes of obesity, including overnutrition and inactivity are also important, and these environmental conditions are often shared in family groups [63, 64, 65]. Overconsumption of energy forces fat cells to enlarge and sometimes to proliferate. Some studies have also shown that diets high in saturated fat lead to increases in both the size and the number of fat cells, whereas diets high in unsaturated fat increase only the size of the fat cells [66]. Inactivity appears to be a major contributor to obesity in children [67]. Rose and Mayer reported that large, placid babies ate fewer calories than a smaller, more active control group of infants [68].

Obesity is common among adults, with studies suggesting that 20 to 30 percent of U.S. adults are moderately obese, and 3 to 10 percent are markedly obese [69]. Estimates of prevalence among children are also high, with the frequency of obesity increasing during adolescence. In a study of 3000 11- to 14-year-old junior high school students 16 percent were 120 percent or greater than mean weight for height [22]. The prevalence of obesity in any population necessarily varies according to the definition of excess body weight or body fatness. Obesity in childhood is usually defined as 120 percent or more of ideal weight for height. Children who are 140 percent or more of ideal weight are referred to as morbidly obese or superobese. Ratios of weight to height, such as body mass index (BMI = weight in kg/height in m²) are also helpful. BMI values above 18 to 20 kg/m² reflect obesity in children and adolescents [70].

Táble 16-3. Classification of blood pressure elevation by age group

Age	Significant hypertension (mm Hg)	Severe hypertension (mm Hg)
Newborn		
1st week	SBP > 96	SBP > 106
8–30 days	SBP > 104	SBP > 110
Infant <2 yr	> 112/74	> 118/82
Child		
3–5 yr	> 116/76	> 124/84
6–9 yr	> 122/78	> 130/86
10–12 yr	> 126/82	> 134/90
Teen		
13–15 yr	> 136/86	> 144/92
16–18 yr	> 142/92	> 150/98

Source: Report of the Second Task Force on Blood Pressure Control in Children — 1987. Pediatrics 1987; 79: 1-25.

Table 16-4. Sizes of commonly available blood pressure cuffs

Cuff designation	Width of bladder (cm)	Length of bladder (cm)
Newborn	2.5 – 4	5 – 9
Infant	4 – 6	11.5 – 18
Child	7.5 – 9	17 – 19
Adult	11.5 – 13	22 – 26
Large arm	14 – 15	30.5 – 33
Thigh	18 – 19	36 – 38

Note: Bladder should be long enough to encircle the arm and wide enough to cover 75% of the upper arm.

Skinfold measures are also used in children to estimate the degree of body fatness. Children with triceps skinfold measures above the eighty-fifth percentile are classified as obese. Combinations of four or more skinfolds summed may be used to estimate total body fat [71, 72, 73]. Table 16-5 provides eighty-fifth percentile values for triceps skinfold measures in children.

Some studies suggest that the prevalence of obesity in U.S. children has been increasing. In the Bogalusa Heart Study, the proportion of 6- to 11-year-olds who were obese increased by more than 50 percent in the 12 years between 1972 and 1984. These data indicated that caloric intake had not increased significantly during this period, so decreased physical activity may have been an important factor in this increase in obesity [74].

Obesity in childhood is associated with a higher prevalence of hyperlipidemia, as well as both systolic and diastolic hypertension [75]. Because of this association serious consideration should be given to the possibility that prevention of obesity in childhood could significantly reduce hypertension and cardiovascular disease among adults. The Muscatine Study, reporting on 4000 school-age children, found that of those children whose body weight was in the upper decile, almost 30 percent had systolic and diastolic blood pressures above the ninetieth percentile [21]. In another study of 2058 high school students, 64 percent of the students with sustained hypertension were obese [56]. Similar findings have been reported for office-based studies. Londe reported that 53 percent of the 74 hypertensive children he identified were

Table 16-5. 85th percentile levels of triceps skinfold measures in children and adolescents

Age (years)	85th percentile triceps skinfold (mm)	
	Male	Female
2	13	13
3	12	12
4	12	12
5	12	13
6	11	12
7	11	13
8	12	15
9	14	17
10	16	19
11	17	20
12	19	20
13	18	23
14	17	22
15	19	24
16	20	23

Source: Data from the Ten-State Nutrition Survey of 1968–1970.

overweight for their age, compared to 14 percent of 74 matched normotensive controls [54].

Higher mean cholesterol levels are also common among obese children and adolescents. In addition, some data suggest that elevated cholesterol levels in overweight children tend to remain elevated, i.e., track better, than in children whose body mass index remains lower [76, 77, 78, 79, 80].

Diet

Many children in the United States consume a diet that falls far short of meeting the dietary guidelines recommended by the American Heart Association (AHA) and reinforced recently by the Expert Panel on Cholesterol in Children and Adolescents of the National Cholesterol Education Program (NCEP) [81, 82].

Information on the usual dietary intake of children comes from a variety of sources. The largest national dietary intake database on U.S. children was developed from the National Health and Nutrition Examination Survey (NHANES II) [83]. Data in this 1976–1980 survey were collected on children aged 4 to 19 years

using a 24-hour dietary recall. Based on these recalls children consumed a mean of 2100 kcal/day, with caloric intake increasing with age. Approximately one-third of calories came from snacks rather than from a particular meal. Lunch and dinner each provided about one-quarter of daily energy, while breakfast provided the least, only 17 percent of calories.

Most U.S. children have an excessive intake of high-fat foods. On the average they consume 36 percent of their calories as fat, compared with the recommended level of 30 percent. This excess intake of dietary fat contributes to childhood obesity and hypercholesterolemia. Data from NHANES II also show that saturated fat intake is higher than recommended and that polyunsaturated fat intake is lower than recommended (Table 16-6).

Dairy products are the greatest source of saturated fat in children's diets. This is not surprising since an ounce of full-fat American cheese or an 8-ounce glass of whole milk each provides 5 grams of saturated fat. The average 10-year-old child following the AHA diet recommendations is usually advised to consume no more than 20 grams of saturated fat per day; thus, three glasses of whole milk and an ounce of cheese would use up the entire day's allotment of saturated fat. Table 16-7 provides a comparison chart for common types of milk and also illustrates the fact that calcium intake is not compromised by the use of lower-fat milk products.

Americans have gradually switched to buying lower-fat milk over full-fat milk. Schools and even fast-food chains are now offering low-fat milk as an alternative to full-fat. Cheese consumption, however, is increasing, probably because people who understand that whole milk is almost 50 percent fat by calories don't understand that full-fat cheese is similar [84] in its fat content.

Consumption of high-fat foods is generally done at the expense of high-fiber foods. American children, like their parents, consume less than optimal amounts of dietary fiber. Mean dietary fiber intake for U.S. children is about 12 grams/day (NHANES II), with the majority derived from fruits, vegetables, and cereals. Al-

Table 16-6.   AHA step 1 diet as compared to typical intake of American children

	NHANES II 1976–1980	AHA step 1 diet for children
	Percent of total calories	(Sufficient calories to promote normal growth and development) Percent of total calories
Fat	36	30
Saturated	13	<10
Polyunsaturated	—	Up to 10
Monounsaturated	—	Remaining
Protein	15	15 – 20
Carbohydrate	50	50 – 55
Cholesterol	280 mg/day	100 mg/1000 kcal up to 300 mg/ day

Table 16-7.   Milk composition comparison chart

	Common designation of type of milk			
Nutrient	Whole	2% milk	1% milk	Skim
Fat (g)	8	4.7	2.6	0.4
Saturated fat (g)	5.1	2.9	1.5	0.3
Percent of calories from fat	48	35	23	4
Protein (g)	8	8	8	8
Calcium (mg)	288	297	300	302
Total calories per 8 oz.	150	125	102	86

though there is no RDA for dietary fiber, the National Cancer Institute (NCI) recommends that Americans consume 20 to 30 grams per day [85]. If the lower level is taken for children, then current consumption may be only 60 percent of optimal. To increase dietary fiber in childrens' diets, there needs to be more emphasis on the consumption of high-fiber breakfast cereals and breads and crackers, as well as an increased intake of fresh fruits and vegetables.

Ellison et al. [86] showed that by simply substituting a cereal-based, low-fat breakfast for their usual bacon and egg breakfast, college students could increase their intake of fiber and decrease their intake of dietary fat (from 85 to 70 grams per day). Consumption of no breakfast at all often reflects a constellation of negative eating habits. Children and adolescents who skip breakfast have been found to have an in-creased frequency of obesity and higher mean serum cholesterol levels compared to children who consume a variety of breakfasts. Children who consume ready-to-eat, high-fiber breakfast cereals were the leanest and had the lowest cholesterol levels in this study [87].

Eating styles of the American family have undergone significant recent changes as more and more wives and mothers have joined the work force. With 60 percent of mothers of children under 6 years of age now working and an even higher percentage of mothers of older children and adolescents, women have turned to the use of ready-made foods and take-out dinners. Frequently such meals are higher in calories, fat, saturated fat, and sodium than foods prepared from raw ingredients at home. Families with young children now eat out at both fast-food and sit-down restaurants in increasingly higher numbers. According to surveys by the American Restaurant Association, children under 6 represent one of the groups whose consumption of restaurant meals is increasing most quickly [88].

Parents often have little control over the type and amount of food that children consume away from home. Since one-quarter of calories are usually consumed at lunch (usually at school) and one-third of calories are consumed as snacks during the day, almost 60 percent of a child's daily energy intake for 5 days of the week may be consumed largely outside the home. This pattern becomes increasingly the case for older children and adolescents and provides another reason to emphasize the need for more nutrition education during the preschool period and throughout the school years, with modification of the current school lunch program to reflect the AHA/NCEP dietary guidelines. (See Chapter 20 for further discussion of school-based intervention).

Cigarette Smoking

Cigarette smoking has been shown to be a major independent risk factor for CHD. The risk of CHD increases with the number of cigarettes smoked and the number of years of smoking. It has been estimated that 30 percent of all deaths from CHD are attributable to smoking, accounting for more than 170,000 deaths each year in the United States alone. Most smokers adopt the habit during adolescence, followed by a lifetime of cigarette consumption. Among young adults of both sexes who are otherwise at low risk of developing CHD, up to three-quarters of CHD cases may be attributable to cigarette smoking [89, 90, 91].

A variety of physiologic changes occur as a result of cigarette smoking that contribute to increased CHD risk. These include altered blood lipid levels, increased carboxyhemoglobin levels, and increased blood viscosity and clotting factor concentrations. In a recent study of child and adolescent smokers (8 to 19 years of age) significant elevations of VLDL, LDL, and triglycerides were found, as well as reductions in HDL and total cholesterol [92]. Overall the effect of increased LDL and decreased HDL results in a more unfavorable lipid profile in

terms of CHD risk. In addition the lipid changes seen in young smokers are greater than those seen in adult smokers.

Even passive smoke has been shown to adversely affect the HDL cholesterol levels of children. In a study of 105 children with at least one smoking parent, HDL cholesterol was significantly lower in passive-smoking children, primarily from exposure to maternal smoke. This study suggests that children with long-term exposure to passive smoke may be at an elevated risk for the development of CHD [93].

Recent surveys in the United States show that the prevalence of daily cigarette smoking by high school seniors has decreased from 27 percent in 1975 to 19 percent in 1986. Currently, however, more young females than males are smokers. Twenty percent of senior girls, compared with 17 percent of senior boys, were daily cigarette smokers in 1986 [94, 95, 96, 97]. A survey of younger adolescents in Ontario found that among 12- to 13-year-olds, 3 percent of boys and 4 percent of girls were regular smokers. This increased to 16 percent of boys and 23 percent of girls by 14 to 16 years of age, an increase of more than fivefold.

Investigators have sought to identify predictors of future smoking in adolescents who have not yet become regular smokers [98]. Such predictors include peer influence (having friends who smoke); having family members who smoke (older siblings and parents); having less educated parents; being more independent and rebellious; having less academic success in school; having an external locus of control (feeling that fate more than self controls destiny); and being less concerned about the health consequences of smoking. Pressure exerted by peers or siblings in a social situation appears to be the most common final pathway to initiation of smoking and usually involves a member of the same sex. Health education programs in schools have used this knowledge to develop successful models of smoking prevention to help students understand the social and psychological factors that influence decisions to smoke and to teach them the social skills needed to resist pressures to smoke.

The decreasing trend of cigarette smoking

among young men and a recent stabilization of the increasing rates of smoking among young women indicate that public health efforts to prevent smoking have had an effect. On the other hand, smoking is still the leading avoidable cause of death in the United States, responsible for over half a million deaths each year from cancer and heart disease alone.

Health care professionals involved in the care of children are urged to take a more active role by being nonsmoking role models, providing smoking prevention messages to children as a part of routine well-child care, helping to counsel parents about smoking cessation, and encouraging school and community antismoking efforts [99].

Exercise

Physical inactivity is an independent risk factor for CHD and has assumed increasing importance in preventive cardiology because of its contribution to the development of obesity, abnormal plasma lipids, high blood pressure, and hyperglycemia, each of which contributes to the risk of CHD [100].

Studies of physical fitness in pediatric populations have demonstrated that children with higher levels of fitness have higher levels of protective HDL cholesterol and significantly less body fat as measured by skinfold thickness. Blood pressure is also significantly lower among physically fit children, even after adjusting for body mass index and sexual maturity ratings [101, 102, 103]. The effect of exercise on HDL cholesterol levels appears to be mediated through an increase in muscle lipoprotein lipase (LPL) concentrations. This results in increased triglyceride clearance and higher HDL cholesterol levels, since free cholesterol produced during triglyceride hydrolysis at the surface of VLDL by LPL is esterified by HDL_3, transforming it into HDL_2 [104] (see Chapter 3).

Surveys suggest that U.S. children have become less physically active and more obese over recent decades. In 1984 less than two-thirds of 6- to 12-year-old boys and only half of similar-aged girls could run or walk a mile in less than 10 minutes, and even fewer could perform just one chin-up. Increased busing of children to schools, decreased physical education during school hours, increased sedentary free-time activities such as watching television and playing video and computer games, and lack of safe play areas for children in urban as well as suburban environments have all contributed to declining levels of physical fitness among our children [105]. U.S. children spend at least 25 hours per week in front of the television, usually simultaneously consuming high-calorie snack foods, while only 36 percent have daily physical education in their schools. Physicians can counsel parents on the need to balance sedentary activities with physically active ones and on the need to provide healthy snack foods for children.

Health professionals caring for children should emphasize the importance of regular daily physical activity beginning at an early age and should be active in efforts to increase physical education and sports activities in schools and communities. The goal should be to develop in the young child a desire for and an enjoyment of physical activity that will persist throughout adult life. Physical activity should help to maintain a more efficient cardiovascular system, a more favorable lipid profile, an ideal level of body fat, and an avoidance of cigarette smoking [106, 107].

Tracking of Risk Factors

Although there is no doubt that we can identify CHD risk factors in children and that they are highly prevalent, the question of how consistently these risk factors track over time has become very important. In this context *tracking* refers to the degree to which a given measurement retains its rank order over time in a percentile distribution of measures among similar-aged children or adults. If the majority of children who have cholesterol or blood pressure values above the ninetieth or ninety-fifth percentile at an early age continue to have high levels throughout childhood and into adult life, intervention at an early age is clearly warranted.

Several longitudinal studies of pediatric populations have studied risk factor tracking [77, 108, 109]. Many of these studies are limited by relatively brief periods of follow-up. The Bogalusa Heart study, however, has followed a cohort of children for 12 years [108, 109, 110]. The results show high levels of persistence in rank order for height, weight, triceps skinfold thickness, systolic blood pressure, and total cholesterol and LDL cholesterol levels. Tracking correlations are lower for diastolic blood pressure and HDL cholesterol and triglyceride levels. Overall, both in this and in similar studies, approximately 70 percent of children with total and LDL cholesterol levels in the top quintile at baseline will still be within the top two quintiles after 12 years of follow-up [77, 110, 111].

HDL cholesterol levels do not track well until after children are 10 years of age. In contrast levels of total and LDL cholesterol at 6 months of age are significantly associated with levels at 7 years of age, with even higher associations from age 1 to age 7. Almost two-thirds of the infants with LDL cholesterol levels at or above the eightieth percentile were still in this top quintile at 7 years of age. It is significant that relative ranking within a peer group tends to stabilize by 2 to 4 years of age. In addition, even though there are marked lipid changes during puberty, especially for white males, this has little effect on their long-term tracking [115].

A similar study of children 8 to 18 years of age who were reevaluated at 20 to 30 years of age also demonstrated that childhood levels of total and LDL cholesterol were good predictors of adult levels, as well as of LDL-to-HDL ratios [112, 113]. HDL cholesterol levels in childhood, however, were not good predictors of adult levels. In this study 62 percent of the children initially in the top decile (above the ninetieth percentile) for total cholesterol levels were found also to be above the seventy-fifth percentile as adults (approximately the 240 mg/dl level). In addition, 80 percent of the children initially in the same top decile for total cholesterol had adult levels above the fiftieth percentile (approximately 200 mg/dl). Since the Adult Consensus Panel of the NHLBI has established a total cholesterol level of 200 to 239 mg/dl as borderline high risk and 240 mg/dl and above as high risk, it would appear that a large proportion of these increased-risk adults can be identified as children.

In a similar manner, there is a high degree of tracking for blood pressure (systolic more so than diastolic) as well as for obesity [109, 110, 114]. Thus, there is strong support for treating children with risk factors for CHD, since the weight of evidence suggests that such increased risk status will track over time and lead to disease in adult life if risk reduction is not achieved.

Clinical Evaluation and Treatment of Cardiovascular Risk Factors in Children

Evaluation

Each child's overall risk profile for CHD should be evaluated in detail after the age of 2 years, preferably before entering school at 5 or 6 years of age. This preschool age is preferable to older ages because patterns of risk usually are set by this time (obesity, lack of activity, elevated total and LDL cholesterol, and sometimes borderline elevated blood pressure levels). In addition this is when lifestyle habits are being formed, when young parents are eager for advice on child care, and when visits to the pediatrician or family practitioner are frequent.

Evaluation of overall risk status should initially include measurement of blood pressure, height, weight, body fatness estimate (by skinfold measurements or calculated body mass index), and total cholesterol in plasma or serum. Patterns of physical activity, diet, and cigarette smoking should be assessed for both the child and the family, since these lifestyles are commonly shared and affect recommendations for treatment. Lipid and lipoprotein measurements should be obtained on the child's parents and siblings, since familial aggregation of hypercholesterolemia is common, reflecting shared heredity, lifestyle, or both.

Although it is our opinion that all children should be screened for elevated blood cholesterol levels as part of the overall examination for risk factors for CHD, it is important to note that this recommendation remains controversial. The NCEP report of the Expert Panel on Blood Cholesterol Levels in Children and Adolescents [82] recommended selective screening based on a positive family history of premature (less than age 55) CVD or a parental history of an elevated (240 mg/dl or higher) blood cholesterol level, while recognizing that such selective screening will miss many children with elevated cholesterol and LDL levels, as noted later in this chapter. The panel justified their decision against universal screening by noting that elevated lipids in childhood do not always track well into adult life; that undue anxiety might be unnecessarily provoked in many children and parents by their being "labeled" as having a problem; and by the cost of such screening and subsequent therapy. We believe that the logic of screening in childhood is sufficiently compelling that the large number of hyperlipidemic children who would be missed by a selective approach is not justified [116, 117]. Only careful long-term follow-up studies evaluating both health and cost outcomes will provide the information needed to resolve this controversy with certainty.

Detailed initial review and an annual update of the family history are essential: (1) for determination of the familial nature of risk factors, (2) for assessment of the family history's contribution to the child's risk status, and (3) for determining the degree of therapeutic aggressiveness indicated to reduce the child's risk status.

BLOOD PRESSURE

Measurement of blood pressure in children must be performed with careful attention to technique. The most common errors include using a cuff of inappropriate size, overinflation of the cuff, too rapid deflation, using the fifth Korotkoff sound for diastolic pressure instead of the fourth in children under 13 years of age, and trying to measure blood pressure in a noisy room or with a crying, uncooperative child. Table 16-4 provides guidelines for choice of cuff size with children. A good rule of thumb is to use a bladder whose length completely encircles the arm and whose width covers at least 75 percent of the length of the upper arm.

Since the definition of blood pressure elevations in childhood is based on percentile distributions of blood pressure in normal populations of children, it is essential to plot blood pressure values on appropriate grids (Figures 16-1 and 16-2). Values in the ninetieth to ninety-fifth percentile range for the age and the sex of the child are considered to be borderline elevated, while values above the ninety-fifth percentile are considered to be significantly elevated. Consideration of the child's height, weight, and maturation stage aid in interpretation of the blood pressure results, since children who are tall, heavy, and more sexually mature than their peers will have higher blood pressure levels as well. Children with persistently elevated blood pressure above the ninety-fifth percentile should be evaluated for the possible presence of underlying renal or cardiovascular disease, as well as for medication effect.

Middle and late adolescence is a common time for the clinical expression of familial essential hypertension. Such adolescents present with borderline elevated blood pressure, and a review of the family history usually reveals a parent and several other close relatives with hypertension.

CIGARETTE SMOKING

Determination of the smoking status of the child and other family members is an important part of CHD risk assessment. Children of smoking parents are more likely to smoke cigarettes themselves, so that family counseling is critical. Pediatricians are frequently the only doctors with whom young parents interact; thus, they have the opportunity and the responsibility to motivate parents to quit smoking when the child is young. Explanations of the adverse effects of passive smoking and the role-modeling effect of parental smoking should be emphasized repeatedly. Referrals of parents and older smoking adolescents to smoking cessation programs and provision of printed materials to help them quit need to be a part of routine pediatric practice.

For children of elementary school age the pediatrician can provide a powerful antismoking message, particularly at each well-child assessment. The physician's reinforcement of non-smoking at each visit can help to counterbalance any negative prosmoking influences exerted by family or friends. Part of the pediatrician's antismoking campaign should be the maintenance

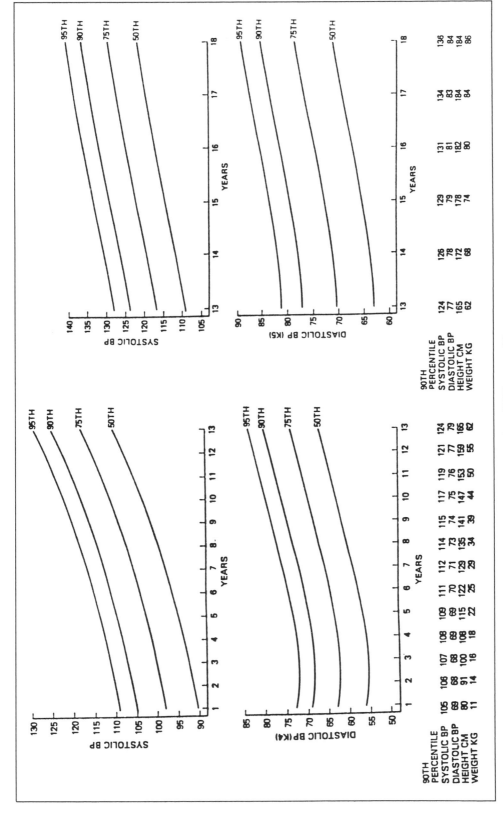

Figure 16-1. Age-specific percentiles of boys' BP measurements. K4 = DBP < age 13 years; K5 = DBP age > 13 years. (Adapted from Ped.79(1):1, 1987).

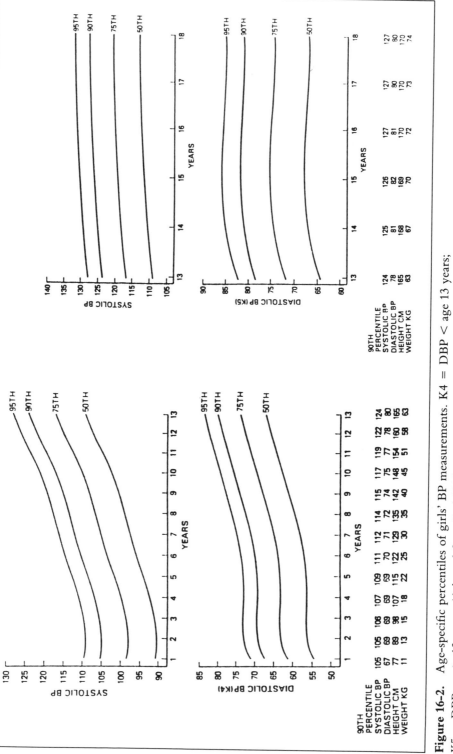

Figure 16-2. Age-specific percentiles of girls' BP measurements. K4 = DBP < age 13 years; K5 = DBP age > 13 years. (Adapted from Ped.79(1):1, 1987.)

of a nonsmoking office environment and perhaps prominently displayed antismoking posters in the waiting and examination rooms [118].

The transition from elementary school to junior high school and from the first to second years of junior high school are times when there is a rapid increase in smoking onset rates. The pediatrician needs to be especially aware of this and step up nonsmoking messages before and during this high-risk period. Such messages should provide information on the harmful effects of cigarette smoking and make children aware of the addictive qualities of nicotine. Pediatricians and other health care workers can also point out the misleading nature of cigarette advertisements, either during office visits or through participation in school health education activities.

Adolescents who are experimenting with cigarettes or who are regular smokers will not always be easy for pediatricians to identify, especially if they are concealing this fact from their parents. The physician who has good communication skills and is able to gain the adolescent's confidence in a one-on-one counseling session may be able to accurately assess the teenager's smoking status or at least determine if the child has experimented with cigarettes. With adolescents it is less helpful to emphasize the long-term adverse health effects of smoking. They may understand these effects but consider them only as very remote possibilities. A more effective strategy for this age is to talk about the more immediate negative effects of smoking, such as bad breath, yellow-stained fingers, hair and clothing that smell like smoke, lack of stamina for sports, wrinkles, increased heart rate, increased blood pressure, and shortness of breath. The use of a spirometer or an ecolyzer in the office setting is another way of emphasizing the nonsmoking message with older children and adolescents.

Helping the child resist peer pressure to adopt the cigarette habit is an essential component of smoking prevention programs for youth. The school appears to be a very effective site for providing large numbers of children with a smoking-prevention program. The pediatric office, however, can also apply the same techniques of reviewing high-pressure situations with young adolescents and helping them to practice refusal responses. Thus, the child gains the social skills needed to avoid yielding to peer pressure to smoke.

Pediatricians should encourage activities for children that tend to preclude cigarette smoking, such as regular physical activity, participation in a variety of in-school and after-school activities, and keeping up with school work. The physician can also praise children's achievements and emphasize their good qualities, to raise their sense of self-esteem and further "immunize" them against pressures to smoke.

WEIGHT STATUS

Determination of weight status for height and estimating (or measuring) degree of body fatness is important in evaluating and treating the hyperlipidemic child, since overfat children need more intensive therapy to reduce caloric intake and increase physical activity.

Height and weight should be plotted on standard NCHS growth charts (Figures 16-3 and 16-4). Determination of the percentile zones for each measure and comparison of the height percentile with the weight percentile give the first indication if the child is overweight for height. A child whose weight is two or more percentile zones above height may be overweight for height (e.g., a child whose height is tenth to twenty-fifth percentile and whose weight is seventy-fifth to ninetieth percentile for age and sex).

Measurement of subcutaneous fat with skinfold calipers adds valuable information to simple height and weight measures by helping the clinician to determine if the overweight child is also overfat. In cases of significant obesity physical inspection is enough to answer this question, but skinfold measures are helpful as baseline determinations and as follow-up measures during subsequent treatment.

PHYSICAL ACTIVITY

Pediatricians in the usual practice setting are rarely able to measure maximal oxygen uptake by treadmill or bicycle ergometer or to determine physical fitness through a series of fitness tests. Such determinations usually require spe-

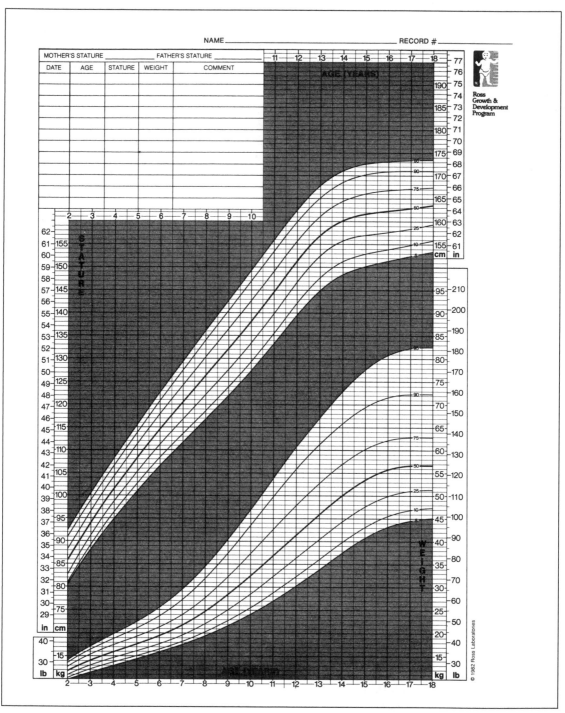

Figure 16-3. Height and weight chart for boys, 2 to 18 years old (NCHS). (Source: Adapted from Hamill PVV, Drizd TA, Johnson CL, Reed RB, Roche AF, Moore WM. Physical growth: National Center for Health Statistics percentiles. Am J Clin Nutr 1979; 32: 607–29. Data from the National Center for Health Statistics (NCHS), Hyattsville, MD.

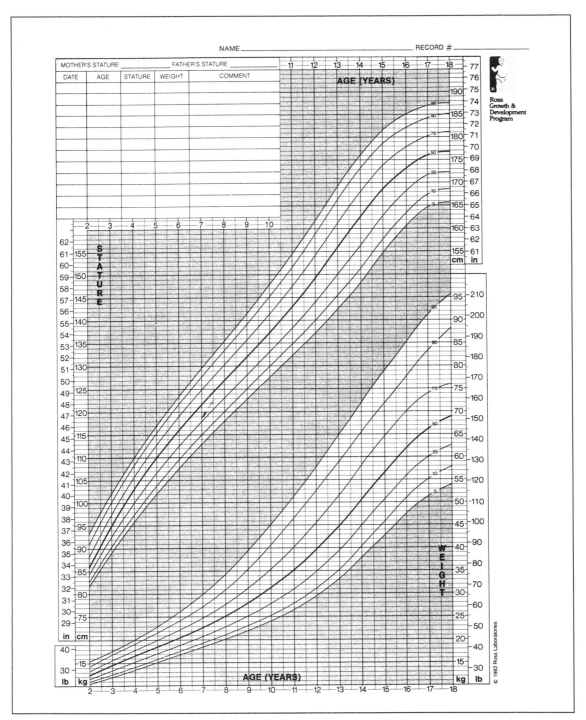

Figure 16-4. Height and weight chart for girls, 2 to 18 years old (NCHS). (Source: Adapted from Hamill PVV, Drizd TA, Johnson CL, Reed RB, Roche AF, Moore WM. Physical growth: National Center for Health Statistics percentiles. Am J Clin Nutr 1979; 32: 607–29. Data from the National Center for Health Statistics (NCHS), Hyattsville, MD.

cial referral, and it may be difficult to justify the cost for most healthy children. Pediatricians instead usually rely on estimating a child's level of physical activity through a series of questions directed at the parent and the child.

For school age children one might use the following categories:

• Inactive children have school gym only and no other planned physical activities.
• Average active children have school gym and also moderate, relatively unstructured after-school and weekend physical activities three or four times a week.
• Highly active children have school gym and also are involved in vigorous and usually structured activity on an almost daily basis.

Evaluation of barriers to physical activity is also important. Children may go directly from school to a babysitter or a grandparent; they may live in a dangerous neighborhood and not be able to play outdoors; or they may not be able to afford the variety of dance and gymnastic programs available to more affluent families.

LIPIDS AND LIPOPROTEINS

Guidelines for evaluating and treating the child with elevated serum cholesterol in pediatric practice have only recently begun to be formulated. The physician who chooses to screen either all patients or only those with a positive family history is still faced with the need to know what to do next after obtaining that initial cholesterol result. The following is a practical guide for the pediatrician in that situation.

Serum Cholesterol. The decision as to how to proceed after a single total cholesterol test may be made on the basis of (1) the degree of elevation of that single value, (2) the presence of other CHD risk factors in the child, and (3) the nature of the child's family history for premature onset CHD or major CHD risk factors.

A single normal serum cholesterol value (below the seventy-fifth percentile, or about 170 mg/dl) in a child with normal blood pressure, normal weight for height, normal activity, nonsmoking, and with a negative family history does not require further follow-up at this time other than routine care. Evaluation should be repeated every 3 to 5 years unless family history or the child's risk status changes. If the child has other risk factors, or if the family history is positive, the initial measurement should be a fasting lipoprotein profile (Figure 16-5).

A single elevated serum cholesterol value in a child should be repeated, preferably within one week of the initial test. Variation between the first and the second test results could be the result of laboratory technical error or of patient day-to-day physiologic variability or abnormal physical state (fever, dehydration). Repeat cholesterol values obtained after 2 or more weeks may reflect dietary changes instituted after the initial result was reported. If the average of the two baseline cholesterol measures is still above the seventy-fifth percentile, a complete lipoprotein profile should be determined from a capillary or venous blood sample after a 12-hour fast.

Evaluating the Lipoprotein Profile. The simplest lipoprotein profile consists of a total cholesterol value, an HDL cholesterol value, and a triglyceride value. The physician can then calculate the LDL cholesterol value from Friedewald's formula (LDLC = TC − HDLC − TG/5), where TG/5 is an estimate of VLDL cholesterol. Ratios of LDL cholesterol to HDL cholesterol and TC to HDL cholesterol can also be calculated. More sophisticated laboratory reports provide the calculated LDL cholesterol, as well as the ratios and population distribution percentiles, or risk scores. Pediatricians should be wary, however, of extrapolating adult risk scores to pediatric age groups.

With each of the lipoprotein values available, the next step is to compare the patient's values with a distribution of values derived from a normal population of children, using age, sex, and race-specific reference values if mean values differ significantly between these groups. Normal values are available in tabular and in grid form from several large epidemiologic studies of children, such as those derived from the LRC Population Study (Table 16-1) and the Bogalusa Project (Figure 16-6).

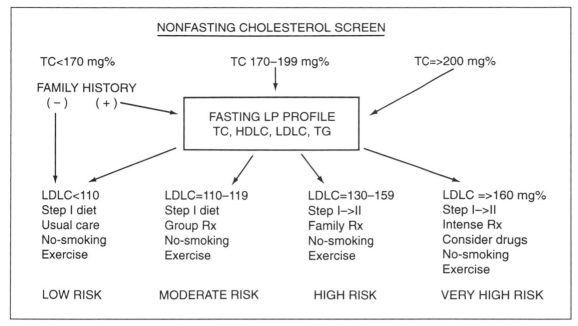

Figure 16-5.   Algorithm for screening and evaluation of serum cholesterol in children >2 years old.

The most important information from the lipoprotein profile can be summarized as follows:

- Does this child have an LDL cholesterol above the seventy-fifth or the ninety-fifth percentile?
- Does this child have an HDL cholesterol below the fifth or the twenty-fifth percentile?

In addition the physician should determine whether the triglycerides are elevated above the ninety-fifth percentile. If so, the pediatrician should make a mental note to ask whether the child was truly fasting and whether the ratio of LDL to HDL is over 3.0 or the TC to HDL ratio is above 4 to 6 (>4 for children under 10; >6 for older children and adolescents). Higher ratios signal increased risk status.

A small percentage of children have elevated total cholesterol levels due to high levels of HDL cholesterol. These children do not need dietary intervention unless their LDL cholesterol is also elevated above the seventy-fifth percentile.

Apoliproprotein A1 and B levels can also be measured as part of the lipid evaluation. These may be especially helpful in families with a strong history of premature onset CHD. In these cases children with normal levels of LDL cholesterol may have elevated apoliproprotein B, and a diagnosis of hyperapobetalipoproteinemia may be made. Such a condition reflects an increased risk of future CHD despite the normal LDL cholesterol levels.

Abnormal Lipoprotein Profiles. By comparing the patient's lipoprotein profile with normal reference values, the pediatrician can first determine if the LDL cholesterol level or triglycerides are elevated and if the HDL cholesterol level is depressed. Abnormal lipoprotein levels in children and adolescents may be the result of an inherited disorder (single gene or polygenic); an underlying disease state; medications or drugs (prescription or self-administered); overnutrition (high-saturated-fat diet), with or without obesity; or pregnancy. It is important to initially rule out underlying disease states such as hypothyroidism, nephrotic syndrome, liver disease, and others outlined in Table 16-8. Physical findings usually suggest such a contributing cause, which laboratory tests will confirm. The incidence of asymptomatic liver, kidney, or thyroid disease diagnosed after a lipid abnormality is noted is low;

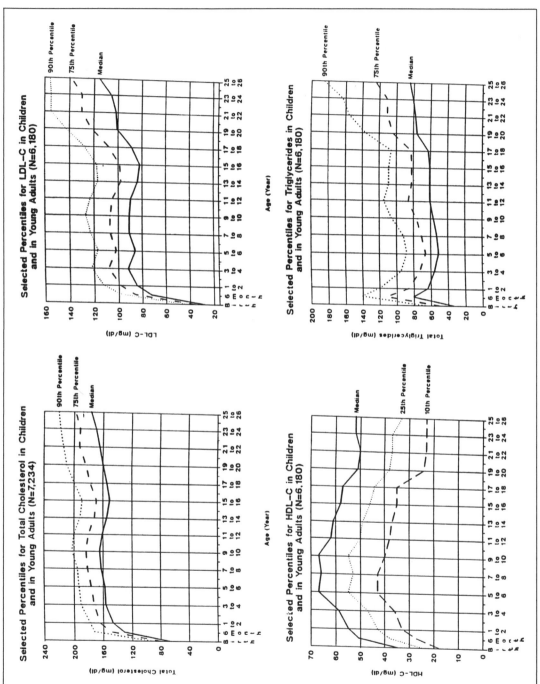

Figure 16-6. Lipid and lipoprotein grids. (Source: Bogalusa Heart Study).

Table 16-8. Secondary causes of hyperlipoproteinemia

Type	Lipid elevated	Secondary causes
Type I	Chylomicrons	Diabetes mellitus, dysgammaglobulinemia, systemic lupus erythematosus
Type IIA	LDL	Nephrotic syndrome, hypothyroidism
Type IIB	LDL VLDL	Obstructive liver disease, multiple myeloma, porphyria
Type III	IDL	Hypothyroidism, dysgammaglobulinemia
Type IV	VLDL	Diabetes mellitus, nephrotic syndrome, pregnancy, hormone use, alcohol excess, glycogen storage disease, Gaucher's disease, Niemann-Pick disease
Type V	Chylomicrons VLDL	Diabetes mellitus, nephrotic syndrome, alcoholism, myeloma, idiopathic hypercalcemia

in our clinical population it is about 1 percent.

The contribution of medications should be evaluated. Steroids used as anti-inflammatory agents, in oral contraceptives, or illegally in sports are common. Anticonvulsant therapy, thyroid hormone replacement, and tobacco and alcohol use may all alter lipoprotein concentrations. (See Chapter 3.)

Familial Dyslipidemias. Children with abnormal lipoprotein profiles may or may not have relatives with similar patterns. Familial aggregation occurs not only because of shared genes but also because of shared environments. Families share diet, exercise routines, and even cigarette smoking habits.

Inherited familial lipid disorders due to a single gene defect, as described in Table 16-2, are usually apparent after the pediatrician takes a family history and determines the lipid profiles of siblings, parents, and grandparents. Premature CHD is often common in relatives in these families, especially in males who also have one or more of the other major risk factors, such as hypertension or cigarette smoking. At times, however, if the older affected relatives are female, nonsmokers, and normotensive, a history of premature CHD may not be present even in the face of total cholesterol levels above 300 to 400 mg/dl in affected individuals.

In families where (1) the lipid abnormalities clearly run on one side of the family, (2) the lipid levels are very high (two to three times normal), and (3) most of the relatives have had their lipids determined, evaluation of the family and genetic patterns is possible. Often, however, much of this information is not available and one can only make an educated guess as to if this condition is a single-gene familial inherited disorder, a polygenic inherited familial disorder, or familial based on environmental factors.

FAMILY HISTORY

The family history may provide valuable information to the clinician evaluating a child's risk of premature cardiovascular disease. The NCEP Expert Panel on Children and Adolescents has proposed that a family history of premature CVD (manifested under the age of 55) should be the primary criterion for deciding whether or not to measure cholesterol in children over 2 years of age [82]. Several studies, however, have recently reported that 50 percent or more of hypercholesterolemic children would be missed if such a criterion were used [116, 117, 119, 120].

Family history is essential in assessing the familial nature of risk factors and in determining the genetic pattern. It also helps to estimate the degree of increased cardiovascular risk for a particular child and therefore guides decisions regarding treatment. For these reasons it is essential to obtain as detailed and accurate a family history as possible on all children with high risk profiles and to update this history annually.

In considering the family history, certain questions emerge:

• Which relatives should be surveyed?
• What diseases and conditions should be ascertained?
• What age of onset of disease is premature?
• What constitutes a positive family history?

Recommendations vary as to the answers to these questions. A review of family history studies in the recent literature shows the variety of definitions used and the lack of consensus.

In the ideal situation both first-degree relatives (parents, siblings) and second-degree relatives (grandparents, blood-related aunts and uncles) would be surveyed. Occurrence of risk factors for atherosclerotic disease would be determined (hypercholesterolemia or other lipid abnormality, hypertension, cigarette smoking, diabetes, obesity), and occurrence and age of diagnosis/treatment of CVD (MI, angina pectoris, sudden cardiac death, stroke, peripheral vascular disease, coronary angioplasty, coronary artery bypass surgery) would be assessed.

The definition of "positive" family history varies. In their 1989 statement the Academy of Pediatrics Committee on Nutrition suggests that a premature MI in a first- or second-degree relative (under age 50 in men, age 60 in women) or the presence of hypercholesterolemia in such a relative be considered a positive family history [121]. In their previous 1983 statement, the definition was broader and also included hypertension, obesity, diabetes, and gout [122]. The NCEP guidelines described above use age 55 as the cutoff for the definition of a positive family history [82], and include a broad array of indicators of CVD.

A workable definition of positive family history and one that I prefer to use in our Preventive Cardiology Center is as follows: a positive family history is the presence of a first- or sec-ond-degree relative with a major CHD risk factor (e.g., total cholesterol >240 mg/dl; hypertension treated with medication) or who has been diagnosed/treated for CVD (heart attack, angina pectoris, sudden cardiac death, stroke, peripheral vascular disease, bypass surgery, or angioplasty), with onset before 55 years of age.

Even positive family histories can be further characterized from weakly to strongly positive, depending on whether first- or second-degree relatives are affected, how many relatives are affected, the age of onset, and the level of severity of disease or risk factor.

SUMMARY RISK PROFILE

Based on an assessment of the child's lipid profile, blood pressure, cigarette smoking status, body fatness or weight for height status, usual level of physical activity, and family history, the physician can characterize the child's overall risk profile as normal, borderline high risk, or high risk. Scoring systems have been suggested for such classification, but it may be more useful for the physician to go over a risk profile sheet such as that provided in Table 16-9, with the family and indicate which risk factors are elevated and which are not. Both the positive and the negative should be emphasized as a baseline for treatment recommendations. Even children who have seriously abnormal lipid profiles are often nonsmokers and have normal weight and blood pressure; these factors should be praised and encouraged while stressing the need to improve the lipid profile.

Treatment of Cardiovascular Disease Risk Factors in Childhood

NUTRITION ASSESSMENT

It is worthwhile and not difficult for the practicing pediatrician to make an objective assessment of the child's diet by means of one or two questionnaires, which the parent or the child can complete before an annual check-up. A simple food frequency check sheet asks the individual to check off how many times per week or month certain foods are eaten (Figure 16-7). Food frequency questionnaires are usually given to obtain qualitative information on the child's

Table 16-9. Sample cardiovascular disease risk factor score sheet for children over 2 years of age.

| | Risk of developing heart disease as an adult | | |
	Low	Moderate	High
Total blood cholesterol (TC) level (mg/dl)	170 and below	170–199	200 and above
LDL cholesterol level (mg/dl)	Below 110	110–129	130 and above
HDL cholesterol level (mg/dl)	45 and above	35–44	Below 35
Weight status	Underweight; below mean for height	Average; 100–119% of ideal	Overweight; >120% of ideal
Cigarette smoking	Never smokes	Experiments	Regular smoker
Exercise	Active sports participation	Gym plus play	Gym at school only
Family history	Rare CHD (not in parent or grandparent)	Grandparent, aunt, uncle had CHD before age 55 First- or second-degree relative has high blood pressure or high serum cholesterol (>240 mg/dl)	Parent had CHD before age 55
Blood pressure (for age/sex)	<75th %	75th–95th %	>95th %*

*95% for SBP for children age 2–13 years is 110–130 mm Hg; 95% for DBP for children age 2–13 years is 55–85 mm Hg. In older teens BP >130/85 is > 95th %.

usual diet; however, some are semiquantitative and can be analyzed to provide quantitative data on dietary intake [123]. These questionnaires are usually beyond the realm of ordinary clinical practice.

Three-day food records are useful and can also provide quantitative data on nutrient intake. They can also simply be used as a guide for the pediatrician to review the kinds of meals that are usually served in the child's home. They can be mailed, with simple instructions, to a parent to fill out a week before the child's appointment. If the diet record is to be analyzed quantitatively, the parent needs a significant amount of instruction in recording everything consumed as well as in accurately estimating portion sizes.

These dietary questionnaires can help the pe-diatrician to assess the dietary contribution to problems such as high serum cholesterol or triglyceride levels, obesity, or borderline hypertension and to begin dietary counseling in the areas most in need of change (e.g., too many fast-food meals, too much cheese, frequent salty snacks).

DIETARY PRESCRIPTION AND COUNSELING

Both diet and exercise are key components in the prevention and treatment of cardiovascular risk factors in childhood. For children over 2 years of age, adherence to a diet variously called the "prudent diet," the AHA or NCEP step 1 diet, or the "30 percent fat" diet will help to lower serum total and LDL cholesterol, reduce excess weight gain, and avoid excess sodium

Patient's Name_____   Date _____

"How often do you eat the following foods?"

	Number of SERVINGS PER DAY	SERVINGS PER WEEK	*(check mark)* SELDOM	NEVER
FOOD				

MILK & DAIRY PRODUCTS:
Cheese (type)_____
Milk (type)_____
Yogurt_____
Ice milk_____
Other Dairy_____

MEAT & MEAT ALTERNATES:
Beef, hamburger_____
Pork, ham_____
Bacon, _____
Veal_____
Luncheon meat_____
Poultry_____
Eggs_____
Fish _____
Shellfish_____
Dried beans, peas_____
Other _____

VEGETABLES & FRUIT:
Vegetables_____
Fruit or juice_____

FATS:
Margarine_____
Butter_____
Cream cheese_____
Mayonnaise_____
Vegetable oil_____
Lard_____
Ice cream_____
Chips_____
Fried foods_____
Nuts_____
Other_____

BREAD & CEREALS:
Bread (type)_____
Cereal (type)_____
Pasta_____
Potatoes_____
Rice_____
Other_____

SWEETS & ALCOHOLIC BEVERAGES:
Candy (type)_____
Baked goods (type)_____
Soft drinks (type)_____
Alcohol (type)_____
Other _____
Other _____

Figure 16-7.   Sample food frequency form.

intake, which may contribute to the development of hypertension. The essential elements of the step 1 diet are listed in Table 16-10. This diet may be further modified to reduce caloric intake if the child is obese, to increase caloric intake if the child is underweight, to reduce sodium if indicated, and to increase fiber intake to increase satiety, reduce constipation, and reduce serum cholesterol (especially soluble fiber such as that found in oat bran and psyllium).

DIETARY TREATMENT OF DYSLIPIDEMIA IN CHILDREN

The great majority of preadolescent children requiring treatment for a lipid abnormality are those with elevated total cholesterol due to a high LDL cholesterol level (above the seventy-fifth percentile for age). Elevated triglyceride levels are more commonly seen in adolescence, since even familial hypertriglyceridemic disorders often are not expressed until the second decade. Low HDL cholesterol levels in the fifth to twenty-fifth percentile range for age are commonly seen in children with elevated cholesterol levels, especially those with familial dyslipidemias or obesity. A much smaller number have elevated triglycerides or low HDL cholesterol, alone or in combination. And even fewer have the rarer lipid disorders, characterized as type I, III, or V. Finally there are some children with hyperapobetalipoproteinemia, where the LDL cholesterol level is normal or borderline high, but the apo-B level is above the ninety-fifth percentile for age (approximately > 110 mg/dl).

The initial treatment of children with abnormal lipid profiles consists of diet modification [82, 124, 125]. Children with elevated LDL cholesterol, elevated apo-B, and low HDL cholesterol are placed on a step 1 diet containing a normal caloric intake (unless the child is obese) but having reduced fat calories, as described in Table 16-10. The greatest emphasis is placed on reducing saturated-fat intake to less than 10 percent of calories. Physicians should know the most common sources of saturated fat in children's diets and be able to offer suggestions regarding alternative low-fat foods as the first step in recommending a low-fat diet (Table 16-11) (see Chapter 9 for further discussion of dietary intervention).

In some cases it may be necessary to count grams of saturated fat consumed to comply with the goal of 10 percent or less of calories from saturated fat. A child consuming 1800 calories per day should eat no more than 20 grams of saturated fat (1 gram of fat = 9 calories; 9 × 20 = 180 calories, or 10 percent of the 1800-calorie daily total). Charts of saturated fat content of foods are available so the parents can see which foods to include in the child's diet and which ones to limit. For example, 8 ounces of whole milk contains 5 grams of saturated fat (one-quarter of the child's allowance for the

Table 16-10. Recommended step 1 and 2 diets for reducing blood cholesterol levels in children over 2 years of age

Nutrient	Step 1	Step 2	Practical tips
Fat, total (%)*	< 30	< 30	Reduce all fat intake; use vegetable oils and
Saturated fat (%)	< 10	< 7	margarine; use skim or 1% milk and lowfat
Polyunsaturated (%)	10	10	dairy products; avoid fried foods; use lean
Monounsaturated (%)	10–15	10–15	meats, fish, and poultry.
Cholesterol (mg/dl)	< 300	< 200	Limit eggs to 2 or 3 per week.
Carbohydrate (%)	50–60	50–60	Eat more whole-grain cereals/bread, fruits, vegetables; fewer sweets.
Protein (%)	15–20	15–20	Eat less animal protein; more vegetable protein.
Fiber (g/day)	25	25	Eat whole-grain cereals/bread; fruits/vegetables with peel; oat bran.

*Percentages are percent of total calories.

Table 16-11.   Sources of saturated fat in children's diets — from high saturated fat content to low

Food item	Grams of saturated fat/ serving
Ice cream, 1 cup 10% fat	9
Hamburger, 3 oz., fast food	8
Hot dog, 2 oz.	7
Butter, 1 tablespoon	7
Pizza with cheese, 1 slice	6
Cheese, 1 oz. American or Swiss	6
Parmesan cheese, 1 tablespoon	5
Milk, 1 cup whole	5
Beef, pork, veal, 3 oz. lean	5
Ice milk frozen dessert, 1 cup	4
Heavy cream, 1 tablespoon	4
Milk, 2% low fat, 1 cup	3
Bacon, 2 slices crisp	3
Egg, 1 medium	3
French fries, 10 medium	3
Peanut butter, 2 tablespoons	3
Cheese, part-skim mozzarella, 1 oz.	3
Cream cheese, 1 tablespooon	3
Margarine, 1 tablespoon	2
Mayonaise, 1 tablespoon	2
Cupcake, chocolate frosted	2
Brownie, frosted	2
Potato chips, 10	2
Chicken, dark meat, 3 oz.	2
Chicken, light meat, 3 oz.	1
Milk, 1% low fat, 1 cup	1
Bagel, 1 medium	0
Baked potato, 1 medium	0
Marshmallows, 5	0
Milk, skim, 1 cup	0
Sorbet, 1 cup	0

Note: Hamburger, cheeseburger, meat loaf, full-fat dairy products, cheese, beef, hot dogs, ham, lunch meats, eggs, cookies, cakes, doughnuts, butter, pork, and white bread and rolls together account for over 60 percent of the saturated fat in a child's diet. The average 10-year-old child on an 1800-calorie step 1 diet should consume less than 20 g saturated fat per day.

day), whereas skim milk contains less than 1 gram per 8 ounces, allowing the child much more freedom to include other low- to moderately-low-fat products in the diet.

Consumption of increased amounts of complex carbohydrates and dietary fiber should also be stressed. Increasing the soluble fiber content of the diet (oat bran, psyllium, etc.) can boost the cholesterol-lowering effect of the low-fat diet in many cases. This can usually be accomplished by encouraging high-soluble-fiber cereal consumption (with low-fat milk) at least five mornings a week. Fresh fruits and vegetables, whole-grain breads, and beans are also good dietary sources of fiber. If the serum triglyceride level is increased, reduction of simple sugars in the diet and achievement of ideal body weight should be stressed as well.

It is essential that caloric intake be maintained to support normal growth. Since fat is calorically more dense than protein or carbohydrate, a reduction in dietary fat must be accompanied by an increase in carbohydrate to make up for the loss of fat calories. Most children like complex carbohydrates (e.g., potatoes, bread, pasta, rice), so this is usually not a problem. Calcium levels are slightly higher in low-fat and skim milk than in regular milk, so calcium intake need not be compromised on the step 1 diet. Intake of other minerals and vitamins will be adequate if a good variety of foods from all food groups is consumed.

Further reduction of saturated fat intake to 7 percent of calories may be necessary to achieve lipid goals. The step 2 diet can be prescribed after 6 to 12 months on the step 1 diet and should be given an adequate trial before medications are considered. Patients who do not comply with the step 1 diet, however, will be even less compliant with the more restrictive step 2 diet. Thus, step 2 should be recommended only when compliance with step 1 is adequate, but the lipid response is insufficient.

Children with normal levels of LDL cholesterol but low levels of HDL cholesterol are also treated with a step 1 diet if their ratio of LDL to HDL is above 3. The diet reduces LDL levels so that the ratio is reduced to a lower risk level. Increased physical activity also helps to raise HDL, as does reducing obesity and avoiding cigarette smoking.

Similarly children with normal to borderline elevated LDL levels but high apo-B levels (above 110 mg/dl) should be treated with a step 1 diet to reduce their LDL level further and thus reduce the level of apo-B as well.

All children should be encouraged to increase their level of regular aerobic physical activity to at least 30 minutes 4 or more days a week at a level that makes the child sweat. Charts can be provided so children can monitor their progress, and appropriate rewards for this behavior can be negotiated to reinforce compliance.

It is not uncommon in clinical practice to see HDL cholesterol levels higher at the end of an active summer of sports camp and then lower during the more sedentary winter months, especially in cold weather areas. Children should be encouraged to participate in one team sport or dance/gymnastics class each season in addition to school gym, recess, and after-school play. Families should be encouraged to share sports activities as much as possible.

SAFETY OF THE STEP 1 DIET IN CHILDHOOD

Since a prudent, step 1 diet has been recommended by the AHA, the American Health Association, and others for all healthy children over 2 years of age, it is appropriate to consider the safety of such a diet, especially as it concerns normal childhood growth and development [126]. Several key points should be emphasized with respect to the adequacy of the diet.

Calories. Total caloric intake should not be reduced. Since fat is a major component of calorie-dense foods, however, a reduction in total fat intake must be compensated for by an increase in calories derived from other food sources, such as complex carbohydrates. Children in countries whre a low-fat diet is consumed as the normal diet (e.g., Japan, Italy, Israel) grow and develop normally. Previous short stature among prewar Japanese was due to low protein intake rather than low-fat intake.

Vitamins. Nutrition experts who have analyzed the step 1 diet have determined that the intake of vitamins on this diet is adequate. The vitamin E content of the step 1 diet is higher because of increased consumption of polyunsaturated fats. Complex carbohydrates (cereals, breads, etc.) are also often supplemented with vitamins and minerals.

Minerals. Mineral intake similarly is not deficient on the step 1 diet. Low-fat milks have as much (and slightly more) calcium as full-fat milk. Cereals and other complex carbohydrates are often supplemented with iron.

Essential fatty acids. Essential fatty acids are plentiful in the step 1 diet because of increased consumption of vegetable oils.

Hormone synthesis. Endogenous hormone synthesis does not depend on dietary sources of cholesterol since various organs of the body synthesize all the cholesterol needed for the production of hormones. Again, children in countries that routinely consume a low-fat diet have normal puberty and hormonogenesis.

Myelin synthesis. In a manner similar to hormone synthesis, the body easily manufactures all the cholesterol needed for myelin production and normal development of the nervous system. Intelligence and other nervous system functions are certainly not deficient in countries such as Japan and Israel, where children routinely eat a low-fat diet from the time of weaning.

In addition to the above issues there have been concerns that a low-fat diet may promote cancer. The bulk of evidence suggests that it is the incubating cancer that is responsible for the association of very low serum cholesterol levels and cancer in some epidemiologic studies, rather than vice versa. In contrast populations that habitually consume high-fat diets have increased rates of a variety of human cancers, particularly of the breast and colon.

When a reduced-fat diet is prescribed medically for a child with an elevated serum cholesterol or other dyslipidemia, it is important that the parents and the child are adequately counseled with respect to achieving the goal and avoiding problems, specifically insufficient caloric intake. Parents who are advised simply to cut out fat and cholesterol from the diet are likely to reduce caloric intake without compensating with increased calories from other sources. Case reports have documented such parental dietary overrestrictions and the inadequate growth that can occur as a result [127, 128]. Regular medical supervision is needed to monitor the progress of children for whom a low-fat diet has been prescribed as a part of the medical treatment of dyslipidemia, especially in the early phases of treatment.

The goals of dietary treatment should be discussed with the parents. For children with a baseline level of LDL cholesterol between 110 and 129 mg/dl the goal is to reduce it to below 110 mg/dl. For children with a baseline LDL level above 130 mg/dl, the goal is to reduce it initially to below 130 mg/dl and ideally to below 110 mg/dl [82]. This may or may not be feasible with dietary intervention alone, depending on the severity of the child's hypercholesterolemia. Gradual achievement of dietary goals over a 6- to 12-month period may be easier for parents and children to accept and may prevent overzealous restrictions.

PHARMACOLOGIC THERAPY OF DYSLIPIDEMIA

Medications may need to be prescribed in the treatment of children and adolescents with lipid abnormalities. This occurs most commonly when the child inherits one of the more severe genetic forms of dyslipidemia, and in less severe cases when the goals of therapy have not been achieved after a year or more of compliant dietary treatment, and the presence of other risk factors places the child at a very high risk for the development of premature CHD. Criteria have been suggested for initiating drug therapy in hypercholesterolemic children such as those summarized in Table 16-12. In addition children

Table 16-12. Criteria for initiation of pharmacologic therapy for children and adolescents with dyslipidemia

I. LDL cholesterol above 190 mg/dl (or above 160 mg/dl if the child also has two or more other risk factors) after one year of compliance with a reduced-fat diet (progressing from step 1 to step 2).

II. There is a family history of premature onset of CHD (parent, grandparent, or blood-related aunt/uncle with CHD onset before 55 years of age).

III. The child is at least 10 years of age and is otherwise healthy and shows every evidence of normal growth and development.

Sources: Kwiterovich, P. Beyond cholesterol. Baltimore: Johns Hopkins University Press, 1989; 286. NCEP Report of the Expert Panel on Blood Cholesterol Levels in Children and Adolescents [82].

whose LDL cholesterol is still above the ninety-fifth percentile after dietary treatment for a year or more (progressing from a step 1 to step 2 diet and increasing soluble fiber intake to maximally tolerated levels), especially in the face of a positive family history or other coexisting risk factors (elevated blood pressure, obesity, cigarette smoking, low HDL or high triglyceride level), may be considered for pharmacologic treatment [129]. The bile acid sequestrant agents cholestyramine and colestipol are currently the drugs of choice for initiating therapy. Although not approved by the FDA for the treatment of hypercholesterolemia in children, they have been used for more than two decades and have been reported to be both effective and safe if monitored carefully. There are also reports of pediatric use of almost all the other cholesterol-lowering drugs currently FDA-approved for use in adults. Clinical trials of some of these drugs are currently in progress in pediatric populations or planned for the future.

Cholestyramine or colestipol are begun at a low dose of one-half to one packet (or bar) (1 packet contains 4 g of cholestyramine or 5 g of colestipol) per day and increased to one to two packets twice a day. Higher doses are not well tolerated in children, the common side effects being constipation, gas, and an upset stomach. Cholestyramine may interfere with the absorption of other medications as well as fat-soluble vitamins, so vitamin supplementation and attention to the timing of other medication doses may be needed (see Chapter 12 for further information on the use of these agents).

For severely affected hypercholesterolemic children a combination of cholestyramine with nicotinic acid or an HMG CoA reductase inhibitor can lower serum cholesterol to almost normal levels. Since there is only limited pediatric experience with drugs other than the bile acid sequestrants, such therapy should be undertaken under the supervision of a lipid specialist.

LONG-TERM FOLLOW-UP

The follow-up of children with lipid disorders depends on the nature and severity of the dyslipidemia as well as the presence and need for treatment of other coexisting risk factors. Children on dietary treatment alone should be monitored at least quarterly with repeat lipid measurements and assessment of growth and dietary compliance.

If a reduced fat intake has resulted in reduced caloric intake not compensated for by increasing complex carbohydrate calories, the child will lose weight. This should be corrected through further dietary counseling. In some cases an increasing intake of monounsaturated fat is needed to keep up caloric intake if the child is unable to eat enough complex carbohydrates to compensate. Such situations are not common, but they must be detected and corrected as soon as possible.

In the usual clinical course, when the patient is compliant with the step 1 diet, total cholesterol and LDL cholesterol levels will drop 10 to 20 percent. The subsequent course, however, will be up and down, and long-term monitoring and follow-up are needed to reinforce the diet and maintain the goals of therapy. Parents and children need to understand the natural history of lipid levels through childhood, particularly the pubertal dip seen especially in white adolescent boys and the subsequent increase in total and LDL cholesterol and the decrease in HDL cholesterol (in boys), seen later in adolescence and in early adult life.

Parents also need encouragement to reduce their own risk of cardiovascular disease. Programs that treat families have an advantage in being able to follow and treat both children and parents in a single clinical setting. More than 90 percent of children with cholesterol levels of 200 mg/dl or above referred to our clinical center have at least one parent who also has hypercholesterolemia. Family-oriented screening, counseling, and treatment are indicated in almost all cases.

Children treated with both diet and medication need more intensive follow-up and monitoring to assess lipid levels and also to detect side effects of drug treatment. Children with severe lipid disorders also need baseline studies of cardiovascular status using electrocardiograms, exercise treadmill tests, and possibly other measures, as well as periodic reassessment.

It is important to maintain a supportive atmosphere yet avoid the creation of undue anxiety. There are children with severe lipid abnormalities in whom there is a risk of CHD onset early in adult life (or in some cases even in adolescence). However, the majority of children evaluated and treated for lipid abnormalities will be completely healthy — the goal is to reduce their risk of future cardiovascular disease. They must be reassured of their healthy status now but made to appreciate our desire to help them avoid disease in the future and to live long and healthy lives.

References

1. Drash A. Atherosclerosis, cholesterol and the pediatrician. J Pediatr 1972; 80:693–6.
2. Kannel WB and Dawber TR. Atherosclerosis as a pediatric problem. J Pediatr 1972; 80:544–54.
3. McMillan GC. Development of arteriosclerosis. Am J Cardiol 1973; 31:542–6.
4. Williams CL and Wynder EL. A blind spot in preventive medicine. JAMA 1976; 236:2196–7.
5. Mitchell SC, ed. Symposium on prevention of atherosclerosis at the pediatric level. Am J Cardiol 1973; 31:539–41.
6. Williams CL. Preventing heart attacks: a pediatric priority. New York Med Quart 1987; 7(3):96–100.
7. Davidson DM, Doyle EJ Jr. Family-directed preventive cardiology. J Fam Pract 1984; 18:57–64.
8. Wynder EL, Berenson GC, Strong WB, et al. Coronary artery disease prevention: cholesterol — a pediatric perspective. Prev Med 1989; 18(3):323–409.
9. Strong WB and Dennison BA. Pediatric preventive cardiology: atherosclerosis and coronary heart disease. Pediatrics in Review 1988; 9(10):303–14.
10. Nora JJ. Identifying the child at risk for coronary disease as in an adult: a strategy for prevention. J Pediatr 1980; 97:706–714.
11. Enos WF, Holmes RG, Beyer J. Coronary disease among United States soldiers killed in action in Korea: preliminary report. JAMA 1953; 152:1090–3. [Reprinted as Landmark Article; JAMA 1986; 256:2859–62.]
12. McNamara JJ, Molot MA, Stremple JF. Coronary artery disease in combat casualties in Vietnam. JAMA 1971; 216:1185–7.

13. Holman RL. McGill HC, Strong JP, Geer JC. The natural history of atherosclerosis: the early aortic lesions as seen in New Orleans, in the middle of the 20th century. Am J Pathol 1958; 34:209–35.

14. Strong JP, McGill HC Jr. Pediatric aspects of atherosclerosis. J Atherosclerosis Res Op 1969; 9:251–65.

15. McGill HC Jr, Eggen DA, Strong JP. Atherosclerotic lesions in the aorta and coronary arteries of man. In: Roberts JC Jr, Straus R, eds. Comparative atherosclerosis. New York: Harper & Row, 1965; 311–26.

16. Stary HC. Evolution and progression of atherosclerosis in the coronary arteries of children and adults. In: Bates SR, Gangloff EC, eds. Atherogenesis and aging. New York: Springer, 1987; 20–36.

17. Newman WP III, Freedman DS, Voors AW, et al. Relation of serum lipoprotein levels and systolic blood pressure to early atherosclerosis: the Bogalusa Heart Study. N Engl J Med 1986; 314:138–44.

18. Berwick DM, Cretin S, Keeler E. Cholesterol, children and heart disease. New York: Oxford University Press, 1980.

19. Williams CI. Pediatric risk factors for major chronic disease. St. Louis: Warren Green, 1984.

20. Berenson GS, ed. Causation of cardiovascular risk factors in children: perspectives on cardiovascular risk in early life. New York: Raven, 1986.

21. Lauer RM, Shekelle RB. Childhood prevention of atherosclerosis and hypertension. New York: Raven, 1980.

22. Williams CL, Carter BJ, Wynder EL. Prevalence of selected cardiovascular and cancer risk factors in a pediatric population: the "Know Your Body" project. New York, USA. Prev Med 1981; 10:235–50.

23. Lauer RM, Connor WE, Leaverton PE, et al. Coronary heart disease risk factors in school children: the Muscatine Study. J Pediatr 1975; 86:697–706.

24. Morrison JA, Glueck CJ. Pediatric risk factors for adult coronary heart disease: primary atherosclerosis prevention. Cardiovasc Rev Rep 1981; 2:1269–75.

25. Golubjatnikov R, Paskey T, Inhorn SL. Serum cholesterol levels of Mexican and Wisconsin school chiliden. Am J Epidem 1972; 96:36–9.

26. Puska P, Vartianen E, Pallonen U. The North Karelia Youth Project. Prev Med 1981; 10:133–48.

27. Kromhout D, Haar F, Hautvast JGAJ. Coronary heart disease risk factors in Dutch school children. Prev Med 1977; 6:500–13.

28. Wynder EL, Williams CL, Laakso K, Levenstein M. Screening for risk factors for chronic disease in children from fifteen countries. Prev Med 1981; 10:121–32.

29. Kafatos AG, Panagiotakopoulos G, Bastakis N. Cardiovascular risk factor status of Greek adolescents in Athens. Prev Med 1981; 10:173–86.

30. Tell GS, Vellar O, Monrad-Hansen HP. Risk factors for chronic diseases in Norwegian school children. Prev Med 1981; 10:211–25.

31. Knuiman JT, Hermus RJJ, Hautvast JGAJ. Serum total and high-density lipoprotein cholesterol concentrations in rural and urban boys from 16 countries. Atherosclerosis 1980; 36:529–37.

32. Williams CL, Carter BJ, Wynder EL, Blumenfeld TA. Selected chronic disease "risk factors" in two elementary school populations: a pilot study. Am J Dis Child 1979; 133:704–8.

33. Wilmore HJ, McNamara JJ. Prevalence of coronary heart disease risk factors in boys, 9-12 years of age. J Pediatr 1974; 84:527–33.

34. Gotto AM Jr, Pownall HJ, Havel RJ. Introduction to the plasma lipoproteins. Methods Enzymol 1986; 3:128–35.

35. Brown MS, Goldstein JL. How LDL receptors influence cholesterol and atherosclerosis. Sci Am 1984; 25:58–62.

36. Brown MS, Goldstein JL. Lipoprotein receptors in the liver: control signals for plasma cholesterol traffic. J Clin Invest 1983; 72:743–8.

37. Brown MS, Goldstein JL. A receptor-mediated pathway for cholesterol homeostasis. Science 1986; 34:232–5.

38. Blankenhorn DH, et al. Beneficial effects of combined colestipol niacin therapy on coronary atherosclerosis and coronary venous bypass grafts. JAMA 1987; 257:3233–40.

39. Consensus Conference Panel. Lowering blood cholesterol to prevent heart disease. JAMA 1986; 253:2080–4.

40. Christensen B, Glueck C, Kwiterovich P. Plasma cholesterol and triglyceride distribution in 13,665 children and adolescents: the prevalence study of the LRC Program. Pediatr Res 1980; 14:194–202.

41. U.S. Department of Health and Human Services. Cardiovascular profile of 15,000 children of school age in three communities, 1971-1975. Public Health Service, National Institutes of Health, National Heart, Lung and Blood Institute. DHEW publ. no. (NIH) 78–1472, 1978.

42. Lipid Research Clinics Program. Population studies data book. Vol. 1. The Prevalence Study. U.S. Department of Health and Human Services, Public Health Service, National Institutes of Health, National Heart, Lung and

Blood Institute. DHHS publ. no. (NIH) 80–1527, 1980.

43. Rensicow K, Kotchen JM, Wynder EL. Plasma cholesterol levels of 6,585 children in the United States: results of the know your body screening in five states. Pediatrics 1989; 84(6):969–76.

44. Berenson GS, Srinivasan SR, Cresanta JL et al. Dynamic changes of serum lipoproteins in children during adolescence and sexual maturation. Am J Epidemiol 1981; 113:157–70.

45. Stanbury JB, Wyngaarden JB, Fredrickson DS, et al. The metabolic basis of inherited disease, 5th ed. New York: McGraw-Hill, 1989.

46. Goldbourt U, Neufeld HN. Genetic aspects of arteriosclerosis. Arteriosclerosis. 1986; 6:357–63.

47. Report of the Second Task Force on Blood Pressure Control in Children — 1987. NHLBI. Pediatrics 1987; 79(1):1–25.

48. Lauer RM, Burns TL, Clarke WR. Assessing children's blood pressure. Consideration of age and body size: the Muscatine Study. Pediatrics 1985; 75:1081–90.

49. Feinlieb M, Garrison RJ, Havlik R. Environmental and genetic factors affecting the distribution of blood pressure in children. In: Lauer RM, Shekelle RB, eds. Childhood prevention of atherosclerosis and hypertension. New York: Raven, 1980; 271–9.

50. Dustan HP. Mechanisms of hypertension associated with obesity. Ann Intern Med 1983; 98:860–4.

51. Page, LB. Dietary sodium and blood pressure: evidence from human studies. In: Lauer RM, Shekelle RB, eds. Childhood prevention of atherosclerosis and hypertension. New York: Raven, 1980; 291–303.

52. Bricker JT. Blood pressure measurement and interpretation in children. Applied Cardiology 1985; 13:29–38.

53. Prineas RJ. Standards of measurement for children's blood pressure. Hypertension 2:Suppl 1:1980; I:18–24.

54. Londe W, Bourgougnie JJ, Robson AM, Goldring D. Hypertension in apparently normal children. J Pediatr 1971; 78:569–73.

55. Kilcoyne MM, Richter RW, Alsup PA. Adolescent hypertension. 1. Detection and prevalence. Circulation 1974; 50:758–64.

56. Levine LS, Levy JE, New MI. Hypertension in high school students. Evaluation in New York City. NYS J Med 1976; 76:40–4.

57. Clarke W. Woolson R. Schrott H, Lauer RM. Tracking of blood pressure, serum lipids and obesity in children: the Muscatine Study. Circulation 1976; 54:Supp 2:23–8.

58. Williams CL, Arnold CB, Wynder EL. Chronic disease risk factors among children: the "Know Your Body" Study. J Chron Dis 1979; 32:505–13.

59. Report of the task force on blood pressure control in children. Pediatrics 1977; 59 (Suppl): 797–820.

60. Report of the Second Task Force on Blood Pressure Control in Children — 1987. Pediatrics 1987; 79:1–25.

61. Borjeson M. The etiology of obesity in children. A study of 101 twin pairs. Acta Pediatr Scand 1976; 65:279–87.

62. Mayer J. Overweight: causes, cost and control. Englewood Cliffs, NJ: Prentice-Hall, 1968.

63. Garn SM, Clark DC, Guire KE. Growth, body composition and development of obese and lean children. In: Winick M, ed. Childhood obesity. New York: Wiley, 1976.

64. Garn SM, Clark DC. Trends in fatness and the origins of obesity. Pediatrics 1976; 57:443–56.

65. Garn SM, Bailey SM, Cole PE. Synchronous fatness changes in husbands and wives. Am J Clin Nutr 1979; 32:2375–7.

66. Martin RJ, Ramsay T, Hausman GJ. Adipocyte development. Ped Annals 1984; 13:448–52.

67. Dietz WH, Gortmaker SL. Do we fatten our children at the TV set? Pediatrics 1985; 75:805–12.

68. Rose HE, Mayer J. Activity, caloric intake, fat storage and the energy balance of infants. Pediatrics 1968; 41:18–23.

69. Abram S, Carroll MD, Najjar MF, Robinson MF. Obese and overweight adults in the United States. Vital and health statistics. NCHS series 11, no. 230. U.S. Department of Health and Human Services. USDHHS publ. no. (PHS) 83–1680, 1982.

70. Benn RT. Indices of height and weight as measures of obesity. J Prev Soc Med 1970; 24:64–8.

71. Frisancho AR. Triceps skinfold and upper arm muscle size norms for nutritional status. Am J Clin Nutr 1974; 27:1052–8.

72. Seltzer CC, Mayer J. Greater reliability of the triceps skinfold over the subscapular skinfold as an index of obesity. Am J Clin Nutr 1967; 20:950–4.

73. Durwin JV, Womersley J. Body fat assessed from total body density and its estimation from skinfold thickness. Measurements on 481 men and women aged from 16 to 72 years. Br J Nutr 1974; 32:77–9.

74. Shear CL, Freedman DS, Burke GL, et al. Secular trends of obesity in early life: the Bogalusa Heart Study. Am J Pub Health 1988; 78:75–7.

75. Fripp RR, Hodgson JL, Kwiterovich PO. Aerobic capacity, obesity and arteriosclerotic risk factors in male adolescents. Pediatrics 1985; 75:813–8.

76. Voors AW, Harsha DW, Webber LS. Cluster-

ing of anthropometric parameters, glucose intolerance and serum lipids in children. Atherosclerosis 1982; 2:346–55.

77. Orchard TJ, Donahue RP, Kuller LH, et al. Cholesterol screening in childhood: does it predict adult hypercholesterolemia? The Beaver County Experience. Pediatrics 1983; 103:687–91.

78. Webber LD, Cresanta JL, Voors AW, Berenson GS. Tracking of cardiovascular disease risk factor variables in school-age children. J Chron Dis 1983; 36:647–60.

79. Freedman DS, Shear CL, Srinivasan SR, et al. Tracking of serum lipids and lipoproteins in children over an 8-year period: the Bogalusa Heart Study. Prev Med 1985; 14:203-16.

80. Clarke WR, Schrott HG, Leaverton PE, et al. Tracking of blood lipids and blood pressures in school age children: the Muscatine Study. Circulation 1978; 58:626–34.

81. Weidman W, Kwiterovich P Jr, Jesse MJ, Nugent E. Task Force Committee of the Nutrition Committee and the Cardiovascular Disease in the Young Council of the American Heart Association. Diet in the healthy child. Circulation 1986; 74:1411A–4A.

82. National Cholesterol Education Program. Report of the Expert Panel on Blood Cholesterol Levels in Children and Adolescents. U.S. Department of Health and Human Services, Public Health Service, National Institutes of Health, 1991, USDHHS publ. no. (NIH) 91–2732.

83. National Center for Health Statistics, Carroll MD, Abraham S, Dresser CM. Dietary intake source data: United States 1976–80. Vital and health statistics. NCHS series II, no. 231. Hyattsville, MD: U.S. Department of Health and Human Services, Public Health Service, National Center for Health Statistics. USDHHS publ. no. (PHS) 83–1681, March 1983.

84. Human Nutrition Information Service. U.S. Department of Agriculture, 1991.

85. National Cancer Institute. Diet, nutrition & cancer prevention: the good news. Bethesda, MD: U.S. Department of Health and Human Services, Public Health Service. USDHHS publ. no. (NIH) 87–2878, 1987.

86. Ellison RC, Morris DH, Donahue RO, et al. Effects of changing type of breakfast on total dietary fat and cholesterol intake and blood cholesterol (abstract). 2nd Int. Conf. on Preventive Cardiology, Washington, DC, June 18, 1989.

87. Resnicow KL, Cohn L, Reinhardt J. The relationship between breakfast habits, plasma cholesterol and quetelet index in 530 school children (abstract). ADA annual meeting, Kansas City, MO, October 23, 1989.

88. National Restaurant Association. Crest Special Study, 1988.

89. U.S. Department of Health and Human Services. The health consequences of smoking: cardiovascular disease. A report of the Surgeon General. U.S. Department of Health and Human Services, Public Health Service, Office on Smoking and Health. USDHHS publ. no. (PHS) 84-50204, 1983.

90. Slone D, Shapiro S, Rosenberg L, et al. Relation of cigarette smoking to myocardial infarction in young women. N Engl J Med. 1978; 298:1273–6.

91. American Heart Association. Cigarettes and cardiovascular diseases: A statement for health professionals. Dallas, 1985.

92. Craig WY, Palomaki BS, Johnson AM, Haddow JE. Cigarette smoking — associated changes in blood lipid and lipoprotein levels in the 8- to 19-year-old age group: a meta analysis. Pediatrics 1990; 85(2):155–8.

93. Moskowitz WB, Mosteller M, Schieken RM, et al. Lipoprotein and oxygen transport alterations in passive smoking preadolescent children. Circulation 1990; 81(2):586–92.

94. Green DL. Teenage smoking. Immediate and long-term patterns. Washington, DC: U.S. Government Printing Office, 1979. U.S. Department of Health and Human Services, National Center for Health Statistics. USDHHS publ. no. (PHS) 85-1232, 1984.

95. The National Center for Health Statistics and Health. USDHHS publ. no. (PHS) 85-1232, 1984.

96. Gritz ER, Brunswick AF. Psychosocial and behavioral aspects of smoking in women. In: Health consequences of smoking for women. A report of the Surgeon General. Part III. Washington, DC: U.S. Government Printing Office, 1980.

97. Johnston LD, O'Malley PM, Bachman JG. Drug use by high school seniors — the class of 1986. Rockville Md.: U.S. Department of Health and Human Services, 1987. USDHHS publ. no. 87-1535.

98. Mittlemark MB, Murray DM, Luepker RV. Predicting experimentation with cigarettes: the childhood antecedents of smoking study (CASS). Am J Pub Health 1987; 77:206–8.

99. AHA Committee on Atherosclerosis and Hypertension in Childhood. Coronary risk factor modification in children: smoking. Circulation 1986; 74:1192A–4A.

100. Chandrashekhar V, Anand IS. Exercise as a coronary protective factor. Am Heart J 1991; 122:1723–39.

101. Tell GS, Vellar OD. Physical fitness, physical activity and cardiovascular disease risk factors

in adolescents. the Oslo Youth Study. Prev Med 1988; 17:12–24.

102. Durant RH, Linder CW, Mahoney OM. Relationship between habitual physical activity and serum lipoprotein levels in white male adolescents. J Adolesc Health Care 1983; 4:235–40.

103. Fripp RR, Hodgson JL, Kwiterovich PO, et al. Aerobic capacity, obesity and atherosclerotic risk factors in male adolescents. Pediatrics 1985; 75:813–8.

104. Thompson PD. What do muscles have to do with lipoproteins? Circulation 1990; 81:1428–30.

105. Jopling RJ. Health related fitness as preventive medicine. Ped in Rev 1988; 10:141–8.

106. Strong WB, Wilmore JH. Unfit kids: an office-based approach to physical fitness. Contemp Pediatr 1988; 5:33–48.

107. AHA Committee for Atherosclerosis and Hypertension in Childhood. Coronary risk factor modification in children: exercise. Circulation 1986; 74:1189A–91A.

108. Webber LD, Cresanta JL, Voors AW, Berenson GS. Tracking of cardiovascular disease risk factor variables in school-age children. J Chron Dis 1983; 36:647–60.

109. Freedman DS, Shear CL, Srinivasan SR, et al. Tracking of serum lipids and lipoproteins in children over an 8-year period: the Bogalusa Heart Study. Prev Med 1985; 14:203–16.

110. Webber LS, Srinivasan SR, Berenson GS. Tracking of serum lipids and lipoproteins over 12 years into young adulthood. The Bogalusa Heart Study (abstract). Circulation 1988; 78:suppl II:481.

111. Toda A, Okuni M. Tracking of blood lipids in school age children. J Jap Ped Soc 1987; 91:32–45.

112. Clarke WR, Schrott HG, Leaverton PE, et al. Tracking of blood lipids and blood pressures in school age children: the Muscatine Study. Circulation 1978; 58:626–34.

113. Lauer RM, Lee J, Clarke WR. Factors affecting the relationship between childhood and adult cholesterol levels: the Muscatine Study. Pediatrics 1988; 82:309–18.

114. Lauer RM, Clarke WR, Beaglehole R. Level, trend and variability of blood pressure during childhood: the Muscatine Study. Circulation 1984; 69:242–9.

115. Freedman DS, Srinivasan SR, Cresanta SR, et al. Cardiovascular risk factors from birth to seven years of age: Bogalusa Heart Study. IV.

Serum lipids and lipoproteins. Ped 1987; 80:Suppl, Part 2:80:789–96.

116. Garcia RE, Moodie DS. Routine cholesterol surveillance in childhood. Pediatrics 1989; 84:751–5.

117. Griffen TC, Cristoffel KK, Binns HJ, McGuire PA. Family history evaluation as a predictive screen for childhood hypercholesterolemia. Pediatrics 1989; 84(2):365–73.

118. Perry CL and Silvis GL. Smoking prevention: behavioral prescriptions for the pediatrician. Pediatrics 1987; 79(5):790–9.

119. Davidson DM, Bradley BJ, Landry SM, et al. School-based blood cholesterol screening. J Ped Health Care 1989; 3:3–8.

120. Medici F, Puder D, Williams C. Cholesterol screening in the pediatric office. In: Williams CL, Wynder EL eds. Hyperlipidemia in childhood and the development of atherosclerosis. Ann NY Acad Sci 1991; 623:200–5.

121. American Academy of Pediatrics. Committee on Nutrition. Indications for cholesterol testing in children. Pediatrics 1989; 83(1):141–2.

122. American Academy of Pediatrics, Committee on Nutrition. Towards a prudent diet for children. Pediatrics 1983; 71:78–80.

123. Willett WC, Reynolds RD, Cotrell-Hoehner S, et al. Validation of a semi-quantitative food frequency questionnaire: comparison with a 1-year diet record. J Amer Diet Assoc 1987; 87:43–7.

124. Williams CL and Spark A. Guidelines for evaluation and treatment of children with elevated cholesterol. In: Williams CL, Wynder EL eds. Hyperlipidemia in childhood and the development of atherosclerosis. Ann NY Acad Sci 1991; 623:239–52.

125. Wiliams CL. Strategies for implementing an AHA step 1 diet in children. In: Williams CL, Wynder EL eds. Hyperlipidemia in childhood and the development of atherosclerosis. Ann NY Acad Sci 1991, 623:253–62.

126. Dwyer J. Diets for children and adolescents that meet dietary goals. Amer J Dis Child 1980; 134:1073–80.

127. Pugliese MT, Weyman-Daum M, Moses N, Lifshitz F. Parental beliefs as a cause of non-organic failure to thrive. Pediatrics 1987; 80:175–8.

128. Lifshitz F, Moses N. Growth failure. AJDC 1989; 143:537–42.

129. Hoeg J. Pharmacologic and surgical treatment of dyslipidemic children and adolescents. In: Williams CL, Wynder EL eds. Hyperlipidemia in childhood and the development of atherosclerosis. Ann NY Acad Sci 1991; 623:275–84.

17

The Prevention-Oriented Practice

LEIF I. SOLBERG
THOMAS ERLING KOTTKE
MILO L. BREKKE

EDITORS' INTRODUCTION

In a time of ever increasing medical care costs, the physician is under increasing pressure to see more patients in less time, a situation that most physicians find frustrating. As fine as one's counseling skills and motivation to practice prevention are, it all comes to naught if the environment in which the physician practices does not support his or her efforts. Fortunately there are now office practice systems that foster prevention rather than hinder it. In this chapter Dr. Solberg and his colleagues describe one such system in which an integrated office approach brings together patient, physician, nurse, and other office personnel in a cost- and time-efficient manner that makes counseling for risk factor modification simply another routine aspect of a well-run practice.

The preceding chapters have described in considerable detail the rationale and techniques physicians should use in dealing with the cardiovascular disease prevention needs of individual patients. A major problem that has been documented by numerous studies is the inconsistency of physicians' efforts to reduce tobacco use and blood cholesterol levels and to improve exercise and nutrition among their patients, thus making these efforts relatively ineffective. Although their efforts at control of diabetes and hypertension have been more effective, even these more traditional "diseases" suffer from incomplete use of behavioral and dietary change techniques and from failures of monitoring and follow-up.

Although physicians often do care about prevention and would like to apply the effective techniques described in this book, an important barrier to using them in daily medical practice is that a busy practice has many distracting factors. These problematic factors include the need for time efficiency, cost concerns, the need to first address the problems and expectations of the patient being seen (which are rarely primarily prevention), and the traditional emphasis on diagnosis and treatment.

When physicians are asked why they do not include prevention activities more consistently in their practices, they usually emphasize the lack of patient motivation or acceptance, time pressures, conflicting recommendations, and inadequate reimbursement [1, 2, 3]. There is reason to doubt that lack of patient interest is a serious issue, and the other barriers need not be problems if the intervention is well designed to be efficient and cost-effective for the practice.

Many studies have demonstrated that physician preventive behavior can change. The classical approaches to producing change through direct education and training clearly are not sufficient, since even if such approaches do produce improved knowledge, attitudes, and skills, they are not enough to overcome the practice barriers described above. Individual (but not group) feedback after performance audits has had some effect, but it is expensive and the changes produced generally have been small and/or temporary. Reimbursement changes, even though

desirable, may not come quickly, and there is little evidence that such changes will make much difference unless they are substantially greater than seems likely.

Evidence suggests that "the environment in which clinicians practice is the most important determinant of behavior" [4]. Of major importance are the use of reminders, identification of prevention needs for specific individuals, and easily available staff support for necessary follow-up, education, behavior change, and monitoring [4, 5, 6, 7]. These are all aspects of practice organization that may be the most amenable to incorporation.

The key to producing the necessary changes in the practice environment is to develop self-sustaining systems that will encourage, support and even require more appropriate physician and staff prevention behaviors [8, 9, 10, 11]. These systems must involve the physicians themselves, not only because of the unique respect patients accord physician advice, but because physicians are the focus of most patient encounters and usually have ultimate control over practice content (and management). The systems must also reinforce the necessary consistent processes of risk identification, motivation, support, follow-up, and reinforcement, which are essential to patient behavioral changes. In other words, the patient must feel the importance that the medical care system attaches to these changes by ensuring that every encounter possible is used to monitor and reinforce them.

Aside from the need to establish systems to support the physician's role in prevention, there is an equal need for these systems to facilitate the invaluable roles of support staff. If it is accepted that physicians are not motivated, trained, or economically appropriate to be the only source for the important tasks of prevention (screening, detailed teaching and behavior modification, providing follow-up and tracking), then it is important to establish systematic methods by which ancillary personnel (nurses, receptionists, and other staff) can play an important role in the process. It is equally important to ensure that physicians do not lose involvement and control over the activities they may delegate to others, including systems to make sure that patients periodically visit the physician for reevaluation of progress, remotivation, and modification of treatment plans.

These points can be more clearly understood by considering risk factors such as hypertension and diabetes, where there has probably been the most physician involvement and the most success in recent years. Aside from physician acceptance of the importance of controlling these conditions, the greatest advances in their control have probably stemmed from the availability of physician-acceptable treatment modalities (i.e., medications) and from the nearly universal systematic screening that takes place as a routine part of office encounters. On the other hand, physician practices are commonly criticized for underutilization of thorough education and behavioral change techniques as well as consistent follow-up, processes that require integration with other professionals and staff for effective action.

Finally it is important for physicians accustomed to one-on-one encounters to understand that it has been organization and a systems approach that has led to greater efficiency and effectiveness in some areas of medical practice and in most other types of business. Semmelweiss and Lister may have discovered the benefits of asepsis, but it was only many years later that this idea led to the phenomenal success of surgery when it became an organizational requirement with systematic application and reinforcement by hospital systems. Such organizational systems changes are not easy to introduce or sustain, particularly in medical practice [12, 13].

Although Ford may have been the father of the modern system of assembly line production, it was Deming and Juran who taught the Japanese to study and modify the systems of manufacturing so that great improvements in quality, efficiency, and work life could take place [14, 15, 16]. American industry, including many service-based businesses, and recently many health care organizations are now discovering the same principle. This chapter explains how to make process improvements in the systems of medical practice as applied to the prevention of cardiovascular disease. It builds on

and details the concepts introduced in a recent monograph [17].

Essential Processes of a Systematic Office Cardiovascular Risk Reduction Program

Although every practice should make its own decisions about the specific policies and procedures it wishes to use in its office prevention system, it is useful to consider these procedures in relation to the separate steps or processes needed to operate an integrated and effective program. To facilitate these decisions, this chapter provides specific alternative examples of and recommendations on how to conduct these processes in a practical way. Individual practices may choose other approaches or modifications to these processes for their own legitimate reasons.

In brief the processes that require specific decisions are the following:

- Screening
- Recording/chart labeling
- Rescreening
- Provider reminders
- Provider interventions
- Education/assistance
- Follow-up
- Outreach

The important considerations, options, and suggestions for each of these processes are discussed next. This discussion is followed by a brief description of an example patient encounter with the system and flow charts of that process.

Screening
WHO?
Our assumption is that at least every adult patient (age 18 and over) should be screened to identify CHD risk factors. Unlike adults, children normally have many required well-visits for screening, although many of the cardiovascular risk factors are either less prevalent or their meaning is more controversial than in adults. Individual practices may want to lower the gen-

eral age for this prevention system or to make use of the existing well-visits for those factors that they wish to screen and intervene in (see Chapter 16).

WHEN?

Our assumption is that the screening will focus on patients actually presenting to the office, although family members of patients found to be at risk may be advised to come in for screening. It has been customary to make use of complete examination visits for whatever risk screening is done, but we strongly advise against relying on that approach since it results in screening only a minority of the patients in any practice. In addition, patients who choose to come in for routine examinations are also more likely already to be aware of their risks and to have lower levels of risk.

If screening each patient seems too imposing, especially at the start when virtually all patients will not have been screened before, it may be necessary to use some approach to reduce this potential bottleneck. For example, one could screen only those patients with prescheduled appointments (i.e., not same-day appointments), those who are not in a hurry, or those who have appointments on the hour. Once most patients have had an initial screening, it is best to move to a system that includes screening as a part of every visit.

HOW?

The only way we know that does *not* work is to rely on the physicians to do the screening. They need to focus on the problem that brought the patient to the office and forget or lack time to consistently screen. Moreover, it is probably best to screen for all relevant risk factors simultaneously, a task done best by office staff.

There are at least three approaches to this initial complete screening, although rescreening at subsequent office visits will generally be done best as a part of the vital-signs measurement before the physician encounter.

- *Questions by the person taking vital signs,* probably using a form to remember everything to ask.

- *Questionnaire* completed by the patient, either in the waiting room or in the exam room. Figure 17-1 provides an example of such a questionnaire. Notice that it includes questions about family history, documentation of preexisting tests, and clarification of risk factors. The advantages of this approach are that the patient may be more honest about answers on a questionnaire and that it doesn't take up much office staff time.

- *Patient-interactive computer.* This has the advantages of the questionnaire, but it requires space and is expensive. However, it can provide in summary form consistent data about all the patients who have been screened, so interventions can be designed for the specific types of patients and risk factors found most commonly in that practice. It also facilitates tracking and follow-up and can include built-in programs to provide patient-specific education, risk appraisals, and instructions.

There are many existing programs for the computer approach. Computerized health risk appraisals that include computation of individualized estimates of the effect of a respondent's risks on survival are available from the Communicable Disease Center (CDC) in Atlanta.* McPhee has developed and tested a simpler program designed primarily to provide the physician with current risk factor patterns on individual patients [18]. Although this program was designed to identify cancer-screening needs, it could just as well be used for cardiovascular risk factors.

Regardless of which approach is used to identify risk factors from the patient's knowledge, it is obviously necessary to obtain additional information from the medical records and from tests in the office. For example, the patient's memory of when tests were last performed and exactly what the results were is not usually very reliable. It is usually necessary for the nurse to verify this information from the record (if it is contained there).

*Contact the Carter Center, Emory University, Atlanta, Georgia.

CARDIOVASCULAR RISK QUESTIONNAIRE

Name: _____   Date: _____

1. Have any close relatives (parents, grandparents, siblings, children) had any evidence of disease of the heart or blood vessels (high blood pressure, heart failure, heart attack, angina, blockage of the arteries, stroke, or aneurysm)? Please list below, and circle any disease/event with onset before the age of 55 years.

   Relative   Disease
   _____
   _____
   _____

2. Have any of your relatives had diabetes? _____ Yes _____ No

3. Have any of your relatives had high cholesterol? _____ Yes _____ No

4. Do you have any of the above problems (#1-#3)? _____ Yes _____ No

   If so, which ones? _____

5. Do you use tobacco? (If no, go to question #6) _____ Yes _____ No

   a. If so, what type? _____

   b. How much and how often? _____

   c. Have you tried to quit? _____ Yes _____ No

   How many times? _____

   What was the longest quit? _____

6. Did you ever use tobacco regularly? _____ Yes _____ No

   If so, when did you quit? _____

7. Do you know your cholesterol level? _____ Yes _____ No

   If so, what was the most recent reading? _____

8. Do you exercise regularly enough to sweat, three or more times a week? _____ Yes _____ No

   If not, how much and what type of exercise do you get? _____ When? _____

9. How much interest (1=lowest to 10=highest) do you have in changing your risk factors? (Tobacco use, high blood pressure, high cholesterol, overweight, lack of exercise) _____

   If more than one factor, which one do you most want to change? _____

Figure 17-1. Cardiovascular risk questionnaire form. (Source: Reproduced from Solberg LI, Kottke TE. Reducing your patients' cardiovascular risks through effective office visits. Kansas City, MO: AAFP, 1991, with permission from the American Academy of Family Physicians, 8880 Ward Parkway, Kansas City, MO 64114. This form may be reproduced or modified for use in patient care by an individual medical practice without permission. However, it may not be distributed or sold without the express written permission of the AAFP.)

Blood pressure and blood cholesterol levels must be measured during the visit. It is easy enough to measure the blood pressure as part of visit preparation; in most clinics this is already part of routine practice. Cholesterol measurement, however, is a much more complicated issue. If the patient has had a cholesterol level measured within the past five years and it was within acceptable limits, no repeat test is necessary. However, if the test was abnormal or was last performed more than 5 years ago, there must be some way to obtain a blood sample for cholesterol during the visit, ideally without the physician having to order it. The alternatives for the nurse are as follows:

- Draw the sample before the physician visit (this probably makes sense only if it is possible to do a finger prick for a capillary sample).
- Place a check on the fee slip or initiate an order slip (whichever is the usual way to order lab tests in the practice). The physician can then countermand the order if desired or can order any additional blood tests to be done at the same time (sparing the patient from two sample collections during one office visit).

In either case, it is helpful to have a card or paper that the nurse can give to the patient to explain why the test is being done and what can be expected for follow-up (see the example in Figure 17-2). This card standardizes the explanation and spares the nurse from having to take a lot of time to explain.

A suggested protocol for screening is diagrammed in Figure 17-6 on page 479.

Recording/Chart Labeling

Once the initial screening information has been collected, it is necessary to record it in such a way that the provider can quickly review it and that at subsequent visits office staff can quickly and easily determine whether initial screening has already taken place.

Both of these objectives can be achieved by inserting into the record either the computer printout or questionnaire used in screening or a separate form for maintaining a status report on risks. The latter form can be limited to the

---

NOKOMIS CLINIC

We believe your cholesterol level is an important measure of your risk of developing heart and blood vessel disease. Fortunately, you can reduce your risk by lowering your blood cholesterol if it's too high.

We would like to use a simple blood test today to measure your blood cholesterol. We will inform you of the result by postcard or phone call. If your cholesterol is higher than ideal, we will help you take steps to lower it.

Thank You
The Nokomis Clinic Physicians

Figure 17-2. Cholesterol test explanation. This form may be reproduced or modified for use in patient care by an individual medical practice without permission. However, it may not be distributed or sold without the express written permission of the AAFP. (Source: same as for Figure 17-1.)

---

cardiovascular risks discussed in this book or may include other risks and screening tests (e.g., seat belt use or cancer screens). Although using the initial screening form has appeal for simplicity, it is difficult to update, which usually means adding to it or replacing it with a new form at each rescreening. Therefore, we recommend having the nurse transfer the risk status information to a permanent risk form (see Figures 17-3, 17-4, and 17-6).

In addition to the risk form in the record, it helps office staff prepare for subsequent office visits if a discrete label or mark is affixed to the record to indicate that initial screening has taken place. If this mark includes the year, it also facilitates recognition of rescreening needs.

Rescreening

It is essential to keep the risk status information up to date; otherwise, it will be unreliable, un-

NAME_____   ©NOKOMIS CLINIC, Ltd.

PREVENTION CARD

ITEM	FREQ	STATUS									
		Prior	1987	1988	1989	1990	1991	1992	1993	1994	1995
✓ Health Evaluation											
Risk Appraisal											
Tobacco (#/day)	yearly										
Alcohol (#/day)	yearly										
Exercise (#/wk)	yearly										
Seat Belts (%)	yearly										
✓ Td	10 yrs										
Flu	yr. 65+										
✓ Blood Pressure	yearly										
✓ Weight	yearly										
Breast	yearly										
Pelvic											
✓ Cholesterol											
Stool Blood											
Pap											
Sigmoidoscopy											
Mammogram											

Figure 17-3.   Prevention card form. This form may be reproduced or modified for use in patient care by an individual medical practice without permission. However, it may not be distributed or sold without the express written permission of the authors.

CARDIOVASCULAR PROGRESS RECORD
(CPR)

For: _____
            Patient's Name

Personal Hx _____   Family Hx _____

Date						
Weight						
Blood Pressure						
Tobacco Use Amount						
Total Cholesterol						
HDL/LDL						
Triglycerides						
Exercise						
Diet						

Change in History						
Interest in Change						
Problems for Change						
Tobacco Category*						

Treatment Plan						
Educational Materials						
Follow-Up						
Return						
Provider						

* W = Winner (has quit)   H = Help needed to stop soon   N = No interest in quitting
  S = Stop on own soon   L = Later will quit, not now   O = Omitted discussion of quitting

Figure 17-4. Cardiovascular progress record (CPR). (Source: Reproduced from Solberg LI, Kottke TE. Reducing your patients' cardiovascular risks through effective office visits. Kansas City, MO: AAFP, 1991, with permission from the American Academy of Family Physicians, 8880 Ward Parkway, Kansas City, MO 64114. This form may be reproduced or modified for use in patient care by an individual medical practice without permission. However, it may not be distributed or sold without the express written permission of the AAFP.)

useful, and unused. Two types of rescreening need to be considered in the initial establishment of the system, and both are usually performed as part of preparing for the physician encounter. This is easily accomplished if the risk status form described above has been set up well. The types of rescreening are the following:

- *Review at each office visit.* The goal of this task is to see whether the patient has complied with recommended actions and follow-up plans from previous visits, e.g., noting at an acute visit for other problems that the patient had failed to return for a repeat test of an abnormal cholesterol level or for an appointment for dietary counseling. Again, the physician should not be relied on to do this review.
- *Periodic rescreening.* The goal of this task is to ensure that information about changeable risks is updated at whatever intervals the practice management decides are appropriate and practical. If different intervals are chosen for the various risk factors, the staff probably needs to use the shortest interval for the rescreening. For example, if it is decided that cholesterol levels should be checked every 5 years but smoking or exercise status every 2 years, it is probably easiest to review everything every two years. This should be done by repeating the approach used in the initial screening. (See Figure 17-6.) However the questions need to be phrased differently to reflect the fact that this is a follow-up. For a questionnaire example of rescreening, see Figure 17-5.

Providing Information to and Reminding the Provider at a Visit

It is necessary to have an explicit and obvious way to remind the physician during normal office visits of the need to make an issue of the patient's cardiovascular risks and to provide the physician with the information needed to effi-

---

**UPDATE SCREENING QUESTIONNAIRE
FOR CARDIOVASCULAR RISKS**

Name: _____ Date _____

   We are interested in learning whether there have been any changes in your cardiovascular risk factors since you were last screened for them with a questionnaire similar to this one in _____.

1. Since then, have you become aware of any additional close blood relatives who have developed diseases of the heart or blood vessels? Please list them and their ages: _____

_____

2. Have any close blood relatives been found to have diabetes or high cholesterol? _____

3. Have you developed any of the above problems? _____

4. Do you use tobacco? _____ If yes, how much? _____

5. How much exercise do you get? _____

6. In the last year, have you made any changes in exercise, diet, tobacco use, or stress levels? _____

Figure 17-5. Update screening questionnaire form. This form may be reproduced or modified for use in patient care by an individual medical practice without permission. However, it may not be distributed or sold without the express written permission of the authors.

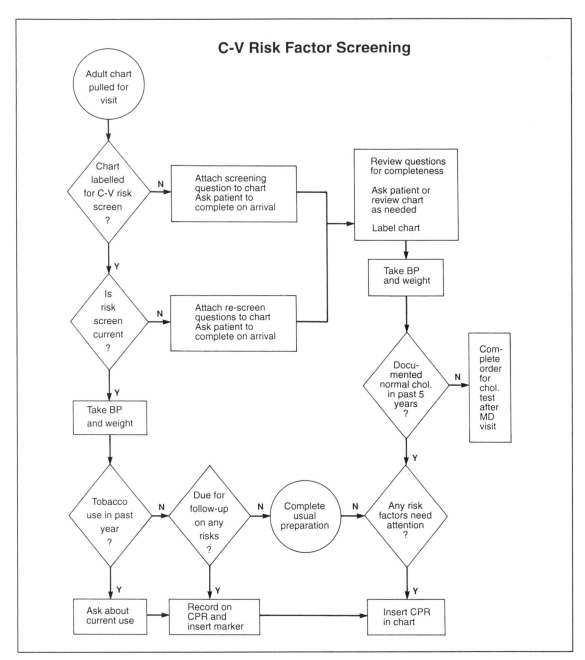

Figure 17-6.   Flow chart of risk factor screening. This form may be reproduced or modified for use in patient care by an individual medical practice without permission. However, it may not be distributed or sold without the express written permission of the authors.

ciently intervene in a maximum of 3 minutes. Although some physicians' practices or some less busy days may permit systems that require more time during a visit for other reasons, our experience has been that 3 minutes is the maximum time that most physicians are able to consistently add to visits for reasons other than those that initiated the visit. It is also clear that for the patient behavior change required for most of these cardiovascular risk factors to occur, it is essential for the physician (and staff) to evidence strong interest and to provide help by raising these issues at every possible opportunity.

These necessities, plus the physician's tendency to focus on the main purpose of the visit, require that a prominent (i.e., unavoidable) reminder be provided about any risk factors needing attention. The information needed by the physician for intervention must be very clear and not require looking through the chart to assemble what is needed for the encounter. The following alternatives are available to meet these requirements.

CHART LABELS

Chart labels help staff to know which patients need screening and rescreening, but they are not enough to catch the physician's attention. Existing labels, even of payment or smoking status, often are not seen (e.g., they may be covered by charge slips). In addition, such labels of a permanent status do not address the physician's need to know what is needed on that day's visit. Research studies have found temporaroy labels to be useful, but to prevent them from becoming obscured, they might need to be placed directly on the progress note for that day's visit.

CHART MARKERS

Colored markers (like long book marks) may be the best answer, particularly because they can be placed in that part of the chart in which the pertinent information is recorded, and they can be easily added, removed, or moved. Markers can be placed in the chart by the nurse during preparation as s/he notes that the physician needs to address some risk factor.

INFORMATION FORM

If the system uses an updated computer printout at each visit to summarize risk status, that printout on the chart cover or in the chart itself can also serve as a reminder. Similar forms filled out by hand are more difficult to use in this way since they will probably be permanently attached to the chart.

Regardless of which approach is chosen to address the need for reminding physicians, it is essential to have a summary form to provide the physician with all the information needed to perform intervention functions. Unless there is a computer terminal in every exam room or the system permits a computer-updated form to be given to the physician at every visit, the office needs to consider two paper alternatives.

SEPARATE PREVENTION CARD AND FLOW SHEET

The prevention card (see Figure 17-3) serves to quickly inform the physician about the most recent assessment of each risk factor as well as whether those results were within an acceptable range. The advantage of this system is that it permits the combination of cardiovascular risk factors with those for cancer and other problems. It is necessary, however, to have a flow sheet or progress summary sheet separate from the prevention card on which to follow the efforts to change or manage these risk factors, since it is difficult to construct one form that will accomplish both purposes. A flow sheet is needed for the following reasons:

- to quickly scan the current status of all risk factors that are being followed because they were problems
- to be able to easily compare serial data over time to understand what interventions were associated with success or problems in an individual patient
- to obtain the same types of data over time
- to facilitate communication and coordination between different physicians and between physicians and other providers

We have developed a specialized flow sheet for smoking that can be kept separate from the chart or in it [9] and that can also serve as a physician reminder by being attached to the outside of the chart during visits. It has worked very well for practices interested enough to make the effort to use it consistently. For multiple risk factors, however, it is probably necessary to go to separate forms, as described above, or to the combined form.

COMBINED FORM

The combined form — the cardiovascular prevention record (CPR) — is illustrated in Figure 17-4. It is intended to serve the functions of both prevention card and flow sheet for cardiovascular risks. Like the prevention card, the CPR is started by staff when a patient is first screened, and like the flow sheet, it is used by both staff and physicians to record in a summary way the key points needed to follow those problems. If more details are needed than can easily be noted on this form, a separate progress note is made. Most of the time, however, no separate note is necessary.

Regardless of which approach is taken, if these forms are kept current, the staff can easily determine if there is a risk factor that needs attention during that day's visit and flag the form/chart for the physician's attention. Some examples of the need for flagging are when the nurse notices any of the following:

- First screening identifies one or more risk factors.
- Rescreening indicates a new risk factor or redevelopment of an old one thought to have been resolved (e.g., patient has started smoking again).
- Smoking was stopped less than 1 year ago.
- The patient has not followed up on diagnosis or treatment recommended at a previous contact.
- Too much time has elapsed since a risk factor was last addressed.

Some of these nurse determinations are easier if the whole practice agrees on a general approach, so the staff person does not need to remember the unique wishes of a particular physician. For example, it can be stipulated that a diastolic pressure greater than 90 or a cholesterol level greater than 200 needs attention. In fact, the whole system benefits from having as much specific agreement and standardization as possible.

Provider Intervention

This section describes the activities performed by the physician during visits for reasons other than specific management of cardiovascular risk factors. Therefore, it focuses on what can be accomplished in the 3-minute interval described previously (probably all that will be regularly available as add-ons to visits for other reasons). It is understood that in visits specifically oriented toward risk factor modification more time can be devoted to such intervention. (For an in-depth discussion of physician-delivered intervention see Chapter 7.) The physician can accomplish the following objectives in this time period:

- Identify at least one outstanding risk to address. If the patient uses tobacco, that problem should usually be addressed since it is the single most important risk factor and since its change requires repeated reinforcement on as many occasions as possible.
- Convey clearly to the patient what the problem is and what changes are needed (e.g., dietary change for lipid problems).
- Maintain a supportive rather than a confrontational approach, accepting the patient's decisions while maintaining the importance of risk factor change. Avoid preaching and guilt-raising tactics and congratulate any positive changes.
- Focus on specific negotiated plans rather than on trying to persuade a patient to change an opinion.
- Make use of other staff and/or community resources and convey support for those people and programs.
- Provide self-help materials.
- Document patient interest and plans on the flow sheet.
- Be willing, if necessary, to avoid dealing with

many risk factors at once or to defer a complete response to any single risk factor until a later visit.

Figure 17-7 is a flow chart that diagrams this interaction.

Assistance with Education and Behavior Change

If the patient has a risk factor that requires medication (e.g., diabetes, hypertension), it is likely that the physician will need to be actively involved in follow-up visits. Even in these cases, however, it is possible to develop protocols that permit most of the follow-up visits to be performed by a nurse [19]. Moreover, patients seeing the physician for these problems usually require more time and detailed information than most physicians are able or willing to provide. Counseling about the specifics of problem solving for diets, medication use and side-effects, exercise programs, and smoking cessation barriers is often best delegated to a nonphysician staff person like a nurse or patient educator. However, the physician must always be active in the loop.

The flow sheet, or CPR, facilitates this shared care of these patients. So does a physician attitude of support for this arrangement. The counselor does need to undertake some assessment of the factors related to the problem at hand, partially by interview and partially by specialized questionnaires and forms such as those noted in the other chapters of this book.

Figure 17-7. Flow chart of provider/patient risk interaction. This form may be reproduced or modified for use in patient care by an individual medical practice without permission. However, it may not be distributed or sold without the express written permission of the authors.

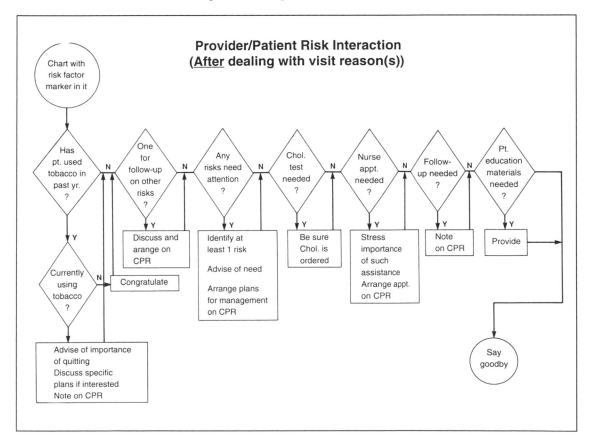

It is also necessary for the counselor to consider outreach to other family members for risk screening or involvement in helping the patient to make changes.

The specifics of counseling are beyond the scope of this chapter, but the focus should be on assisting patients to develop their own solutions to the problems faced in making change. Other important features of successful counseling involve expecting personal habits to change slowly and providing prolonged frequent follow-up. (See Chapter 7 on counseling.)

Some of these education and counseling goals can be met or facilitated by groups, either in the practice or through existing community groups. Many patients are not willing to use a group approach, however, and individualized visits will be necessary.

Follow-up

Two types of followup are important: after a critical visit and during normal visits for other reasons.

AFTER A CRITICAL VISIT

Follow-up after a critical visit is particularly important when a patient has recently quit smoking, has agreed to quit in the near future, or has agreed to take some specific action to lead to quitting. The best follow-up is to have a return visit with the physician. However, both physicians and patients seem reluctant to arrange this, so it may be nearly as helpful to have a system in place that ensures that the patient is contacted at the critical time by an office staff member. If the physician notes this on the flow sheet (CPR) and discusses it with the patient, the staff person can be alerted to schedule the call by a note on the charge slip or by flagging the chart for staff attention after the visit (perhaps by using a chart marker). The recently quit smoker should be called in 1 to 3 weeks and the promised quitter about 3 to 6 days after a planned quit date. The emphasis of the call should be on assessing how the task of quitting is going and whether additional help is needed. It also serves as a reminder of the physician's interest in the patient's risk factors.

With risk factors other than tobacco use, there may be less need for a prearranged follow-up, but individual patients may benefit from a call that can be arranged by the physician in much the same way if the flow sheet is marked clearly. In either case, when the patient has been called, it is important for the staff person to document that action on the flow sheet along with any new information about status or plans.

Figure 17-8 diagrams staff follow-up for both cholesterol results and the provider/patient interaction.

DURING ROUTINE VISITS

Since tracking patients to ensure that they have complied with recommended actions is expensive and makes many physicians uncomfortable, it is important to take advantage of every office visit to check on progress and compliance. Using the forms regularly and keeping them updated make this a relatively simple task for the office staff. When a chart is being prepared for a visit or when the patient is being placed in an examination room, it is easy to review the CPR (or equivalent) to see whether there is a need for updating risk screening or for reinvolving the physician in addressing change in some risk factor. Again, this can be highlighted for the physician by simply inserting the special chart marker.

Outreach

Although it is not customary for medical practices to look beyond the immediate patient, it is particularly important to be more proactive for the best management of the cardiovascular risks discussed in this book. There are at least two reasons for this: risk screening and risk management.

RISK SCREENING

Because genetics and/or a shared environment contribute to most cardiovascular risk factors, people who live with the patient are at greater risk of having the same problem. A patient who has been found to have cardiovascular risks should be advised to have other family members checked for the same risk factors (e.g., hypertension, hyperlipidemia). This good medical practice can also become a practice builder if

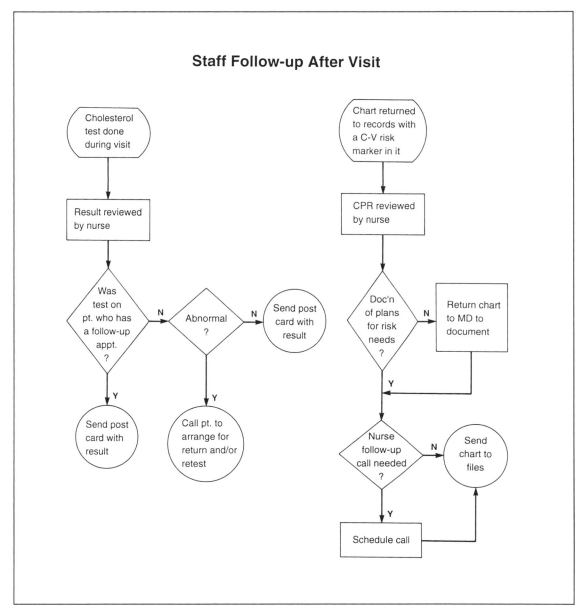

Staff Follow-up After Visit

Figure 17-8. Flow chart of follow–up by staff. This form may be reproduced or modified for use in patient care by an individual medical practice without permission. However, it may not be distributed or sold without the express written permission of the authors.

those family members do not already have a medical care relationship elsewhere. A form such as that shown in Figure 17-9 can be used to notify patients of their results.

RISK MANAGEMENT

Even if other family members do not have risk problems, the lifestyle changes required of the patient are often facilitated by having those who share diets or living space made aware of the patient's needs, as well as the ways in which they can be most supportive of the necessary changes. If they share the risk factor, it is particularly important that they at least cooperate with the person trying to make changes.

In either case, having a nonphysician counselor or staff person involved in the patients' care makes it more likely that these other individuals will become involved. For example, a patient who is planning to return for follow-up with the nurse can be requested to bring along other family members to the same appointment.

Finally, there is the issue of outreach to those in the community or practice population who are not regular users of medical services. The practice should consider advertising special risk-screening days or using signs, posters, and brochures in the office to encourage patients to have their family and friends screened as well. Undertaking a prevention program as an entire clinic or practice makes this type of action more feasible.

Example of the System in Action

Although each practice (clinic) will have its own variations in the way that it chooses to develop and implement the system of essential processes described here, it may be helpful to illustrate how one clinic implemented such a program, using visits by a hypothetical patient.

The Case of Mr. Jones

Mr. Jones is a 45-year-old manufacturing supervisor who is married and has three children, ages 15 to 20. He has become more concerned about his health since turning 40 but tends to go to the physician only when necessary. His father had a heart attack at age 58 and his father and grandmothers have hypertension. He smokes one pack of cigarettes a day, eats a fairly high-fat diet, is moderately overweight, gets almost no exercise, and considers himself stressed by work and his children. Although he has been told that he has mild hypertension, he usually has his blood pressure medicine refilled by phone, avoiding going to the physician as much as possible because he "doesn't have time." Although his physician told him once that he should quit smoking and lose weight, nothing more specific was offered or done, so he figures that it can't be that important.

One day (after his clinic had set up a system like that described here), Mr. Jones went in to be treated for a skin rash and was surprised at how differently he was treated.

The receptionist asked him to complete a short questionnaire (like Figure 17-1) while he was waiting to see the doctor.

As the nurse was getting him ready for the physician, she reviewed his completed questionnaire and his chart and showed him how she was recording all the cardiac risk factors he had on a special form in the chart (Figure 17-3). Since there was no indication that he had ever had his cholesterol measured, she told him that the physician would want that done after their visit, and she completed an order form for that test. Then she attached a red sticker to his chart, wrote the year on it, and left a big red book mark in the chart at the page of the CPR form (Figure 17-4).

After the physician took care of his rash, she said that she noted the chart marker, said that she was very concerned about his heart (without even listening to it), and pointed out all the risk factors he had. She indicated that it was very important that they work together to reduce these risks. Was he willing to work on stopping smoking, since that was clearly the most important changeable risk? And was he willing to schedule a return visit in the next few weeks with both the physician and her nurse to start work on these problems?

Although Mr. Jones was a bit shocked at this turn of events, he agreed that he would like to

Nokomis Clinic, Ltd.

During your recent clinic visit, your cholesterol was measured.

Your blood cholesterol level is:_____

☐ **This is a high level.** Please make an appointment soon with your physician and nurse. It is not possible to deal adequately with this problem by telephone.

☐ This is an acceptable level. *CONGRATULATIONS!* It should be rechecked in five years.

Comments: _____
_____

- -

=============== **Other Tests** ===============

The following other test results are also available now: _____

_____
_____
_____
_____

Those results that are circled are abnormal. You should do the following about them:

_____
_____

Figure 17-9. Cholesterol report postcard. This form may be reproduced or modified for use in patient care by an individual medical practice without permission. However, it may not be distributed or sold without the express written permission of the authors.

at least try to stop smoking and would make a return visit in the week after his promised quit date in two weeks.

He was given a booklet on smoking cessation and another on cardiac risk factors, had his blood tested for cholesterol level, and made his follow-up appointment (Figure 17-7).

Three days later, he received a phone call at work from a clinic nurse. She said that his cholesterol had come back high and they would be discussing this on his return visit. (She had known to do this because the lab technician had left her the chart, as was always done after screening cholesterols were completed, and the CPR had documented the previous plans) (Figure 17-8). Mr. Jones was especially impressed because he usually never heard about test results unless he called in.

At the next visit, the nurse asked him how his quitting smoking had gone (how did she know?) and even congratulated him when he reported that so far he had done it. Mr. Jones's physician congratulated him too, and they talked briefly about whether he needed any additional help. Then she told him that he had a number of other problems, none of which was terrible by itself, but that when taken together needed sustained attention. She said that the main first step was not new medications but to slowly change many of his lifestyle behaviors. To accomplish that, he would need to learn some things and to have help solving the problems confronting anyone making such changes. Since her nurse had the time, experience, and knowledge to best provide that learning and help, she wanted Mr. Jones to plan to meet with her (the nurse) three to six times before returning to the physician to reevaluate his situation. Since there was a possibility that his insurance wouldn't cover the necessary counseling and teaching, having the nurse provide them also made it possible for the costs to be lower. Then she introduced Mr. Jones to Nurse Smith.

Ms. Smith led him to her office and asked a lot of questions about his habits, his interest in making changes, support from his family, etc. She said that since his wife did much of the food shopping and preparation, it would be important for her to come with him to at least two

of the next visits. Besides, she said, his family would need to know what changes were necessary, how to be most helpful to him, and perhaps to have their own cardiac risks assessed.

Over the next year Mr. Jones gradually made many changes. He noticed that if he came to the office for other acute problems, the office staff and other physicians always seemed to know how he was doing, to ask about it, and to express their support, even when he made slips. And once when he missed a follow-up appointment, the need to make another was brought up when he came in later for an ankle injury.

Mr. Jones and his family were so impressed with the obvious importance that the whole clinic attached to these problems and the coordinated way in which they helped him that he realized the need to change and recommended the clinic to anyone who asked about where to get medical care.

Essential Processes to Initiate and Sustain the Program

Just as more traditional office systems (e.g., appointments, charging, lab tests) require that work and attention be devoted to setting up and maintaining those systems, the office that wants to have an efficient and effective cardiovascular risk reduction program needs to address the following processes to support that program [8, 11, 20]:

- policy establishment
- coordination
- implementation plan
- orientation and training
- resources
- evaluation and modification
- maintenance

Policy Establishment

It is not likely that the type of system described in the first half of this chapter will even be possible unless it is set up to include all (or at least most) of the physicians and all of the staff at a group practice. We and others have demonstrated that even the most dedicated physician will not be able to sustain a complex approach to patient care that involves cooperation from staff members and reminders to the physician unless it is set up as a deliberate clinic policy with support and attention from the practice as a whole.

There are several aspects to obtaining this necessary long-term policy and support.

FORMAL DECISION

In a one-physician practice all that is required is a commitment by that physician to establish such a program. However, groups larger than one or two physicians usually have a management body that meets regularly and makes policy decisions for the practice. This management body needs to decide whether such a program fits within the resources and priorities of the practice group and, if so, to formally establish it. It may be wise to decide first to set up a pilot program in one section or office of a large clinic, expanding it to the rest of the clinic if it proves to be feasible and successful.

SUPPORT

This program requires leadership with the authority to manage it. The people who will provide this leadership will need to be named and backed by the practice management. They will also require access to resources, including staff time. The management group must identify these people and resources.

FOLLOW-UP

At the time that the policy and support are identified, it is probably wise to also establish a regular interval for reports back to management on the progress and needs of the program (e.g., at every management meeting).

Coordination

As noted, the program needs leadership. Clinical programs like this one generally need both a physician coordinator and a staff coordinator. The reasons for each are suggested by the job descriptions for these people.

PHYSICIAN COORDINATOR

The responsibilities of the physician coordinator include the following duties:

- to obtain and maintain management support for the program
- to meet regularly with the staff coordinator to develop, assess, and modify the program, as well as to problem solve and develop strategies
- to orient other physicians and encourage their understanding and cooperation

STAFF COORDINATOR

The responsibilities of the staff coordinator include the following duties:

- to develop the original plan for specifics of the program and strategies for establishing it (with the physician coordinator)
- to prepare a written description of the program
- to order and maintain necessary supplies
- to plan and conduct necessary orientation, training, and retraining
- to conduct periodic evaluations and feedback
- to focus attention on the program and to keep spirits up about it until it becomes an automatic and permanent part of the practice

Even in small practices it is likely that the two coordinators will need more support in the form of a committee or task force, at least during the initial start-up phase. Such a group ideally should include a representative of each area that will be involved in the process (e.g., reception, medical records, lab).

Implementation Plan

Each of the seven essential program processes described above needs to be reviewed by the coordinating team to decide how best to implement those processes in that practice. As long as these process objectives are accomplished, there is no problem with modifying the way the process is performed to suit the desires and needs of the individual clinic. However, it is necessary to remember that whatever alternatives are developed must avoid relying on human memory as much as possible and must consider systematic ways of performing the tasks.

One good way of ensuring that the plan will be integrated and understandable is to start by constructing a flow chart of the whole process (like that in Figure 17-7). Once this is down on paper, it will be easier to change or simplify it, to identify the tasks and the people who will be involved, and to plan for training and resources. It is particularly important to be clear about the role of the physicians in this plan.

The final element in the plan is to set a date and place to begin implementation. If the organization is large, it is probably best first to establish a pilot test in one department, branch, or site. After that has run for a time and data have been collected about how the system is working, modifications can be made and the system expanded to other areas.

Orientation and Training
ORIENTATION
Everyone (physicians and staff) should have an opportunity to learn what is planned and why. This can usually be accomplished in a short general meeting or two. Participants will need an opportunity to ask questions and to see that modifications are made for significant problems or additions that they bring up.

TRAINING
Each person with a role/task in the system needs to learn exactly what he or she is expected to do. Since the staff know their jobs better than anyone else, this should be a two-way conversation with a chance to make changes if necessary. Ideally the system and tasks should be described in writing so they can be referred to in the future.

RETRAINING
After the system has been operating for a time and some evaluation data have been collected, needs for additional training will become apparent. Remember that as staff turnover occurs, it will be necessary to orient and train new people to the system as well as to the other aspects of their jobs. It is rarely a good idea to rely on

the new person's predecessor or coworker to conduct this training, since, as in the childhood game of telephone, the message becomes distorted as it is passed from one person to the next.

Resources
The materials needed for the system operation (questionnaires, chart markers, and forms) can be copied from those in this text or modified and printed to suit the desires of an individual clinic. Someone must take charge of that task as well as maintain supplies and reorder as needed. In addition, the materials need to be in the places where they will be accessible. Other materials — patient education booklets, posters, and signs — need to be created or ordered from the various sources noted throughout this book and stocks maintained. Finally, it is helpful to compile a list of referral resources for those patients who want or need programs or instruction not available in the clinic.

Evaluation and Readjustment
It is common to leave out the critical step of evaluation and readjustment in establishing any system, perhaps in the belief that it is too time-consuming to collect data about how the system is functioning. Just ask yourself how many times your office has started a new program, only to see it gradually decline into a state of dysfunction or disappearance. If you have invested the time and energy needed to get something started, isn't it worthwhile to spend a little more to ensure its continuance and improvement?

Without evaluation, feedback, and system modification, the weaknesses that can kill systems are allowed to survive and grow. Furthermore, without evaluation and feedback, much of what good systems are accomplishing often goes unnoticed and uncelebrated, thus robbing participants of the reinforcement to continue good work.

AUDIT
One simple but valuable evaluation tool is a survey of physicians and staff as to how the system is working and whether they are satis-

fied with it. It's only a little more trouble to include a few patients in this survey. Besides indicating how the system is working, such a survey also reminds everyone about it and tells them that someone thinks it is important. This survey can be done in person or with a few simple questions on paper.

Even more useful is collection of data on the functioning of the process and on its outcomes. This doesn't require a formal research project. If the data can't be gathered in 1 hour, the audit is probably unnecessarily complex. For example, a coordinator can look at 10 to 15 charts waiting to be refiled after visits and get a fairly good idea of the extent to which charts are being labeled, forms are being initiated by staff, and physicians are discussing and documenting risk factor management with those patients. Once there is a rough idea of whether various components of the system are being used, it can be decided whether additional, more detailed data need to be collected.

REACTION

Once some opinions and data have been gathered, the coordinating group can decide whether there is a need for modifications in the system, retraining of some individuals, asking for help, or simply allowing more time to pass. It is wise to build into the original plan some specific dates for this reassessment following collection of monitoring data.

REAUDIT

Whether modifications are made or not, there should be periodic repetitions of the audit process, followed by reassessments. Some would call this type of approach "closing the loop." In modern quality improvement jargon, this repeating cycle of *Plan-Do-Check-Act* is called the PDCA, or Shewhart, cycle after the man who described it as an essential part of the continuous quality improvement approach [15].

Maintenance

As suggested above, new programs or processes tend to decline unless either they have enormous reinforcement built into them or a lot of attention is paid to sustaining them until they have become institutionalized and part of the normal way of operating. The audit process discussed here is one way to reduce the likelihood of decline over time. However, there are other steps that should be taken.

FEEDBACK

Reporting the results of audits and surveys to individuals and to the group as a whole can attract attention to the system and emphasize its importance. In addition, by emphasizing successes, feedback can help to create a good aura surrounding the program.

SPIRIT BUILDING

The clinics that were able to sustain the Doctors Helping Smokers system were usually those that celebrated its presence in various ways. This can range from parties to T-shirt days (where everyone wears a special T-shirt associated with the program) to contests to community publicity.

Summary

Although the approach described above may sound complicated, it is necessary and easier than it may appear. The main incentive to undertake this approach is the realization that without it, important preventive services are simply not going to be provided consistently or effectively. A secondary incentive may be the understanding that if a clinic can introduce and maintain this system for cardiovascular risk factors, it can expand the system to include any other prevention activities it desires and have a model that can be applied to any other aspect of the clinic's activities. In that sense, it may very likely make the difference between a clinic that thrives or one that declines in the future.

References

1. Gemson DH, Elinson J. Prevention in primary care: variability in physician practice patterns in New York City. Am J Prev Med 1986; 2:226–34.
2. David AK, Bolt JS. A study of preventive health attitudes and behaviors in a family practice setting. J Fam Pract 1980; 11:77–84.

3. Henry RC, Ogle KS, Snellman LA. Preventive medicine: physician practices, beliefs, and perceived barriers for implementation. Fam Med 1987; 19:110–3.

4. Battista RN, Mickalide AD. Integration of preventive services into primary care: a conceptual framework for implementation. In: Goldbloom RB, Lawrence RS, eds. Preventing disease: beyond the rhetoric. New York: Springer, 1990; 466–73.

5. Pommerenke PA, Weed DL. Physician compliance: review and application to cancer detection and prevention. Am Fam Phys 1991; 43:560–8.

6. Inui TS, Belcher DW, Carter WB. Implementing preventive care in clinical practice. I. Organizational issues and strategies. Med Care Rev 1981; 38:129–54.

7. Belcher DW, Berg AO, Inui TS. Practical approaches to providing better preventive care: are physicians a problem or a solution? In: Battista RN, Lawrence RS, eds. Implementing preventive services. New York: Oxford University Press, 1988; 27–48.

8. Kottke TE, Solberg LI, Brekke ML. Beyond efficacy testing: introducing preventive cardiology into primary care. Am J Prev Med 1990; 6: suppl 1:77–83.

9. Kottke TE, Solberg LI, Brekke ML. Initiation and maintenance of patient behavioral change: what is the role of the physician? J Gen Int Med 1990; 5:Suppl:S62–7.

10. Solberg LI, Maxwell PL, Kottke TE, et al. A systematic primary care office-based smoking cessation program. J Fam Pract 1990; 6:747–54.

11. Kottke TE, Solberg LI, Brekke ML, Maxwell PL. Smoking cessation intervention strategies for the clinician. Qual Life Card Care 1990; 86–93.

12. Freeman WL. Implementing COPC: achieving change in a small organization. In: Nutting PA, ed. Community-oriented primary care: from principle to practice. U.S. Department of Health and Human Services, USDHHS publ. no. (HRSA)PE 86-1, 1987.

13. Tornatsky LG, Eveland JD, Boylan MG, et al. The process of technological innovation: reviewing the literature. National Science Foundation 1983; NSF 83-7.

14. Berwick DM. Continuous improvement as an ideal in health care. N Engl J Med 1989; 320:53–60.

15. Walton M. The Deming management method. New York: Dodd Mead, 1986.

16. Tufo HM, Rothwell MG, Frymoyer JW. Managing the quality of care for low back pain. In: Frymoyer JW, ed. The adult spine: principles and practice. New York: Raven, 1991.

17. Solberg LI, Kottke TE. Reducing your patients' cardiovascular risks through effective office visits. Kansas City, MO: AAFP, 1991.

18. McPhee SJ, Bird JA. Implementation of cancer prevention guidelines in clinical practice. J Gen Int Med 1990; 5:Suppl:S116-21.

19. Solberg LI, Johnson JM. Physician and nurse: a manual for collaboration. Minneapolis: University of Minnesota, 1981.

20. Solberg LI, Maxwell PL, Kottke TE, et al. Doctors helping smokers — an office manual. Minneapolis: University of Minnesota, 1989.

III

INTERVENTION: THE PUBLIC HEALTH PERSPECTIVE

18

Community Intervention and Advocacy

BETI THOMPSON
MICHAEL PERTSCHUK

EDITORS' INTRODUCTION

In this chapter and those that follow we expand our horizons beyond the individual physician–patient relationship and examine prevention of CHD from the perspective of the community. Physicians and other health care workers have considerable influence in their communities and can play an important role in the modification of risk factors on a large scale. In fact much of the accelerating pace of smoking and diet modification in this country has to do with changes occurring at work sites, in schools, and in public places. Individual change is made much easier when the environment in which one works or plays supports such change. In this chapter the authors describe the rationale for a community approach and the manner in which community change can be brought about. Of particular interest is a description of ways in which a physician can be a more effective advocate for community change — by working with the media and with political groups.

Technological advances and public health efforts have resulted in dramatic improvements in control of acute diseases, and thereby have increased life expectancy. While acute diseases are on the decline, however, the incident rates of many chronic diseases are increasing [1]. This is particularly true in the case of CHD, which in 1930 surpassed infectious diseases as the major cause of death in the United States [2, 3]. Although CHD mortality has declined since 1950, with two-thirds of the decrease occurring since 1970 [2, 3], CHD still accounts for 37 percent of deaths in the United States [3]. Rates of certain types of cancer are increasing, most notably lung cancer, which increased two- to fourfold for older male smokers (aged 49 and above) in the past 25 years and four- to sevenfold for older female smokers in the same time period, while there were no changes in lung cancer rates during that time for non-smokers [4]. Similarly breast cancer rates have increased 23 percent in the past fifteen years [5].

Much of the risk for chronic disease is behavioral and can be controlled. For example, the most important cancer risk factors are related to diet, smoking, and sexual behavior; these lifestyle behaviors account for up to 70 percent of all cancers [6, 7]. Lifestyle behaviors are similarly important in the prevention of CHD, much of which is attributed to the behavioral factors of diet, smoking, and uncontrolled hypertension [2, 7].

Changing behavioral factors can have a significant effect on disease morbidity and mortality. The decrease in CHD rates over the past three decades is attributed as much to modification of lifestyle behaviors as to improved treatment [2]; some studies suggest that risk factor modification accounts for more of the decrease [2, 8] (see Chapter 2). In terms of cancer reduction, the National Cancer Institute (NCI) estimates that a reduction in smoking prevalence to 15 percent could reduce cancer mortality by 8 to 15 percent by the year 2000 [9].

There is a long history of experimental studies designed to modify selected health risk behaviors. These experiments have largely followed a medical model, with individuals targeted for behavior change. Many lifestyle behaviors (e.g., diet, hypertension management, weight control) have been focal points for intervention, with efforts around smoking cessation providing a good example of the changing emphasis in such intervention campaigns. For both CHD and cancer a primary target of behavior change has been smoking cessation. In the more than 25 years since smoking has been recognized as a primary preventable cause of disease and death, numerous studies have been conducted on the best methods of assisting individual smokers in stopping their habit [10]. As a result many smoking cessation programs have been developed, with the majority focusing on clinical settings [11]. Similarly screening for hypertension has become standard practice for physicians; in addition, workplaces, health fairs, and other community organizations provide hypertension screening opportunities.

The success rates of such programs have been determined in randomized trials in which individuals are assigned to an intervention or to a comparison condition. Based on the difference in the targeted health behavior rates between the two groups, programs are assessed as being efficacious or not. The focus is on individual change. The efficacious programs, however, have not been very effective because they have not been able to reach large numbers of people. In general, such programs rely on volunteers to participate in small group sessions. Clinical programs are limited in the numbers of people that can be reached. In an attempt to expand the reach of efficacious interventions, smoking cessation programs have been applied at worksites; unfortunately the participation rates among smokers is quite small, with large worksites reporting participation by only 4 to 10 percent of their smokers [12]. These findings, along with evidence that long-term abstinence from smoking is rather low [13, 14], indicate that there are limitations to the ability of individually addressed smoking cessation programs to achieve large-scale reductions of smoking prevalence in the general population.

The past two decades have seen a change in the manner in which smoking is viewed. Increasingly, smoking is being perceived not as an individual problem but as a public health problem. One implication of this approach is that smoking control activities are expected to occur in many of the natural settings in which smokers congregate. Smoking control policies have been implemented in a variety of public and private places, including hospitals, worksites, schools, and restaurants. These settings also frequently provide venues for smoking cessation activities. Smoking control is no longer an individual matter but an activity that is pervasive in numerous and varied community channels [14].

Dietary habits also are no longer considered purely individual matters. The Food and Drug Administration and the U.S. Department of Agriculture have produced a report recommending food and nutrition labeling reform. This report has already become part of the rule-making process for regulation of the food industry [15]. As with smoking, a number of natural settings where eating occurs have taken actions that promote healthier diets. Many restaurants offer "heart healthy" choices, and a popular fast-food restaurant chain has introduced a lean hamburger. Other fast-food restaurants provide nutrition information for their products. Increasingly healthy food options are becoming integral to many natural settings.

In recognition of the need to involve diverse community channels, a relatively new orientation — a community approach — to widespread behavioral change around health risk behaviors has gained some prominence among health promotion researchers. A community approach has a greater capability to reach large numbers of people. Organizing an entire community around a health promotion project or effort necessarily involves more people than individual or small group recruitment activities. The reach is further enhanced when messages about the behavior change are widespread throughout the community, making it difficult to avoid exposure to change messages.

Community approaches involve various community individuals, groups, organizations, and institutions, providing a greater base for support of behavior change. Over time the un-

healthy behavior is no longer seen as merely an individual problem; rather, the community takes on some of the responsibility. Examples of this can be found in alcohol control projects, in which communities have organized themselves to use policy approaches to change the social and physical environment in which alcohol is made available. This extends the focus to include key factors external to the person as well as to individual variables. Most importantly, behavior change strategies can be integrated into the community and its institutions so that change endures over time. Interventions conducted through community groups and organizations are likely to become part of the community's resources and services.

This chapter provides an overview of community approaches to health promotion. Special attention is given to the role of the health care provider in community organizing for health promotion. The three major sections of this chapter include a rationale for a community approach to health promotion, followed by principles and examples of organizing communities for health promotion, and conclude with a section that defines appropriate roles and responsibilities of health care providers in community efforts.

Rationale for a Community Approach

The Social Context of Behavior

The public health model posits an interaction among the host (the recipient of an illness), the environment (the setting in which the illness occurs), and the agent (the cause of the illness). Health risk behaviors can fit into such a model. Smoking and poor dietary intake can be seen as agents of disease affecting the people who indulge in those habits. Another major principle linked to the public health perspective of behavior change is the recognition that behavior is greatly influenced by the environment in which it occurs. For example, the preponderance of fast-food restaurants with their generally high-fat products makes it easy to engage in poor dietary habits. The increasing number of smoke-free settings places constraints on smokers. Changing the specific health risk behavior without changing the environment may result in difficulty in maintaining behavior change, since an individual is likely to revert back to the undesired behavior when encountering familiar situations.

Cues and constraints related to health risk behavior can be accounted for by societal norms. Norms — shared rules and expectations for behavior [16] — produce a complex system of formal and informal guides for the appropriateness of specific behaviors. Norms are likely to vary over time and by locality. Individuals are greatly influenced by the normative environment in which their behaviors occur. Smoking provides good examples of this interaction between an individual and the environment. A smoker often responds to environmental cues when deciding to smoke or not to smoke. A work break, the end of a meal, and exiting from a smoke-free facility are examples of situations that provide cues to smoke, while attendance at a religious service or working in designated nonsmoking areas are examples of cues that inhibit smoking. Changing the environment in which people act involves changing the rules about acceptable behavior. For example, smoking prevalence is steadily decreasing as increasingly more public areas ban or restrict smoking [4, 17]. Similarly attention to the relationships between diet and disease have resulted in "official" recommendations to lower fat and increase fiber [7]. Many food products reinforce that standard by labeling their products as low in fat or cholesterol and high in fiber. The community approach to health promotion is cognizant of the importance of norms; indeed, the approach is based on the notion that long-term behavior change is best achieved by changing norms for the behavior.

Physicians have long been involved in norms around health promotion activities, both as advisers to individual patients and as public health advocates. Physicians are important policy makers in our society and have regular opportunities to offer health promotion messages to their patients, since the vast majority (76 percent) of people visit a physician annually [18]. In addition to the ability of physicians to affect individuals' health habits, they can be powerful proponents of health promotion activities. Through their professional associations, e.g., the American Medical Association (AMA), the American Academy of Family Physicians, physicians present a formidable lobby to persuade policy makers to approve policies to control tobacco use, promote hypertension and cholesterol screening, and provide labeling standards for food products. Other physician organizations, such as Doctors Ought to Care (DOC), regularly lobby at the national, state, and local level to restrict tobacco use. Physician involvement in health promotion can also be influential at the community level. The next section provides a conceptual framework for working with communities to effect widespread health-risk behavior change.

Conceptual Framework

The social environment within which behavior occurs can be viewed as a system with interdependent parts that act to maintain the environment. It is based on some degree of cooperation and consensus on social norms [19, 20]. The system includes many components, or subsystems, that carry out the activities required to keep the system viable. Among these subsystems are the political, economic, and educational institutions that ensure governance of, resources for, and socialization into the system (Figure 18-1). The system is more than the sum of its parts; rather, by combining the components and all the relationships among them, it becomes a unique structure [21]. Individuals who live within the system are subject to systemic norms and generally act within its normative context, including the manner in which they make choices about health-related behaviors.

Communities can be considered systems, and by being viewed as such, some insights for changing the environment that affects health behaviors are apparent. Social change may occur when parts of the system are in conflict or when they are no longer adequate to serve the needs of the constituents [22]. Similarly external effects or changes in the broader societal system (e.g., at the national level) can have an impact

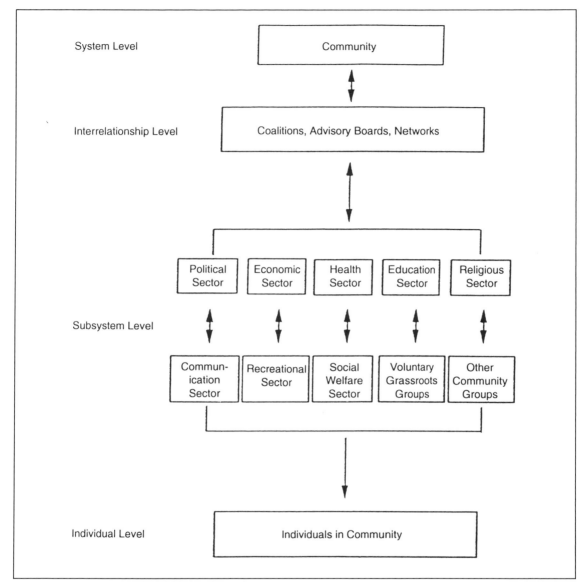

Figure 18-1.   A systems view of community.

on the local community system. In a systems perspective changes in any part of the system can be expected to reverberate throughout the system and result in adjustments or responses that will ultimately affect the entire system. Social norms change along with the system to provide new rules of conduct to help maintain the newly configured system [16].

Tobacco use provides a good example of emerging norms within a system. Recognition of the dangers of smoking and of inhaling second-hand smoke have led to restrictions in public smoking. As this secular trend accelerates, new rules for smoking must be developed, since smokers find it is no longer appropriate to light up in all settings. The effect of these changes is evident in many of the subsystems or components of the system, with some components pushing for tobacco use and others pushing against tobacco use.

Within the political subsystem the legal right of the tobacco industry to manufacture, sell, and advertise its products supports the rights of individuals to buy and use tobacco. Through such support, the tobacco industry can further develop and promote its products. In addition the tobacco industry has become expert in its utilization of the communication subsystem to relay messages about the acceptability of tobacco use [23, 24, 25, 26]. Finally, at an individual level, the addictive nature of tobacco [27] essentially guarantees that the tobacco industry will have a substantial number of consumers for its products. Addiction thus proves profitable and thereby involves the economic subsystem.

The pushes for continued use of tobacco are modified by forces that push against the use of tobacco. Despite its support for some aspects of tobacco use, the political sector has also acted to impose restrictions on tobacco use. Areas of particular impact include restraints in the distribution and promotion of tobacco products to minors [4, 28, 29]. The establishment of fairly high excise taxes on tobacco products has some effects on the economic sector; in addition, because cigarette taxes are considered "sin" taxes [30, 31], a message about the behavior is disseminated through the system. The economic sector may also affect the prevalence of smoking since estimates note about a 2-percent drop in adult smoking prevalence for every 8-cent increase per package of cigarettes [29, 32, 33]. Finally, the health sector has been instrumental in pushing against the use of tobacco by publishing thousands of studies linking tobacco use with disease.

Slowly systems at the national, state, and local levels are moving away from supporting continued tobacco use in favor of increasing restrictions on the use of tobacco products. Some of the ways in which this has been manifested include the restriction of tobacco advertising to nonelectronic media [34], the implementation of restrictions on smoking in public places in 41 states [35], the enactment of cigarette taxes by all states [4], and many local restrictions on tobacco sales and use [36].

These environmental changes have an effect on individual smoking habits. The release of the 1964 Surgeon General's Report on smoking, for example, was the beginning of a continuing decline in smoking prevalence [4]. The action by the Federal Communications Commission to create the fairness doctrine required equal-time advertisement for electronic antismoking messages to match prosmoking advertisements; there is some suggestion that this led to decreases in smoking prevalence [37]. The recent addition of numerous state acts restricting public smoking adds to the inconvenience of smoking, as does taxation, which, as previously discussed, appears to reduce prevalence.

As the forces toward restrictions of tobacco use multiply, a synergy develops among them. Synergy is the cooperation among various parts of the system or, more specifically, the way the components of the system relate to each other. When relations are oriented toward a common goal, the synergy makes the net effect of the forces together more than the sum of the parts. In the case of tobacco use the synergy of the various forces supporting tobacco restrictions should lead to a social norm that tobacco use is nonacceptable.

Dietary behavior is also likely to be influenced by emerging norms around both healthy eating and nutrition labeling. The 1988 Surgeon General's Report on Nutrition and Health [38] was a compilation of the many scientific studies that indicated that consumers were eating an unhealthy diet. The following year the National Research Council's report on reducing the risk of chronic disease through dietary change recommended dietary changes related to long-term health [39]. In 1990 the Institute of Medicine of the National Academy of Sciences released its report, requested by the government, recommending that nutrition labeling be made mandatory on packaged foods, that certain nutrient information be included on food labels, that standardized serving sizes be set, and that a comprehensive education program be launched to familiarize consumers with the labeling schemes to assist them in making wise food choices [40]. The political and health sectors are thus involved in effecting change around dietary habits.

The food industry, part of the economic sector, has taken advantage of the recommendations and is producing packaged foods that make claims to be cholesterol free, high in fiber, low in fat, and low in sodium. Consumers have responded to this new trend by demanding foods that are both convenient and healthful [15]. Unfortunately the vagaries of current food-labeling practices often leave consumers confused or with inadequate information [15].

As the push from the political and health sectors toward healthier food choices meets the interests of food manufacturers in the economic sector, there is likely to emerge a norm that requires not only accurate and complete food labeling but also public education concerning the content of food. This, in turn, is likely to lead to a greater awareness of the types of food purchased and consumed. The synergy among the three sectors — political, health, and economic — should lead to norms that promote healthier eating.

Within the conceptual framework of a systems orientation, there are general principles of community organization, as well as examples of studies that have utilized that strategy for health promotion activities. The next section reviews selected community studies and presents principles of community organization and partnership.

Organizing Communities for Health Promotion

Community Study Experiences

For the past 20 years increasing attention has been paid to community organization as a means of achieving large-scale change in both primary prevention and treatment of chronic health problems [41, 42, 43]. Experts have argued that community organization could change the community setting to support healthier lifestyles [41, 42, 43, 44]. That change would be translated to reductions in individuals' health-risk behavior, which in turn would lead to decreases in chronic disease morbidity and mortality.

In the past 15 years a number of major health-promotion initiatives have used a community approach to change behavior [45, 46, 47, 48, 49,

50, 51, 52]. Most of these efforts addressed multiple risk factors related to cardiovascular disease, with the goals of changing smoking, dietary, and screening behaviors. All described themselves as community projects and used different community institutions, organizations, groups, and individuals in the delivery of the interventions. Most emphasized public education through mass media, schools, and other organizations. The majority of these projects recognized the need to change the social context of their communities, arguing that the environment has a significant influence on facilitating or inhibiting the adoption of new behaviors [44, 50, 52, 53, 54, 55]. Community organization was seen as a means to achieve social context changes and normative changes.

Most large-scale health risk behavior interventions have been incorporated in multimodal health behavior change protocols aimed at lowering cardiovascular mortality and morbidity [56]. One of the best known large-scale American studies was the Multiple Risk Factor Intervention Trial (MRFIT) [57, 58], in which 12,866 men at high risk for CHD were randomized into special-intervention and usual-care groups. The intervention group received intensive efforts to modify CHD risk factors, including control of hypertension, blood cholesterol, and smoking. After 6 years, all risk factor levels were reduced substantially more in the intervention group [59]. A number of other large-scale studies (e.g., the Oslo study [60, 61], the Veterans Administration Study [62]) have examined the relationship between health risk behaviors and CHD. Although MRFIT and other CHD-control studies were large-scale, they were not community studies, since the interventions were targeted for a select group of high-risk adults that could not be related to a specific source population. Nevertheless, from those studies much was learned about a multiple risk factor approach that was subsequently applied to the new generation of community studies.

An early community trial was the Stanford Three-Community Study [54], in which the purpose of the research, as in the MRFIT trial, was to reduce cardiovascular risk. Three communities were assigned to media-only, to media and face-to-face intervention, or to control strategics. The results of the study indicated that it was possible to change a community's health behavior [54]. The Stanford Three-Community Study was encouraging for its results but very expensive in terms of time and resources for large-scale application. Subsequently three more such studies — the Stanford Five City Project, the Minnesota Heart Health Program (MHHP), and the Pawtucket Heart Health Program (PHHP) — were funded by the National Heart, Lung and Blood Institute (NHLBI) to further investigate the concept of changing behavior in an entire community. All three of these studies have utilized community organization techniques to ensure extensive participation by members of the communities. Early results from one of the projects, the Stanford Five City Project, indicate small changes in the overall cardiovascular risk factor behaviors in the community [63].

The Australian North Coast Program was similar to the Stanford Three-Community Study [64] in that it also emphasized cardiovascular health. Three towns were assigned to a control, a media-only, or a media plus community programs group. Media messages were given in three stages: to raise awareness, to give information, and to stimulate action. In the media plus community programs group, the community was organized to produce workshops, support systems, clinics, and other agencies to deliver smoking cessation programs, with physicians asked to disseminate self-help quit kits. In addition physical fitness and stress management were emphasized. Independent random samples of community residents suggest that behavior changes did occur on a community level.

The Swiss National Study [65] was also concerned with reducing cardiovascular risks. Communities in this study were randomized to intervention and control. In the intervention communities citizen groups were formed to integrate interventions for affecting health-related factors such as smoking, blood pressure, lipid levels, and exercise into existing community

structures. In addition, the media were used to promote programs, and public policy issues (e.g., no-smoking areas) were raised. A 4-year follow-up showed significant differences in cardiovascular risk factors. This study is notable for its utilization of existing resources and community infrastructure to achieve change.

The Finnish North Karelia Project [52, 66] is a well-evaluated long-term project with the primary goal of reducing cardiovascular risk factors. Two neighboring counties in Finland were nonrandomly assigned to treatment or control conditions. The treatment group received intensive intervention ranging from education and point-of-purchase advertising to televised demonstrations of how to reduce smoking, serum cholesterol, and hypertension. The project used community organization strategies and established a number of social support systems. The North Karelia study, though a nonrandomized trial, demonstrates the value of multichannel saturation. By the 10-year follow-up, men in the intervention group demonstrated a 28-percent decrease in smoking, a 3-percent decrease in mean serum cholesterol, a 3-percent decrease in systolic blood pressure, and a 1-percent decrease in mean diastolic blood pressure; all of the changes were statistically significant [52, 66]. The results of this program are very encouraging, especially its demonstration that intensive multimodal intervention can be effective.

The community studies reviewed here have a number of implications for other interventions. All the studies have addressed health behavior change in the context of cardiovascular risk factor modification. Although the actual rates vary with the specific studies, the results have been encouraging in that the significant differences in behaviors that were detected seem to be community-wide. The Stanford study showed that an extremely intensive intervention could achieve good results. The Australian study showed that less intensive intervention could also produce significant differences in behavior change. Both the Finnish and the Swiss studies have contributed greatly to our knowledge of community interventions since they deal with multimodal methods of achieving cardiovascular risk factor modification. All these studies, however, are limited by small numbers of communities or a lack of randomization. Even the three NHLBI heart health programs currently underway involve small numbers of communities and not all have randomized the communities, making it difficult to generalize results.

In summary past community studies have had some success in achieving health behavior change. More important they suggest that there is a great potential for community interventions, especially when those interventions are designed to tap into existing community structures and resources. The most cost-effective approach is one that uses existing community resources and structure to implement change. The MHHP study, for example, took 3 years to develop a system with community leaders to disseminate risk factor reduction information and programs within the community. The advantage of that approach, however, is that such a system will provide ongoing program delivery for an indefinite time; indeed, the majority of the MHHP activities were adopted by community groups and organizations when federal funding ended [67].

At least partly as a result of the increasing interest in community studies, it became necessary to develop firm theoretical underpinnings for the process of community organization, that is, the basic approach to organizing communities. These are reviewed in the next section.

Models of Community Organization

Effective community interventions must be based on strong theoretical underpinnings. Root [68], in a comment on the Symposium on Community Organization for the 1980s, notes that

The importance of community organizations in planning is nowhere more evident than in the case of providing community-based services. The hostility which has met efforts . . . has put service planners on notice that they must work with communities if they hope to introduce productive, community-based facilities (p. 14).

While Root recognized the need for the use of community organization theory in practice, Rothman notes that such theories are not easily identified [69, 70]. In an attempt to consolidate the literature, Rothman describes three different types of community organization methods. These are (1) the locality development method, (2) the social planning approach, and (3) the social action approach.

The *locality development model* proposes that community intervention is best achieved through the participation of a wide spectrum of people at the local community level in goal determination and action [69]. The *social planning approach* relies on expert planners to design plans to deliver services to members of the community. It differs from the locality development method in the extent to which community participation occurs; rather than enlisting the help of community leaders in decisions about project components, the intervention is placed on the community. The *social action approach* is oriented toward social justice for disadvantaged segments of the community. This approach is generally concerned with empowerment and resource redistribution. Rothman's threefold typology of community organization theory has been applied in a number of community studies [46, 50, 51].

Rothman acknowledges that his model proposes three ideal types and that in reality interventions are likely to include aspects of more than one type. In a recent update of his work, he urges change agents to be fully aware of the potential uses of all the models and to select the processes or parts of the model that may be successfully applied to the particular situation [71]. Physicians, for example, may be likely to use the social planning approach because of their status in the community; however, they could equally well be the catalyst for organizing a diverse group of community residents around an issue (locality development or social action). In sum, from a model perspective, there is no evidence that any one model is superior to another; therefore, the best approach is likely to be an eclectic one.

Community Partnership

Regardless of the type of model followed in the organizing of a community, a number of basic principles are critical to the success of any organizing effort. An important element of community organization is the establishment of partnership with the community. The principle of participation states that large-scale behavioral change requires the people heavily affected by a problem to be involved in defining the problem, planning and instituting steps to resolve the problem, and establishing structures to ensure that the desired change is maintained [43, 72, 73]. Ownership is closely related to the principle of participation and means that local people must have a sense of responsibility for and control over programs promoting change, so they will continue to support the programs after the initial organizing effort [69, 74, 75]. The basic premise underlying both the principles of participation and ownership is that change is more likely to be successful and permanent when the affected people are involved in initiating and promoting it. In addition to the general principles, a number of additional factors are important to the successful development of partnership. These tenets, which follow, are critical for effective and long-lasting community involvement.

COLLABORATION

The first "rule" is that it is important to have real collaboration, not merely representation. A true partnership means that the community members are involved in the whole project and have significant decision-making capability.

COMMUNITY STRUCTURES

It is also critical to build on existing community structures rather than replace them or add new structures, which are unlikely to be sustained after external funding expires. It is equally important to work with a community, not in competition with it or with agencies within it. It is unwise to create a structure that can be perceived as a threat to existing groups.

LONG-TERM PLANNING

To address a community problem requires long-term planning as opposed to short-term problem solving. For a long-term effect attention must be paid to underlying factors that influence behavior. For example, the task of educating smokers to help them to become nonsmokers is substantially easier when the community is structured to promote smoke-free environments. Smoke-free workplaces and public areas, widespread availability of cessation opportunities, and enforcement of rules restricting access to tobacco products by minors all contribute to reinforcing the basic smoke-free message and to strengthening educational efforts.

FACILITATING AND INHIBITING FACTORS

Another guideline requires that care be taken to recognize community inhibiting and facilitating factors to ensure that the solutions developed are suitable for a community. Communities differ in values, norms, and structures, and those differences are vital to the manner in which partnerships must be established and in which intervention activities are chosen. Similarly there may be unique opportunities in a community that will make community organization and interventions easier.

MULTIDIMENSIONAL ASPECT

The approach should be multidimensional, that is, it must involve all major community sectors in a variety of ways. It is insufficient to change a single sector of the community and expect the entire community to change. Similarly one activity in a community sector is not likely to have a widespread effect. For example, implementation of a restrictive worksite policy may push some smokers toward smoking cessation, but more are likely to quit if the policy is accompanied by readily available cessation programs, incentives to achieve cessation, and perhaps a friendly competition to encourage participation.

DIVERSE INVOLVEMENT

To establish a strong partnership, major components of a community must be involved, not just those groups already concerned with, say, the smoking problem. For a nonsmoking norm to spread to an entire community, representation of a target audience and others not historically involved in tobacco control must be solicited. In addition to spreading the influence of the partnership, such diverse involvement is more likely to have an effect on all the key sectors that are involved in cuing and constraining behavior.

SHARED RESPONSIBILITY

Finally, there must be shared responsibility for the problem, rather than defining it as a problem for a target group alone. It is now clear that many unhealthy behaviors affect many people, not merely those who engage in the behavior. Within the partnership there must be recognition that all parties must work together and take responsibility for addressing the problem.

Essential Features of Community Organizing

Given the conceptual framework and the principles underlying community organization, the next question is pragmatic: how can organizers help make change happen in a community? What are the premises for stimulating community change? Such stimulation requires the identification of a health promotion issue and the activation of community groups and individuals to deal with that issue. A basic plan for action follows and is depicted in Table 18-1.

UNDERSTANDING THE COMMUNITY

Stimulation for change requires that the organizers have a thorough understanding of the community. It is important to know the community through community analysis. This helps the organizers plan for appropriate contacts, coalitions, and task forces. Important areas of information about the community include demographic facts about the inhabitants, the kinds of political and economic systems that characterize the community, and the names of health-related organizations, educa-

Table 18-1. Essential features of community organizing

Community analysis
Geographic description
Demographic description
Local health behavior patterns
Community climate
Community culture
Community leadership
Local organizations
Unique factors

Community stimulation
Problem identification
Model for involvement
Information dissemination
Setting of priorities

Community advisory group
Select a model
Recruit members
Provide resources and assistance
Facilitate activities

Maintenance of change
Coordinate with existing structures
Plan for longevity
Facilitate maintenance activities

tional groups, and civic associations. The organizers must discover what religious and civic groups exist and how they fit into community life. It is also essential to identify sources of mass and local communication.

A number of community characteristics may inhibit or facilitate a community's ability to be stimulated and/or its willingness to accept change. Among these are (1) the complexity of the structures of the components of the community (e.g., accessibility to key individuals and the formality of organizational structures influences activation of specific organizations); (2) a sense of external control (are individuals or groups fatalistic or do they believe they can shape their worlds?); (3) involvement in community life (what are voting rates? membership rates? are there citizen boards? what kinds of informal involvement occur?); and (4) community reactions to issues (do groups or individuals support or ignore seatbelt laws, helmet laws, etc.?).

A community analysis can identify the important characteristics to be examined, and a force field analysis can identify restraining and driving forces that may affect the success of the community stimulation efforts.

COMMUNITY ANALYSIS

A community analysis is an invaluable tool in helping the organizers understand the community. Not only can it be used to identify facilitating and/or inhibiting conditions, it can also generally be used to characterize the community. Critical components of characterization include (1) a geographic description, (2) demographic description, (3) local health behavior patterns, (4) community climate, (5) community culture, (6) community leadership, (7) community organizations, and (8) any other components that may be unique to a particular community.

FORCE FIELD ANALYSIS

A force field analysis is a process in which all the facilitating and inhibiting forces acting on a desired change are identified and weighed in terms of their importance to achieving the change. Subsequently the forces are evaluated as to who, if anyone, has control over those items; then reasonable plans can be made regarding appropriate actions to be taken.

STIMULATION COMPONENTS

Once the community has been carefully characterized and a force field analysis has identified and rated facilitating and inhibiting forces, community stimulation for change can begin. Stimulation of the community is the process whereby the community is (1) made aware of a condition that exists within the community that has negative implications for the community; (2) identifies that condition as a priority for community action; (3) institutes steps to change the condition; and (4) establishes structures to ensure that the desired change is maintained.

Problem identification requires that the organizers make the community aware of the extent of the condition, the consequences resulting from the condition, and possible solutions. Awareness and consequences involve making

knowledge about the condition available to the community. It is vital that the community realize that solutions exist; without that realization, a community is unlikely to attempt to effect change.

The methods for imparting knowledge to the community vary by community and by segments within it. For example, in homogeneous communities with a single governing body, the best way to foster awareness may be a top-down approach. Community leaders and key influentials can be invited to participate in a series of informational seminars and meetings in which the condition, its consequences, and solutions are discussed by scientific experts and credible organizations. Heterogeneous communities, especially those with factions that distrust the governing body, may respond more favorably to a bottom-up approach. Meetings with members of grass-roots organizations, neighborhood coalitions, ethnic groups, and/or other small groups may provide the necessary involvement to gain momentum toward action from a number of diverse constituencies. In some communities it may be necessary to combine the approaches. The community analysis must be the tool by which the communities are appropriately characterized so that the approach used is the one that maximizes involvement for that community.

The manner in which the information is disseminated is only one part of the awareness process. The materials used to define the problem as an issue are also important. Techniques used in the past include community events (e.g., the Great American Smoke-out), competition (such as the Memphis weight-loss program and Quit-to-Win smoking cessation contests), media events (e.g., newspaper campaigns, television campaigns), and community meetings. A combination of all these is probably important for initial stimulation. Additional methods should be used if appropriate for particular communities.

Once the problem has been identified, the community must set priorities for tackling that problem. It is desirable for the community to establish some type of advisory board or coalition of community members to set goals and objectives for changing the condition. Since a basic premise of community organization is that the community "owns" the project, the organizers can have only limited input into this process.

Ideally the community advisory board should be representative of the various constituencies in the community. Organizers can use a number of options to facilitate the process of forming a board. Once there has been some activity in the community concerning the condition (e.g., newspaper articles, discussion at the city council or other community-wide group) the organizers can call a large, open town meeting in which volunteers are solicited to sit on such a board. Alternatively the organizers can attend a number of small group meetings and encourage representatives of those groups to network and bring pressure for an advisory board on governing bodies. A similar tactic could be taken for key community organizations that might be appropriate to spearhead a movement. Again, the actual methods to be used will vary by community and should be selected only after a careful community analysis.

After a mechanism is in place to set priorities for changing the community condition, the organizers must provide the community advisory board with the concrete assistance necessary to accomplish the community change. For changes in health behaviors, the community board and its subgroups need access to the latest theories and technologies for modifying risk behaviors. The organizers should provide a list of these resources and an evaluation of their efficacy to the community board. The community board can facilitate a network of communication among community agencies. In addition resources within the community must be identified and tapped to help provide health behavior change services.

The key role of the organizers at this stage is to be facilitators. The community advisory board must be brought into the structure of the entire project. It must be informed of the expectations of other project staff at the different organizational levels. A procedure for a working relationship must be established.

To ensure the longevity of the change, struc-tures to maintain the change must be built into or accessed in the community. For a smoking project, nonsmoking policies must be maintained; services to smokers attempting to quit must continue; referrals must be made for those experiencing relapse. For a hypertension control project, screening centers or activities must be maintained, follow-up systems for tracking people at risk must be instituted, and public education concerning the risks of hypertension must be ongoing. Again, the organizers must act as facilitators in this process and relay to the community those technologies and procedures that are most likely to be effective.

It is evident that the process of organizing a community for health promotion change presents a significant challenge in terms of time, energy, and other resources. It is a process that can only rarely be done by one individual; usually, groups of community people work in concert to achieve the goals of health promotion. The health care provider plays an important role in that process.

The Role of the Health Care Provider in Community Organizing

Health care providers are in unique positions to affect health behavior change. The vast majority (76 percent) of Americans report visiting a physician within the last year, with many of them (59 to 85 percent) reporting repeat visits within the year [1]. Even low-income and minority group members report high levels of physician visits within the past year (74 percent of people with a family income of less than $10,000 per year, 68 percent of Hispanics, and 73 percent of blacks) [1]. If all these patients were given routine advice and assistance regarding prevention of health risk behavior, the public health impact would be enormous [1, 18].

Individual Actions
EFFICACY OF PHYSICIAN INTERVENTION
Physician assistance has been demonstrated to be efficacious in the field of tobacco control. A review of 28 major physician trials around smoking cessation found that simple advice re-

sulted in smoking cessation rates of 5 to 10 percent, and those interventions that were more intensive (providing cessation materials, follow-up of decisions to quit) produced quit rates of 20 to 25 percent [10, 76]. The physician smoking cessation studies indicate that physicians can be instrumental in changing patients' health behaviors without consuming an inordinate amount of time [1]. Indeed, the NCI-initiated physician training program demonstrates that simple office procedures and physician messages (Table 18-2) are easily integrated into the majority of practices. The smoking cessation experience can be expanded to include other health risk behaviors. (See Chapter 7 for an overview of physician-delivered intervention and Chapter 17 for a discussion of setting up an office system to facilitate physician-delivered intervention.)

LOCAL EXPERTS
Health care providers can be local advocates in a number of areas. Where health risks pose problems for communities or for the public health, a local physician, dentist, or other health care professional can provide expert testimony as to the ill effects of such behaviors and may contribute to legislative efforts to control such behaviors. DOC members, for example, reg-

ularly testify as to the deleterious effects of billboard advertising of tobacco products on the youthful onset of tobacco use [24]. In a medium-sized community in the state of Washington, a pharmacist, concerned about alcohol and tobacco billboards, was instrumental in convincing the city council to ban all billboard advertising [77]. Because the opinions of health professionals are highly valued in this society, their voices are usually heard.

HEALTH CARE ENVIRONMENTS
Health professionals can also be influential by modifying the environments in which they practice. Hospitals and medical offices, for example, should be smoke-free. Materials on healthy behaviors should be available for patients. Wall posters advocating good dietary habits, exercise, nonsmoking, and hypertension control confirm the health professionals' commitment to healthy behaviors. Patients who encounter an environment that actively promotes good health and prohibits unhealthy behaviors (e.g., smoking) on the premises, who receive advice, counsel, and other assistance from the health care provider, and who are followed in terms of their progress in modifying health-risk behavior will receive a consistent message about the importance of behavior change.

Mandates of Health Professional Organizations
The role of the physician in regard to individual patients is critical to health behavior change; however, many other opportunities exist for physician involvement in influencing healthy behaviors. Health care providers can be influential policy makers and advocates in the promotion of health. That such activities are within the purview of the disciplines is seen in the proactive positions many health professional groups are adopting around health risk behaviors. The AMA, for example, has recognized smoking as a "serious health problem" since 1964 [78] and has advocated education around smoking since 1969 [79]. The American Dental Association as early as 1964 urged its membership to educate patients about tobacco use and recently hosted its first national dental sym-

---

Table 18-2.   Smoking cessation tips for health care providers

Office standards for patient smoking cessation
Select an office smoking-cessation coordinator.
Create a smoke-free office.
Identify all smoking patients.
Develop patient smoking-cessation plans.
Provide follow-up support.

Tips to help patients stop smoking
ASK about smoking at every opportunity.
ADVISE smokers to stop.
ASSIST patients in stopping by setting a quit date, providing self-help materials, and prescribing nicotine replacement therapy if indicated.
ARRANGE follow-up visits to foster maintenance and prevent relapse.

Source: Glynn TJ, Manley MW. How to help your patients stop smoking. National Cancer Institute, U.S. Department of Health and Human Services. USDHHS publ. no. (NIH) 89-3064, 1987.

posium on smoking cessation [80]. The American Pharmaceutical Association has recommended that pharmacies not sell tobacco products [81].

A number of health organizations have made recommmmendations concerning dietary behavior [15]. Two of the major health voluntary organizations, the American Cancer Society (ACS) and the American Heart Association (AHA), as well as the National Institutes of Health (NIH) have made dietary recommmmendations to the public. The AMA has consistently updated its recommmmendations on dietary behavior to reflect the increasing scientific base of information on diet and health relationships [82].

Community Actions
MEDIA ADVOCACY

There is little doubt that the mass media shape society's dominant health beliefs, attitudes, and behaviors. The news media inform, interpret, and help determine public policy agendas, including those that shape the environments in which health behaviors evolve. The media know the importance of a physician advocate for any commercial product. Similarly the media regard physicians as a potent resource. Examples abound in the area of tobacco control. Whether it is C. Everett Koop challenging the Tobacco Institute's denial of the addictive nature of smoking, Reed Tuckson, former health commissioner of Washington, D.C., challenging tobacco companies' targeting of inner city blacks and Hispanics with billboards promoting alcohol and tobacco, or Secretary of Health and Human Services Louis Sullivan taking a tobacco company to task for developing a product specifically for blacks, it is clear that physicians as advocates can be effective in calling attention to the promotion of such unhealthy behaviors.

Utilizing the media to call attention to either healthy or unhealthy behaviors has much promise as a force for change. Media advocates can use mass media as a resource for advancing a public health initiative (e.g., dietary change, hypertension screening, smoking cessation). Media advocacy takes an activist approach to the media, viewing media as resources to be

Table 18-3. Steps for media advocacy

Delivering the news
Controlled-message channels
    Letters to the editor
    Op-ed columns
    Public service announcements
    Paid advertisements
Uncontrolled-message channels
    Newspapers
    Radio
    Television
    Magazines

Approaching the media
Build media relationships.
Initiate stories.

Dealing with the media
Be flexible and spontaneous.
Seize the initiative.
Stay focused.
Make it local and relevant.
Make news.
Frame the issue.

aggressively pursued. Relatively simple steps can be followed to become a successful advocate (Table 18-3).

Delivering the News. Mass media are classified in many different ways, but for advocates it is useful to think of controlled and uncontrolled channels. *Controlled channels* can be used for messages that are developed by the advocate or targeted to a specific population; they take time to create, however, and may be expensive. Common channels for such messages include letters to the editor, opinion-editorial columns, public service announcements, and paid advertisements for radio, television, newspapers, and magazines. Table 18-4 provides some guidelines for producing pieces for free channels.

Uncontrolled channels are those that are operated by the media themselves, who provide access because they believe a story is newsworthy. These kinds of messages are likely to have high visibility and credibility. Two paths, hard news and soft news, provide access to uncontrolled channels. The *hard path* consists primarily of news coverage that is characterized by intramedia competition, controversy, and investigative reporting. The *soft path* provides access

Table 18-4. Guidelines for producing information for free channels

Make your point quickly.

Use statistics sparingly.

Use your position to give the letter credibility.

Avoid offensive or accusatory language.

Stay with one subject per letter.

Use recent newsworthy events as a hook.

Give enough background so the reader has pertinent information.

Be consistent if your group conducts a letter-writing campaign.

Avoid form letters.

Concentrate on local angles.

through the relatively new health or lifestyle sections of newspapers and health segments on electronic media. Hard news has more visibility, but soft news often contains more in-depth coverage of an issue.

Approaching the Media. A key factor in approaching the media is to build relationships with media representatives prior to the time when there is a story to be told. Meeting an investigative reporter over breakfast or lunch presents a good opportunity to acquaint the reporter with the advocate's general background and availability as a source of information on the issue. While it is a breach of journalistic ethics for reporters to openly support groups that have public causes, reporters rely on dependable sources for good, reliable news and information; therefore, reporters soon learn to go to the advocate for newsworthy comments related to stories about the cause. To be trusted by the media, it is important for the advocate not only to be credible but to appear credible by maintaining a professional appearance and demeanor in public.

As the list of media contacts grows, it is important to keep careful notes and records of the information given to particular reporters. In that way identification of news reporters who have or have not received background information on the story can be made, so the time spent with a news reporter on a particular story can be maximized.

When initiating a story, it is important for the advocate to provide three basic pieces of information to the news reporter: (1) what the story is; (2) why the story is significant; and (3) how the story can be independently verified. It is crucial to be absolutely honest in the information given; in addition, it is important to properly footnote or reference the material. A good avenue for disseminating information to news reporters is through news releases, which are an inexpensive method for making news available to the media and also convenient for the media. Table 18-5 summarizes some criteria for good press releases.

Dealing with the Media. A number of factors are critical in dealing with the media. The following guidelines will help an advocate use the media to best advantage.

- Be flexible, spontaneous, opportunistic, and creative. While it is necessary to be well-versed in a subject, it is also important to take advantage of breaking news and reframe it to benefit the public health cause. A news story on national mobilization to prevent a small number of deaths due to product tampering can provide an opportunity to note how lethargic the community is in confronting the hazards of alcohol.
- Seize the initiative and do not be intimidated. Public health media advocates have science and credibility on their side. Confidence and the willingness to engage the media aggressively lead to successful media advocacy.
- Stay focused on the issues. Arguments in media situations often lead to personal ani-

Table 18-5. Guidelines for news releases

Write as though you are the reporter — answer the questions of who, what, where, when, and how.

Write with clarity and conciseness but maintain an interesting angle.

Label your news releases for either immediate release or release at a different time.

Provide a contact name and telephone number.

Adhere to the favored news release format for the targeted outlets.

mosity and turn the discussion away from the issue. Staying calm and focused on public health disarms the opponent. Similarly keep responses short and to the point rather than long and complicated.

- Make it local and keep it relevant. National statistics are often meaningless to people within a community, but local statistics can be very persuasive. Local role models, not necessarily the advocate, should also be used to promote the public health cause.

- Make news. The media search for angles and hooks that make a story newsworthy; specific desirable characteristics include timeliness, local appeal, human interest, conflict, someone of prominence, unusual aspects, and the credibility of the source. Information must be presented in an interesting manner to appeal to reporters. For example, rather than speak about the total number of deaths associated with smoking in a year, the advocate might note how many people die of smoking-related diseases in one hour.

- Frame and seize the symbols of debate. While the health professional is accustomed to having science frame an issue, media compress facts and arguments into labels and symbols. Physicians who practice media advocacy can become adept in evoking affirmative societal symbols in arguing for healthy behaviors and policies. Building on values that are central to Americans, messages around individual autonomy, freedom from harmful environmental influences, physical strength and well-being, family welfare, and social accountability of those who market harmful products can be presented. The advocate must project positive symbols such as "medical defenders of community health," community health leaders, spokespersons for clean air, health scientists, and health advocates for infants, children, women, minorities, the family, and the poor. In building on such sumbols, advocates are perceived by the public as promoting solid American values.

The image of a health care provider as a media advocate is foreign to many physicians; however, with a little training and practice, the art of media advocacy can be mastered. Throughout this country, public health advocates — physicians prominent among them — have learned to work with the media. Some have begun to learn the art of media advocacy and have displayed great creativity in gaining access to the media and alerting and informing the public of health risks and policy implications. The public believes its health professionals, whether interacting with them personally or observing them through mass media; thus, health professionals have great potential as media advocates.

COLLABORATION WITH HEALTH VOLUNTARY GROUPS

At a minimum, physicians must advise and counsel patients on the hazards of unhealthy behaviors. Examples include providing advice on smoking cessation, hypertension screening and control, cholesterol screening, the benefits of exercise, and good dietary habits. Physicians who counsel their patients to change unhealthy behaviors must also be aware of available resources that may be useful to the patient in change attempts. The majority of communities in this country have health behavior change resources that are available either free or for little cost.

Selecting an organized program for assistance in changing health behaviors is often a highly individual matter. A host of for-profit dietary change programs are available in most communities. Similarly exercise opportunities range from local community-sponsored recreation activities to private health clubs. Physicians must become familiar with both the realm of available resources and an assessment of the relative value of each for a particular patient. In the smoking cessation area, for example, the cessation rate is fairly similar across program modalities; thus, the smoker's level of addiction and preference can be used to identify the most appropriate form of assistance. With an understanding of the patient's needs and a list of what is available, the physician can determine what modality the patient would prefer and benefit from and can then steer the patient to the appropriate cessation service provider.

By far the greatest effort to change unhealthy behaviors has been made by the three national major health voluntary organizations. These are the ACS, the American Lung Association (ALA), and the AHA. In 1964 the three voluntary organizations joined together to form the National Interagency Council on Smoking and Health to facilitate coordination of their activities around smoking control. While coordination has occurred, many of their efforts have also remained separate. In general the voluntary organizations stressed the public health education approach to disease control in the 1960s and the 1970s [4]. In the late 1970s and in the 1980s the voluntary organizations began supporting legislative movements such as the nonsmokers' rights movement and the trend toward health promotion at the worksite, and began marketing smoking policy and cessation services to businesses [4]. The ACS has focused attention on smoking cessation and breast cancer screening and recently has embarked on a program promoting dietary change. The ALA is actively involved in smoking cessation and prevention. The AHA has been extremely successful in making the public aware of the need for regular hypertension screening, as well as simple behavior changes (e.g., maintaining appropriate weight, exercising, reducing salt intake) that may help prevent hypertension. This group has also been active in informing the public of the need for cholesterol screening and monitoring.

Health professionals can become involved with the health voluntary groups in many ways. Physicians, for example, have participated in the ACS's Great American Smoke-out by organizing activities, staffing informational booths, and providing nicotine replacement therapy prescriptions for their smoking patients. Physicians have joined in "healthy heart" activities sponsored by the AHA by disseminating information, making presentations to groups at worksites, and sponsoring poster contests in schools that increase both youth and adult awareness of the importance of activities that are likely to prevent heart disease.

COORDINATION WITH OTHER COMMUNITY SECTORS

At least four community sectors provide opportunities for health care provider involvement (see Table 18-6). Within the political sector physicians and other health care providers can identify harmful health situations that need to be controlled. For example, they can press for ordinances restricting environmental pollution, the distribution of harmful substances, and access to controlled substances (e.g., tobacco and alcohol) by minors, as well as lobby for health promotion community resources (e.g., exercise trails, swimming pools, health care facilities).

The educational sector can benefit from health professional involvement. Presentations to students at all grade levels can point out the advantages of lifestyle behaviors that, if adopted in youth, can endure through adulthood. Presentations to colleagues can draw other health care providers into participation in communitywide health promotion activities. Finally, by practicing the health behaviors that are promoted, health care providers become good role models for youth to emulate.

Table 18-6. Physician roles for coordination with other community sectors

Sector	Role
Political	Identify harmful situations. Lobby for health promotion measures.
Educational	Make presentations to students. Make presentations to colleagues. Provide a good role model.
Economic	Lobby for financial incentives and reimbursement for health promotion counseling to patients.
Associations	Incorporate health promotion components in continuing medical education. Provide association support for community efforts.

Within the economic sector, health care providers can work toward the provision of financial incentives to promote healthy behavior. Some insurance companies, for example, already provide reduced rates for nonsmokers. Similar arguments can be made for extending insurance discounts to worksites that are smoke-free. Health insurance companies might also be lobbied to provide incentives for subscribers to participate in health promotion programs (e.g., reimbursement for smoking control, weight control, or exercise classes). Health care providers can also push for reimbursement for health promotion counseling given to patients.

Health care providers can play an active role in their local or regional associations by pushing for policies to incorporate health promotion components in continuing medical education seminars for all types of health care providers. Such associations may be convinced to support local community efforts (e.g., special health promotion events and activities) either by resolution, member involvement, or financial support.

Summary

Changing health-risk behaviors is no longer simply a matter of convincing individuals to change their behavior. While much progress has been made in individual interventions around behavior change, it is not likely to generate a large public health effect. For widespread and long-term change, it is necessary to involve large numbers of people in change activities. One way to do this is the community approach, wherein communities form partnerships with health professionals, scientists, or other researchers to address a public health problem. Past community studies support this type of approach.

A systems view of social change necessitates involving diverse community sectors in the change effort. Models of community organization for health promotion change emphasize outside involvement in different ways; nevertheless, all the models emphasize the importance of community partnership and ownership of the health promotion effort.

Community organizing for change requires a good understanding of the community. This can be achieved through a community analysis in which critical components of a community are characterized and assessed for their potential contribution to the health promotion effort. Once the community is understood, it must be stimulated to take action around health promotion.

Health care providers can take on many roles in a community effort for health promotion. As individual providers they can give efficacious advice and counseling to their patients, become local experts in health issues, and modify their facilities to reflect positive messages and environments for patients. At a community level health care providers can become media advocates for health promotion and collaborate with local, regional, or national health voluntary groups to promote their activities. In collaboration with other community services, health care providers can work with the political sector around ordinances to safeguard the public; with the educational sector, to inform the public; with the economic sector, to provide incentives to encourage healthy behaviors; and with their local or regional associations, to incorporate health promotion in ongoing activities.

By working in concert with communities, a great deal of interdependence and synergy is gained between the health care provider and the community. The interdependence between health professionals and community health promotion efforts occurs on two levels: the individual level and the societal level. Health professionals who see the devastating effects of health-risk behaviors depend on their patients to take actions that will preserve and maintain health. Patients depend on their physicians for advice and counseling about appropriate health behaviors. When individuals heed physician advice, health benefits are realized. The physician benefits from having a healthier clientele. At the societal level, physicians depend on social norms to reinforce healthy behaviors, while society as a whole benefits from a strong, influential group that works toward health promotion.

The synergistic effect of messages from health professionals, other health promotion activities, and the community is found in the repeated and pervasive messages to individuals to modify their behavior. In addition the health care environment promotes healthy behaviors as the community standard. To the extent that the environment expands beyond the health care setting, in part through political activities of health care provider groups and associations, community members are further cued to adopt healthy behaviors. As physicians' and other health care providers' advice and activities become normative medical practice, the societal norm around health promotion becomes stronger.

In conclusion health care providers are central to the health of the community. Their efficacy can expand beyond the clinic and contribute greatly to the overall health of the community. By becoming involved in a community organization effort around health promotion, health care providers serve their own, their community's, and society's interests.

References

1. Glynn TJ, Manley MW, Cullen JW, and Mayer WJ. Cancer prevention through physician intervention. Sem Oncol 1990; 17:1-7.
2. Levy RI. Causes of the decrease in cardiovascular mortality. Am J Cardiol 1984; 54:7C-13C.
3. Feinleib M. The magnitude and nature of the decrease in coronary heart disease mortality rate. Am J Cardiol 1984; 52:2-6C.
4. U.S. Department of Health and Human Services. Reducing the health consequences of smoking: 25 years of progress. A report of the Surgeon General. U.S. Department of Health and Human Services, Public Health Service, Centers for Disease Control, Center for Chronic Disease Prevention and Health Promotion, Office on Smoking and Health. USDHHS publ. no. (CDC) 89-8411, 1989.
5. U.S. Department of Health and Human Services. Cancer statistics review 1973-1986. U.S. Department of Health and Human Services, Public Health Service. USDHHS publ. no. (NIH) 89-2789, 1989.
6. Doll R, and Peto R. The causes of cancer: quantitative estimates of avoidable risks of cancer in the United States today. JNCI 1981; 66:1191-1303.
7. U.S. Department of Health and Human Services. The Surgeon General's report on nutrition and health. U.S. Department of Health and Human Services, Public Health Service. USDHHS publ. no. (PHS) 88-50210, 1988.
8. Levy RI, Moskowitz J. Cardiovascular research: decades of progress, a decade of promise. Science 1982; 217:121-9.
9. National Cancer Institute. Cancer control objectives for the nation: 1985-2000. U.S. Department of Health and Human Services, National Institutes of Health, National Cancer Institute. NCI monograph 2, 1986.
10. Schwartz JL. Review and evaluation of smoking cessation methods: the United States and Canada, U.S. Department of Health and Human Services, USDHHS publ. no. (NIH) 87-2940, 1987.
11. Lichtenstein E, Mermelstein R. Review of approaches to smoking treatment: behavior modification strategies. In: Matarazzo JD, Herd JA, Miller NE, and Weiss SM, eds. Behavioral health: a handbook of health enhancement and disease prevention. New York: Wiley, 1984; 695-712.
12. Omenn GS, Thompson B, Sexton et al. A randomized comparison of worksite-sponsored smoking cessation programs. Am J Prev Med 1988; 4:261-7.
13. Fiore MC, Novotny TE, Pierce JP, et al. Methods used to quit smoking in the United States: do cessation programs help? JAMA 1990; 263:2760-9.
14. U.S. Department of Health and Human Services. The health benefits of smoking cessation: A report of the Surgeon General. U.S. Department of Health and Human Services, Public Health Service, Centers for Disease Control, Center for Chronic Disease Prevention and Health Promotion, Office on Smoking and Health. USDHHS publ. no. (CDC) 90-8416, 1990.
15. Earl R, Porter DV, Wellman NS. Nutrition labeling: issues and directions for the 1990s. J Am Diet Assoc 1990; 90:1599-601.
16. Robertson I. Sociology. New York: Worth, 1977.
17. Bureau of National Affairs. Where there's smoke: problems and policies concerning smoking in the workplace. Washington, DC: Bureau of National Affairs, 1986.
18. Ockene JK. Physician-delivered interventions for smoking cessation: strategies for increasing effectiveness. Prev. Med. 1987; 16:723-37.
19. Ashby WR. General systems theory as a new discipline. General Systems 1958; 3:1-6.

20. Boulding KE. General systems theory — the skeleton of science. In: Shafritz J, Whitbeck P, eds. Classics of organization theory. Oak Park, IL: Moore, 1978; 121-31.

21. von Bertalanffy L. General systems theory: a critical review. General Systems 1962; 7:1-20.

22. Moore WE. Social change. Englewood Cliffs, NJ: Prentice-Hall, 1963.

23. Warner K. Selling smoke: cigarette advertising and public health. Presentation at the annual meeting of the American Public Health Association, October 1986.

24. Tye J, Warner K, Glantz S. Tobacco advertising and consumption: evidence of a causal relationship. J Public Health Policy 1987; 8:492-508.

25. White L. Merchants of death: the American tobacco industry. New York: Beech Tree Books, Morrow, 1988.

26. Leventhal H, Glynn K, and Fleming R. Is the smoking decision an informed choice? Effect of smoking risk factors on smoking beliefs. JAMA 1987; 257:3373-6.

27. U.S. Department of Health and Human Services. The health consequences of smoking: nicotine addiction. A report of the Surgeon General. U.S. Department of Health and Human Services, Public Health Service, Centers for Disease Control, Center for Chronic Disease Prevention and Health Promotion, Office on Smoking and Health. USDHHS publ. no. (CDC) 88-8406, 1988.

28. Tobacco-Free America Project. State legislated actions on tobacco issues. Washington, DC: Tobacco-Free America Project, October 1988.

29. DiFranza JR, Norwood BD, Garner DW, Tye JB. Legislative efforts to protect children from tobacco. JAMA 1987; 257:3387-9.

30. Harris JE. Increasing the federal excise tax on cigarettes. J Health Econ 1982; 1:117-20.

31. Tobacco Institute. Tax burden on tobacco. Washington, DC: Tobacco Institute, 1988.

32. Lewit EM, Coate D. The potential for using excise taxes to reduce smoking. J Health Econ 1982; 1:121-45.

33. Warner KE. Smoking and health implications of a change in the federal cigarette excise tax. JAMA 1986; 255:1028-32.

34. Whiteside T. Selling death: cigarette advertising and public health. New York: Liveright, 1971.

35. U.S. Department of Health and Human Services. The health consequences of involuntary smoking. A report of the Surgeon General. U.S. Department of Health and Human Services, Public Health Service, Centers for Disease Control. USDHHS publ. no. (CDC) 87-8398, 1986.

36. Pertschuk M, Shopland DR. Major local smoking ordinances in the United States. U.S. Department of Health and Human Services, Public Health Service, National Institutes of Health, National Cancer Institute. USDHHS publ. no. (NIH) 90-479, September 1989.

37. Warner K. Cigarette advertising and media coverage of smoking and health. New Eng J Med 1985; 312:384-8.

38. U.S. Department of Health and Human Services. The Surgeon General's report on nutrition and health. Washington, DC: Government Printing Office, 1988.

39. Food and Nutrition Board. Diet and health: implications for reducing chronic disease. Washington, DC: National Academy Press, 1989.

40. Porter DV, Earl RO, eds. Nutrition labeling: issues and directions for the 1990s. Report of the Committee on the Nutrition Components of Food Labeling. Food and Nutrition Board, Institute of Medicine. Washington, DC: National Academy Press, 1990.

41. Blackburn H. Research and demonstration projects in community cardiovascular disease prevention. J Public Health Policy 1983; 4:398-421.

42. Farquhar JW. The community-based model of lifestyle intervention trials. Am J Epidemiol 1978; 108:103-11.

43. Green LW. The theory of participation: a qualitative analysis of its expression in national and international health politics. Advances in health education and promotion. Vol. 1. Greenwich, CT: JAI Press, 1978; 211-36.

44. Green LW, Raeburn J. Contemporary developments in health promotion. In: Bracht N, ed. Health promotion at the community level. Newbury Park, CA: Sage, 1990; 29-44.

45. Abrams DB, Elder JP, Carleton RA, et al. Social learning principles for organizational health promotion: an integrated approach. In: Cataldo ME, Coates TJ, eds. Health and industry: a behavioral medicine perspective. New York: Wiley-Interscience Publications, 1986; 28-51.

46. Carlaw RW, Mittelmark MB, Bracht N, Luepker R. Organization for a community cardiovascular health program: experiences from the Minnesota Heart Health Program. Health Educ Q 1984; 11:243-52.

47. Cohen RY, Stunkard A, Felix MR. Measuring community change in disease prevention and health promotion. Prev Med 1986; 15:411-21.

48. Elder JP, McGraw SA, Abrams DB, et al. Organizational and community approaches to community-wide prevention of heart disease: the first two years of the Pawtucket Heart Health Program. Prev Med 1986; 15:107-17.

49. Farquhar JW, Fortmann SP, Maccoby N, et al. The Stanford Five-City Project: design and methods. Am J Epidemiol 1985; 122:323-34.

50. McAlister A, Puska P, Salonen JT, Toumilehto J, Koskela K. Theory and action for health pro-

motion: illustrations from the North Karelia Project. Am J Public Health 1982; 72:43-50.

51. Mittelmark MB, Luepker RV, Jacobs DR, et al. Education strategies of the Minnesota Heart Health Program. Prev Med 1986; 15:1-17.

52. Puska P, Nissinen A, Tuomilehto J, et al. The community-based strategy to prevent coronary heart disease: conclusions from the ten years of the North Karelia Project. Annu Rev of Public Health 1985; 6:147-93.

53. Tarlov AR, Kehrer BH, Hall DP, et al. Foundation work: the health promotion program of the Henry J Kaiser Family Foundation. Am J Health Promotion 1987; Fall:74-80.

54. Farquhar JW, Wood PD, Breitrose H, et al. Community education for cardiovascular health. Lancet 1977; 1:1192-5.

55. Farquhar JW, Maccoby N, Wood PD. Education and communication studies. In: Holland WW, Detels R, Knox G, eds. Oxford textbook of public health, vol. 3. Oxford: Oxford University Press, 1985; 207–21.

56. U.S. Department of Health and Human Services. The health consequences of smoking: cardiovascular disease. A report of the Surgeon General. U.S. Department of Health and Human Services, Public Health Service, Office of the Assistant Secretary for Health, Office on Smoking and Health. USDHHS publ. no. (PHS) 84-50204, 1984.

57. Hughes GH, Hymowitz N, Ockene JK, et al. The Multiple Risk Factor Intervention Trial (MRFIT). V. Intervention on smoking. Prev Med 1981; 10:476-500.

58. Kuller L, Neaton JD, Caggiula A, Falvo-Gerard L. Primary prevention of heart attacks: the Multiple Risk Factor Intervention Trial. Am J Epidem 1980; 112:185-99.

59. Cutler JA, Neaton JD, Hulley SB, et al. Coronary heart disease and all-causes mortality in the Multiple Risk Factor Intervention Trial: subgroup findings and comparisons with other trials. Prev Med 1985; 14:293-311.

60. Hjermann I, VelveByre K, Holme I, Leren P. Effect of diet and smoking intervention on the incidence of coronary heart disease: report from the Oslo Study group of a randomised trial in healthy men. Lancet 1981; 2:1303-10.

61. Holme I, Hjermann I, Helgeland A, Leren P. The Oslo Study: diet and antismoking advice. Additional results from a 5-year primary preventive trial in middle-aged men. Prev Med 1985; 14:279-92.

62. Dayton S, Pearce ML, Hashimoto S, et al. A controlled clinical trial of a diet high in unsaturated fat in preventing complications of atherosclerosis. Circulation 1969; 40:suppl 2:1-63.

63. Fortmann SP, Sinkleby MA, Flora JA, et al. Ef-

fect of long-term community health education on blood pressure and hypertension control: the Stanford Five-City Project. Am J Epidem 1990; 132:629-46.

64. Egger G, Fitzgerald W, Frape G, et al. Result of large scale media antismoking campaign in Australia: North Coast "Quit for Life" Programme. Br Med J 1983; 286:1125-8.

65. Gutzwiller F, Schweizer W. Intervention on smoking: an individual and collective challenge. In: Schettler FG, Gotto AM, Middethoff G, Haberniehr AJ, Jurutlea AJ, eds. Atherosclerosis: proceedings of the Sixth International Symposium. New York: Springer, 1983.

66. Puska P, Nissinen A, Salonen JT, Tuomilehto J. Ten years of the North Karelia Project. Results with community-based prevention of coronary heart disease. Scan J Soc Med 1983; 11(3):65-8.

67. Bracht N. Personal communication, 1990.

68. Root L. Theory, practice, and curriculum: issues emerging from the symposium on community organization for the 1980s. Soc Dev Issues 1981; 5:10-6.

69. Rothman J. Three models of community organization practice. In: Cox FM, Erlich JL, Rothman J, Tropman JE, eds. Strategies of community organization. Itasca, IL: F. E. Peacock, 1979; 86-102.

70. Rothman J, Erlich JL, Teresa JG. Changing organizations and community programs. Beverly Hills, CA: Sage, 1981.

71. Rothman J, Tropman JE. Models of community organization and macro practice perspectives: their mixing and their phasing. In: Cox FM, Erlich JL, Rothman J, Tropman JE, eds. Strategies of community organization: macro practice. 4th ed. Itasca, IL: F. E. Peacock, 1987.

72. Green LW, McAlister AL. Macro-intervention to support health behavior: some theoretical perspectives and practical reflections. Health Educ Q 1984; 11:322-39.

73. Vandevelde M. The semantics of participation. In: Kramer RM, Specht H, eds. Readings in community organization practice. 3rd ed. Englewood Cliffs, NJ: Prentice-Hall, 1983; 95-105.

74. Kahn S. A guide for grassroots leaders: organizing. New York: McGraw-Hill, 1982.

75. Kettner P, Daley JM, Nichols AW. Initiating change in organizations and communities: a macro practice model. Monterey, CA: Brooks/Cole, 1985.

76. Kottke TE, Battista RN, DiFriese GH, et al. Attributes of successful smoking cessation interventions in medical practice. JAMA 1988; 259:2883-9.

77. Goltz B. Personal communication, 1990.

78. Lundberg GD. In the AMA, policy follows science: a case history of tobacco. JAMA 1985; 253(20):3001-3.

79. Rosenberg J. The AMA tackles smoking: "a strong stand." NY State J Med 1983; 83:1363-5.

80. McCann D. Tobacco use and oral health. J Am Dent Assoc 1989; 118:19-25.

81. Smith MC, Fincham JE. The role of the pharmacists in smoking cessation counseling. University, MS: University of Mississippi, Department of Health Care Administration, 1989.

82. Council on Scientific Affairs. American Medical Association concepts of nutrition and health. JAMA 1979; 242:2335-8.

19

Worksite Intervention

GLORIAN SORENSEN
JAY HIMMELSTEIN

EDITORS' INTRODUCTION

Because much of our lives is spent working, the potential for the worksite to be an effective force for risk factor modification is great. Smoking policies, the food served in company cafeterias, and company-sponsored screening and fitness programs can all play important roles in promoting the goal of a population free of CHD. Increasingly businesses themselves are taking an active role in this process, as they perceive prevention as a way of holding down spiraling health care costs. In this chapter Drs. Sorensen and Himmelstein describe the advantages and disadvantages of using the worksite for health promotion and some of the particular problems that must be addressed.

With increasing numbers of businesses seeking to respond to rising health care costs, health care providers have found a new partner in their efforts to reduce the population risk of CHD. Worksites provide an opportunity to apply a variety of risk reduction approaches with adults not previously labeled as patients who may have limited contact with the medical establishment. In addition health promotion efforts can be tailored to the unique setting of each worksite. Seventy percent of adults between 18 and 65 years of age are employed [1]. Even a small intervention effect in this large segment of the population has the potential to produce substantial changes in health behaviors associated with increased risk of CHD in the employed population [2, 3]. This target population includes many individuals with low income and education levels who may not be reached through other intervention channels. Interventions addressing multiple risk-related behaviors, such as smoking, diet, and exercise, can be offered in worksites repeatedly over time, thus increasing the likelihood of motivating change in persons who are at various points of readiness for such change [4].

The worksite also provides a vehicle for helping individuals to reduce CHD risk through changes in the work organization and environment. For example, CHD risk may be reduced by eliminating or reducing exposures to certain hazardous substances or work conditions [5]. Risk of CHD has also been associated with high job demands and a lack of control over job decisions [6, 7]; redesigning jobs and the structure of the work organization may be a viable means of risk reduction. Restrictions on smoking in the workplace can reduce exposure to environmental tobacco smoke for smokers and nonsmokers alike and also provide support to smokers for quitting smoking [8, 9]. Such changes in the environment may also influence the social norms influencing health-related behaviors, thus facilitating behavior change [10].

This chapter examines approaches that health care providers can use in the worksite to promote the reduction of CHD risk. Assessment and planning are the necessary first steps in responding to the unique needs of each worksite setting. The effectiveness of these efforts can be enhanced by participation of workers and management. We describe three major elements of a comprehensive corporate health program, similar to those described by Walsh [11], including medical care aimed at the individual, public health strategies aimed at modifying the exposures and health outcomes of groups of workers, and management approaches aimed at the organization. We also discuss how these intervention efforts can be integrated into a worksite's overall approach to health and safety. Throughout this chapter we seek to introduce the health care professional to the context and culture of the worksite, which holds substantial potential as a site for interventions to reduce CHD risk.

Health Promotion in the Worksite

The number of health promotion programs in worksites has increased in recent years. Most of these programs are aimed at individual behavior change. Results of the first National Survey of Worksite Health Promotion Activities found that 65.5 percent of responding worksites had one or more types of health promotion activity [12]. Overall prevalence by type of activity showed the most common type of program to be smoking cessation (36 percent), followed by health risk assessment (30 percent), back problem and back care (29 percent), stress management (27 percent), exercise/fitness (22 percent), on-the-job accident prevention (20 percent), nutrition education (17 percent), blood pressure treatment and control (17 percent), and weight control (15 percent). The frequency of these activities increased with worksite size and varied by industry type.

Health promotion objectives are generally compatible with worksites' long-term goals of survival, profitability, and productivity [13]. With the growing cost of health care, worksites may view health promotion efforts as a mechanism to reduce costs associated with absenteeism, insurance claims, and disability [14]. Few systematic studies have provided evidence that health promotion is a cost-effective means of decreasing health care costs [15], although the evidence for tangible benefits is beginning to accumulate. A recent study conducted at the Du Pont Company compared 41 intervention sites and 19 control sites with 29,315 and 14,573 hourly employees, respectively. Over 2 years blue-collar employees at intervention sites experienced a 14-percent decline in disability days compared to a 5.8-percent drop in control sites. Savings due to lower disability costs at intervention sites offset program costs in the first year and provided a return of $2.05 for every dollar invested in the program by the end of the second year [16]. Similar results have been reported by others [17, 18, 19, 20].

Recent evidence also suggests that a comprehensive health promotion program may have other benefits for employers, including improved attitudes of employees toward the company and lowered health care costs. The Johnson & Johnson Live for Life Program provides a case in point. Four Johnson & Johnson companies offered the Live for Life Program, which targets the entire worksite population as well as the worksite environment. Three Johnson & Johnson companies acted as a control group and offered employees only an annual health screen. Compared to the attitudes of employees in the control companies, there were significant improvements in the attitudes of employees of companies that received the health promotion program, including attitudes about organizational commitment, supervision, working conditions, job competence, pay and fringe benefits, and job security [21]. In addition this study, based on all employees at the site and not just participants, also showed significant reductions in corporate health benefits costs and utilization for inpatient services [22]. The mean annual per-capita in-patient cost over 5 years increased significantly less in the sites receiving the health promotion programs than in the comparison sites. Health promotion sites also had smaller increases in hospital days and admissions, although there were no significant reductions in outpatient or other health costs. Similar results were found by Blue Cross-Blue Shield of Indiana [18, 23, 24].

Employers' priorities may lead them to perceive a variety of benefits from health promotion and education programs. For some employers, the major motivation for sponsoring health promotion efforts may be the potential savings that result from healthier employee lifestyles; in such cases, accurate estimates of cost savings can improve the program's chances of adoption [25]. Other employers may be interested primarily in programs as a means to improve employee morale or the company's public image and may be especially responsive to employee requests when offering programs [26]. Prospective employees may be attracted to the worksite as a place of employment by the availability of health education programs.

Health promotion programs offered at the worksite also offer several distinct advantages to the employee. Such programs are accessible and convenient, may cost less than programs sought elsewhere, and offer the advantage of attempting health behavior changes with the support of coworkers [25].

A major obstacle to the success of programs aimed exclusively at the individual is their lack of attention to conditions in the work environment and in the structure of work that are also associated with increased CHD risk. This chapter presents a model for health promotion that builds on these programs aimed primarily at individual risk reduction and individual behavior change. Integrating such programs into a more comprehensive strategy of changes in the worksite organization and environment has several distinct advantages.

Barriers to Worksite Health Promotion Efforts

A thorough analysis of the worksite can inform providers of potential pitfalls to avoid [13, 14] (Table 19-1). Several barriers may exist from the management perspective. Some managers may think that health promotion is outside the mission of their organization or that reduced risk of CHD and other chronic diseases is an unlikely result of changes in either health behaviors or the worksite environment. Other managers may be concerned about the potential consequences of programs, believing, for ex-

Table 19-1.   Advantages of and barriers to worksite health promotion

Advantages	Barriers
For the employer	
• Possible improved employee morale and productivity	• Resistance to change and other management attitudes
• Possible reduction in health care costs	• Concern about potential consequences
• Enhanced recruitment and retention of employees	• Participation costs
• Corporate image	• Competing priorities
For the employee	
• Access and convenience	• Perceived inappropriate interference in personal life
• Reduced cost	• Confidentiality
• Participation with co-workers	• Diversion of attention from competing issues
• Social and environmental support for behavior change	• Release time and other logistics of program delivery
For the provider	
• Access to large numbers of people	• Logistics of program delivery
• Ability to target underserved groups	
• Opportunity for long-term, repeated interventions	
• Social support for the intervention message	
• Possibility of changes in the environment and in social norms	

Source: Sorensen, Glasgow, Corbett [25].

ample, that health programs or policies would provide only negligible economic benefits or would increase conflict between management and employees. Others may be concerned that spending work time on health issues diminishes productivity or that such programs are not worth their cost.

Competing priorities present another barrier to health promotion efforts. These include other health-related programs or company concerns with economic stability or labor issues. Employers may also be willing to promote individual health behavior change but unwilling to consider the important accompanying changes in the worksite environment and organizational structure [25]. Health care providers can play an important role in addressing these barriers by educating employers about the benefits of health promotion and alternative strategies for incorporating health promotion efforts into long-term corporate goals. Understanding

these obstacles can also be useful in tailoring programs to the individual work setting.

Employees may also perceive barriers to health promotion and education efforts. For example, some employees may view health behaviors as issues of private concern outside management's purview. Some workers have expressed concern that health promotion efforts may divert attention from occupational health issues, particulary worksite hazards perceived as more serious to worker safety [27, 28]. These concerns underline the importance of integrating efforts aimed at individual change with simultaneous changes in the worksite organization and environment. Workers also need assurance of the confidentiality of individual medical records. Inconvenient timing and location of program offerings often reduces participation rates; this potential problem can be prevented by effective planning [25].

Unions and the workers they represent typically have been quite supportive of some efforts to promote worker health within the worksite while resistant to other efforts. A priority for unions is the reduction of potential worker exposure to hazardous substances or work conditions, factors often beyond the control of the individual worker. In their efforts to protect the health of the labor force, they may seek to increase employer responsibility and liability for worker health. Unions sometimes are less supportive of program or policy efforts aimed at changing individual health behaviors that may be perceived as outside the employer's mandate [25, 28, 29]. For this reason union participation in setting the agenda for the health issues to be addressed in the worksite and in decision making about any health promotion and health protection effort is crucial to the success of these programs [30].

Additional challenges to health promotion and health protection programs result from the organizational structure specific to the workplace. As would be expected, businesses and organizations are structured in a manner that attempts to maximize profits for owners and stockholders. In general, health promotion and health protection are not seen as profit centers within an organization, and managers responsible for these areas are usually not in positions of power. Those responsible for health promotion or health protection in any particular workplace usually are patched in to an already existing organizational structure. For example, a nurse involved in health promotion often reports to the personnel department and has little opportunity to make an impact on organizational change. Frequently a safety officer or others responsible for health protection report to an engineering department and also have quality control obligations. A combination of inefficient reporting relationships and lack of decision-making power by those responsible for health promotion and health protection programs may limit their impact in the workplace [31]. By building a strong interdisciplinary team, it may be possible to garner the support of decision makers from different areas within the organization.

In summary health care providers can provide leadership as worksites seek to address barriers to health promotion efforts. For management they can translate the benefits of health promotion into means to achieve other corporate goals. Ultimately the effectiveness of health promotion programs depends as well on responding to employee and union concerns. The health care provider along with other influential people at a worksite can help to facilitate employee and union participation in planning, promoting, and implementing health promotion efforts.

The Health Care Provider and Worksite Interventions

The health care provider can play a crucial role in the planning, implementation, and maintenance of health promotion and education programs in the worksite. To be most effective, the provider must consider public health functions and management interventions in addition to the provision of medical care to individuals. However, health care providers frequently have little training in these areas and must, therefore, work as part of a multidisciplinary team to achieve these goals.

The members of the health team vary from worksite to worksite. The organization of this team also may differ, although a similar structure is often observed. Larger workplaces with more than 1000 employees are likely to have a plant medical department consisting of a consulting physician, nurses, and allied health personnel who deal with a full range of health care problems. In these situations the medical department may be responsible for the development and delivery of health promotion programs. Traditionally the medical department is part of the personnel and benefits department within the organization.

Responsibility for control of workplace exposures to chemicals and physical hazards usually belongs to the safety department, which often consists of safety specialists and industrial hygienists, professionals responsible for compliance with health and safety regulations in the workplace. The safety department frequently reports to plant engineering, making coordination with the medical department somewhat cumbersome. Larger corporations may also have a corporate function responsible for the overall coordination of benefits, including specialists in health insurance and disability coverage. Thus, larger companies may employ in-house most of the multidisciplinary team needed for delivery of comprehensive approaches to worksite risk reduction. The organization of this team within the worksite, however, seldom facilitates an effective coordinated effort with shared goals.

Indeed, such an organized effort for offering comprehensive approaches to health promotion and protection is likely to be found only in the largest of corporations. More often these functions are fragmented or nonexistent. This is especially true at worksites that employ fewer than 250 workers. Approximately 35 percent of U.S. workers are employed at worksites with fewer than 500 employees [32], worksites that usually lack comprehensive approaches to health and safety. For these worksites medical care may be delivered by a part-time contract physician, local emergency departments, or free-standing clinics, or it may not be offered at all. In these situations there may be no medical input on a managerial level, and a public health perspective for the worksite may never have been addressed.

Smaller companies provide additional challenges because they often use more informal decision-making and communication processes than do larger companies. As a result health promotion programs, if offered, often are inconsistent and fragmented and focus only on individual change. Cholesterol screening, for example, may be offered without available medical follow-up and without any other environmental supports for changing nutritional patterns. Smoking cessation information may be available, but there may be little support for restricting smoking in the workplace.

In smaller companies, therefore, it is necessary for health care providers to think expansively about their potential role in the worksite and to involve others to develop a multidisciplinary team for the design and implementation of worksite health promotion programs. In general this team should include health care providers currently involved in the worksite (e.g., the plant nurse), in-house staff responsible for safety and personnel, a representative from upper-level management who can ensure that management-level interventions can be implemented, and representatives from the workforce. In addition community health nurses, local hospitals, and representatives from voluntary organizations such as the American Cancer Society (ACS) and the American Heart Association (AHA) may provide valuable assistance in program content and follow-up. In this team context, it is the health care providers' responsibility to ensure the accuracy of program content and to follow through on detected risk factors or newly diagnosed cardiovascular disease.

In summary, CHD prevention in worksites requires a collaborative effort among physicians, other health care providers in the company, if available, and representatives of other company departments. The health care provider's role is likely to depend on the size of the worksite and the types of roles filled by others in the company.

Theoretical Perspectives on the Process of Health Behavior Change

The effectiveness of worksite health promotion and education efforts can be enhanced by incorporating principles from a variety of theoretical perspectives. (Chapter 7 describes theories of individual change, and Chapter 18 describes public health approaches.) Several theoretical models have particular relevance to worksite interventions, as described briefly here, including community organization, social learning, social marketing, and diffusion of innovations.

Community organizing strategies provide methods for adapting a given intervention model to an individual worksite by involving workers in the planning process, in setting priorities, and in making decisions about the intervention [33,

34, 35]. The tailoring of the program to fit the needs of the worksite can best be achieved when both workers and management participate in planning and implementing the program from the very beginning [36]. Through this process, it is possible to build worksite "ownership" of health promotion efforts and the worksite's capacity to carry out programs, thereby enhancing the likelihood that programs are maintained over time [37].

Social learning theory provides an important underpinning to many aspects of health promotion and education efforts [38, 39, 40]. (See Chapter 7 for an in-depth discussion of this theory.) One of the principles of this theory, termed *reciprocal determinism,* notes that personal factors and the environment interact in a reciprocal and interactive manner to influence behavior [41]. Following the concept of reciprocal determinism, a supportive environment can be established through promotion of environmental changes such as policies that restrict smoking or encourage labeling of healthy foods in cafeterias. When individual changes are implemented with support from changes in the environment, they are more likely to be maintained [42]. Effective health education programs depend as well on the personal factors that affect behavior, including an individual's ability to symbolize the meanings of behavior, to foresee the outcomes of behavior patterns, to learn by observation, to self-regulate behavior, and to analyze and influence personal experiences [38].

Several other key concepts influence the development of worksite health promotion efforts. Worksite representatives can be taught skills to implement the program themselves. Development of such skills will increase their perceived self-efficacy, that is, the confidence they have in themselves to perform the necessary activity to implement the program. Health care providers can provide training in such skills, or they can help worksite representatives find other sources for learning outside the workplace. Role models are another important source of information for developing self-efficacy. Role models can be observed through programs such as group classes or contests, or

they can be members of a worker planning committee. Health care providers can model desired behaviors, facilitate changes in the worksite environment that support health behavior changes, and support workers' feelings of self-efficacy related to these changes.

Social marketing principles are increasingly being applied in worksite health education endeavors. Social marketing experts stress the need to communicate incentives for or benefits of adopting the desired behavior that build on the existing motives, needs, and values of the target group. Commercial marketers have long understood that people are more likely to attend to and remember messages that meet their needs or that support values in which they believe [43, 44]. The key for the health care provider, then, is to define the benefits of the desired behavior. These benefits can be identified by a thorough analysis of the targeted audience [45]. The experience of commercial advertisers makes clear that, in many cases, a health promotion program should emphasize benefits that are not related to health per se but to universal and more salient human desires for acceptance, security, or status. In addition, pretesting of intervention materials to assess the concepts, message content, design, and distribution strategies is likely to enhance their effectiveness during full-scale implementation [46].

The *diffusion of innovations model* suggests that a variety of factors influence whether an individual or organization adopts, implements, and maintains an innovation such as a health behavior or a health promotion program [47, 48, 49]. These factors that influence the fit between the organization and the innovation include the extent to which the innovation is consistent with the past experience and values of the adopting individual or organization, organizational support for the innovation, the difficulty and complexity of implementing the innovation, its cost, and the extent to which the innovation can be tried on a limited basis or adapted to the setting. Thus, according to the diffusion theory, an innovation is not adopted at the same time by all adopters [50]. By understanding the characteristics of early adopters, health care providers can direct early intervention messages toward this target group. Early adopters are likely to encourage others to adopt the innovation. Later messages can then be tailored with that target audience in mind.

Figure 19-1 incorporates key elements from these theoretical perspectives [39, 51]. Intervention efforts are aimed simultaneously at individuals, groups, and the worksite environment, thus providing multiple supports for behavioral and organizational changes. By applying community organization strategies, health care providers can work with others at the worksite to organize and mobilize employees in planning, promoting, and implementing interventions. In addition, behavior change strategies are designed to accelerate the process of change for individuals at various stages of readiness for behavior change and thus target promotion, action, and maintenance of behavior change. Figure 19-1 can be used as a checklist to make sure that a comprehensive program addresses the concerns of persons in various stages of their readiness to make changes. For some activities several boxes may be checked. For example, a health fair may motivate some employees to think about making dietary changes while also

providing social support for changes others have already initiated.

Implementing Health Promotion and Education Efforts in Worksites

Three steps should be considered in the process of implementing health promotion and education efforts in worksites. First, an assessment of the worksite is conducted to identify the needs, concerns, and culture of the worksite that may affect program and policy adoption. Second, on the basis of this assessment, the program is planned and promoted, with participation from diverse sectors in the worksite. Third, programs are implemented that target individuals, groups, and the worksite environment/organization. Program maintenance strategies are discussed as part of each step.

Assessment of the Worksite

A worksite can be viewed as a small community with its own corporate culture and ways of getting things done. For health promotion efforts to succeed, the factors unique to each worksite setting need to be taken into account in estab-

Figure 19-1. Theoretical model for worksite intervention. (Adapted from Abrams, Elder, Carleton, et al. [39] and Lefebre, Flora [45].)

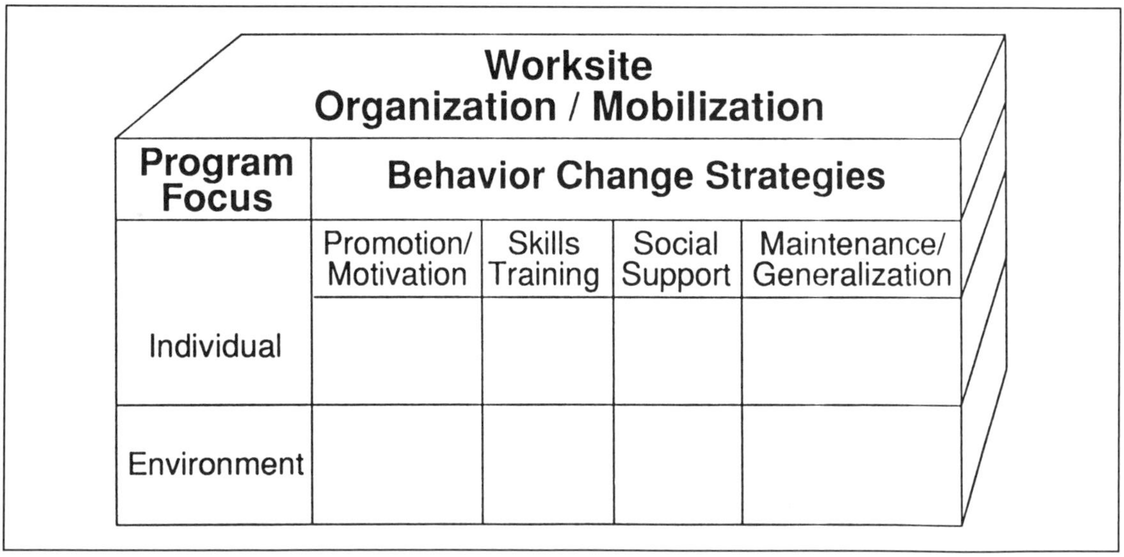

Program Focus	Behavior Change Strategies			
	Promotion/ Motivation	Skills Training	Social Support	Maintenance/ Generalization
Individual				
Environment				

Worksite Organization / Mobilization

lishing priorities, planning and implementing programs, and initiating policies and practices that influence worker health.

The techniques used to assess the problems and needs of a worksite in relation to disease prevention are analogous to those used by clinicians to evaluate and treat individual patients. The problem-oriented medical record (POMR), pioneered by Weed [52], structured the method that clinicians use to collect and analyze data about patients' medical problems. His SOAP approach described four stages for data collection and analysis. *Subjective* data about the problem are collected by interviewing the patient and other sources. *Objective* data are collected through the clinician's own observations and through laboratory or other testing. Based on the subjective and objective data, an initial *assessment* is made of the patient's problem(s). Finally *plans* are made for each identified problem. These plans may include specific treatments, further data collection, or scheduling follow-up evaluations. A similar approach can be applied with the worksite as "patient." Of course, the problem that is diagnosed in this case is not a disease; rather, the worksite's priorities and concerns are identified to lay the foundation for effective health promotion efforts. Using this familiar strategy may provide a useful tool for clinicians to gain an understanding of the unique needs of the worksite setting.

SUBJECTIVE DATA

Subjective data are likely to include interviews with key contacts such as the plant manager, the personnel manager, the union president, the shop steward, and on-site health care providers. The provider needs to know the level of interest and concern about cardiovascular disease in the particular workplace, the competing priorities the worksite is seeking to address, and worker and management perceptions about health promotion and protection in general. For example, do the representatives see heart disease as an important problem? Have they lost employees to cardiovascular impairment or premature death? What do they think about workplace-based programs? Have previous programs been implemented for health promotion? Were they satisfied with the results of these programs? These interviews also provide an opportunity to learn more about positions of authority and decision-making processes in a particular worksite, information vital for the planning and implementation phases. The worksite analysis should also provide information about the potential barriers to implementing a program in a given worksite.

Surveys of employees can be an additional source of subjective data. Surveys can provide information about employee needs and priorities, assess the worksite culture and receptivity to health promotion efforts, and be used as a baseline measure for later evaluations of program effectiveness. To ensure that the survey provides an unbiased view of the worksite, it should be distributed to a representative sample of all employees or to all employees, rather than to a group of volunteers who are willing to complete it. A high response rate can best be achieved if the survey has the endorsement of both labor leaders and upper-level management and if it assures confidentiality of the responses [25].

OBJECTIVE DATA

Objective data can provide additional direction for health promotion planning. Objective data can be used to assess medical care costs and health care utilization, evaluate potentially hazardous situations and substances in the workplace, identify resources available for health promotion and protection, and analyze the business and organizational climate that may assist in tailoring health promotion activities to the context of the particular worksite.

Medical care costs and utilization rates collected from archival sources can identify priority areas to address in a health promotion program. These data can also provide important information about the effects of the program once it is initiated. A review of medical costs and utilization data may illustrate the absolute magnitude of costs and cost trends and highlight those conditions that account for a disproportionate share of costs. Further analysis may identify groups (e.g., employees versus their families) that account for a substantial share of medical care costs and the medical benefits that are used most often. Health data are an indicator of the health- and illness-inducing conditions within the work setting as a whole [53]. This information can also set expectations about whether a health promotion program might realistically be able to affect medical care costs.

It is important to keep in mind that while insurance data may provide some useful information, they are often difficult to obtain and sometimes difficult to interpret [14]. For example, health insurance information does not always separate employee from dependent costs. Furthermore, the occurrence of conditions with long latency periods, such as cancer and CHD, might not reflect current exposure or future incidence. Some worksites may also choose to examine the rates of absenteeism, tardiness, and turnover but should keep in mind that these outcomes may be determined by factors other than those that can be changed through health promotion efforts.

An assessment of potential occupational hazards includes determining the presence of hazardous substances, as through a review of material safety data sheets; an assessment of the potential for exposure, including where hazardous substances are used, the number of workers potentially exposed, and the potential routes for exposure; and an evaluation of workers' knowledge of the application of safe practices and procedures. A workplace walkthrough can be conducted to assess the general working environment. Occupational hazards are generally classified into physical, chemical, psychologic, and biologic hazards. Potential physical hazards include noise, heavy material handling, and extremes of environmental temperature. The presence or absence of physical hazards may have considerable implications for health promotion programs. For example, the adoption of an exercise program is more relevant where workers are employed in a well-controlled and comfortable environment with no physical stress than where individuals are working at their maximum metabolic expenditure 8 hours a day. Environmental temperature extremes

may place additional stress on the heart, especially in those situations where people already have coronary disease. Similarly numerous chemical hazards have been associated with the development of both cancer and CHD. Identification of the use of potentially harmful substances and the conditions of their use is necessary in planning chronic disease prevention programs. Where appropriate, health care providers should request consultation to document that potential exposure is adequately controlled.

The resources available for implementing health promotion efforts are also among the objective data collected. Within the worksite these resources include the prior programs offered by the worksite, the staff currently available to conduct programs, support available from top management and union officials for health promotion efforts, the budget allocated for programs and other initiatives, and the internal communication channels available to the provider [14]. The community provides further resources for the worksite's efforts. Outside vendors are often available to sponsor a variety of programs. Many communities also have a consortium that addresses worksite health promotion issues. Such a group may be sponsored by the local chamber of commerce or business groups and can provide an important network for health care providers in worksites [25].

ASSESSMENT

An organizational assessment may include collection of information on company history, the formal statement of goals, the actual working goals, formal and informal organizational structure, labor-management relations, and regional economic trends. Information can be collected by review of internal and external written material as well as by interview and direct observation (Table 19-2). The content most relevant to the health and safety consultation includes the following areas.

Company History. Basic information should be collected on the company's product and management history. More detailed information should be collected on product or management

Table 19-2. Sources for business information

Direct observation of plant operations
  Raw materials, product flow, and inventory
Interviews
  All personnel in health and safety organization,
    including safety committee members
  Management responsible for personnel, benefits,
    and manufacturing
  Union officials
  Sample of workers
Written materials
  Annual reports
  Business periodicals, trade journals
  Wall St. Journal (check index for company name),
    local newspapers and business magazines
  Dun and Bradstreet review of company
  IRS 1000 document (for public-stock companies
    only)
  Government statistics for industry
  Bureau of Labor Statistics
  Commerce department reports
  Previous reports or consultations regarding health
    and safety
  Internal memos

Source: Snyder et al. [31].

changes that may have coincided with changes in injury rates reflected in the OSHA log or workers' compensation costs. Such changes include changes in company ownership, management team, organizational structures, product line or volumes, and profitability for various products. For example, a change in an OSHA regulation may affect a company's, sometimes an entire industry's, health and safety practices.

STATED GOALS

Long- and short-term goals of publicly held companies can be easily obtained from archived materials such as annual reports or business periodicals. In addition stated goals of the company with respect to health and safety should be sought from interviews and internal documents. Examples of stated goals include "30-percent reduction in workers' compensation costs within 1 year" or "20-percent increase in productivity."

Working Goals. The actions of a company may not be consistent with its formal or stated goals. Hatten and Hatten [54] illustrate how the work-

ing strategy of a company can be analyzed by examining each functional area (e.g., marketing, production/operations, finance, human resources, and health and safety). This functional analysis approach used during a health and safety audit can help determine how the practices of each functional area affect workers' health and safety.

Organizational Structure. Since top management cannot implement every program by itself, it must delegate this power to others. The manner by which this power is delegated determines who has the authority to institute changes in work practices and policies. Understanding the organizational structure is critical to the health care provider's ability to bring about change. The health care provider must identify and have access to persons with sufficient authority to facilitate the acceptance and implementation of recommendations, policies, and programs.

All personnel with health and safety responsibilities should be identified and their reporting points in the organization determined. Unfortunately not all companies have organizational charts, and those that exist may not accurately reflect the true reporting structure. Therefore, the health care provider should request a formal or informal organization chart, then verify it through interviews and observation. The differences among various employees' perceptions of the organizational structure can also be useful information.

REGIONAL CONSIDERATIONS
Information regarding the local unemployment rate, make-up of the labor pool, and competition from other area employers should be sought. These factors affect the nature of the work force in terms of education, skill level, and organizational commitment and may have significant effects on health and safety programs.

Based on a working understanding of the company provided by these data, the health care provider can begin planning health promotion efforts. Because the recipient of these efforts is now an entire organization rather than an individual, it is often useful to develop strategies for gaining ongoing input from workers in planning and implementing such efforts.

Enhancing Program Planning and Promotion Through Worker Participation

Two models have generally been applied in delivering worksite health promotion programs. First, in the *vendor-delivered model,* an outside vendor has the primary responsibility for delivering predesigned interventions to worksite employees. This model uses the worksite as a location for implementing discrete educational packages, without reference to the specific setting in which they are implemented [55, 56]. Second, in the *participatory model,* which is derived from principles of community organization and social marketing, the program is tailored to the worksite setting according to the needs and interests of the worksite and its employees [51]. It is possible for an outside provider to use a participatory model. In such a case the provider acts as a partner with the worksite, using worker input to plan, promote, implement, and evaluate health promotion programs. Worker participation increases the likelihood that the program will influence informal networks of employees and in turn encourage the initiation and maintenance of healthy lifestyle changes. Workers also are more likely to participate in programs when they are involved in planning and implementing those activities. Participation rates in health promotion programs generally are quite small, indicating the limitations of aiming programs only at individuals and also underlining the importance of worker participation in program planning and development [57, 58] (see also Chapter 18).

One mechanism for providing worker participation is through a planning committee representing management and workers [25, 59]. This planning committee can serve the following functions:

- as a catalyst for the support and involvement of other workers in health promotion efforts

- as a source of information about ways to tailor programs to fit the worksite needs
- as a liaison between management and workers at the worksite and program providers, including voluntary health organizations and service vendors
- as a clearinghouse of information for employees on health information and community resources
- as a coordinator in sponsoring health promotion activities
- as a support for ongoing program implementation

Although health care providers may not always be directly responsible for organizing the planning committee, their support and direction can enhance the effectiveness of the planning committee's efforts. For example, the health care provider at the worksite can provide leadership in establishing the planning committee. The planning committee is likely to include several key players, including a member of management who is well respected by employees and who has decision-making authority; at least one representative of labor/union interests, preferably elected by the work force; and other peer opinion leaders from each of the primary market groups one hopes to influence, also chosen by employees. Members should be chosen who are interested in health promotion, have the respect of workers, are able to influence fellow workers, and are able to communicate effectively with others. Planning committees addressing specific health issues are most effective when they include persons representing opposing views; for example, a committee planning a smoking policy should include smokers and nonsmokers in proportion to their numbers in the worksite. To ensure that the committee remains actively involved in program activities, members should be selected for defined terms and recognized and rewarded for their contributions. Program efforts can be effectively facilitated by a worksite coordinator, an employee of the worksite primarily responsible for health promotion activities.

The health care provider can also help to ensure that the mission of the planning committee is clearly delineated and that the committee is given sufficient authority to fulfill its roles. Some committees may be established with a specific issue in mind, such as the establishment of a worksite smoking policy. Other committees may function more broadly in addressing a variety of health issues. For those committees, one of their first tasks may be the development of an integrated plan for health promotion efforts, based on the worksite analysis described previously. The plan should establish priorities for health issues to be addressed and define the type of intervention activities and the tasks necessary to implement the intervention, the persons responsible for implementing the activities, and a timeline for their completion. Committee members can help design publicity and facilitate use of internal lines of communication, such as word of mouth, in promoting the program. To increase its effectiveness, the planning committee needs to receive ongoing training about the health promotion efforts and effective committee functioning.

Implementing the Intervention

As already described, three avenues within the worksite can be employed to reduce the risk of CHD among workers. First, interventions can be aimed at individuals, including those who are at high risk for CHD as well as the population as a whole. Second, interventions can target groups of workers, as through direct education approaches promoting changes in risk-related behaviors. Finally, risk can be reduced by changing the worksite environment to reduce potential exposures that may increase risk or by altering the organization of work. Sample programs are shown in Table 19-3. An effective comprehensive program designed to reduce CHD risk integrates all three of these levels.

The objectives of programs that target individuals and groups may include building program awareness, motivating behavioral change, building skills to make the change, and providing assistance to maintain the change, as shown in Figure 19-1. Changes in the worksite environment can facilitate these changes by establishing cues supportive of change and building

Table 19-3. Worksite interventions: selected examples

Interventions that target individuals
   Employee assistance programs
   Health screening programs
   Health risk appraisals
   Medical evaluations

Interventions that target groups
   Incentives and contests
   Worksite-wide events and campaigns
   Group programs/classes

Interventions that target the worksite environments and organization
   Cafeteria programs
   Smoking policies
   Exposure reduction efforts
   Job redesign

social support for the change. For each intervention target described next, several examples illustrate these program objectives.

INTERVENTIONS THAT TARGET INDIVIDUALS

Interventions aimed at individuals can be offered on a voluntary basis to interested workers or integrated into existing health care services, such as required medical evaluations (preplacement, return-to-work after disability, and routine surveillance exams). Clinical interventions described in earlier sections of this book can be readily applied to the worksite setting and are most effective when they are integrated into interventions that target groups and the worksite environment.

A wide variety of voluntary health screening programs have been offered to individuals at their place of work [60, 61, 62, 63]. Cardiovascular risk screening might include a personal and family medical history, blood pressure monitoring, cholesterol and lipid screening, and exercise and fitness testing. The workplace provides a setting where a large number of persons can be screened relatively rapidly and at low cost. Follow-up monitoring and referral can be made available through the worksite. Some barriers to care, such as direct patient fees or the physical accessibility of medical care, also are obviated [64, 65]. Identification of high CHD risk within the workplace also permits assessment of the work context, with the possibility of identifying and alleviating job conditions that may be associated with heightened risk [53].

Hypertension screening is a common type of screening conducted in worksites. In a review of eight studies of worksite hypertension screening programs, Taylor and colleagues [65] found that from 5 to 29 percent of screened individuals were found to be hypertensive and that many of these were previously undiagnosed cases. In addition, of the hypertensives receiving treatment, fewer than 50 percent were found to be under control. One potential negative side effect noted by several studies is an increase in absenteeism among newly identified hypertensives, perhaps because being newly labeled as a hypertensive encourages adoption of the "sick" role [66, 67].

Follow-up is an important element of risk factor screening. In the worksite it is possible to integrate screening with other interventions. For example, smokers may be referred to a smoking cessation class or encouraged to quit smoking through a worksite quit-smoking contest. Individual workers also may be directed to self-help materials, aimed especially at individuals who are ready to initiate health behavior changes but who do not choose to participate in group programs. These materials can be useful in motivating behavior change and in building the skills needed to make these changes. These materials may be most effective when used in conjunction with other intervention strategies. For example, a recent meta-analysis of worksite smoking cessation studies showed that sole reliance on bibliotherapy or other self-help methods resulted in relatively low quit rates [68].

When a large number of individuals are being screened, use of computerized health risk appraisals (HRAs) can be an efficient method for collecting data about cardiovascular risk factors as well as a means of motivating individuals to make needed behavior changes [20]. A recent study of worksites found that 29.5 percent of all worksites offer health risk assessment activities, including questionnaires and health/physical exams [12]. HRAs are a systematic means of collecting information on individual and family health history, risk factors such as blood pressure or serum cholesterol levels, and health-related behaviors. HRAs vary in cost, complexity, and validity; most construct an estimated life expectancy or risk score by comparing a person's health profile to morbidity and mortality statistics associated with known risk indicators [25]. Despite their advantages HRAs are not without problems. The validity of the risk and life expectancy calculations used for most HRA assessments is unknown [69]. Users of HRAs need to assess the match between their target population and the population used in developing the HRA; for example, some databases are based on data from white males, whose risk profiles differ markedly from women and minorities. Many HRAs also base their recommendations on 10-year mortality estimates, which may be an inappropriate outcome measure for employees under 40 years of age. As a result, recommended changes may focus on alcohol consumption and exercise rather than on smoking or eating patterns that are important to long-term mortality. It is also important that the reading level of the HRA match that of the target audience [70].

Routine medical evaluations in the worksite are an opportunity to provide screening for cardiovascular risk and to deliver health promotion messages to the working well. In the United States, more than 50 percent of all new hires are required to have some sort of preemployment examination, and many industries are required to offer periodic testing either because of exposure to hazardous substances (e.g., lead, asbestos) or because of potential danger to the public resulting from impaired workers (e.g., transportation workers, airplane pilots) [71]. These examinations can be potentially useful for health promotion purposes because they are frequently the only direct contact with a clinician for the generally young and healthy working population. They can be especially important in situations where the effects of a workplace exposure, such as to lead or asbestos, may be heightened by concurrent behavioral risk factors such as smoking.

In the United States, where no national health

insurance system exists and obtaining health insurance is directly linked to employment, required medical examinations are increasingly being seen by employers as a way of controlling health care costs through selection screening [72]. Employees therefore approach employer-sponsored required medical examinations with increasing and appropriate caution. There is great concern among workers that the personal risk factor information obtained in such examinations may be used against the worker in hiring and promotion and not solely for the purpose of improving and protecting the workers' health status or safety in the workplace. For example, personnel department knowledge of hypertension and hypercholesterolemia in a 50-year-old executive under consideration for hiring or promotion might affect the hiring decision, even though such practices are prohibited by law [73]. Knowing this, employees might be less than revealing about their risk factors and health concerns in these settings.

In theory a number of safeguards are in place to protect the confidentiality of workers' medical records [74] and to guard against the misuse of personal risk factor information obtained in required medical evaluations [73, 71]. In practice, however, the protection of workers' rights may be difficult in those situations where medical personnel are directly employed by the company or have financial interests in the success of the employer. The ethical responsibilities of the health care professional have been summarized in the code of ethical conduct for physicians who provide occupational medical services. According to this code, the physician should

treat as confidential whatever is learned about individuals served, releasing information only when required by law or by overriding public health considerations, or to other physicians at the request of the individual according to traditional medical ethical practice; and should recognize that employers are entitled to counsel about the medical fitness of individuals in relation to work, but are not entitled to diagnoses or details of a specific nature [75].

Given worker concerns about the confidentiality of individual health data, health care providers may find it useful to take several precautions. If the data are collected by outside vendors contracted by the workplace, their relationship with the employer should be clarified before any health screening is done. For example, Who will have access to individual test results? Where will the test results be kept? How will the test results be communicated to the employees? Addressing these issues in writing prior to health screening is likely to be reassuring to all the participants. Particular care should be taken in ensuring the confidentiality of required examinations, such as Federal Aviation Administration examinations for airplane pilots, Department of Transportation exams for truck drivers, and urine drug testing for illegal drugs. Despite the protection outlined above, when information is collected by the employer or its agents, the potential and the perception exist that the information collected may be misused to affect future employment options.

INTERVENTIONS THAT TARGET GROUPS

Interventions that target groups of workers and possibly their families may be aimed at motivating behavior change, building skills to make the changes, and maintaining the behavior change. These programs, which generally focus on reducing CHD risk through changes in health-related behaviors, are designed to maximize their effect across all workers in an organization. The program's impact is a function of both the proportion of workers who participate and the proportion of participants who actually change their behavior. Programs aimed at persons ready to make behavior change tend to have low rates of participation [25]. Programs reaching large numbers generally produce lower rates of behavior change than do more intensive direct education programs that attract smaller numbers. Thus, intervention programs providing intensive assistance to small numbers of workers ready to initiate behavior change need to be offered in conjunction with strategies likely to attract larger numbers of workers still contemplating behavior change [25, 76, 77].

Large numbers of workers may be attracted

by programs that use incentives or contests that may promote or motivate behavior change as well as assist in its long-term maintenance. Incentive programs offer the advantages of requiring little professional time to administer them. Three approaches are commonly used: guaranteed incentives or awards, contests within a worksite, and challenges or contests between worksites (or departments or sites of a given company) [25]. Guaranteed incentives are used to reinforce behavior changes such as losing weight [26, 78] or quitting smoking [79]. Such incentives may also include health insurance cost reductions for nonsmokers or cash benefits for quitters as inducements for change. A contest within a worksite may include, for example, a lottery drawing among participants who achieve specified goals for a given month. Participants' goals and performance (e.g., number of minutes of exercise per week) can be posted in the worksite to draw attention to and reinforce healthy behaviors. Finally, competition between worksites has been used effectively by several community heart disease prevention programs [81, 82]. Such competitions are most effective in worksites where employees strongly identify with their companies [83, 84].

Other worksite-wide events can be used to motivate change in large groups of workers. Health fairs, summer barbecues featuring healthy foods, and road races are activities that may attract large numbers of workers and stimulate interest in behavior change. Educational materials provided at the event can be used to provide information and teach skills [51].

Other group programs are aimed especially at workers ready to make behavior changes. Participants can be taught general behavioral principles such as gradual behavior change based on goals derived from baseline data, performance feedback, and coping skills training. In addition, programs can identify potential pitfalls (e.g., Brownell [85]) and focus on relapse prevention strategies (e.g., Marlatt and Gordon [86]). Programs can be offered as single sessions or as a series of sessions; each session should be flexible in length, since in some worksites only short break periods are available [51]. Participation in more time-consuming alternatives

may be limited unless employees are given time off from work to participate and training activities can be conducted at the worksite. Health care professionals are often instrumental in advocating for work time to participate in programs, a factor that can significantly enhance participation rates. Although health care providers are likely to teach some classes, they can also arrange for classes to be taught by others, such as voluntary health agencies, e.g., the AHA, the ACS, the American Lung Association (ALA), or university-based programs in the local community. These agencies can also provide training for onsite personnel to instruct these classes, which may be a useful means of building the worksite's ability to offer programs on an ongoing basis.

INTERVENTIONS THAT TARGET THE WORKSITE ENVIRONMENT AND ORGANIZATION

Efforts that target individual behavior change must be integrated with changes in the worksite environment and in the structure of work to maximize the potential for CHD risk reduction in the worksite. Environmental and organizational changes underline the fact that employer actions are an integral component of a comprehensive approach to workers' health [28]. Changes in the worksite environment and the organization of work may contribute to CHD risk reduction in three ways. First, environmental changes can provide support for workers seeking to make changes in health behaviors, such as smoking or diet. Such environmental changes include cafeteria or point-of-choice food selection programs and smoking policies. Second, other environmental changes can directly reduce potential exposures to substances or conditions associated with increased risk of CHD. Several environmental toxins are linked to increased risk of CHD. In addition, exposure to environmental tobacco smoke can be eliminated or diminished by policies restricting or banning smoking. Third, CHD risk can be diminished by changes in the work organization, including redesigning jobs to increase job control and to decrease psychological stressors at work. Health care professionals can facilitate each of these types of change.

Environmental strategies that promote healthy eating at the worksite provide opportunities for dietary changes while also removing barriers to following a healthy diet [87]. Cafeteria and point-of-choice labeling programs are the most common types of worksite nutrition environmental programs [88]. Labeling of healthy foods in worksite cafeterias and vending machines can enhance direct education efforts by exposing a large number of workers each day to messages about healthy eating [51, 89, 90]. Some labeling programs have included incentives to encourage individuals to select recommended items [91, 92]. Changes in the worksite's catering policy may also support long-term changes in eating patterns; such changes may stress the addition of healthy food options to catered company events [87].

Smoking policies are useful in supporting workers' efforts to quit smoking while also reducing nonsmokers' exposure to environmental tobacco smoke [93, 94, 95]. An increasing number of worksites are adopting policies that restrict or ban smoking at the worksite [12]. Several studies have found that a nonsmoking policy may encourage workers to quit smoking [96, 97], although not all studies addressing this relationship have reached similar conclusions [98, 99, 100]. The announcement of a smoking policy may also stimulate participation in smoking cessation classes [56, 101].

Few studies have objectively measured changes in exposure to environmental tobacco smoke. Only a total ban on smoking can ensure the reduction in exposure to environmental tobacco smoke. The effects of partial smoking restrictions on air quality hinge on the type of ventilation system in place. Unless smoking areas are fully vented to the outside, environmental tobacco smoke is likely to be recirculated throughout the worksite [8]. Workers are likely to respond most favorably to restrictions on smoking when such policies are uniformly implemented and when the policy is announced with sufficient lead time. Gaining worker input in planning such policy changes can help to ensure that employees perceive such changes not as limitations on their privileges but as benefits that promote their health.

In addition to smoking restrictions the worksite can use other policy approaches to assist workers in quitting smoking. For example, several workers in the process of quitting might be permitted to arrange for the same shifts, rest periods, and locker areas to provide support for one another and to avoid contacts with smokers during this crucial period. By redesigning the work environment for nonsmokers, businesses may reinforce alternatives to smoking, for example, by removing cigarette machines and locating smoking areas away from halls and gathering areas [102].

The worksite also provides the opportunity for reducing exposures to occupational factors associated with the genesis of heart disease. Numerous case reports have associated specific chemical and physical agents with an increased risk of heart disease; epidemiologic studies have confirmed several of these associations [5]. Table 19-4 summarizes some of the reported associations and the relative strength of the evidence supporting those associations.

For several of the exposures listed in Table 19-4, such as carbon disulfide, the nitrates, arsenic, lead, cadmium, and halogenated solvents, the correlation with heart disease is strong enough that consideration should be given to ruling out previous or current exposures in all patients with CHD. As a corollary to this, risk screening in the workplace must inquire about occupational exposures that may be contributing to cardiovascular risk. When such risk factors are identified, they can usually be modified or eliminated through a combination of workplace changes (such as product substitution or process redesign), employee education, and the appropriate use of personal protective devices such as respirators. Unlike lifestyle risk factors, the modification or elimination of exposure risk factors is highly dependent on the interest and the willingness of the employer to make changes in the work environment.

The physical and psychosocial demands of jobs may also be related to cardiovascular risk. Several studies have shown a relationship between highly demanding physical jobs and *de-*

Table 19-4. Some occupational hazards associated with cardiovascular disorders

Hazard	Cardiovascular effect	Strength of evidence
Carbon monoxide	Atherosclerosis	Weak
Carbon disulfide	Atherosclerosis	Moderate
Certain aliphatic nitrates	Coronary spasm	Strong
	Atherosclerosis	Weak
Arsenic	Coronary heart disease	Moderate
Lead, cadmium	Coronary heart disease secondary to nephrotoxicity	Moderate
Noise	Transient high blood pressure	Strong
	Long-term high blood pressure	Absent
Shift work	Coronary heart disease	Weak
Halogenated solvents	Arrhythmia	Moderate
Chronic hand-arm vibration	Vibration white finger	Strong

Source: Levy BS, Wegman DH. Occupational health: recognizing and preventing work-related disease. Boston: Little, Brown, 1988; 422.

creased cardiovascular mortality [103]. Few jobs in today's mechanized society, however, require work at metabolic rates that lead to cardiovascular conditioning [104]. There is significant concern, on the other hand, that workers with untreated CHD may experience coronary events as a result of physical overload at work. Strenuous exercise can cause cardiac dysfunction and death in persons with underlying heart disease. In fact, it has been demonstrated that over 90 percent of exercise-related deaths occur in persons who had previous cardiac disease [105]. Overall it is likely that the benefits of active physical demands in the workplace outweigh the cardiovascular risk [106]. Nevertheless, patients with major risk factors, premonitory symptoms, or known coronary disease should be counseled and closely monitored with regard to workplace physical demands [107].

Job characteristics and the social milieu of the worksite also have been associated with increased risk of CHD, as described in Chapter 11. Recent research indicates that risk of CHD is highest among workers whose jobs are highly demanding but that allow little opportunity for control over those demands [6, 7]. Risk may be lowered by redesigning jobs to increase workers' control over the decisions affecting their work. Low decision latitude may also be associated with more medical problems,

more psychological stress, increased absenteeism, and lower job satisfaction, relationships that may convince management of the need for making such changes. A program of company-wide job redesign may include broadening workers' skills through job rotation, the availability of flextime, task redesign, increased training, and higher levels of autonomy. Also, management can be trained to work with a less authoritarian style and to promote teamwork [53].

In some companies job stress is addressed through employee assistance programs (EAP), which provide free counseling for employees who experience stress on the job. While such programs may provide useful approaches to reducing the stress of some workers, their long-term effectiveness may be limited unless the organizational determinants of job stress are addressed. Job redesign and management training are examples of such an organizational approach.

Health care providers can facilitate the process of job redesign. Aggregate health data collected during the assessment and planning phases can provide the rationale for needed organizational changes. With the participation of workers and management, health care professionals can contribute to defining what is psychologically, physiologically, technically, and economically feasible for a given worksite [53].

Summary

In general worksite health promotion has targeted the individual rather than the organization or the workplace environment for intervention. This chapter has sought to find a balance in targeting both domains for change. Finding that balance requires integrating health promotion efforts with occupational health and safety concerns in the worksite. In addition, a comprehensive health and wellness program is not complete without also addressing how jobs are structured within the corporate culture.

An exclusive focus on individual lifestyle factors runs the risk of deflecting attention away from potentially serious health hazards and effects of the work environment. Ignoring the employer's responsibility for worker health also threatens the credibility of health care providers with workers, whose primary health concerns may be their exposure to hazardous substances on the job or the stressors associated with their work [28, 108]. A focus on individual behavior change may also lead to blaming the victim and may take on a moralistic tone [109].

Effective application of the participatory strategies described in this chapter will help to ensure that workers and management jointly establish priorities for health promotion and health protection efforts, including those aimed at making necessary changes in the work environment. Worker input in the planning process may facilitate participation from worker groups least likely to attend programs but often at high risk for CHD. Some evidence suggests that people who participate in wellness programs may be healthier than those who do not [19, 109]. In addition blue-collar workers have generally been less likely to participate in programs than white-collar workers, perhaps due to scheduling or conflicting priorities [109, 110, 111].

A comprehensive program that targets individuals, groups, the worksite environment, and the organization of work may be effective in reducing CHD risk in the worksite. Input from management, workers, and union representatives can be used to tailor efforts in response to the unique needs, risks, and priorities of the individual worksite. The health care provider plays a crucial role in assessing individual and organizational risk factors, motivating and educating individuals to make needed health behavior changes, promoting changes in environmental and organizational factors associated with increased risk, and offering leadership and direction for the integration of efforts across multiple channels.

References

1. U.S. Bureau of the Census. Statistical abstract of the United States. Washington, DC: U.S. Government Printing Office, 1986.
2. Terborg JR. The organization as a context for health promotion. In: Oskamp S, ed. Social psychology and health: the Claremont Symposium on Applied Social Psychology. Newbury Park, CA: Sage, 1988.
3. Rose G. Strategy of prevention: lessons from cardiovascular disease. Br Med Jour 1981; 282:1847–51.
4. Terborg JR. Health promotion at the worksite: a research challenge for personnel and human resources management. Res Pers Hum Resour Manage 1986; 4:225–67.
5. Theriault GP. Cardiovascular disorders. In: Levy BS, Wegman DH, eds. Occupational health: recognizing and preventing work-related disease. 2nd ed. Boston/Toronto: Little, Brown and Co., 1988.
6. Karasek RA, Theorell T, Alfredsson L, et al. Job psychological factors and coronary heart disease. Adv Cardiol 1982; 29:62–7.
7. Karasek RA, Theorell T, Schwartz JE, et al. Job characteristics in relation to the prevalence of myocardial infarction in the U.S. HES and HANES. Am J Public Health 1988; 78:910–8.
8. U.S. Environmental Protection Agency. Environmental tobacco smoke: a guide to workplace smoking policies. Public review draft. U.S. Environmental Protection Agency. Washington, DC, 1990.
9. U.S. Department of Health and Human Services, Public Health Service, Centers for Disease Control. The health consequences of involuntary smoking: a report of the Surgeon General. USDHHS publ. no. (CDG) 87-8398, 1986a.
10. Sorensen G, Pechacek T, Pallonen U. Occupational and worksite norms and attitudes about smoking cessation. Am J Public Health 1986; 76(5):544–49.
11. Walsh DC. Corporate physicians: between medicine and management. New Haven: Yale University Press, 1987.

12. Fielding JE, Piserchia PV. Frequency of work-site health promotion activities. Am J Public Health 1989; 79:16–20.

13. O'Donnell MP, Ainsworth T. Health promotion in the workplace. New York: Wiley, 1984.

14. Sloan RP, Gruman JC, Allegrante JP. Investing in employee health: a guide to effective health promotion in the workplace. San Francisco: Jossey-Bass, 1987.

15. Warner KE, Wickizer TM, Wolfe RA, et al. Economic implications of workplace health promotion programs: review of the literature. J Occup Med 1988; 30(2):106–12.

16. Bertera RL. The effects of workplace health promotion on absenteeism and employment costs on a large industrial population. Am J Public Health 1990; 80(9):1101–5.

17. Jones RD, Bly JL, Richardson JE. A study of a worksite health promotion program and absenteeism. J Occup Med 1990; 32:95–9.

18. Reed RW, Mulvaney D, Bellingham R, Huber KC. Health promotion service: evaluation study. Indianapolis: Blue Cross-Blue Shield of Indiana, 1985.

19. Baun WP, Bernack EJ, Tsai SPA. A preliminary investigation: effect of a corporate fitness program on absenteeism and health care cost. J Occup Med 1986; 28:18–22.

20. Blair SN, Piserchia PV, Wilbur CS, Crowder JH. A public health intervention model for work-site health promotion. JAMA 1986; 225:921–6.

21. Holzbach RL, Piserchia PV, McFadden DW, et al. Effect of a comprehensive health promotion program on employee attitudes. J Occup Med 1990; 32:973–8.

22. Bly JL, Jones RC, Richardson JE. Impact of worksite health promotion on health care costs and utilization: evaluation of Johnson and Johnson's LIVE FOR LIFE Program. JAMA 1986; 256:3235–40.

23. Gibbs JO, Mulvaney D, Hanes C, Reed RW. Worksite health promotion: five-year trend in employee health care costs. J Occup Med 1985; 27:826–30.

24. Mulvaney D, Reed R, Gibbs J, Henes C. Blue Cross and Blue Shield of Indiana: five year payoff in health promotion. Corp Comment 1985; 5:1–6.

25. Sorensen G, Glasgow R, Corbett K. Involving worksites and other organizations. In: Bracht N, ed. Organizing for community health promotion: a guide. Newbury Park, CA: Sage, 1990.

26. Brownell KD. Weight control at the workplace: the power of social and behavioral factors. In: Cataldo ME, Coates TJ, eds. Health promotion

in industry: a behavioral medicine perspective. New York: Wiley, 1986; 143–61.

27. Levenstein C. Worksite health promotion (editorial). Am J Public Health 1989; 79(1):11.

28. Green KL. Issues of control and responsibility in workers' health. Health Educ Q 1988; 15(4):473–86.

29. Brown ER, McCarthy W, Marcus A, et al. Workplace smoking policies: attitudes of union members in a high-risk industry. J Occup Med 1988; 30(4):312–20.

30. Marcus AC, Baker DB, Froines J, et al. The ICWU cancer control and evaluation program: research design and needs assessment. J Occup Med 1986; 28(3):226–36.

31. Snyder T, Himmelstein JS, Pransky GS, Beavers JD. Business analysis in occupational safety and health consultation. J Occup Med 1991; 33:1040–5.

32. U.S. Small Business Administration. The state of small business: a report to the President. Washington, DC: US Government Printing Office, 1984.

33. Carlaw R, Mittlemark M, Bracht N, Luepker R. Organization for a community cardiovascular health program: experiences from the Minnesota Heart Health Program. Health Educ Q 1984; 11(3):243–52.

34. Orlandi MA. The diffusion and adoption of worksite health promotion innovations: an analysis of barriers. Prev Med 1986; 15:522–36.

35. Wallack L, Wallerstein N. Health education and prevention: designing community initiatives. Intern Q Com Health Ed 1987; 7(4):319–42.

36. Farquhar JW, Fortmann SP, Maccoby N, et al. The Stanford Five City Project: an overview. In: Matarazzo J, Weiss SM, Herd JA, Miller NE, Weiss SM, eds. Behavioral health: a handbook of health enhancement and disease prevention. New York: John Wiley & Sons, 1984.

37. Minker M. Improving health through community organization. In: Glanz K, Lewis FM, Rimer BK, et al., eds. Health behavior and health education: theory, research, and practice. San Francisco: Jossey-Bass, 1990.

38. Bandura A. Social foundations of thought and action: a social cognitive theory. Englewood Cliffs, NJ: Prentice-Hall, 1986.

39. Abrams DB, Elder JP, Carleton RA, et al. Social learning principles for organizational health promotion: an integrated approach. In: Cataldo MF, Coates TJ, eds. Health and industry: a behavioral medicine perspective. New York: Wiley, 1986; 28–51.

40. Parcel GS, Eriksen MP, Lovato CY, et al. The diffusion of school-based tobacco-use prevention programs: project description and baseline data. Health Educ Research 1989; 4:111–24.

41. Perry GL, Baranowski T, Parcel GS. How individuals, environments and health behavior interact: social learning theory. In: Glanz K, Lewis FM, Rimer BK, et al., eds. Health behavior and health education: theory, research and practice. San Francisco: Jossey-Bass, 1990.

42. Bandura A. Social learning theory. Englewood Cliffs, NJ: Prentice-Hall, 1977.

43. Flay B. Mass media linkages with school-based programs for drug abuse prevention. J School Health 1986; 56:402–6.

44. Brehony KA, Frederiksen LW, Solomon L. Marketing principles and behavioral medicine: an overview. In: Frederiksen LW, Solomon LJ, Brehony KA, eds. Marketing health behavior: principles, techniques, and applications. New York: Plenum, 1984.

45. Lefebre RC, Flora JA. Social marketing and public health intervention. Health Educ Q 1988; 15(3):299–315.

46. Manoff RK. Social marketing. New York: Praeger, 1985.

47. Basch CE, Sliepcevich, EM. Innovators, innovations and implementation: a framework for curricular research in school health education. Health Educ 1983; 14:20–4.

48. Murray DM. Dissemination of community health promotion programs: the Fargo-Moorhead Heart Health Program. J School Health 1986; 56:375–81.

49. Rogers EM, Shoemaker FF. Communication of innovations: a cross-cultural approach. New York: Free Press, 1971.

50. Rogers EM. Diffusion of innovations. 3rd ed. New York: Free Press, 1983.

51. Sorensen G, Hunt MK, Morris D. Promoting healthy eating patterns in the worksite: the Treatwell Intervention Model. Health Educ Res 1990; 5(4):505–15.

52. Weed LL. Medical records, medical education, and patient care: the problem-oriented record as a basic tool. Cleveland: The Press of Case Western Reserve University, 1969.

53. Karasek R, Theorell T. Healthy work: stress, productivity, and the reconstruction of working life. New York: Basic Books, 1990.

54. Hatten K, Hatten ML. Strategic management. Englewood Cliffs, NJ: Prentice Hall, 1987.

55. Rost K, Marcus M, Haire-Joshu D, Fisher EB. Employee direction of health promotion programs: preliminary findings from the Working Hearts Program. Unpublished manuscript, 1990.

56. Sorensen G, Hsieh J, Hunt MK. Worker participation in a worksite nutrition intervention program: experiences from the Treatwell Program. Am J Health Promotion (in review).

57. Omenn GS, Thompson B, Sexton B, et al. A randomized comparison of worksite-sponsored smoking cessation programs. Am J Prev Med 1988; 4:261–7.

58. Fiore MC, Novotny NE, Pierce JP, et al. Methods used to quit smoking in the United States: do cessation programs help? JAMA 1990; 263:2760–9.

59. Kizer, WM. The healthy workplace: a blueprint for corporate action. New York: Wiley, 1987.

60. Brownstein PM, Herd JA. Practical indices of compliance in cardiovascular risk reduction programs. In: Cataldo MF, Coates TJ. Health and industry: a behavioral medicine perspective. New York: John Wiley & Sons, 1986; 210–30.

61. Alderman MH, Melcher LA. Occupationally sponsored, community provided hypertension control. Occup Med 1983; 25:465–70.

62. Drazen M, Nevid JS, Pace N, O'Brien RN. Worksite based behavioral treatment of mild hypertension. J Occup Med 1982; 24:511–4.

63. Ruchlin HS, Melcher LA, Alderman MH. Work-related hypertension care programs. J Occup Med 1984; 26:45–9.

64. Alderman MH, Davis TK. Blood pressure control programs on and off the worksite. J Occup Med 1980; 22:167–70.

65. Taylor CB, Agras WS, Sevelius G. Managing hypertension in the workplace. In: Cataldo, MF, Coates TJ. Health and industry: a behavioral medicine perspective. New York: Wiley, 1986; 193–209.

66. Haynes RB, Sackett DL, Taylor DW, et al. Increased absenteeism from work after detection and labelling of hypertension patients. New Engl J Med 1978; 299:741–4.

67. Baer L, Parchment Y, Kreeshaw M. Hypertension in health care providers. Effectiveness of worksite treatment programs in a state mental health agency. Am J Public Health 1981; 71:1261–3.

68. Fisher KJ, Glasgow RE, Terborg JR. Worksite smoking cessation: a meta analysis of long-term quit rates from controlled studies. J Occup Med 1990; 32:429–39.

69. Wagner EH, Beery WL, Schoenbeack VJ, Graham RM. An assessment of health hazard/health risk appraisal. Am J Public Health 1982; 72, 347–52.

70. Bibeau D, Mullen K. Evaluating health promotion technology: health risk appraisals. Paper presented at the annual meeting of the American Public Health Association, New Orleans, 1987.

71. Himmelstein JS. Worker fitness and risk evaluations in context: In: Himmelstein JS, Pransky

GS, eds. State of the art reviews. Occup Med 1988; 3(2):169–78.

72. Rothstein MA. Medical screening and the employee health cost crisis. Washington, DC: BNA Books, 1989.

73. Americans with Disabilities Act Employment Provisions, Code of Federal Regulations (CFR) 29. Office of Federal Register, National Archives and Records, Administration. Washington, DC: U.S. Government Printing Office, 1991.

74. Access to employee exposure and medical records. Code of Federal Regulations (CFR) 29, Part 1910.20. Office of Federal Register, National Archives and Records Administration. Washington, DC: U.S. Government Printing Office, 1990.

75. American Occupational Medical Association. Code of ethical conduct for physicians providing occupational medical services adopted by the Board of Directors. J Occup Med 1976; 18:(8)Cover.

76. Nathan PE. Johnson & Johnson's Live for Life: a comprehensive positive lifestyle change. In: Matarazzo JD, Weiss SM, Herd JA, Miller NE, Weiss SM, eds. Behavioral health: a handbook of health enhancement and disease prevention. New York: John Wiley & Sons, 1984; 1064–70.

77. Stachnik TJ, Stoffelmayr BE. Work-site smoking cessation program: a potential for national impact. Am J Public Health 1983; 73; 1395–6.

78. Forster JL, Jeffrey RW, Sullivan S, Snell MK. A worksite weight control program using financial incentives collected through payroll deduction. J Occup Med 1985; 27:804–8.

79. Shepard DS, Pearlman LA. Health habits that pay off. Business Health 1985; 2:37–41.

80. Elder J, McGraw S, Rodrigues A, et al. Evaluation of two community-wide smoking contests. Prev Med 1987; 16:221–34.

81. King AC, Flora JA, Fortmann SP, Taylor CB. Smokers' challenge: immediate and long-term findings of a community smoking cessation contest. Am J Public Health 1987; 77, 1340–1.

82. Pechacek T, Freutel J, Arkin R, Mittelmark M. The Quit and Win Contest: a community-wide incentive program for smoking cessation. Paper presented at the World Congress on Behavior Therapy, Washington, DC, 1983.

83. Brownell KD, Felix MRJ. Competitions to facilitate health promotion: review and conceptual analysis. Am J Health Promotion 1987; 77:28–36.

84. Klesges RC, Glasgow RE. Work-site smoking control programs. In: Cataldo M, Coates TJ, eds. Health promotion in industry: a behavioral medicine perspective. New York: Wiley, 1986; 231–54.

85. Brownell KD. The LEARN Program for weight control. Philadelphia: University of Pennsylvania, 1988.

86. Marlatt GA, Gordon JR. Relapse prevention: maintenance strategies in the treatment of addictive behaviors. New York: Guilford, 1985.

87. Glanz K, Mullis RM. Environmental interventions to promote healthy eating: a review of models, programs and evidence. Health Educ Q 1988; 15:395–415.

88. Glanz K, Seewald-Klein T. Nutrition at the worksite: an overview. J Nutr Educ 1986; 18,2:Suppl:S1–S12.

89. Wilbur CS, Zifferblatt SM, Pinsky JL, et al. Healthy vending: a cooperative pilot research program to stimulate good health in the market place. Prev Med 1981; 10:85–93.

90. Zifferblatt SM, Wilbur CS, Pinsky JL. Changing cafeteria eating habits. J Am Diet Assoc 1980; 76:15–20.

91. Cincirpini PM. Changing food selections in a public cafeteria. Behav Modif 1984; 8:520–39.

92. Mayer JA, Brown TP, Heins JM, Bishop DB. A multi-component intervention for modifying food selections in a worksite cafeteria. J Nutr Education 1987; 19:277–80.

93. Eriksen MP. Workplace smoking control: rationale and approaches. Adv Health Educ Promot 1986; 1(A):65–103.

94. Rosenstock IM, Stergachis A, Heaney C. Evaluation of smoking prohibition policy in a health maintenance organization. Am J Public Health 1986; 76:1014–5.

95. Walsh DC, McDougall V. Current policies regarding smoking in the workplace. Am J Indust Med 1988; 13:181–90.

96. Sorensen G, Rigotti N, Rosen A, et al. Effects of a worksite non-smoking policy: evidence for increased cessation. Am J Public Health 1991; 81(2):202–4.

97. Millar WJ. Smoke in the workplace: an evaluation of smoking restrictions. Ottawa: Minister of Supply and Services, 1988.

98. Becker DM, Conner HF, Waranch HR, et al. The impact of a total ban on smoking in the Johns Hopkins Children's Center. JAMA 1989; 262(6):799–802.

99. Biener L, Abrams DB, Follick MJ, Dean L. A comparative evaluation of a restrictive smoking policy in a general hospital. Am J Public Health 1989; 79:192–5.

100. Rigotti NA, Pikl BH, Cleary P, et al. The impact of banning smoking on a hospital ward: acceptance, compliance, air quality, and smoking behavior (abstract). Clin Res 1986; 34, 833A.

101. Martin MJ. Smoking control — policy and

legal methods (letter). West J of Med 1988; 148:199.

102. Schilling RF, Gilchrist LD, Schinke SP. Smoking in the workplace: review of critical issues. Public Health Reports 1985; 100:473–9.

103. Kristensen TS. Cardiovascular diseases and the work environment. A critical review of the epidemiologic literature on nonchemical factors. Institute of Social Medicine, University of Copenhagen, Denmark. Scand J Work Environ Health 1989; 15:165–79.

104. Fine L. Cardiovascular disease. In: Levy BS, Wegman DH. Occupational health: recognizing and preventing work-related disease. 1st ed. Boston: Little, Brown and Co., 1983.

105. Ragosta M, Crabtree J, Sturner WQ, et al. Death during recreational exercise in the state of Rhode Island. Med Sci Sports Exerc 1984; 16:339.

106. Friedewald VE Jr, Spence DW. Sudden cardiac death associated with exercise: the risk-benefit issue. Methodist Hospital, Sid W. Richardson Institute for Preventive Medicine, Houston, Texas. Am J Cardiol 1990; 66:183–8.

107. Tempte J. Cardiovascular conditions and worker fitness and risk. In: Himmelstein JS, Pransky GS, eds. State of the art reviews. Occup Med 1988; 3:241–54.

108. Walsh DC. Toward a sociology of worksite health promotion: a few reactions and reflections. Soc Sci Med 1988; 26:569–75.

109. Conrad P. Wellness in the workplace: potentials and pitfalls of worksite health promotion. Milbank Q 1987; 65:255–75.

110. Pechter K. Corporate fitness and blue collar fears. Across the Board 1986; 23:14–21.

111. Sloan RP, Gruman JC. Participation in workplace health promotion programs: the contribution of health and organizational factors. Health Educ Q 1988; 15:269–88.

20

School Intervention

MICHAEL P. ERIKSEN

EDITORS' INTRODUCTION

Chapter 16 described the rationale for intervention in childhood to modify risk factors for CHD. In this chapter Dr. Eriksen addresses the workplace of the child — the school. The logic for intervention in the school is even clearer than that for the worksite, because habits developed here last for a lifetime. Studies of school-based approaches to risk-factor modification are described, and barriers to such change are discussed. Dr. Eriksen points out how the health care worker can play an important role in this setting. All of us, whether or not directly involved in the care of children, should be interested in this topic and should make every effort to support such change.

Schools are the major organizational sites for improving the health of children [1]. While other organizations provide access to pediatric populations (Girl Scouts, 4-H clubs, Little League), none provides the opportunity to reach as large a population of children for as many years as do schools [2]. More than 50 million children attend private and public schools, 5 to 8 hours a day, 5 days a week, 36 weeks a year [3].

Schools have long been used to protect and promote the health and well-being of children and adolescents. In the 1880s Horace Mann advocated the teaching of health subjects in public schools and the development of standards for school buildings [4]. In 1850 Lemuel Shattuck, a leader in education and public health, observed that

Every child should be taught early in life, that to preserve his own life and his own health and the lives and health of others is one of the most important and constantly abiding duties. Everything connected with health, happiness, and long life depends upon health [4].

This acknowledgement of the schools' importance in protecting and promoting the health of children resulted in a comprehensive framework of school health programs in the early 1900s. That model had three components: school health services, health instruction, and a healthful school environment. Today's school health services include health examinations, screening programs, communicable-disease control, and correction of remediable problems. Health instruction includes planned instruction to influence health-related knowledge, attitudes, and practices and incidental instruction to help shape a student's health awareness and beliefs. The school environment includes the actual physical environment and practices as well as cognizance of their influence on the mental health of students [5]. The three-component model has guided the development of school health programs throughout the twentieth century and has been the framework of cardiovascular disease interventions as well as interventions in other acute and chronic diseases.

Recently a variety of additions have been suggested to complement the triadic model of school health. These focus on physical education, food services, counseling, health promotion programs for faculty and staff, and the integration of those services with school and community programs [2]. Despite the existence of this expanded model of school health, most school-based efforts to influence student health have relied on school health education. Before 1980 the goal of most school health education programs was similar to that of other academic programs, that is, to impart knowledge with the expectation that increased knowledge would lead students to adopt positive health behaviors. When student health behaviors did not change, the focus of school health education programs needed to be evaluated and a new approach developed. The new approach places less emphasis on knowledge acquisition and more on skills development, social influences, and behavioral competencies, with the goal of intervening before risk behaviors become established [6].

Despite the fact that schools represent the best opportunity to reach children and adolescents, school-based programs still have a number of problems. First of all they do not influence the high-risk adolescents who have already dropped out of school. Not only are these adolescents untouched by school-based interventions, their risk behaviors often exceed those of their peers who are still in school. This is true of smoking [7, 8] and may also be the case for other cardiovascular risks. Second, the majority of existing school-based programs have not been developed for or evaluated among such special populations as children of minority, rural, and poor families and those at low-achieving scholastic levels [9].

School-based Approaches and Their Efficacy

The contemporary burden of cardiovascular disease in America has its roots in childhood. In fact the atherosclerotic process may actually begin early in life, not becoming symptomatic for decades [10, 11]. Although there are clearly genetic and other unalterable determinants, a large proportion of adult cardiovascular disease is attributable to risky behaviors that are often established in early childhood. The estimate is that, by age 12, at least one modifiable risk factor for CHD exists in 36 to 60 percent of children in the United States [12]. Although few prospective studies document the extension of cardiovascular risk factors of children into adulthood, there is some evidence that cardiovascular risks tend to track over time (see Chapter 16) [13, 14]. Despite the absence of definitive prospective studies, the general belief is that psychosocial conditions of childhood contribute to behaviors that are associated later with adult behavioral risk factors and may ultimately lead to cardiovascular disease morbidity and mortality [6]. The adult behavioral risks that often begin in childhood (cigarette smoking, poor dietary habits, and lack of exercise) are all difficult to modify once they are fully established. Thus, programs designed to prevent the establishment of cardiovascular risk factors through school-based interventions should be one of the most efficient approaches to preventing cardiovascular disease.

In attempting to prevent the establishment of risk behaviors, we should rely less on the traditional armamentarium of behavior modification techniques (because the behaviors often have yet to be established) than on the psychosocial factors that lead to the actual development and adoption of risk behaviors. School-based prevention programs provide the perfect opportunity for this type of etiologic approach, not only because they can influence the precursors of risk behaviors in a child (cognitions and beliefs), but also because the school environment can help shape the child's future behaviors [15]. It is unrealistic to expect school health education programs to achieve their objectives of smoking prevention or improved nutrition if the school environment sends out conflicting messages [2].

Smoking

Cigarette smoking, one of the most injurious of cardiovascular risks, is also one of the most preventable. As noted in previous chapters, 30 percent of CHD is estimated to be attributable to smoking, but stopping smoking is relatively difficult to do; 50 million Americans continue to smoke, and only about 6 percent of smokers quit in a given year. The majority (90 percent) of adults who smoke begin smoking while in their teens [16], and the rates of adolescent smoking have not declined as have those of other age groups. Recently the previously observed rate of decline in teenage smoking has stalled, particularly among teenage girls, who now smoke more than their male counterparts [9]. Because the risk of smoking is so serious and the behavior so prevalent, smoking prevention programs are often the focus of school-based interventions. Unfortunately the problem is even greater for teenagers not in school, with high school dropouts having smoking rates double that of their counterparts in school [7, 8].

School-based programs have had generally positive, albeit modest, results [17, 18], the most successful being programs that delay the onset of smoking, which is important in terms of reducing the likelihood of an individual becoming a heavy smoker as an adult [19]. These programs have had little effect, however, on helping regular smokers quit [20], and they also have had difficulty in reaching high-risk and minority youth [9]. To achieve better results, a panel of experts assembled by the National Cancer Institute (NCI) concluded that, at a minimum, a smoking prevention program should offer information about the social consequences and short-term physiological effects of tobacco, information on the social influences that lead to smoking, and training in refusal skills [9]. They further recommend that these components be offered at least in two five-session blocks during separate school years between the sixth and ninth grades, although the preferred method is to offer smoking prevention instruction in all grades.

SOCIAL INFLUENCES

A number of the elements recommended by the NCI Expert Panel on Smoking Prevention [9] are consistent with what has become known as the social-influences approach. Social-influences programs emphasize the short-term consequences of a specific behavior, as well as the social influences (tobacco advertising, peer pressure, etc.) that lead to the behavior in question. Correspondingly social-influence interventions often include critiquing advertising and other social influences, role playing, and practicing peer resistance skills. The social-influences approach is frequently described as the most effective model for prevention of adolescent smoking, and it is, in fact, the only program with demonstrated results [21]. With up to 5 years of follow-up, these programs have consistently demonstrated the ability to delay the onset of smoking [22]. Recent evidence suggests, however, that the benefits in early adolescence may disappear entirely by the time a student graduates from high school [7].

Some educators question the value of the social-influences model of prevention and wonder whether it may have an untoward effect on those already at risk. In a recent series of letters [20, 23] the authors noted that these programs may benefit only subsets of adolescents. In an evaluation of Project ALERT, a multirisk-factor prevention program, only the smoking behavior of experimental smokers (who had smoked one or two cigarettes in the last year and none in the past month) was improved, with no effect shown on nonsmokers and a possibly negative effect on regular cigarette users. Based on results such as these, some critics question the utility of the widespread diffusion of social-influence programs in the schools [23]. Proponents argue, however, that these programs do affect the majority of students, those who are not yet confirmed users (experimenters and nonsmokers). Most social-influence programs are intended to prevent smoking, not to achieve smoking cessation, which is a behavior that may require more intensive treatment [20].

SCHOOL SMOKING POLICIES

Because there is some evidence that even the best smoking prevention program may not sustain its benefit for students into their senior year of high school [7], the establishment of school environments that support smoking prevention and nonsmoking as the norm are often recommended [24]. Accordingly a growing number of school districts are establishing restrictive smoking policies for students and faculty [18]. In 1986 nearly half of all school districts prohibited students from smoking, 10 percent prohibited smoking among teachers, and 2 percent prohibited any type of tobacco use by anyone at any time during school hours. School no-smoking policies are becoming ever more restrictive [25].

Although, of course, one goal of smoke-free schools is to protect students from the adverse effects of second-hand smoke [26], a more important reason is the expectation that restrictive smoking policies, coupled with smoking-prevention learning activities, are effective in achieving and sustaining the prevention of students' smoking. There is some evidence that this occurs. A recent study in California showed that in schools with the most restrictive smoking policies and a strong emphasis on prevention fewer students used tobacco [27]. Recognizing the importance of school smoking policies, the NCI recommended establishment of restrictive smoking policies by schools as one of the essential elements of school-based tobacco-use prevention programs [9].

Schools are an ideal setting for achieving smoking prevention or at least to deter the onset of smoking. Through tobacco-free policies, appropriate health norms of students can be reinforced and modeled in the school environment. Unfortunately this is rarely the case. Most school-based smoking prevention efforts are didactic one-shot efforts, and they do not reflect contemporary behavior-change strategies [28]. Similarly although most school districts restrict students' tobacco use, relatively few restrict or prohibit tobacco use by teachers and administrators [18].

Diet

Dietary recommendations are a major component of national chronic disease prevention strategies, particularly on cancer and cardiovascular disease. National recommendations include reducing total- and saturated-fat consumption, increasing the consumption of fruits, vegetables, and whole-grain products, and reducing alcohol, sugar, and salt intake. Although these recommendations are for adults, they seem to be appropriate as well for children over the age of 2 years [29]. Like those of adults, the dietary practices of children tend to be at variance with the recommendations. One study of 10-year-old children showed that their total-fat, saturated-fat, and sodium consumption exceeded recommended levels [30].

The food preferences of children and adolescents mirror those of their community and their culture [30]. There is good evidence that parents have a powerful influence on their children's eating behavior, an influence that is probably even greater than it is in the case of cigarette smoking [31]. Although parents usually select most of their children's food, these selections take into account the needs and the expressed demands of children [32]. These demands are often shaped by the advertising of foods on television, commercials that make up half of all advertising directed at children and that promote sugar-filled foods almost exclusively [6].

Like American adults children tend to consume over one-third of their calories in fat. In an analysis of school lunches, done as part of a cardiovascular disease prevention program, total fat accounted for 38.8 percent of the total calories children consumed at lunch, nearly 30 percent above the recommendations of the National School Lunch Program [29]. These results were consistent with the findings of other school-based heart disease prevention programs [30] and showed little change even after the U.S. Department of Agriculture published guidelines in 1983 for reducing the fat, sugar, and sodium content of school lunches [29].

Schools have a great opportunity to influence the dietary behavior of American youth, both through health education and lunch programs. Nutrition education programs alone may be effective in improving students' knowledge, attitudes, and short-term behaviors, but to be maintained these changes must be reinforced and supported by the school environment [11]. Because 60 percent of public school students participate in school lunch programs and consume 25 percent to 33 percent of their total daily calories at school [3, 29], cafeteria and school lunch interventions are a common component of comprehensive school-based nutrition programs. The National School Lunch Act of 1946, an integral part of comprehensive school health services, currently provides 27 million lunches and 3 million breakfasts daily [33]. When Ellison and colleagues [34] tested the influence of an environmental nutrition program aimed at changing the food buying and preparation practices of school food service workers, even without a corresponding educational component, they found 15 to 20 percent less sodium and 20 percent less saturated-fat intake among the students. Thus, through school lunch programs alone, schools can significantly influence schoolchildren's diet.

Exercise

In adults, lack of physical activity is related to obesity, hypertension, high blood lipid levels, and early death from CHD. As shown in a review of studies of the health effects of a sedentary lifestyle [35], physical activity and CHD are inversely related, the level of risk being similar to that associated with hypertension, hyperlipidemia, and cigarette smoking. National surveys of adult physical fitness indicate that only a minority of adults (8 to 20 percent) engage in regular physical activity at a level likely to maintain cardiorespiratory fitness [14]. Unfortunately physical inactivity in adulthood often has its roots in childhood [36, 37].

The fitness level of American children is often decried in reports in various media. However, because of differences in definition and research methods, the actual state of physical fitness is difficult to assess. Most observers have concluded that the current generation of children is not as fit as the previous one, today's youth having more body fat than children in the 1960s [11, 14] (see Chapter 16). Yet according to national survey data, more than half of fifth- to twelfth-grade students engage in "appropriate" physical activity, which is defined as activity involving large-muscle groups at an intensity requiring at least 60 percent of cardiovascular capacity for 20 minutes at least three times a week [38]. But most of this activity occurs outside school physical education programs.

The data suggesting that children's physical

inactivity is associated with adult cardiovascular disease are limited. Accordingly a major value of physical activity in youth is the extent to which it will lead to physical activity in adulthood, which strongly correlates with protection from CHD. Consequently the goal of school-based physical education programs should be, at least partially, to create favorable attitudes, experiences, and skills to increase the likelihood that children will carry on physical activity as adults [14]. At least 80 percent of 10- to 18-year-olds are enrolled in physical education programs at school [38], but these programs often emphasize sports competition among the best athletes and often do not focus on health-related fitness that will, hopefully, lead to greater activity by adults. Schools can reach the largest number of children with structured physical education programs, but they must shift the emphasis away from motor-skills development and sports competition to health-related fitness and participation by all students, which will be more likely to lead children to maintain health-related fitness activities as adults.

The Comprehensive Approach

In addition to programs aimed at specific risk factors, some programs have combined risk factors and targeted cardiovascular health among elementary school students [29, 39, 40, 41], high school students [42], and minority populations [43]. Most notable among these is the current National Heart, Lung and Blood Institute-funded cooperative agreement called CATCH: The Child and Adolescent Trial for Cardiovascular Health [6]. This study's overall goal is to determine the effect of school-based intervention on promoting healthy behavior and reducing the risk of cardiovascular disease among elementary school students with programs that promote exercise, healthy diet, and fitness. Interventions focus on school curricula and environment and on fostering parental involvement [6].

In the CATCH program the interventions that are used are based on social-psychological principles that have been effective among different age groups and for different risk factors. This application of a common conceptual framework applied to both home and school should act synergistically to reduce cardiovascular risk and serve as a model for the primary prevention of chronic heart disease in children.

The CATCH program represents a comprehensive approach to cardiovascular disease prevention in schools. Not only does it target multiple risk factors, but it directs interventions at the individual, the teacher, and the school environment. This integration of organizational and individual change is most likely both to reduce cardiovascular risks of children and to help the schools maintain these programs. Parcel and his colleagues proposed a four-step model to plan, initiate, and maintain change in school health programs by (1) obtaining institutional commitment, (2) altering health policies and practices, (3) altering roles and actions of staff, and (4) providing positive student learning activities [2].

Institutional commitment, essential for the adoption, implementation, and maintenance of a program, can either start with school administrators and be transferred to teachers and staff (top-down) or start with the program implementors and spread to administrators (bottom-up) [2]. Clearly alterations in policies and practices are essential to a comprehensive approach to school health in which individual and organizational factors are blended. School smoking policies, cafeteria programs, and physical fitness programs all are structural elements that can either support and reinforce or contradict and challenge a school health promotion program. In-service training, technical assistance, and feedback on performance all have been shown to be effective in changing the roles and the actions of staff members in such a way as to create more successful school health programs [40]. Finally, with the preceding three steps in place, effective student learning activities can be implemented.

A supportive and reinforcing school environment increases the likelihood that students will develop health-promoting skills and attitudes [24]. Student activities should be based on sound behavioral and learning theory and, whenever possible, be those that have already been shown to be effective in achieving positive outcomes [2]. In addition to smoking prevention policies and healthy cafeteria menus, the school environment can play a direct role in promoting students' health. Nearly 80 percent of state governments regulate a variety of aspects of the school environment including sanitation, heating, lighting, access for handicapped students, and emergency procedures [44].

PARENTAL INVOLVEMENT

While schools can be instrumental in promoting the health of school-aged children, they cannot be expected to do the job alone. A supportive and reinforcing family and home setting is particularly important in encouraging children to establish healthy behaviors [45, 46]. Reviewing the literature of the role of families in influencing health-related behaviors, Perry and colleagues [47] concluded that children can influence their parents' health behavior, that parents are often difficult to recruit to traditional health education classes, and that more flexible learning methods are needed that can be used at home.

The relationship of home and school-based programs has been examined in several studies. In one of these [48] conducted in San Diego among Mexican-American and Anglo-American families, each of whom had a child in the fifth or sixth grade, half of the more than 200 families were randomized to a year-long education program designed to change dietary and exercise habits with classes held in local schools, while the other half were assigned to a control condition. After 1 year, positive changes had occurred in the intervention families' dietary practices, but their cardiovascular fitness levels had not changed significantly. The authors concluded that involving families in health education programs using school-based resources is effective and that this is a promising area for future research.

In another study [46] the benefits of school-based programs were compared with those aimed directly at the home environment. Conducted in Minnesota and North Dakota, the study compared the results of a five-week school-based program for third graders with that of a 5-week program of written information sent to the homes of third graders; both programs required parental involvement. Eighty-six percent of eligible parents participated in the home-based program, and 71 percent completed the 5-week course. Students in the home-based program had better health outcomes than did those in the school-based program. The study showed that a large number of parents are willing to participate in home-based programs, and that this type of parental participation can initiate changes in the eating patterns of young children as well as the parents.

Identifying and Removing Barriers to School-based Interventions

Although we are beginning to establish a scientific basis for identifying programs that seem to work under specific conditions, school health promotion programs still face a tough struggle [20]. Funds for school health education are scarce and schools are under considerable pressure to implement certain programs, especially those that target drug education and prevention, or risk losing designated federal funds. Evaluated programs based on tested behavioral theories have the best chance of reducing adolescent health risks and contributing to the creation of a healthy school environment.

The barriers to school-based smoking prevention programs, which are also barriers to other cardiovascular disease prevention programs, include overcrowded curricula, overburdened teachers, desire for broad programs, desire for local adaptation of programs, inadequate funding, and lack of teacher training [9]. Teacher training and full program implementation have been identified as being particularly important in school health programs [19]. Considering these barriers, we must be realistic in assessing what can be accomplished and the time and the effort required to meet program objectives and overcome these problems.

In the development of a strategy to overcome barriers to the successful implementation of school health programs, a consideration of diffusion theory should be of value [6, 19, 42].

Diffusion theory posits that the characteristics of the innovation and those of the eligible adopting individual and organization determine the speed at which an innovation spreads through a social system. Thus, according to diffusion theory, a school-based cardiovascular disease prevention program should fit community norms and existing school policies and practices, involve all relevant community resources and agencies, and be low-cost and relatively simple to implement. It is also useful to partition the diffusion process into four stages: dissemination, adoption, implementation, and maintenance [28]. By doing so, interventions can be directed at each step of the diffusion process and potential obstacles overcome.

Among the many other barriers to successful implementation of school programs targeted at coronary disease prevention, one barrier of particular concern is the relative lack of attention directed at high-risk, hard-to-reach youth. With a few notable exceptions [43, 48] most cardiovascular disease prevention programs have been targeted at nonminority, middle-class populations. Although these are important populations because of their size, programs that are effective for this group are not automatically transferable to other populations. Health professionals and schools must be continually alert to providing appropriate programming for high-risk, difficult-to-reach groups, particularly while they can still be reached in the formal school system. Too often children at highest risk leave school and are no longer exposed to potentially valuable interventions.

The Role of Health Care Providers in School-based Programs

Increasingly schools are involving health professionals in their cardiovascular disease prevention programs. This is particularly important because the proportion of children without financial access to medical services is growing. In 1988 15 percent of children aged 10 to 18 did not have health insurance coverage, a substantial increase over previous years [33]. Because of this financial barrier and because of the difficulties of transporting children to medical services, school clinics have recently been established, particularly in junior and senior high schools, to meet the wide-ranging health and psychosocial needs of adolescents [49]. The actual coordination of school health programs with community agencies to improve the health of students is one component of the expanded model of a comprehensive school health program [2].

According to a recent survey by the American School Health Association [44], two-thirds of states provide a legal basis for providing health services at schools. Typical services given by these clinics are immunizations and vision and hearing screenings, but they may have other disease prevention activities, provide nursing care for children with handicaps, and render emergency care. The provision of health services is an obvious and direct manner in which health professionals can become involved in school health programs.

Traditionally, because of heavy clinical responsibilities, physicians and other health professionals have not been involved in public health issues that affect their schools and communities. Rather than allowing elected officials and school board members to set policy on issues that directly affect the health of their community and school populations, health professionals should become actively involved in civic issues in a way that complements their clinical responsibilities. Despite changing environments health professionals continue to be among the most credible and trustworthy voices in the community. This privileged status should be used for the sake of bettering the public health.

Health professionals have the obligation to ensure the availability of exemplary programs in their community school districts and to lend their support to these programs. When such programs address both individual and organizational issues, health professionals are better able to support school initiatives, either directly by providing school health services or indirectly by consultation and technical assistance in the design and implementation of prevention programs. Because of the importance of pediatric cardiovascular risk reduction, this is the time for health professionals, both as parents and as concerned citizens, to become involved in school health programs.

Summary

The existing model of school health programs, which integrates school health services, health instruction, and healthy school environments, has served school health well for most of the twentieth century. Other models have been proposed that expand this framework to include additional components [50, 51] and that view school health in the context of educational achievement [52].

One of the most appealing of these new concepts is the ACCESS model proposed by Stone [5], in which administration, community, curricula, environment, and school services are viewed as integrated elements that facilitate the planning, implementation, and evaluation of school health programs. The administration component includes relevant laws and regulations, available resources, budgets, and teacher training. The community component includes school health advisory boards and community health councils, school boards, community agencies, and parent and family linkages. The environmental component includes school policies and practices that promote healthy behaviors. In the curricular and school services components are the elements traditional to original school health programs. Stone recommends that the administration and community components be established first to provide management and resource support for the others, and that this be followed by the environmental component to set the proper tone for students and school personnel. Once the administrative and environmental structures are in place, the curricular and school service components can function optimally [5].

Recently the National Association of State Boards of Education and the American Medical Association assembled the National Commission on the Role of the School and Community in Improving Adolescent Health, which issued the report [53] "Code Blue: Uniting for Health-

ier Youth." The commission urged schools to play a stronger role in improving the health of adolescents and specifically recommended improved collaboration within and outside schools to ensure help for students with health and other problems that may interfere with their learning.

In reviewing advances in cardiovascular health promotion programs in schools, Stone et al. [11] recommended a series of methods to improve behavioral research in school health. Their recommendations follow the CATCH model, and those most closely related to school health practices are (1) using a theory-based health curriculum, including the identification of psychosocial risk factors; (2) emphasizing curricula based on skills and not only knowledge acquisition; (3) including booster sessions to reinforce more intensive interventions; (4) considering the student's developmental stage in designing health interventions; (5) improving the total school environment; and (6) complementing school-based programs with family- and home-based interventions.

Health care professionals have a myriad of opportunities to influence the school environment to advance the goals of cardiovascular disease prevention. As discussed here, some programs have been shown to influence students' major cardiovascular risk factors of smoking, harmful dietary habits, and physical inactivity. Experts consistently recommend that programs with established effectiveness be implemented and fully maintained as intended. A solid body of research evidence suggests that environmental supports reinforce student learning activities and often have an independent effect on changing student health behaviors.

References

1. Iverson DC, Kilbe LJ. Evolution of the national disease prevention and health promotion strategy: establishing a role for the schools. J School Health 1983; 54:33–8.
2. Parcel GS, Simons-Morton BG, Kolbe LJ. Health promotion: integrating organizational change and student learning strategies. Health Educ Q 1988; 15:435–50.
3. Frank GC. Primary prevention in the school arena: a dietary approach. Health Values 1983; 7:14–21.

4. Means RK. Historical perspectives in school health. Thorofare, NJ: Charles B. Slack, 1975.
5. Stone E. ACCESS: keystones for school health promotion. J School Health 1990; 60:298–300.
6. Perry CL, Stone EJ, Parcel GS, et al. School-based cardiovascular health promotion: the Child and Adolescent Trial for Cardiovascular Health (CATCH). J School Health 1990; 60:406–13.
7. Flay BR, Koepke D, Thomson SJ, et al. Six-year follow-up of the first Waterloo School Smoking Prevention Trial. Am J Public Health 1989; 79:1371–6.
8. Pirie PL, Murray DM, Luepker RV. Smoking prevalence in a cohort of adolescents, including absentees, dropouts, and transfers. Am J Public Health 1988; 78:176–8.
9. Glynn TJ. Essential elements of school-based smoking prevention programs. J School Health 1989; 59:181–8.
10. McGill HC. Morphologic development of the atherosclerotic plaque. In: Lauer RM, Shekelle RB, eds. Childhood prevention of atherosclerosis and hypertension. New York: Raven Press, 1980.
11. Stone EJ, Perry CL, Luepker RV. Synthesis of cardiovascular behavioral research for youth health promotion. Health Educ Q 1989; 16:155–69.
12. Williams C, Carter B, Wynder E. Prevalence of selected cardiovascular and cancer risk factors in a pediatric population: the Know Your Body Project. Prev Med 1981; 10:235–50.
13. Harlan WR. A perspective on school-based cardiovascular disease research. Health Educ Q 1989; 16:151–4.
14. Simons-Morton BG, Parcel GS, O'Hara NM, et al. Health-related physical fitness in childhood: status and recommendations. Ann Rev Public Health 1988; 9:403–25.
15. Parcel GS, Simons-Morton BG, O'Hara NM, et al. School promotion of healthful diet and physical activity: impact on learning outcomes and self-reported behavior. Health Educ Q 1989; 16:181–99.
16. Escobedo LG, Anda RF, Smith PF, et al. Sociodemographic characteristics of cigarette smoking initiation in the United States. JAMA 1990; 264:1550–5.
17. Rundall TG, Bruvold WH. A meta-analysis of school-based smoking and alcohol use prevention programs. Health Educ Q 1988; 15:317–34.
18. U.S. Department of Health and Human Services. Reducing the health consequences of smoking: 25 years of progress. A report of the Surgeon General. U.S. Department of Health and Human Services, Public Health Service, Centers for Disease Control. USDHHS publ. no. (CDC) 89-8411, 1989.
19. Best JA, Thomson SJ, Santi, et al. Preventing cigarette smoking among children. Ann Rev Public Health 1988; 9:161–201.
20. Ellickson PL, Bell RM. Response: drug abuse prevention programs. Science 1990; 250:740.
21. Pentz MA, Dwyer JH, MacKinnon DP, et al. A multi-component community trial for primary prevention of adolescent drug abuse: effects on drug use prevalence. JAMA 1989; 261:3259.
22. Perry CL, Klepp KI, Sillers C. Community-wide strategies for cardiovascular health: the Minnesota Heart Health Program youth program. Health Educ Res 1989; 4:87–101.
23. Ferrence RG, Kozlowski LT. Drug abuse prevention programs. Science 1990; 250:739–40.
24. Stevens NH, Davis LG. Exemplary school health education: a new change from HOT districts. Health Educ Q 1988; 15:63–70.
25. National School Boards Association. No smoking: a board member's guide to nonsmoking policies for the schools. Alexandria, VA: National School Boards Association, 1987.
26. Olds RS. Promoting child health in a smoke-free school: suggestions for school health personnel. J School Health 1988; 58:269–72.
27. Pentz MA, Brannon BR, Charlin VL, et al. The power of policy: the relationship of smoking policy to adolescent smoking. Am J Public Health 1989; 79:857–62.
28. Parcel GS, Eriksen MP, Lovato CY, et al. The diffusion of school-based tobacco-use prevention programs: project description and baseline data. Health Educ Res 1989; 4:111–24.
29. Parcel GS, Simons-Morton BG, O'Hara NM, et al. School promotion of healthful diet and exercise behavior: an integration of organizational change and social learning theory interventions. J School Health 1987; 57:150–6.
30. Frank GC, Berenson GS, Webber LS. Dietary studies and the relationship of diet to cardiovascular risk factor variables in 10-year old children — the Bogalusa Heart Study. Am J Clin Nut 1978; 31:228–40.
31. Crockett SJ, Mullis R, Perry CL, Luepker RV. Parent education in youth-directed nutrition interventions. Prev Med 1989; 17:475–91.
32. Wadden TA, Brownell KD. The development and modification of dietary practices in individuals, groups and large populations. In: Matarazzo JD, Weiss SM, Herd JA, Miller NE, Weiss SM, eds. Behavioral health: a handbook of health enhancement and disease prevention. New York: Wiley, 1984.
33. Stone EJ, Perry CL. United States: perspectives in school health. J School Health 1990; 60:363–9.
34. Ellison RC, Capper AL, Goldberg RJ, et al. The environmental component: changing school

food service to promote cardiovascular health. Health Educ Q 1989; 16:285–97.

35. Powell KE, Thompson PD, Casperson CJ, et al. Physical activity and incidence of coronary heart disease. Ann Rev Pub Health 1987; 8:253–87.

36. Iverson DC, Fielding JE, Crow RS, et al. The promotion of physical activity in the United States populations: the status of programs in medical, worksite, community and school settings. Public Health Reports 1985; 100:212–4.

37. Riopel DA, Boerth RC, Coates TJ, et al. Coronary risk factor modification in children: exercise. Circulation 1986; 74:1189A–91A.

38. Ross JG, Pate RR. The national children and youth fitness study. II. A summary of findings. J Phys Ed. Rec and Dance 1987; 58:51–6.

39. Butcher AH, Frank GC, Harsha DW, et al. Heart Smart: a school health program meeting the 1990 objectives for the nation. Health Educ Q 1988; 15:17–34.

40. Simons-Morton BG, Parcel GS, O'Hara NM. Implementing organizational changes to promote healthful diet and physical activity at school. Health Educ Q 1988; 15:115–30.

41. Walter HJ. Primary prevention of chronic disease among children: the school-based "Know Your Body" intervention trials. Health Educ Q 1989; 16:201–14.

42. Killen JD, Robinson TN, Telch MJ, et al. The Stanford Adolescent Heart Health Program. Health Educ Q 1989; 16:263–83.

43. Bush PJ, Zuckerman AE, Taggart VS, et al. Cardiovascular risk factor prevention in black school children: the "Know Your Body" evaluation project. Health Educ Q 1989; 16:215–27.

44. Lovato CY, Allensworth DD, Chen F. School health in America: an assessment of state policies to protect and improve the health of students. 5th ed. Kent, OH: American School Health Association, 1989.

45. Cohen RY, Felix MRJ, Brownell KD. The role of parents and older peers in school-based cardiovascular prevention programs: implications for school development. Health Educ Q 1990; 16:245–53.

46. Perry CL, Luepker RV, Murray DM, et al. Parent involvement with children's health promotion: a one year follow-up of the Minnesota Home Team. Health Educ Q 1989; 16:171–80.

47. Perry CL, Crockett SJ, Pirie P. Influencing parental health behavior: implications of community assessments. Health Educ 1987; 18:68–77.

48. Nader PR, Sallis JF, Patterson TL, et al. A family approach to cardiovascular risk reduction: results from the San Diego Family Health Project. Health Educ Q 1989; 16:229–44.

49. Dryfoos JG, Klerman LV. School-based clinics: their role in helping students meet the 1990 objectives. Health Educ Q 1988; 15:71–80.

50. Allensworth DD, Kolbe LJ. The comprehensive school health program: exploring an expanded concept. J School Health 1987; 57:409–12.

51. Allensworth DD Wolford CA. Schools as agents for achieving the 1990 health objectives for the nation. Health Educ Q 1988; 15:3–15.

52. Nader PR. The concept of "comprehensiveness" in the design and implementation of school health programs. J School Health 1990; 60:133–8.

53. National Commission on the Role of the School and Community in Improving Adolescent Health. Code blue: uniting for healthier youth. Alexandria, VA: National Association of State Boards of Education, 1990.

IV

OTHER ISSUES REGARDING THE PREVENTION OF CORONARY HEART DISEASE

21

Cost Effectiveness

NICOLE URBAN

EDITORS' INTRODUCTION

Controlling the cost of medical care is one of the most important issues now facing the United States and other countries. It is hardly possible to open a newspaper without seeing another article on this topic. Prevention is often seen as a panacea in this regard, advocated by politicians and business people alike as a way of reducing the health care burden. Yet prevention-related activities have their own costs, and establishing the true cost-benefit ratio of any given risk-factor modification activity can be difficult. Dr. Urban, a noted health care economist, takes us through some of the technical aspects of assigning costs to health care–related activities and then reviews the cost effectiveness of various strategies for the prevention of CHD. An important distinction is made between cost effectiveness and cost saving, two concepts that are frequently confused. Most physicians would prefer not to have to deal with cost issues, but this is a luxury that is no longer available. Dr. Urban provides us with the information needed to understand some of the forces that affect the practice of medicine and to advocate for intelligent and responsible choices.

Various estimates of the societal costs of CHD and of the cost effectiveness of preventing CHD have been reported in the literature. Their interpretation is facilitated by an understanding of (1) conceptual issues underlying the methods used in estimating costs, (2) the purpose and mechanics of conducting a cost-effectiveness analysis, and (3) some frame of reference or standard of comparison for placing in perspective the magnitude of the reported cost and cost-effectiveness estimates.

The Costs of CHD

The large burden imposed by CHD in the United States has long been recognized [1, 2]. In 1980 Hartunian, Smart, and Thompson reported the economic costs of cancer, heart disease, motor vehicle accidents, and strokes [3], using what has become the standard incidence approach to estimating the costs of illness. They estimated that the economic costs of CHD in the United States were $13.7 billion in 1975 dollars, which included $2.5 billion in direct medical costs and $11.2 billion in lost earnings. Lifetime costs associated with an average case of CHD were estimated to be $20,785, which included $3775 in direct costs associated with treatment and $17,010 in indirect costs (lost earnings) associated with premature mortality. They also reported that an estimated reduction in life expectancy of 9.1 years is associated with each case of CHD. The incidence of CHD in 1975 was estimated to be 659,926 [3].

The reported $13.7 billion ($20,784 per case) is an estimate of the *present value* in *1975 dollars* of the *opportunity cost* of CHD in the United States. The principles that underlie the use of these terms come from basic economic theory. *Opportunity cost* is the value of the opportunities foregone by society. There are two major categories of opportunities foregone as a result of CHD incidence. The first is the value of the resources used to treat CHD, including all the medical services (physician, nursing, and hospital effort), which might have been used to treat other diseases. Conceptually the value of using these resources to treat other diseases is the opportunity cost of their use in treating

CHD; they are referred to as the *direct costs* of CHD. The second category of opportunities foregone is the value of the time lost due to premature death attributable to CHD. Time is a productive resource that can be used in many different ways. The value of time can be measured in several ways, but often the average wage rate is used because it represents what society would be willing to pay for the use of time. Accordingly, in the Hartunian analysis, the *indirect costs* of CHD are measured by the foregone earnings associated with CHD mortality. Another analyst might have included the foregone earnings associated with CHD morbidity as well or chosen another method for valuing the time lost to CHD.

The cost estimate reported by Hartunian and colleagues is of the *present value* of the opportunity cost of CHD. This means that the costs have been specified over time, beginning with a base year (in this case the year of incidence) and that the stream of future costs has been discounted to the base year. The mechanics of discounting are shown in Figure 21-1. A stream of costs over time is specified or estimated, and costs in each year are discounted by multiplying by a factor that is a function of time and the rate of return on investment of a real resource. The factor is $1/(1 + r)^t$, where r is the *real rate of interest* and t is the number of years since the

Figure 21-1.   Discounting a stream of costs over time (discount rate = 5 percent).

Year	Undiscounted Costs	Discount Factor	Discounted Costs
0	$100.00	$1/(1+.05)^0$	$100.00
1	$100.00	$1/(1+.05)^1$	95.24
2	$100.00	$1/(1+.05)^2$	90.70
3	$100.00	$1/(1+.05)^3$	86.36
.	.	.	.
.	.	.	.
.	.	.	.
10	$100.00	$1/(1+.05)^{10}$	61.39
Total	$1,100.00		$872.17

base year. The sum of the discounted stream of future costs is called the *present value* of the costs. It is exactly like investment analysis, in which money invested provides a rate of return, a concept with which most of us are familiar, except that instead of asking "What will my $100 be worth in 5 years if I invest it today at a rate of interest of 5 percent?" we are asking, "How much must I invest today to have $100 five years from now, if the rate of interest is 5 percent?" Discounting lowers the estimate of cost if any of the costs occur in the future. The higher the discount rate and the longer the period over which costs occur, the greater will be the effect of discounting.

The mechanics of discounting are relatively straightforward. What is not so clear is why we discount. The principle underlying discounting is that, other things being equal, people prefer to have things now rather than to have them in the future. This *time preference* reflects uncertainty about the future as well as the fact that something available now can be put to productive use, generating returns that accrue over time. For example, people borrow money to purchase a car because they require the services of the car immediately; they are willing to pay 5 percent, or 10 percent, or even 15 percent annual interest to have the car now rather than wait until they have saved the total purchase price. The rate at which we discount is the price society is willing to pay to have things today rather than to defer consumption for a year; it reflects the real rate of return on investment.

Hartunian and colleagues introduced a method now known as the *incidence* approach to estimating lifetime costs of a disease, which is particularly appropriate for evaluating the benefits of prevention programs. The alternative approach is referred to as the *prevalence* approach. In the former approach, the year of incidence of the disease is taken as the base year for discounting, so that treatment costs as well as the foregone earnings attributable to premature death are discounted to the year of incidence. In the latter approach, treatment costs are not discounted; rather, treatment costs of all *prevalent* cases are counted in the year when they occur; the year of death due to disease is taken

as the base year for discounting, and the foregone earnings are discounted to the year in which death occurs. The incidence approach is more appropriate when prevention interventions are being evaluated, because the investment in prevention is made prior to incidence of the case.

The appropriate discount rate for use in calculating the present value of the cost of CHD is the *real rate of interest,* which measures time preference and the real return on investment but does not reflect inflation. The *nominal* rate of interest, the rate of interest we actually pay, reflects inflation as well as time preference and is higher than the real rate of interest. Conceptually time preference is independent of the relative value of money from one year to the next. Even in the absence of inflation, time preference would exist and discounting would be necessary. In a cost or cost-effectiveness analysis, adjustment for inflation is taken into account not by discounting but by measuring the opportunity cost in *real* rather than *nominal* dollars.

The cost estimate reported by Hartunian and colleagues is of the present value of the opportunity cost of CHD measured in *1975 dollars.* When a stream of costs measured in dollars is specified over time or when costs occuring in different years are being compared some means of adjusting for inflation is needed. When costs are reported in the dollars of the year in which the costs are incurred, we say that they are reported in *nominal* or *current* dollars. This is not generally done in cost-effectiveness analysis, because interest is in the value of the real resources (opportunity cost). To avoid the distortion introduced by inflation, resources are measured in *real* or *constant* dollars, which means that inflation is ignored, and all costs are measured in some arbitrary year's dollars regardless of when they are incurred. In the Hartunian analysis, the value of the resources used to treat CHD and the foregone earnings were measured in 1975 dollars. To make Hartunian's estimates more meaningful today, it is helpful to convert from 1975 to 1989 dollars using the consumer price index (CPI) and the medical care price index (MCPI), published by the Bureau of Labor Statistics [4].

Direct costs per case are converted from 1975

to 1989 dollars using the MCPI, because they measure use of medical services. Indirect costs are converted using the CPI, because they measure foregone earnings. Costs per case of CHD expressed in 1989 dollars are $11,823 in direct costs associated with treatment and $39,205 in foregone earnings, for a total of $51,028 in lifetime costs associated with a case of CHD. Assuming that CHD incidence remained the same between 1975 and 1989, these estimates suggest that the burden of CHD in 1989 was about $33.6 billion annually, of which $7.8 billion was in direct medical costs. Use of 1989 rather than 1975 dollars inflates the cost estimates by a factor of about 2.4. Clearly in interpreting the estimates of costs or cost per unit of effectiveness in a cost-effectiveness analysis, it is important to take into consideration the year's dollars used to measure real resource use.

The Cost Effectiveness of Strategies for Preventing CHD

Estimates of the cost effectiveness of strategies to prevent CHD, summarized in Table 21-1, vary considerably. For example, the cost effectiveness of counseling a patient to quit smoking has been reported to be between $705 and $2058 per year of life saved [5], while the cost effectiveness of treating hypercholesterolemia has been reported to be between $32,000 and $176,000 per year of life saved [6]. How should these estimates be interpreted and compared?

First, all estimates should be converted to constant dollars, to adjust for differences that are attributable to changes over time in the value of the dollar. In the last column of Table 21-1 estimates of the cost effectiveness of the prevention strategies have all been converted to 1989 dollars using the July 1989 MCPI, to be consistent with the estimates reported in Table 21-2 [6]. Second, the purpose and the mechanics of conducting a cost-effectiveness analysis should be understood, so that the methods used to obtain a particular estimate of cost effectiveness can be taken into account. Third, the magnitude of the estimates should be placed in

perspective, to permit judgments about the relative cost effectiveness of various strategies.

When we ask if prevention of CHD is cost effective, we are asking if it is worthwhile, taking into account all the effort and resources that go into it, including costs borne by patients, physicians, and society more generally. Cost-effectiveness analysis is a tool that assists us in making this judgment. It can be used to help us judge the relative cost effectiveness of two or more strategies for preventing and/or treating CHD or the absolute cost effectiveness of a new strategy relative to a baseline, usually representing the status quo. Some baseline or alternative must always be specified, because cost-effectiveness analysis involves comparing incremental, or *marginal,* benefits to incremental, or marginal, costs.

The mechanics of cost effectiveness are summarized in Figure 21-2. An intervention strategy is cost effective if it yields a net marginal benefit worth its net marginal cost, relative to an alternative strategy or baseline [7]. Cost-effectiveness analysis yields a *ratio,* an estimate of the cost per unit of health benefit, which allows comparison of cost effectiveness among various strategies. The numerator of the cost-effectiveness ratio is measured in dollars, and the denominator is measured in units of health benefit, such as lives saved, years of life saved, or years of quality-adjusted life saved. In comparing cost-effectiveness estimates, care should be taken that health benefits as well as dollars are measured in comparable units. In Table 21-1, a few of the estimates are of cost per quality-adjusted year of life saved, but most are of cost per year of life saved without a quality adjustment.

The costs and benefits that are usually counted in a cost-effectiveness analysis, described in 1977 by Weinstein and Stason [7] and discussed with respect to prevention strategies in 1986 by Russell [8], are summarized in Figure 21-2. In the numerator are the dollar costs and savings attributable to the strategy being assessed, relative to a baseline, which might be the status quo or an alternative strategy. These costs include the direct medical (or prevention)

Table 21-1. Cost per year of life saved of strategies to prevent and treat (costs and benefits discounted at 5%)

Strategy	Cost per year of life saved ($)	Year in which dollars are measured	Cost per year of life saved in 1989 dollars
Smoking			
Counseling by physicians [5]	705–2058	1984	985–2877
Follow-up visit [5]	5051	1984	7060
Nicotine gum [11]	4113–9473	1984	5749–13,241
Hypertension [12]			
Propranolol	10,900	1987	12,485
Hydrochlorothiazide	16,000	1987	18,326
Nifedipine	31,600	1987	36,194
Prazosin hydrochloride	61,900	1987	70,898
Captopril	72,000	1987	82,467
Hypercholesterolemia [6]			
High-risk men aged 60+			
cholesterol >300 [16]	32,000	1989	32,000
Cholesterol >315 [15]	91,000	1989	91,000
Cholesterol >265 [13]	77,000–176,000	1989	77,000–176,000
Cholestyramine resin [14]	117,400	1985	154,572
Lovastatin (high-risk men) [25]	6000–53,000	1989	6,000–53,000
Lovastatin (high-risk women) [25]	19,000–160,000	1989	19,000–160,000
Colestipol [14]	63,900	1985	84,132
Oat bran [14]	17,800	1985	23,436
Treatment strategies* [13]			
CABG for left-main disease	4000	1984	5591
Beta blockers following MI	4200	1984	5871
CABG for three-vessel disease	7000–8000	1984	9784–11,182
CABG for two-vessel disease	35,000	1984	48,922
CABG for single-vessel disease	600,000	1984	838,655
CCU admission (20% risk of MI)	33,000	1980	65,780
CCU admission (10% risk of MI)	66,000	1980	131,561
Exercise* [21]	12,623	1985	16,620

*Years of life saved are quality adjusted.

care costs associated with the strategy and its side effects and the savings associated with preventing morbidity and mortality. To the extent that a prevention strategy reduces morbidity and mortality, it results in a dollar savings that may or may not be offset by the dollar costs of the prevention strategy itself. When the numerator is less than zero, the prevention strategy is said to be cost-saving. More often, the numerator is greater than zero; in this case the ratio measures the cost per unit of effectiveness. In the denominator the net health effects are summarized, usually measured in quality-ad-justed years of life. They include the change in life expectancy attributable to the strategy, the change in the quality of life attributable to reduced morbidity, and any change in the quality of life associated with the strategy itself (side effects).

Cost effectiveness is intended to guide resource allocation. In general society should allocate resources in such a way that the strategies with the lowest cost per year of life saved are implemented first. Strategies should be implemented in ascending order until the cost per year of life saved of the next strategy exceeds the

Step 1:   Numerator
Count the marginal costs, including:
(a) direct costs of the new treatment/measure,
(b) costs of treating side effects,
(c) savings attributable to curing/preventing the disease.

Step 2:   Denominator
Measure the marginal effectiveness (benefits), including:
(a) impact on mortality by age (change in life expectancy),
(b) impact on morbidity (change in quality of life):
  (1) side effects of treatment or preventive measure,
  (2) direct effects attributable to curing/preventing the disease.

Step 3:   Present Value
Discount both the numerator and denominator to get costs and benefits measured as present value, using the real rate of return on investment as the discount rate.

Step 4:   Cost-Effectiveness Ratio
Divide the present value of marginal costs by the present value of marginal benefits to express cost effectiveness as the cost per unit of effectiveness.

Step 5: Net Benefits (optional)
Convert benefits (denominator) to dollars by choosing a dollar value to place on a year of healthy life, and express as a difference (benefits–costs) rather than a ratio (costs/benefits).

Figure 21-2.   Summary of cost-effectiveness analysis.

value society places on a year of life. Equivalently one strategy is preferred to another on the basis of cost effectiveness if its cost per year of life saved is lower.

Smoking

The health benefits attributable to a reduction in smoking are well known. As Warner recently pointed out, the benefits of a smoke-free society would be on the order of a gain in life expectancy of 15 years among the nation's 350,000 smokers who each year die of tobacco-related disease, or a gain of between 1 and 2 years for society overall [9]. Manning et al. have estimated the external costs of smoking — the costs that smokers impose on others — to be approximately $.15 per pack of cigarettes [10]. This figure is low relative to the external costs of excess alcohol, estimated to be $1.19 per excess ounce, because smokers tend to cause only their own premature deaths, while drinkers are likely to cause the deaths of others in traffic accidents. In their analysis *each pack* of cigarettes is associated with a medical care cost increase of $.38 and a savings of $1.82 (undiscounted) in pensions due to a reduction in life expectancy of 2 hours and 17 minutes. Manning and colleagues report their estimates in 1986 dollars.

The cost effectiveness of physician counseling against smoking has been analyzed by Cummings and colleagues [5], who conclude that it is at least as cost effective as other preventive strategies and should be done routinely for patients who smoke. They estimate that the cost effectiveness of brief advice during routine office visits ranges from $705 to $988 per year of life saved among men and from $1204 to $2058 per year of life saved among women. Their estimates are based on the assumption that an additional 2.7 percent of smokers would quit as a result of brief advice. The marginal cost effectiveness of a follow-up visit devoted to counseling about quitting smoking, assumed to result in an additional 1 percent of smokers quitting, is estimated to be $5051 per year of life saved [5]. These estimates are reported in 1984 dollars; future costs and benefits were discounted at 5 percent. As shown in Table 21-1, the cost effectiveness of counseling against smoking appears to compare favorably with treatment for hypertension and hypercholesterolemia.

The cost effectiveness of nicotine gum as an adjunct to advice against smoking has been analyzed by Oster and colleagues, who report that the cost per year of life saved by nicotine gum ranges from $4113 to $6465 for men and from $6880 to $9473 for women [11]. Their estimates are based on an assumption that a box of nicotine gum costs $20.18 and that patients who use it and quit use $161 worth of gum, while patients who use it but do not quit use $40 worth of gum. Their estimates are reported in 1984 dollars; future costs and benefits are discounted at 5 percent.

Hypertension

A recent study of the relative long-term cost effectiveness of five drugs used to lower blood pressure, in individuals aged 35 to 64 years with diastolic pressure of 95 mm Hg or greater and no known CHD [12], reports somewhat more favorable cost-effectiveness ratios than had been reported in earlier studies [13]. Therapy was simulated over a 20-year period (1990 to 2010), future costs and benefits were discounted at 5 percent per year, effectiveness was measured in years of life saved, and costs were reported in 1987 dollars. Cost-effectiveness ratios vary from $10,900 for propranolol hydrochloride to $72,000 for captopril. Hydrochlorothiazide, nifedipine, and prazosin hydrochloride were estimated to have cost-effectiveness ratios of $16,000, $31,600, and $61,900, respectively.

Hypercholesterolemia

A recent review of the literature on the cost effectiveness of treating asymptomatic hypercholesterolemia was prepared by the Toronto Working Group on Cholesterol Policy [6]. Eight relevant studies were identified, of which four (Kinosian [14], Oster [15], Taylor [16], and Weinstein [13]) were included in the review because they met the criteria that results were expressed as costs per life year saved, both costs and benefits were discounted (at 5 percent), evidence for efficacy of the intervention program was clear, middle-aged men were included, and

methods could be appraised. All four studies included cholestyramine as it was used in the Lipid Research Clinics Coronary Primary Prevention Trial [17]. One [16] also included dietary therapy as it was used in the Multiple Risk Factor Intervention Trial [16a] and another [14] included oat bran as it was used in a cholesterol-lowering trial [16b], and colestipol as recommended by the manufacturer.

Results of the four studies with respect to the cost effectiveness of cholestyramine for reducing cholesterol in middle-aged men are summarized in Table 21-2. Costs per year of life saved are reported in 1989 dollars. The lowest estimate of cost per life year saved was $32,000, obtained for 60-year-old men with cholesterol levels above 300 (ninetieth percentile), who also smoke heavily, have high blood pressure (ninetieth percentile), and have low HDL cholesterol (tenth percentile) [16]. Estimates below $100,000 were also obtained for men with the risk factors just described and cholesterol above 240 ($32,000 to $71,000) [16]; for men with cholesterol above 290 in combination with smoking, diabetes, and hypertension ($60,000) [15] or smoking alone ($97,000) [15]; and for men with cholesterol above 315 ($91,000) [15].

The Toronto Working Group concluded that the treatment of hypercholesterolemia is generally less efficient than many alternative approaches to reducing CHD mortality and that routine treatment of men with levels of cholesterol below 265 is one of the least cost-effective interventions against CHD [6]. Kinosian and Eisenberg, who specifically sought cost-effective alternatives for treating hypercholesterolemia, concluded that pharmacologic therapy is most cost-effective when low-cost forms are applied to high-risk individuals such as smokers and that a broad public health approach aimed at dietary modification by the general population may be a better approach than a medically oriented campaign that focuses on drug therapy. They reported a cost per year of life saved in 1985 dollars of $117,400 for cholestyramine resin, $63,900 for colestipol, and $17,800 for oat bran [14].

More recently Hay and colleagues [17a] carried out an analysis of the use of lifetime lo-

Table 21-2.   Results of four studies on the cost effectiveness of cholestyramine for reducing serum cholesterol in men

Study	Age	Serum TC (mg/dl)	Other risk factors	Cost per year of life saved in 1989 dollars
Kinosian	45–50	>265	Avg. U.S. profile	A. (packets) 155,000
				(bulk) 77,000
				B. (packets) 143,000
Oster	45–49	265	Avg. U.S. profile	148,000
	45–49	290	Avg. U.S. profile	115,000
	45–49	315	Avg. U.S. profile	91,000
	45–49	290	None	141,000
	45–49	290	Smoker	97,000
	45–49	290	Smoker, diabetic, hypertensive	60,000
Taylor	40	240	Low (see text)	606,000
	40	300	Low	329,000
	60	240	Low	711,000
	60	300	Low	408,000
	40	240	High (see text)	71,000
	40	300	High	38,000
	60	240	High	57,000
	60	300	High	32,000
Weinstein	45–50	>265	Not stated (probably avg. U.S. profile)	176,000

Source: Naylor et al. [6].

vastatin therapy as the intervention for cholesterol lowering for adults between 35 and 55 years of age. For average-risk men with total serum cholesterol levels between 220 and 380 mg/dl the cost per year of life saved in 1989 collars ranged from $9000 to $106,000, depending on age when therapy is begun and initial cholesterol level. For average-risk women the equivalent cost is $35,000 to $297,000. In high-risk men (who smoke and are hypertensive) the cost per year of life saved ranged from $6000 to $53,000. They concluded that there are some 800,000 high-risk men in the United States aged 35 to 55 in whom the net cost of lovastatin therapy would be less than $35,000 per year of life saved.

Similar to the Toronto Working Group, Hall and colleagues also concluded that a population-based strategy that educates the entire population is likely to be more cost effective than an approach that requires screening of the population to identify individuals at high risk [18].

The population-based approach has the advantages that screening of individuals for risk factors is not required and that multiple risk factors can be targeted through the media. They report that such a strategy costs $8000 (1986 dollars) per case of MI prevented, compared to between $12,000 and $26,000 per case prevented for alternative strategies that require identification of high-risk individuals. It should be noted that these estimates are not directly comparable to the estimates summarized in Table 21-1 and reported above because the effectiveness measure is different. Hall and colleagues report costs per case prevented rather than costs per year of life saved.

Although the cost effectiveness of dietary interventions to reduce cholesterol has not been reported, Murray and colleagues described low-intensity interventions designed for use in the general public [19]. Net reductions in total cholesterol of about 4 percent were found at 1-year follow-up in response to classes requiring 8 hours of contact time for a cost of $20. At a conference sponsored by the National Heart, Lung and Blood Institute (NHLBI) in September 1990 on the cost and health implications of cholesterol lowering, Goldman reported that the cost effectiveness of a population approach to cholesterol lowering ranges from a cost saving to a cost of $34,200 per year of life saved, for programs ranging from $4 to $7 in intervention costs per person per year, and from 1 percent to 4 percent in serum cholesterol reductions [20].

Exercise

Hatziandrieu and colleagues [21] recently analyzed the cost effectiveness of exercise as a health promotion activity. They concluded that the cost per quality-adjusted year of life saved through regular exercise such as jogging, estimated to be $12,623 in 1985 dollars using a discount rate of 5 percent, is favorable when compared with other strategies for preventing or treating CHD. They assumed that nonexercisers have a relative risk of CHD of 2.0 for a CHD event and that the direct costs of exercise were $100 annually plus $75 for physician counseling. The indirect cost of exercise, reflecting the value (opportunity cost) of time spent exercising, was assumed to be $4.50 per hour for those who are neutral in their feelings toward exercise, $9 per hour for those who dislike it, and $0 for those who enjoy it, based on an average wage rate of $9 per hour in 1985.

The Cost Effectiveness of Strategies for Reducing CHD Mortality

It is useful to consider the cost effectiveness of efforts to prevent heart disease in the context of efforts to reduce mortality from heart disease more generally. This approach facilitates comparisons among primary, secondary, and tertiary prevention strategies and provides a context for judging the cost effectiveness of primary prevention approaches. Savings in treatment costs attributable to prevention of the disease are appropriately discounted and reflected in the cost-effectiveness ratio for a pri-

mary prevention strategy, so that cost-effectiveness ratios among the various types of strategies are directly comparable.

The evidence regarding the cost effectiveness of alternative strategies for reducing mortality from CHD was reviewed in 1985 by Weinstein and Stason [13]. Evidence in the literature regarding several treatment strategies was examined, including coronary artery bypass surgery (CABG), beta-blocking drugs following an MI, coronary care unit (CCU) use, and emergency care programs, including prehospital cardiopulmonary resuscitation (CPR) and defibrillation. The cost effectiveness of primary prevention strategies was considered as well, including hypertension detection and treatment, hypercholesterolemia detection and treatment, and community interventions targeting hypertension, hypercholesterolemia, smoking, and obesity simultaneously.

Weinstein and Stason summarized the evidence on the relative cost effectiveness of these various strategies by reporting their cost per quality-adjusted life year (QALY) saved in 1984 dollars. Estimates for the treatment strategies they investigated are included in Table 21-1. The most cost-effective strategies are CABG for left-main disease ($4000 per QALY), beta blockers following MI ($4200 per QALY), and CABG in patients with three-vessel disease ($7000 to $8000 per QALY), followed by detection and treatment through dietary change of hypercholesterolemia among 10-year-old children ($23,000 per QALY) and detection and pharmacologic treatment of hypertension among adults ($28,500 per QALY).

Treatment of two-vessel disease by CABG is also relatively cost effective ($35,000 per QALY), particularly when restricted to patients suffering from severe angina ($23,000 per QALY). The addition of mobile CCU care (defibrillation by trained paramedics) to a basic emergency system that includes EMTs and CPR education is in the same cost-effectiveness range as CABG for two-vessel disease ($35,000 per QALY). Admission to a CCU rather than an intermediate-care unit is cost effective relative to the approaches above only if the risk of an MI is at least 20 percent; CABG for single-vessel disease is not cost effective ($600,000 per QALY) unless the patient is suffering from severe angina ($23,000 per QALY). Based on their analysis, pharmacologic treatment of adults by cholestyramine for hypercholesterolemia does not appear to be a cost-effective strategy for the prevention of CHD ($117,400 in 1985 dollars per QALY), relative to the other approaches.

Summary

From the estimates summarized in Table 21-1 and the preceding discussion, it can be concluded that the cost effectiveness of the prevention of CHD depends on the particular prevention strategy chosen. Estimates of cost per year of life saved range from under $1000 to over $150,000 in 1989 dollars, for physician counseling of smokers and pharmacologic treatment of cholesterol above 265 mg/dl, respectively. Treatment strategies vary just as much in their cost effectiveness, from under $5000 to over $500,000 per QALY saved in 1989 dollars for CABG for left-main disease and CABG for single-vessel disease, respectively. What do all these estimates mean?

The goal is efficiency in resource allocation, to attain the greatest benefit in terms of reductions in morbidity and mortality within resource constraints. Efficiency in resource allocation requires knowledge of costs as well as benefits; the condition for efficiency is that marginal benefit equals marginal costs. Each prevention strategy should be pursued if and only if its marginal benefit equals or exceeds its marginal cost.

Cost-effectiveness analysis does not tell us if a particular strategy is cost effective in an absolute sense unless we specify how much society is willing to pay for a unit of health benefit. Cost-benefit analysis, in which health benefits such as years of life are valued and measured in dollars, yields a net *difference* between marginal benefits and marginal costs. If benefits exceed costs, the strategy is judged cost beneficial or cost effective [7]. In cost-benefit analysis, the magnitude of the health benefit is implicit in the calculation of net benefit.

When comparing two strategies relative to the same baseline, we must consider the magnitude of the health benefits of each strategy in judging cost effectiveness. Because the cost per year of life saved can be expected to increase with the number of years of life saved, we would expect to pay more per year of life saved for a program that saved twice as many years of life. If the programs are not mutually exclusive, the one with the lower cost per year of life saved should be implemented first; the more expensive strategy should then be reevaluated relative to the less expensive one to estimate its *marginal* cost effectiveness relative to the new baseline. Only in this way can we assess whether the additional (marginal) life years to be saved using the more expensive strategy are worth their marginal cost.

In judging the value of a prevention strategy, we must remember that prevention can be cost effective without being cost saving. A strategy is said to be cost saving if the numerator of the cost-effectiveness ratio is negative [22]. This would occur if the savings in treatment costs attributable to reduced morbidity and mortality more than offset the costs of prevention. Then, the prevention strategy would actually save money, in addition to reducing morbidity and mortality. That is rarely the case, however, and should not be the criterion for judging a prevention strategy worthwhile [8].

A prevention or treatment strategy may be cost saving without being cost effective, or cost effective without being cost saving. It is cost effective without being cost saving if it does not save money but yields a benefit worth its cost. This is the usual condition. It is cost saving without being cost effective if it saves money but results in morbidity and mortality that are not worth the monetary savings [22]. It is important that this distinction be kept in mind in judging prevention strategies, because in general they yield significant health benefits but do not lead to cost savings. Too often prevention strategies are judged in terms of their potential savings in treatment costs, without adequate consideration given to their impact on health. We should expect each increment in health to come at some marginal cost, regardless of whether the increment in health is the result of treatment or prevention [8].

The unit chosen for measuring health benefit also has important implications for the conclusions that can be drawn from a cost–effectiveness or cost–benefit analysis. Health effects are often measured as deaths averted or years of life saved. The latter takes into account the average age at death, while the former values all deaths equally. The measure of benefit most commonly recommended, however, is the QALY [7, 8, 23]. This measure of health benefit takes into account improvement or degradation in functional health status as well as impact on length of life [24] and facilitates comparisons among treatments and prevention efforts with heterogeneous effects on health. It should be recognized that the method of measurement chosen implies a value judgment. Depending on the nature of the analysis, quality adjustment of life years saved may discriminate against the handicapped, while use of life years saved rather than deaths averted may discriminate against the elderly.

It could be argued that the value of cost–effectiveness analysis lies chiefly in its requirement that all assumptions, including those that reflect implicit value judgments, be made explicit, so that the reasons for different judgments become clear. Regardless of the assumptions the goal that is implicit in every cost–effectiveness analysis is efficiency in the allocation of resources. Resources are allocated efficiently when there exists no reallocation that would result in greater aggregate benefit. As in microeconomic theory more generally the condition for efficiency is that marginal benefit equals marginal cost, a condition that is explicit in cost–benefit analysis.

The question is neither "Is prevention cost effective?" nor "Is prevention more cost effective than treatment?" Overall it can be concluded that some prevention strategies are cost effective and that some prevention strategies are more cost effective than some treatment strategies. However, efficiency in resource allocation will be attained only when the most cost-effective strategies from within the available sets of treatment and prevention strategies are used.

Prevention and treatment are not mutually exclusive. When the best prevention strategies are combined with the best treatment strategies, the best outcome will be realized.

References

1. Rice DP. Estimating the cost of illness. Public Health Services Economic Series #6. Washington, DC: U.S. Government Printing Office, 1966.
2. Cooper BS, Rice DP. The economic cost of illness revisited. Soc Sec Bull 1976; 39:21–36.
3. Hartunian NS, Smart CN, Thompson MS. The incidence and economic costs of cancer, motor vehicle injuries, coronary heart disease, and stroke: a comparative analysis. Am J Public Health 1980; 70:49–1260.
4. U.S. Bureau of the Census. Statistical Abstract of the United States: 1990. 110th ed. Washington DC, 1990. Table no. 761.
5. Cummings SR, Rubin SM, Oster G. The cost-effectiveness of counseling smokers to quit. JAMA 1989; 261:75–9.
6. Naylor DC, Basinski A, Frank JW, Rachlis MM. Asymptomatic hypercholesterolemia: a clinical policy review. Chap. 6. Efficiency considerations: the cost-effectiveness of treating asymptomatic hypercholesteremia. J Clin Epidem 1990; 43:1093–101.
7. Weinstein MC, Stason WB. Foundations of cost-effectiveness analysis. N Engl J Med 1977; 296:716–21.
8. Russell LB. Is prevention better than cure? Washington DC: Brookings Institute, 1986.
9. Warner KE. Health and economic implications of a tobacco-free society. JAMA 1987; 258:2080–6.
10. Manning WG, Keeler EB, Newhouse JP, et al. The taxes of sin: do smokers and drinkers pay their way? JAMA 1989; 261:1604–9.
11. Oster G, Huse DM, Delea TE, Colditz GA. Cost-effectiveness of nicotine gum as an adjunct to physician's advice against cigarette smoking. JAMA 1986; 256:1315–8.
12. Edelson JT, Weinstein MC, Tosteson ANA, et al. Long-term cost-effectiveness of various initial monotherapies for mild to moderate hypertension. JAMA 1990; 263:408–13.
13. Weinstein MC, Stason WB. Cost-effectiveness of interventions to prevent or treat heart disease. Ann Rev Public Health 1985; 6:41–63.
14. Kinosian BP, Eisenberg JM. Cutting into cholesterol: cost-effective alternatives for treating hypertension. JAMA 1988; 259:2249–54.
15. Oster G, Epstein AM. Cost-effectiveness of antihyperlipidemic therapy in the prevention of

coronary heart disease: the case for cholestyramine. JAMA 1987; 258:2381–7.

16. Taylor WC, Pass TM, Shepherd DS, Komaroff AL. Cost-effectiveness of cholesterol reduction for the primary prevention of coronary heart disease in men. From an unpublished cost-effectiveness background paper for the U.S. Preventive Services Task Force. February 1988.

16a. Farrand ME, Mojonniel L. Nutrition in the Multiple Risk Factor Intervention trial. J Am Diet Assoc 1980; 76:347–51.

16b. Anderson JW, Story L, Sieling B, et al. Hypocholesterolemic effects of oat-bran or bean intake for hypercholesterolemic men. Amer J Clin Nutrition 1984; 40:1146–55.

17. Lipid Research Clinics. The Lipid Research Clinics Coronary Primary Prevention Trial results. JAMA 1984; 251:351–64.

17a. Hay JW, Wittels EH, Gotto AM. An economic evaluation of lovastatin for cholesterol lowering and coronary artery disease reduction. Amer J Cardiol 1991; 67:789–96.

18. Hall JP, Heller RF, Dobson AJ, et al. A cost-effectiveness analysis of alternative strategies for the prevention of heart disease. Med J Aust 1988; 148:273–7.

19. Murray DM, Kurth C, Mullis R, Jeffery RW. Cholesterol reduction through low-intensity interventions: results from the Minnesota Heart Health Program. Prev Med 1990; 19:181–9.

20. Tosteson ANA, Weinstein MC, Williams L, Goldman L. Cost effectiveness of population approaches to reduce serum cholesterol levels (abstract). Clinical Research 1991; 39:2.

21. Hatziandrieu EI, Koplan JP, Weinstein MC, et al. A cost-effectiveness analysis of exercise as a health promotion activity. Am J Public Health 1988; 78:1417–21.

22. Doubilet P, Weinstein MC, McNeil BJ. Use and misuse of the term "cost-effective" in medicine. N Engl J Med 1986; 314:253–6.

23. Torrance GW. The measurement of health state utilities for economic appraisal. Health Econ 1986; 5:1–30.

24. Patrick DL, Bergner M. Measurement of health status in the 1990s. Ann Rev Public Health 1990; 11:165–83.

22

Training Program

JUDITH K. OCKENE
IRA S. OCKENE

EDITORS' INTRODUCTION

We come now to the final chapter in this book. If all that precedes this chapter is of value, then it is imperative that we incorporate these views and skills into the training of future physicians and other health care workers. In this chapter we suggest a program to carry out that objective. It is based on programs developed at the University of Massachusetts Medical School under the auspices of the Preventive Cardiology Academic Award Program and the Physician-Delivered Smoking Intervention Project, supported by the National Heart, Lung and Blood Institute (NHLBI) and the National Cancer Institute (NCI), respectively. We have found these approaches to be effective, time efficient, and well accepted by the individuals being trained. It is exceptionally gratifying to see students and house officers not only using these counseling tools in promoting risk-factor change but also incorporating them into their everyday interactions with patients — the best evidence that they find these skills truly valuable.

To help physicians develop the motivation and the skills to carry out prevention interventions, medical education must include clinical and research experiences in prevention. These experiences should help physicians to do the following:

- see prevention as an important part of their routine activities
- understand the remarkable effects that behavioral, psychological, and environmental factors can have on health and on the onset and progression of disease
- learn the basic counseling and behavioral skills, information, and office practice organizational procedures necessary to help patients change unhealthy behaviors and develop alternatives to medication and invasive treatment
- understand the public health aspects of medical care and the key role that the physician can play as part of the larger social structure in promoting positive health attitudes and behavior change
- become aware of the great emphasis that various health care and professional groups such as the U.S. Preventive Services Task Force [1] have placed on counseling as one of the most important prevention interventions physicians can implement

Training physicians in behavioral techniques not only provides them with the skills they need to help patients modify cardiac risk factors but also favorably influences the manner in which they diagnose and treat disability and disease [2, 3].

To broaden the traditional medical model of health and illness to include disease prevention and health promotion, the basic principles, perspectives, and methods of preventive medicine need to be integrated and interwoven into all aspects of mainstream clinical training and practice. An opportunistic approach is necessary, that is, prevention training occurs whenever and wherever the opportunity arises. When such integration takes place, lunch-time conversation is as likely to deal with the importance of a patient's dietary habits or smoking pattern as it

is with his need for diuretics or coronary angioplasty. Integrating behavioral/preventive medicine skills training in this manner helps to demonstrate its utility, break down some of the resistance to such approaches that often is found among traditionally trained physicians [4], and establish a prevention culture. It also reinforces the skills and information learned and promotes the long-term institutionalization of such teaching.

Skills acquisition must not only be integrated, it must also be gradual and begin early in training, to allow for progressive reinforcement and building on previous learning and to emphasize its importance in patient management and care. Effective integration of the teaching of CHD risk factor modification techniques into all aspects of medical training and practice, both on the student and the postgraduate levels, requires that physicians become teaching role models. Role modeling by professors as well as peers is a critical element in teaching prevention; trainees are well attuned to the difference between subjects given lip service and those thought to be truly important. In the absence of such reinforcement the teaching of preventive medicine will fail no matter how many hours of curriculum time are given to the effort; with reinforcement, the desired goal can be achieved with minimal scheduled instruction.

Already existing classes and modalities can be used as vehicles for accomplishing the specific skills training objectives of preventive medicine in an integrated fashion. A more formalized behavioral intervention training session can be included, but this need take only 2 to 3 hours of assigned teaching time. Thus, little extra time is actually necessary for teaching risk factor intervention skills.

Successful institutionalization of a new program into an existing program, besides requiring acceptance and support by pertinent individuals and trainees in the organization, also requires that everyone involved perceives that the benefits of the training and the intervention exceed the costs; that the training is compatible with the overall mission and objectives of the program [5]; and that clinical standards are set in which it is expected that physicians will include what they learn in their practice. Development of each of these factors can facilitate an organization's acceptance, integration, and institutionalization of a prevention program.

Risk-Factor Modification Training Objectives

The physician-trainee needs to develop a preventive perspective toward medical practice, be conversant with and knowledgeable about the concepts and language of prevention, and develop the level of counseling and behavioral skills needed to work with most patients. The training objectives that need to be met to enable physicians to implement risk-factor modification interventions for the prevention of CHD, as well as other preventive interventions, should include the ability to do the following [6]:

- communicate effectively with patients
- assess relevant nonphysical factors (behavioral, psychological, and social) that play a role in the physical disease process and its treatment
- know how to do patient-centered counseling
- know and perform a range of cognitive/behavioral techniques that can be incorporated into a regular outpatient medical encounter
- know how to organize an office practice to facilitate intervention, follow-up, and monitoring of patients for the prevention of CHD
- work effectively with individuals in other prevention-related disciplines and organizations, such as psychology, nutrition, exercise science, Alcoholics Anonymous, the American Heart Association, and the American Cancer Society
- be knowledgeable about available referral resources for interventions appropriate to particular health-related lifestyle problems and know how and when to make an appropriate referral
- be aware of the difficulties and the resistances involved in changing habitual maladaptive behaviors and in adopting and maintaining prevention-related lifestyle behaviors, both for one's patients and for oneself

- be knowledgeable about the fundamental theories and principles of behavior

The objectives listed here constitute a basic core of clinical knowledge and skills appropriate for all well-trained physicians. The integration of such training into already existing experiences helps to ensure the treatment of the patient as a whole person rather than as a disease entity and facilitates the prevention as well as the treatment of disease.

The Preventive Cardiology Academic Award Program: A Focus on Physician Education

The need for additional efforts in the area of CHD prevention was identified in the 1970s by several conferences and reports [7], and the American College of Cardiology included a statement on prevention in its statement of purpose [8]. A group of scientists from the NHLBI Clinical Applications and Prevention Advisory Committee responded to this need by recommending that a program be developed to stimulate individuals to develop curricula in medical schools that would motivate and enable physicians to include prevention in their practice. Thus, in 1978 the first request for applications for the Preventive Cardiology Academic Award (PCAA) was released [9]. The PCAA program was intended to stimulate the development of curricula that would have a significant impact on the opportunities of students, house staff, and fellows to learn both the principles and practice of preventive cardiology.

Currently 60 medical schools have or have had NHLBI-funded PCAAs. The last announcement, which appeared in 1990, focused on training for prevention in minority groups [10]. The PCAA program has contributed significantly to the development of the University of Massachusetts Medical Center's preventive cardiology program.

A directory, *Preventive Cardiology Resources for Physician Education* [11], was published in 1989 to provide a list and a brief description of the wide spectrum of instructional programs and materials developed by grantees of the NHLBI

PCAA programs. This reference guide contains information on preventive cardiology curricula, computer software and audiovisual materials, the set-up and use of preventive cardiology clinics as teaching opportunities, and evaluation strategies. Separate sections describe resources for intervention in smoking, lipids, hypertension, and other risk factors. (See the last section of this chapter for the address to write to for this resources directory.)

Teaching Risk-Factor Counseling Skills

In this section we present examples of how the teaching of risk-factor intervention skills can be integrated into the regular teaching of medical students, residents, fellows, and community physicians. Most of these examples come from our curriculum at the University of Massachusetts Medical School and need to be adapted to the needs of your own programs. Key words to be remembered to make effective teaching happen and work in your program are *flexibility, integration, creativity,* and *compatibility*.

Medical Students
Medical students at the University of Massachusetts Medical School, as at other PCAA sites, participate in a risk factor screening assessment when they first enter medical school. Measurements include a total cholesterol and complete lipoprotein profile; a maximal exercise test; measurement of blood pressure, height, weight, and skin-fold thickness; family history; smoking history; and dietary recall (food frequency questionnaire). Students receive overall risk evaluations and feedback regarding their risk profiles. Students with an elevated risk are provided with individual consultation and follow-up. The class information as a whole is summarized and presented to the students during clinical correlation sessions in biochemistry, nutrition, and preventive medicine. For the latter course the information is used to illustrate epidemiologic concepts. The students' risk profiles thus provide valuable and personalized information for teaching risk-factor assessment and intervention.

At multiple points in the curriculum medical students are also exposed to the teaching of behavioral medicine/risk-factor counseling skills (Table 22-1). In the first year training emphasizes development of the concepts of communication and patient-centered counseling. Communication Skills, which provides instruction in ten 2-hour sessions to students in groups of eight to ten, teaches the conduct of patient-centered interviews to facilitate an understanding of patients and the problems with which they present. During these sessions students are introduced to the idea that physicians need to use a counseling approach to assess disease-related risk factors, to educate patients about the impact of their lifestyle on their health, and to help patients make lifestyle changes. In these small groups patient simulators and role-playing are used extensively. In our experience the use of these methodologies facilitates the process by which students become comfortable with their roles as educators and counselors and also aids in evaluation of the students' skills. Smoking is often the behavior used to model how to assess risk factors, although any lifestyle behavior needing change (e.g., overeating, high-fat diet, lack of exercise) can be used.

First-year students also participate in a Medical Interviewing course. This course includes three 3-hour sessions in which students are exposed to the importance of the physician as an educator and a counselor, as well as to theories of behavior change and the use of the medical interview as a vehicle for helping patients to alter disease-related lifestyle behaviors such as smoking, alcohol abuse, and nonadherence to medication. They are able to practice these skills in small-group sessions. Students are taught that the methodologies used and taught in risk-factor counseling are similar to those taught for taking an adequate patient history of many other medical problems, such as hypertension or diabetes. The emphasis is on the patient and his or her needs, with inquiries into prior treatment and satisfaction and problems encountered with the treatment included in the history, as opposed to the usual physician-oriented (fill in the boxes and obtain the physiologically important data) approach. The five-

Table 22-1. A suggested sequence for teaching risk-factor counseling to medical students

Year	Course	Content related to prevention and counseling
1	Communication Skills	Communication Patient-centered counseling
	Medical Interviewing	Using the medical interview for behavioral counseling
2	Epidemiology and Preventive Medicine	CHD risk factors Module on risk factor alteration, including role play and discussions
3	Medical Clerkship	Relationship of lifestyle to inpatient problems Brief behavioral interventions to be used during medical workup Barriers to inpatient counseling
4	Electives	Preventive and behavioral medicine Cardiac rehabilitation Stress reduction and relaxation program

step counseling intervention technique developed as part of our NCI-funded Physician-Delivered Smoking Intervention Project (PDSIP) is taught, demonstrated, and practiced [12] to help students learn the techniques of counseling. The principles advocated in this approach are applicable to any risk-factor counseling situation. A trainer's manual, a videotape that illustrates five different patient-physician counseling scenarios and runs for a total of 27 minutes, and a slide package that contains 44 slides have been developed by the PDSIP project and are available. Information is provided on how to adapt the training to a particular setting. (See the last section of this chapter for information on how to obtain the training package.)

The patient-centered approach focuses on the physician's use of time-efficient and effective questioning to elicit information from patients and to help them assess the five following areas: (1) personal desire and motivation for change, (2) past experiences with change (e.g., smoking cessation), (3) factors that inhibit change, (4) resources for change, and (5) strategies to use in the negotiated plan for change. (See Chapters 7 and 8 for a discussion of patient-centered counseling.) Students are also taught to rephrase and feed back the relevant information to the patients to help them develop a plan for change

and a plan for subsequent follow-up visits or telephone calls. Thus, the five-step intervention combines the processes of effective questioning with the provision of relevant information to assist patients. The approach also focuses on a third process, eliciting feelings, and is easily integrated into a course that teaches medical interviewing and patient-centered communication skills. (A sample counseling intervention script is shown in Table 7-5 and discussed in that chapter.)

In the second year medical students participate in an Epidemiology and Preventive Medicine course, during which the counseling model is reviewed in the context of examining the relationship of risk factors to disease prevalence. The importance of understanding the whole patient as embedded in a system composed of many interacting factors is emphasized, as is the impact of the environment (economic, social, and political) on the patient.

In the third year of medical school the medical clerkship is used as a vehicle to give students experience in helping patients on the inpatient service as well as in the ambulatory-care clinics to alter their risk factors. The preceptor first leads a discussion of the relationship of lifestyle and other behavioral factors to particular inpatient problems, discusses the use of brief interventions that can be used during and after the medical workup, and then goes to the patient's bedside with the students to demonstrate a counseling interaction. All the problems attendant to inpatient counseling are raised — conflicting demands for the patient's time, the realities of pain and discomfort and the greater attention given to the acute problem by both patient and staff, the problem patient, and the difficulties attendant to the necessary inpatient-outpatient coordination — and methods of resolving these issues are discussed. Here, too, students should be exposed to the prevention-oriented medical culture, in which risk-factor modification is seen by the staff physicians and the house staff to whom the students are exposed as an important and integral part of medical care and as worthy of casual discussion and inquiry as is the state of the patient's platelets or the results of the last magnetic resonance imaging study.

In the fourth year there are no required formal sessions in risk-factor modification. However, students on internal medicine or family practice rotations continue to be exposed to the counseling-oriented risk-factor modification philosophy of the medical center. In addition, specific electives are available in preventive and behavioral medicine, stress reduction, cardiac rehabilitation, and preventive cardiology, with individual research opportunities also available for a number of students.

House Staff

The primary care/general medicine residency program at the University of Massachusetts Medical Center is a good example of the beginning of institutionalization of a new culture in medicine. To achieve our objectives, we have utilized already existing components of the training program that are likely to be in place in other institutions. These include daily bedside attending rounds, morning report, outpatient chart review, weekly grand rounds, daily residents' teaching conferences, journal clubs, and monthly morbidity, mortality, and management conferences (Table 22-2).

We have used other modalities, which may already be in place in some institutions or relatively easy to establish in others. These include

Table 22-2.   Opportunities for teaching risk-factor counseling to house staff

Inpatient rounds
Morning report
Noon conferences
Grand rounds
Lipid clinic
Preventive cardiology elective
Behavioral medicine elective
Journal clubs

elective rotations in lipid clinic, behavioral medicine, the stress reduction program, and the preventive cardiology program, weekly cardiac rehabilitation rounds, outpatient behavioral medicine clinical case conferences, psychosocial rounds, monthly behavioral medicine seminars, and epidemiology seminars.

We use two 1-hour teaching conferences in both internal medicine and family practice, which all residents are required to attend, to teach patient-centered counseling for health behavior change [12]. (Extra sessions accommodate all residents' schedules.) Following the training the residents have individual 20-minute tutorial sessions during clinic time for feedback about their counseling techniques. As with the students the patient-centered approach focuses on the use of effective questioning by the physician to elicit information, focusing on the five noted content areas: the patient's motivation, past experiences, resources, problem areas, and, subsequent to the assessment of these areas, the development of a plan for change and follow-up. The sequence of questions helps patients to identify those skills and resources necessary to make a change and to feel confident of their ability and commitment to do so [13]. Residents also are taught to elicit feelings and to provide information. The five content and three process areas covered in our teaching of the patient-centered counseling approach are evaluated, and we use a special evaluation form to provide residents with feedback.

Videotapes and role playing help the residents develop the required counseling skills. (The training package used with the medical students is also used here.) The hypercholesterolemic, overweight patient with an MI might be used in a script in which house staff play the parts of both patient and physician. This approach helps the residents gain an understanding of the problems faced by the patient. As a result of these 2½ hours of training, residents report significantly improved confidence in their own efficacy for initiating positive health behavior change with their patients and are more comfortable dealing with the need for such lifestyle alterations [14].

This training has been accepted widely by our house staff. Of the 200 residents eligible for training during the period of the original NCI-supported project, 198 were so trained. After termination of the research project, both of the involved departments (internal medicine and family and community medicine) committed themselves to continuing the training, since it had been perceived to be valuable and applicable to a wide variety of physician-patient encounters. In addition all faculty in general medicine and in family medicine have participated in the training, either in special groups or with the residents.

To adapt training to a particular situation, it is important to be creative and flexible and to gain the support of the residency program director and/or the outpatient clinic director and/or department chair (see Table 22-3). Other attending physicians also need to buy into the need for a prevention model and to use it in their own practice of medicine (Table 22-4).

Fellows in Cardiovascular Medicine

Fellows in our training program in cardiovascular medicine are given the same 2½ hours of training as are the residents. Training in this group of neophyte specialists emphasizes counseling for the prevention of cardiovascular disease and the role of the consultant as a teacher of other physicians. In addition specific lectures are given on atherosclerosis, epidemiology, behavioral medicine, cardiovascular risk factors, and risk factor modification as it applies to the patient who already has CHD (secondary prevention).

Within the division of cardiovascular medicine are several physicians who are both leaders in invasive cardiology and ardent proponents of risk factor modification (the present and former directors of the cardiac catheterization laboratories also codirect the preventive cardiology clinic). We have found that this situation gives our efforts toward prevention great credibility, and strongly recommend this form of role modeling. Physicians-in-training expect epidemiologists to talk prevention, but when the director of the interventional cardiology (angioplasty) service stresses the need for risk-factor modification, everyone pays attention.

Electives

A number of electives are available for students in all years. Summer fellowships have allowed students to investigate risk-factor modification programs in depth, and we have sent a number of students to such places as Zuni, New Mexico, and Quito, Ecuador, to work on projects investigating risk-factor changes that occur as native populations urbanize. Students assist in the risk-factor testing program implemented with first-year students and do all the fitness testing as well as participate in research projects. These students form an especially interested and motivated nucleus within their classes.

PREVENTIVE CARDIOLOGY ELECTIVE

This elective, usually one month in duration, gives the trainee an intensive experience in preventive cardiology. The elective can be tailored to the individual's background and needs but is usually divided between the cardiology and behavioral medicine services. The trainee spends time in the preventive cardiology clinic, which includes a lipid management program, sees inpatients who have been referred to the preventive cardiology service, and attends the various conferences in which these patients are discussed.

BEHAVIORAL MEDICINE ELECTIVE

Students, residents, and fellows can elect to be participant/observers in an outpatient behavioral medicine group, the Stress Reduction and Relaxation Program (SRRP), or the individual outpatient behavioral medicine clinic program.

Table 22-3. Logistics for training residents in preventive interventions

1. Be creative and flexible.
2. Be opportunistic. Fit training into whenever there is time.
3. Get support from the residency program director, the clinic director, or the department chair (whoever would be the most influential).
4. Bring together a group of residents to discuss how they think they would best be trained.
5. Bribe! (Food is effective.)
6. Use a noontime or an afternoon conference.
7. Take 30 minutes of clinic time at the beginning of clinic session.
8. Use a Friday afternoon and offer pizza.
9. Speak at morning and noon reports.
10. Schedule an hour (with breakfast) before work rounds begin.
11. Gather all the residents who are on elective rotations and train them together as a group.
12. To market the training session:
    a. Make flyers to post around the hospital announcing the training session.
    b. Place flyers in the residents' mailboxes.
    c. Meet with the chief residents and elicit their support; they can announce the training session at morning report.
    d. If you have residents at outside hospitals, contact the chief residents or clinic directors at these hospitals about the training session. Negotiate time for residents to participate in training.

The "internship" in the SRRP is an effective behavioral adjunct to medical training as well as a resource for learning to manage personal and professional stress. The program is an 8-week course for patients with a wide range of diagnoses. They are referred by their physicians to learn relaxation skills and to enhance their ability to cope more effectively with stress and chronic illness [15, 16]. The physician-participant joins a class of 25 patients, sharing with them both progress and difficulties as they work to change attitude and lifestyle and practicing the same cognitive/behavioral health–enhancing techniques taught to the patients. They themselves often enjoy experiencing the potential personal benefits of the regular practice of such self-regulatory techniques as meditation and yoga used in the group.

In the outpatient behavioral medicine clinic patients are seen individually for help concerning risk-factor change and disease prevention. Students and residents are able to observe and participate in the provider-patient interactions. Trainees in the behavioral medicine elective usually find that they develop a new respect for the ability of people to grow and change, acquire an understanding of the complexity of their patients' life stresses, and realize the level of commitment required to make any lifestyle change, even one thought of as simple. We have found that the experience of seeing patients with serious behavioral and medical problems make lifestyle and attitudinal changes and experience significant symptom reduction is an effective teaching tool. Participants incorporate what they learn into their work with their own patients and into the conduct of their own lives.

This type of elective is ideal for the individual looking for a greater understanding of how people can be helped to change. Participation by physicians-in-training in such patient-oriented behavioral medicine programs has a positive effect on their beliefs about what their patients might be capable of if given encouragement, behavior change skills, and techniques for enhancing self-regulation and self-knowledge.

For students in both the preventive cardiology and the behavioral medicine electives, experiences are also available in our community programs such as the NCI-funded worksite intervention program WellWorks, which includes intervention for smoking, nutrition, and occupational risk; and the NCI-funded community smoking intervention program, COMMIT, which uses all available community channels (e.g. schools, media, hospitals, worksites); and in other group programs such as an asthma self-management group and a group for compulsive

Table 22-4.　Overcoming training barriers

Barriers	Suggestions
For faculty-instructors:	
No awareness or support for training program from directors	Elicit support of the residency and clinic director/ department chair and the chief resident. Provide information and set up individual meetings.
Competing demands for faculty instructor's time	Negotiate with department chair for this training as part of teaching responsibilities. Present benefits of training to the institution, department, and residents. Recommend how to incorporate training into existing curriculum.
Faculty-instructor not confident in ability to carry out training	Consult with colleagues at other institutions who have done risk-factor counseling. Call UMMS project staff for consultation. Reread materials and role play with colleagues. Elicit support of psychology staff to assist with training.
Difficulty in finding time to assess residents' skills	Utilize precepting or clinic time, case review time, or rounds.
Low turnout at conferences	Offer food. Page residents on day of program. Remind them to attend and that food will be provided! Send reminders and express benefits to residents. Develop incentives.
For residents:	
Competing demands for residents' time	Use existing scheduled meeting time, such as noon conference and preceptors' time.
Lack of incentives for residents to complete training	Consider incentive for completing the training, such as a lottery drawing for a gift certificate, award pin, credit toward residency program performance review.
Time for training:	
No standard time for residents to be together for information sharing	Notify residents via letter from department chair, residency director, and chief resident. Utilize faculty preceptors to remind residents of training. Print up and prominently display program reminders. Place training reminder with paycheck.
No available extra time for training in other subjects	Utilize existing training conference time: morning report, grand rounds, residents' teaching conference, clinic chart review. Send out a newsletter with patient progress reports. Schedule a focus group or round table discussion. Serve food.

eaters. For individuals interested in research, particularly if a longer elective or a summer experience (for students) is desired, an individual project can be arranged, and greater experience is provided in the methodologies of preventive cardiology, especially epidemiology.

Although a number of the more research-related activities described here are not available in most institutions, electives tailored around preventive cardiology/lipid clinics, behavioral medicine clinics, and stress reduction programs are all excellent teaching tools that can be easily developed at many medical centers.

Examples of Risk-factor Counseling Training

The following examples are ways in which we use traditional training vehicles to incorporate training in risk-factor counseling.

In the cardiac catheterization laboratory morning conference several patients with multiple risk factors and premature CHD are presented. Treatment and follow-up of these risk factors are discussed, with particular attention to communication with referring physicians, appropriate referrals (behavioral medicine, preventive cardiology clinic, cardiac rehabilitation), and risk-factor control during rehabilitation from cardiac surgery. In these discussions the need not to lose sight of the nonacute but important problem of risk-factor change is emphasized, since it is usual in these settings for such concerns to be subordinate to the more pressing acute problems that have led to catheterization and consideration of angioplasty and surgery.

On bedside rounds patient R.B. is presented. She is a 56-year-old woman with a recent MI who has a 40-year history of cigarette smoking. After establishing rapport with the patient and managing the acute problems related to the infarction, the attending physician demonstrates to the students, residents, and fellows a systematic patient-centered approach to smoking cessation [12]. The link between the patient's infarct and her smoking is established; the level of nicotine addiction is assessed, as is the patient's interest in quitting; and resources for

quitting are determined. The patient is encouraged to develop a plan for cessation that will begin in the hospital, with maintenance to be facilitated during daily rounds. The physician-in-training will conduct the interview on rounds the next day with another patient.

At morning report a 50-year-old farmer with chronic obstructive pulmonary disease is presented. In addition to the usual discussion of diagnosis and treatment, preceptors knowledgeable about occupational and behavioral medicine discuss aspects of the situation appropriate to their own special points of view. Preceptors can also facilitate discussion related to reducing risk of further injury and preventing disease in family members and coworkers and emphasize the importance of recognizing preventable illness and helping patients modify behavior to promote their health.

Residents' daily teaching conferences provide opportunities for in-depth review of relevant clinical areas (e.g., the physiology of nicotine addiction and other addictive behaviors, dealing with anxious patients, treatment of hyperlipidemia, exercise programs, weight reduction, relaxation training).

Grand rounds is used as a major forum for discussion of such topics as preventive cardiology, epidemiology, eating disorders, occupational medicine, alcohol abuse, cigarette smoking, school health programs, nutrition counseling, fitness promotion, behavioral counseling techniques, and stress reduction.

Journal clubs can be used for many purposes, but we have found that they are an ideal forum to teach the epidemiologic underpinnings of cardiovascular risk-factor modification.

The outpatient chart review conference is a particularly suitable place to emphasize the need for adequate communication between physician and patient and to teach the methodologies involved in the long-term care of patients who are not acutely ill. The need for careful follow-up, small steps, and patience are taught in this setting. A review of several patients' charts can be carried out to note whether risk factors were assessed and whether job-related and social stressors and support mechanisms, as they relate to the patients' illnesses, were adequately evaluated. Suggestions for the incorporation of assessments and behavioral intervention approaches in the clinical encounter and for effective referral for further behavioral intervention, when appropriate, can be made.

The Need to Motivate Physicians to Do Prevention

Arousing physician interest in disease prevention is much more difficult than motivating disease treatment. The rewards are distant and nebulous. Few patients thank you for saving their lives after you manage to convert them to a low-fat, low-cholesterol diet. The patient who has stopped smoking or lost weight is proud of that accomplishment and often is grateful to the physician, but for every such patient there are three or four others who do not make such changes and are a source of frustration to both themselves and their physicians. In addition the manner in which reimbursement practices are now structured provides little financial reward for vigorously pursuing lifestyle change.

Physicians need to have realistic expectations about health behavior change outcomes. To the physician with a strong conviction that prevention is better than treatment, successful risk factor modification can be very gratifying. Motivation has to be on an intellectual as well as an emotional level. The ability to think in terms of large numbers of patients as well as the individual patient, a perspective foreign to usual physician practice, is helpful. A 5-percent drop in cholesterol is small when seen from the perspective of the individual physician-patient relationship, but a 5-percent drop in cholesterol is a 10-percent decrease in risk [17], and a 10-percent decrease in risk in a disease that causes 500,000 deaths a year is an annual saving of 50,000 lives. Gratifying indeed, when seen from such a population perspective.

The physician also must understand that once a patient becomes ill, all medicine usually has to offer is palliation. We cure very few adult diseases, and the knowledgeable physician understands that the cost of such therapy is extraordinary. The patient who remains healthy because the physicians successfully assisted him to stop smoking may never appreciate that he is well and active instead of prematurely retired following an MI. However, for the prevention-oriented physician the rewards can be great. Effective training of physicians in preventive cardiology must include, therefore, the development of realistic expectations, the ability to think in epidemiologic terms, and a sense of responsibility for the larger community as well as for the individual patient.

Summary

Teaching risk factor intervention skills is a natural and necessary adjunct to teaching disease treatment. Increasing emphasis is being placed on preventive medicine, particularly at a time of spiraling medical care costs. The physician must be given the tools with which to assist, monitor, and follow individuals who need to make lifestyle changes: the ability to communicate effectively with patients, to assess behavioral and social factors that affect each patient's ability to make changes, to assess the patient's resources, to use behavioral intervention techniques in an effective and time-efficient manner, to organize a practice that helps to facilitate such intervention, and to work effectively with other professionals with special areas of expertise. Training in these areas often can be incorporated into such already existing teaching vehicles as rounds, morning report, chart review conferences, preventive intervention programs, clinics, and electives.

The integration of the preventive and behavioral medicine training experiences of medical students, residents, and fellows into existing training vehicles and hospital programs ensures a better fit between their training and what they are actually called on to do in practice. It is also a way of systematizing essential aspects of effective patient care and providing role models for young physicians in a preventive culture that supports such approaches. Moreover, by making use of existing vehicles, using opportunities for preventive training when appropriate, and ensuring that risk-factor modification is accepted as part of the fabric of normal medical practice and is compatible with the mission of the training programs and of the trainees, training in preventive cardiology and behavioral medicine need not put an extra time burden on the training program. These factors will help to ensure that the benefits of providing training in preventive cardiology outweigh the costs.

Suggested Further Resources and Addresses

For the Physician-Delivered Smoking Intervention Program (PDSIP) trainer's package write:
Judith K. Ockene, Ph.D.
Division of Preventive and Behavioral
   Medicine
University of Massachusetts Medical School
55 Lake Avenue North
Worcester, MA 01655

For *How to Help Your Patients Stop Smoking. A National Cancer Institute Manual for Physicians,* by Thomas J. Glynn, Ph.D., and Marc W. Manley, M.D., M.P.H. (NCI publ. no. 89-3064, March 1989), write:
Office of Cancer Communications
National Cancer Institute
Building 31, Room 10A24
Bethesda, MD 20892

For information on "Train the Trainers" workshops for teaching physician-delivered smoking intervention skills, given by the NCI, write or call:
Marc W. Manley, M.D., M.P.H.
Division of Cancer Prevention and Control
National Cancer Institute
Executive Plaza North, Room 320
9000 Rockville Pike
Bethesda, MD 20892
(301) 496-8577

For the directory *Preventive Cardiology Resources for Physician Education* write:
Elaine Stone, Ph.D.
National Heart, Lung and Blood Institute
7550 Wisconsin Avenue
Federal Building, Room 604A

NIH NHLBI-DECA-PDRB
Bethesda, MD 20205

For the American Academy of Family Physicians (AAFP) Stop Smoking Kit and the Family Physician's Guide to Smoking Cessation write:
American Academy of Family Physicians
1740 West 92nd Street
Kansas City, MO 64114

For *Clinical Opportunities for Smoking Intervention — A Guide for the Busy Physician* write:
National Heart, Lung and Blood Institute
Smoking Education Program
National Institutes of Health
Bethesda, MD 20892

For *Nutrition in Primary Care: How to Help Your Patients Improve Their Eating Habits,* by C. Tziraki, C. Dresser, and A. Lasswell (in preparation), write:
The Division of Cancer Prevention and
   Control
National Cancer Institute
National Institutes of Health
Bethesda, MD 20205

References

1. U.S. Preventive Services Task Force. Report. Guide to clinical preventive services. Baltimore: Williams and Wilkins, 1989.
2. Weiss SM. Behavioral medicine: an idea. . . . In: McNamara JR, ed. Behavioral medicine approaches to medicine: application and analysis. New York: Plenum Press, 1979.
3. Epstein L, Cincirpini R. Behavioral medicine III. Assoc Adv Behav Ther Newslett 1988; 4:7–9.
4. Maistra MM, Drabman RS. The development of behavioral competence in medical setting. In: McNamara JR, ed. Behavioral medicine approaches to medicine: application and analysis. New York: Plenum Press, 1979.
5. Rogers EM. Diffusion of innovations. 3rd ed. New York: Free Press, 1983.
6. Ockene JK, Ockene IS, Kabat-Zinn J, et al. Teaching risk-factor counseling skills to medical students, house staff, and fellows. Am J Prev Med 1990; 6:suppl 1:35–42.
7. Stamler J. Primary prevention of coronary heart disease: the last 20 years. Am J Cardiol 1981; 47:701–6.

8. Brandenburg RO. The mission of prevention. Am J Cardiol 1981; 47:687.
9. Stone EJ. The preventive cardiology academic award program: a focus on physician education. Am J Prev Med 1990; 6:suppl 1:6–13.
10. National Heart, Lung and Blood Institute. Program guidelines: preventive cardiology academic award. November 1989.
11. Stone EJ. Preventive cardiology resources for physician education. NHLBI, June 1989:1–133.
12. Ockene JK, Quirk M, Goldberg RJ, et al. A resident's training program for the development of smoking intervention skills. Arch Intern Med 1988; 148:1039–45.
13. Bandura A. Self-efficacy: toward a unifying theory of behavior change. Psychol Rev 1977; 84:191–215.
14. Ockene JK. Physician-delivered interventions for smoking cessation: strategies for increasing effectiveness. Prev Med 1987; 16:723–37.
15. Kabat-Zinn J. An outpatient program in behavioral medicine for chronic pain patients based on the practice of mindfulness meditation: theoretical considerations and preliminary results. Gen Hosp Psychiatry 1982; 4:33–47.
16. Kabat-Zinn J, Chapman-Waldrop A. Compliance with an outpatient stress reduction program: rates and predictors of program completion. J Behav Med 1988; 11:333–52.
17. Lipid Research Clinics Program. The Lipid Research Clinics Coronary Primary Prevention Trial results: II. The relationship of reduction in incidence of coronary heart disease to cholesterol lowering. JAMA 1984; 251:365–74.

Index